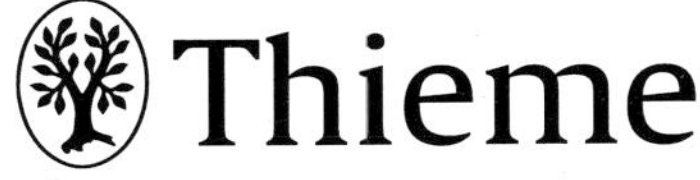

Ultrasound Diagnosis of Fetal Anomalies

Michael Entezami, M.D., Ph.D.

Matthias Albig, M.D.

Adam Gasiorek-Wiens

Rolf Becker, M.D., Ph.D.
Gynecology, Obstetrics, and Perinatology
Center for Prenatal Diagnostics, Kurfürstendamm 199
Berlin, Germany

With contributions by
U. Knoll, L. Schmitz, R.D. Wegner

Translated by Sanyukta Runkel, M.D., Ph.D.

488 illustrations

Georg Thieme Verlag
Stuttgart · New York

Library of Congress Cataloging-in-Publication Data is available from the publisher

This book is an authorized translation of the German edition published and copyrighted 2002 by Georg Thieme Verlag, Stuttgart, Germany. Title of the German edition: Sonographische Fehlbildungsdiagnostik. Lehratlas der fetalen Ultraschalluntersuchungen

Contributors

Ute Knoll, M.D.
Pediatrics, Medical Genetics
Center for Prenatal Diagnostics
Kurfürstendamm 199
Berlin, Germany

Lothar Schmitz, M.D.
Children's Cardiology
Humboldtuniversität Berlin
Campus Charité Mitte
Berlin, Germany

Rolf Dieter Wegner, Ph.D.
Biology, Human Genetics
Center for Prenatal Diagnostics
Kurfürstendamm 199
Berlin, Germany

Translator: Sanyukta Runkel, M.D., Ph. D.
VS-Villingen, Germany

Rüdigerstraße 14
D-70469 Stuttgart, Germany
http://www.thieme.de

Thieme New York, 333 Seventh Avenue,
New York, NY 10001, USA
http://www.thieme.com

Cover design: Martina Berge, Erbach

Typesetting and printing in Germany by
Druckhaus Götz GmbH, D-71636 Ludwigsburg

ISBN 3-13-131861-9 (GTV)
ISBN 1-58890-212-9 (TNY) 1 2 3 4 5

Important note: Medicine is an ever-changing science undergoing continual development. Research and clinical experience are continually expanding our knowledge, in particular our knowledge of proper treatment and drug therapy. Insofar as this book mentions any dosage or application, readers may rest assured that the authors, editors, and publishers have made every effort to ensure that such references are in accordance with **the state of knowledge at the time of production of the book.**

Nevertheless, this does not involve, imply, or express any guarantee or responsibility on the part of the publishers in respect to any dosage instructions and forms of applications stated in the book. **Every user is requested to examine carefully** the manufacturers' leaflets accompanying each drug and to check, if necessary in consultation with a physician or specialist, whether the dosage schedules mentioned therein or the contraindications stated by the manufacturers differ from the statements made in the present book. Such examination is particularly important with drugs that are either rarely used or have been newly released on the market. Every dosage schedule or every form of application used is entirely at the user's own risk and responsibility. The authors and publishers request every user to report to the publishers any discrepancies or inaccuracies noticed.

Preface

Since 1979, ultrasound screening has become part of a routine examination in the antenatal care of pregnant woman in Germany. Ongoing technical developments have improved the diagnostic possibilities dramatically. In particular, improved ultrasound image quality, with higher resolution, and development of vaginal ultrasound and color Doppler imaging have enabled ultrasound examination to become a standard and accepted clinical procedure, especially in pregnancy care.

There is a wide spectrum of possible fetal malformations, which on the whole occur rarely. One major problem is diagnosing a fetal anomaly from a large number of normal findings and evaluating it correctly for the clinical outcome of the pregnancy.

This book should help practitioners responsible for antenatal care (obstetricians and midwives) to interpret the findings and their possible consequences for the fetus and the mother and offer the appropriate clinical management. This is further supported by the extensive photo documentation of ultrasound findings. The main aim is to provide *one* textbook that reviews not only the frequent anomalies but also lists a range of rare syndromes that may be diagnosed by a detailed screening or can be considered as differential diagnosis. This book is not intended to replace the many excellent textbooks on ultrasound diagnostics that are already available. It is basically a reference work that can be used for orientation and illustration of findings in a quick and effective way in the daily clinical practice.

The introduction deals briefly with ultrasound screening in Germany: the 10/20/30 weeks' concept. The following chapters deal with fetal malformations systematically, according to the organs affected. The next chapters describe the chromosomal aberrations and frequent ultrasound findings diagnosed in the clinical practice. Selected syndromes and associations are also dealt with as well as fetal hydrops, prenatal infections, placenta disorders, and multiple pregnancy. The appendix summarizes syndromes, chromosomal disorders, and differential diagnosis of the second screening in a tabulated form, thus allowing a clear overview. In the last part of the book the normal fetal measurement charts are shown.

We hope this book serves its intended purpose and is a helpful reference for the daily clinical practice in pregnancy care.

Berlin,
Summer 2003

M. Albig
R. Becker
M. Entezami
A. Gasiorek-Wiens

Contents

Chromosomal Disorders and their Soft Markers 177

Selected Syndromes and Associations 235

Introduction

1 Ultrasound Screening

General Considerations

Perinatal mortality is considered to be an indicator of the quality of antenatal care and perinatal medicine. It is defined as intrauterine fetal death with a fetal weight of at least 500 g, or as neonatal death within the first 7 days after birth. At present, the perinatal mortality rate in Germany is six per 1000 live births. Intrauterine fetal deaths account for two-thirds of perinatal deaths. The most relevant factors for perinatal mortality are congenital fetal malformations, insufficiency of the uteroplacental circulation, and very premature birth. Ultrasound examination in pregnancy is thus of the utmost importance, as fetal malformations and placental insufficiency can be diagnosed early in pregnancy.

As early as 1979, Germany was the first country in the world to introduce ultrasound screening programs into routine antenatal care. Initially, two ultrasound examinations were recommended—between 16 and 20 weeks and 32 and 36 weeks of gestation. From 1995, three ultrasound examinations were offered: at 8–11 weeks ("first screening"), at 18–21 weeks ("second screening"), and between 28 and 31 weeks of gestation ("third screening").

First Screening (8–11 Weeks)

The aim of this examination is to confirm the presence of a *viable intrauterine pregnancy*, to verify the *expected delivery date* by measuring the crown–rump length, and to identify *multiple gestations*. In addition, even at this gestational age, *early signs of fetal malformations* should also be looked for.

In recent years, the *nuchal translucency* measurement has been increasingly used to evaluate the risk of a chromosomal anomaly. The optimal time to perform nuchal translucency measurement is between 11 and 13 weeks of gestation. After this, the predictive value of this measurement decreases.

Accurate measurement of nuchal translucency is a demanding task requiring sufficient time, clinical practice, and experience. False measurements result when the amnion is mistaken for the skin surface, giving abnormally high values.

A rigid upper limit of 2.5 or 3.0 mm is not useful, as the age of the mother has to be taken into account for the evaluation of the risk of chromosomal anomaly. The risk of Down syndrome is evaluated as one in 498 in a fetus of a 20-year-old mother with a crown–rump length of 55 mm and nuchal translucency of 2.5 mm, whereas the same fetal measurements in a 45-year-old mother raise this risk to one in 27. The best time to perform the first screening for early detection of fetal malformations appears to be 12–13 weeks of gestation. Earlier ultrasound does not allow detailed examination of the fetus to the same extent.

The *basic examination* should include—in addition to measurements of crown–rump length—head and abdominal circumferences and nuchal translucency, evaluation of extremities, stomach, bladder, fetal body contours, and fetal heart. Using the zoom function of the ultrasound apparatus, it is often possible to obtain a four-chamber view of the heart. The great vessels can only be reviewed using color flow mapping (CFM). This method is also necessary for exclusion of a single umbilical artery. The extremities can be viewed very well at this gestational age of 12–13 weeks. An overall view of the fetus at this early gestational age is more easily obtained than at later stages.

Although abdominal sonography is sufficient in most cases, vaginal sonography is often necessary when the mother is obese or the uterus is retroverted.

For reasons of safety, *Doppler flow* examinations in the first trimester should be reserved only for urgent indications. Color flow mapping requires comparatively less energy than the Doppler velocity waveform assessment.

At least 15 min are required for a thorough first trimester screening when normal findings are present.

The first screening examination is ideal for determining zygosity in multiple gestations (see section 15.1).

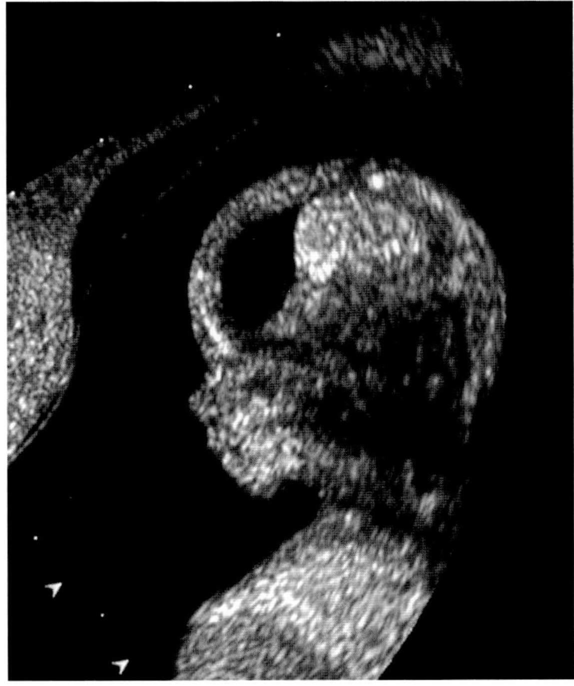

Fig. 1.**1** **First screening: early pregnancy, 8–11 weeks.** Normal fetal profile 12 + 4 weeks (vaginal sonography, 10 MHz).

1

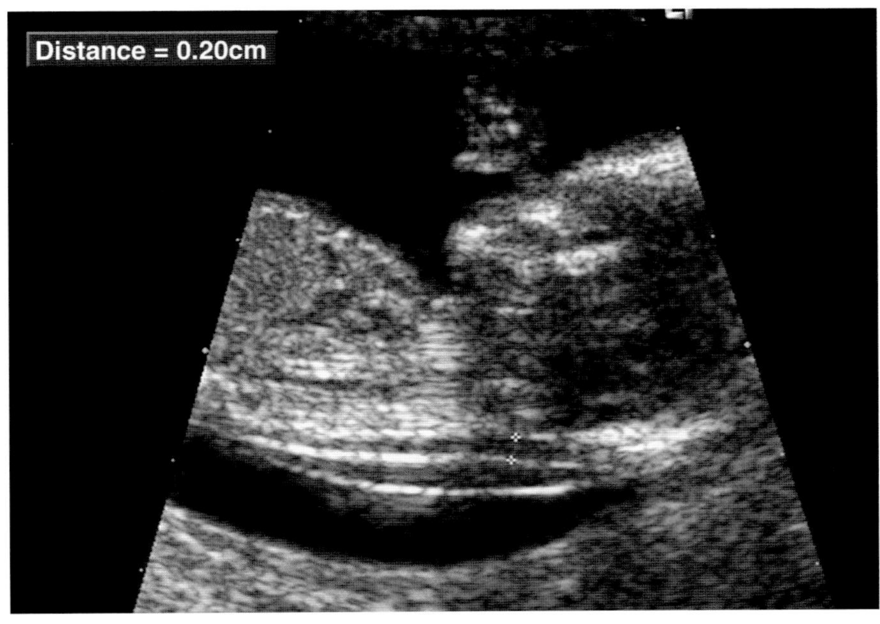

Fig. 1.**2** **First screening: early pregnancy, 8–11 weeks.** Longitudinal section of a fetus of 12 + 5 weeks, showing nuchal translucency as well as the amnion.

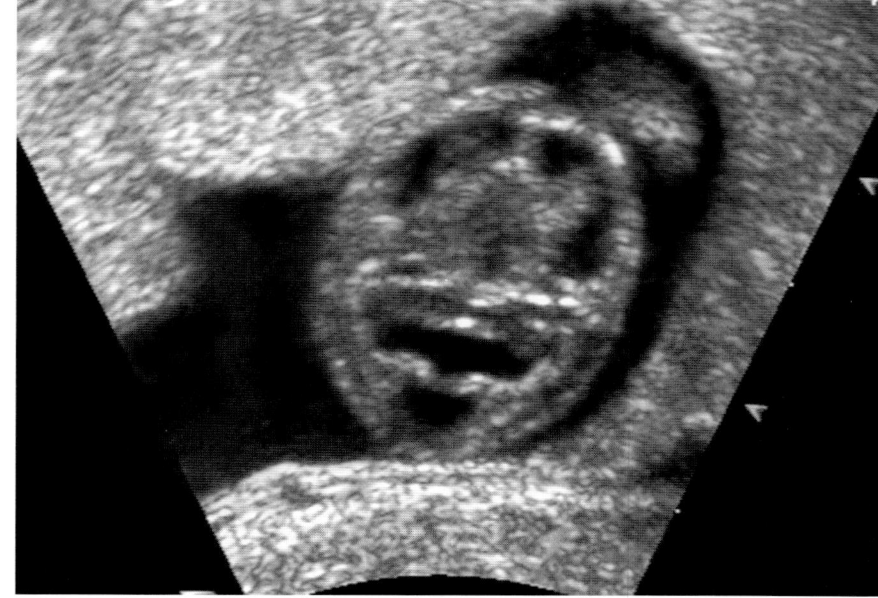

Fig. 1.3 **First screening: early pregnancy, 8–11 weeks.** Cross-section of the fetal head at 9 + 5 weeks, showing the lateral ventricle, choroid plexus, and posterior fossa of the skull (vaginal sonography, 10 MHz).

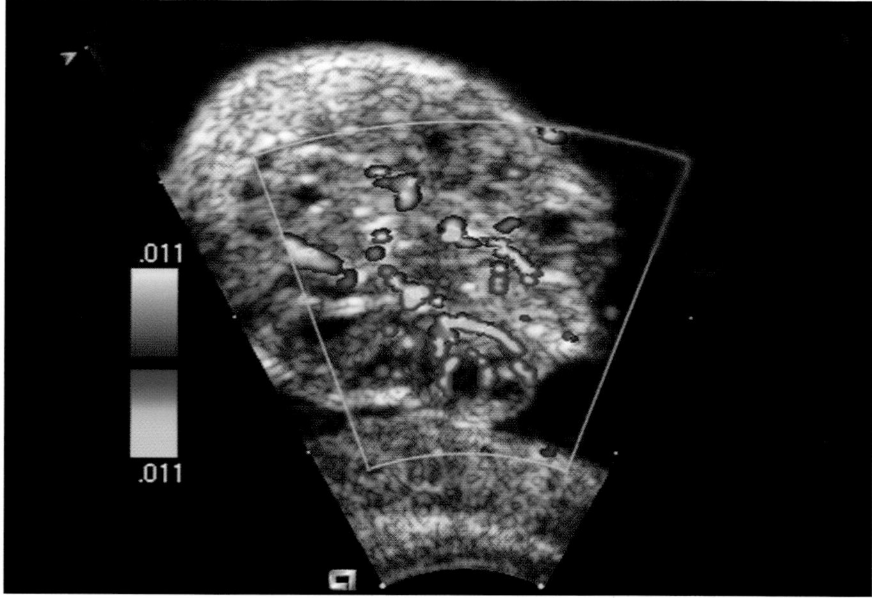

Fig. 1.4 **First screening: early pregnancy, 8–11 weeks.** Cross-section of the fetal head at 12 + 3 weeks, depicting the hyaloid artery supplying the lens of the eye.

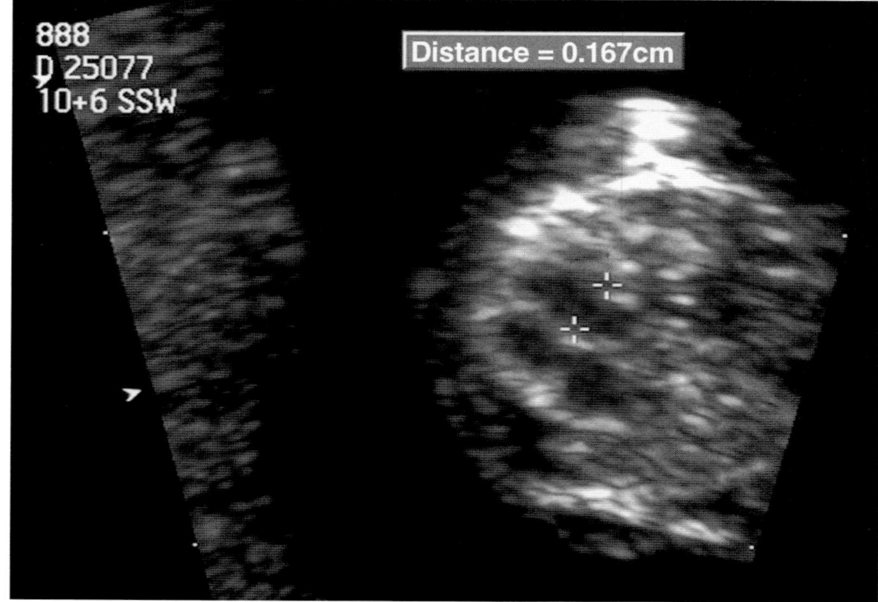

Fig. 1.5 **First screening: early pregnancy, 8–11 weeks.** Cross-section of the fetal thorax at 10 + 6 weeks at the level of the heart. The four-chamber view is clearly visible. The width of the left ventricle measures 1.67 mm (vaginal sonography, 10 MHz).

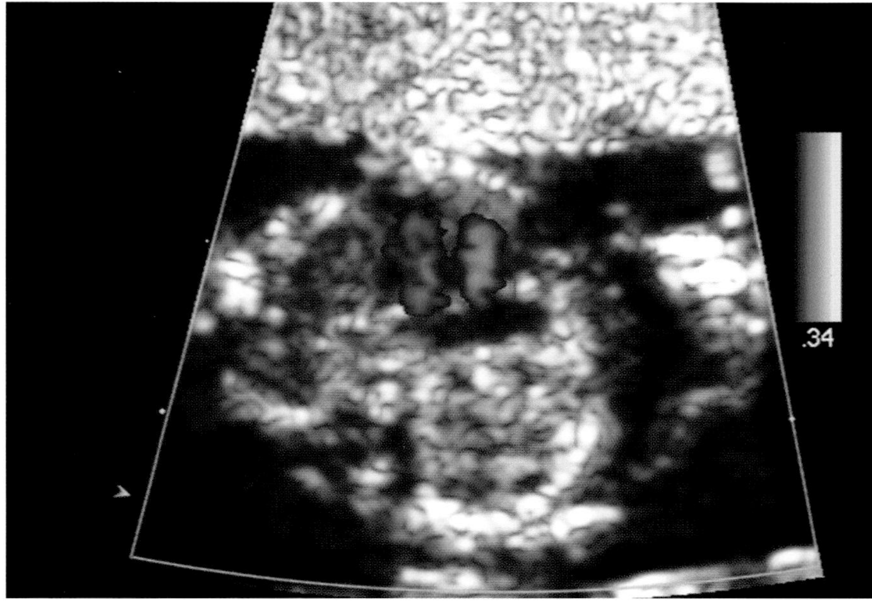

Fig. 1.6 **First screening: early pregnancy, 8–11 weeks.** Cross-section of the fetal thorax at 13 + 1 weeks at the level of the heart. Apical view of the four chambers of the heart using Doppler sonography (color Doppler energy). Depiction of diastolic blood flow through the tricuspid and mitral valves into the ventricles.

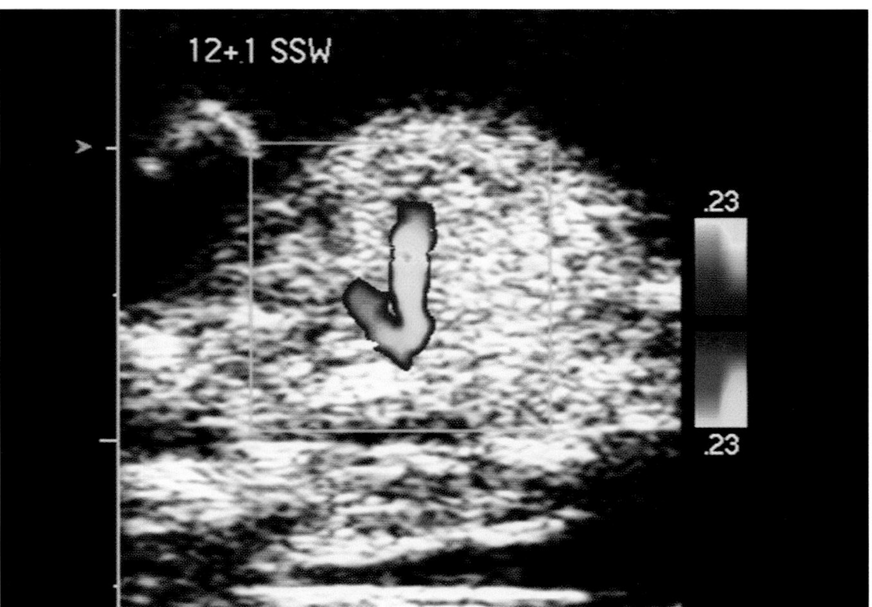

Fig. 1.7 **First screening: early pregnancy, 8–11 weeks.** Cross-section of the fetal thorax at 12 + 1 weeks in the region of the outflowing vessels. Blood flow into the aortic arch and the ductus arteriosus (Botallo's duct) is demonstrated.

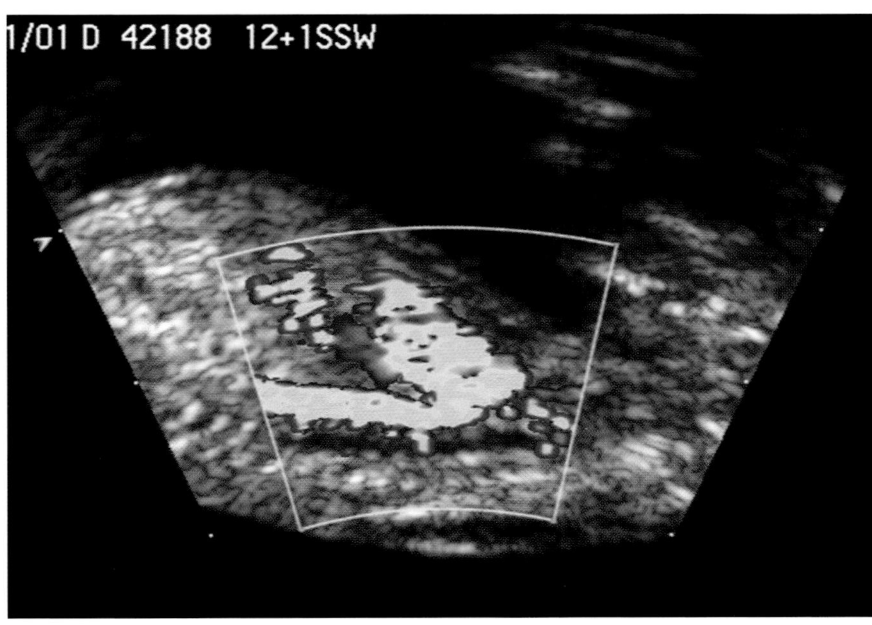

Fig. 1.8 **First screening: early pregnancy, 8–11 weeks.** The fetal aortic arch at 12 + 1 weeks is demonstrated using color Doppler sonography. The three vessels arising from the aortic arch are clearly seen.

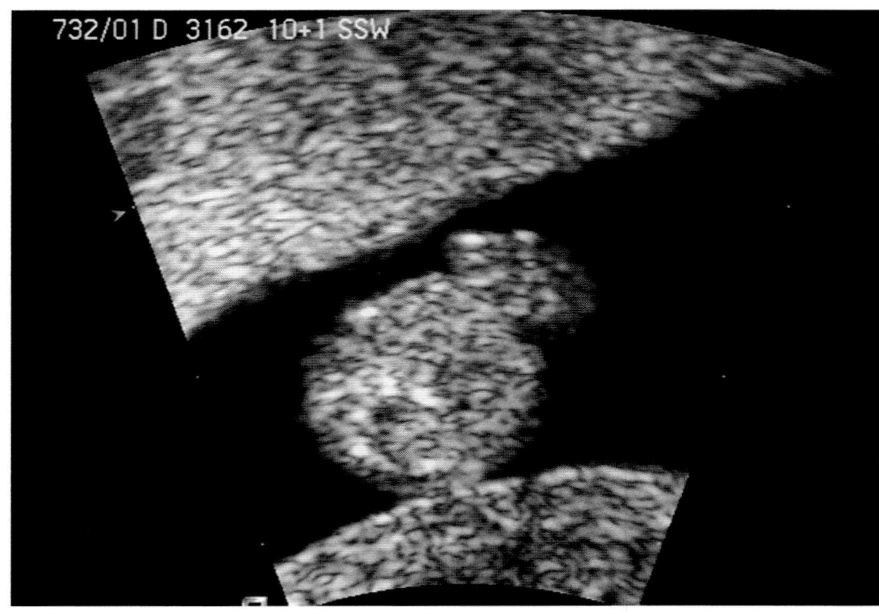

Fig. 1.**9** **First screening: early pregnancy, 8–11 weeks.** Cross-section of the fetal abdomen at 10 + 1 weeks at the region of the navel, showing a “physiological omphalocele.”

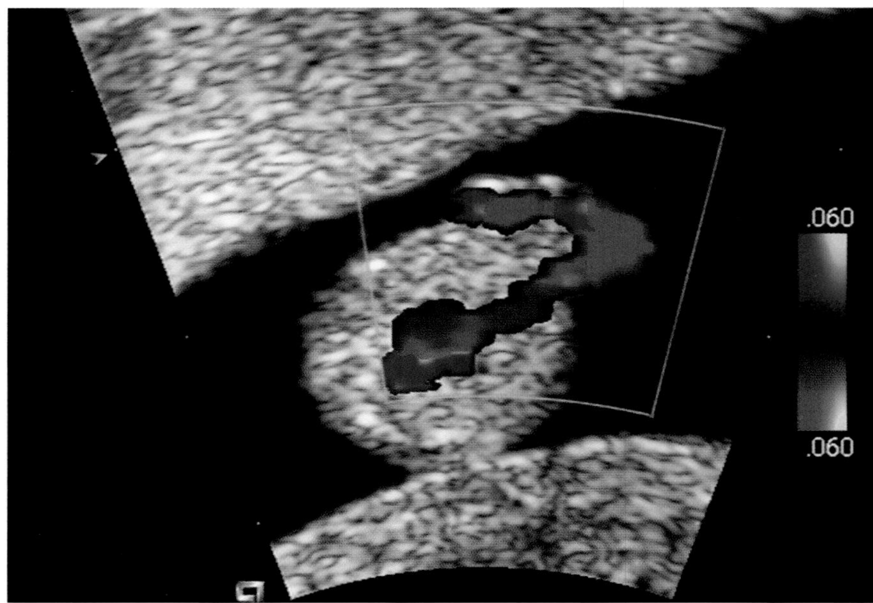

Fig. 1.**10** **First screening: early pregnancy, 8–11 weeks.** Same as the previous figure, with the use of color Doppler sonography. Protrusion of the intestines through the base of the navel is clearly visualized next to the umbilical vessels.

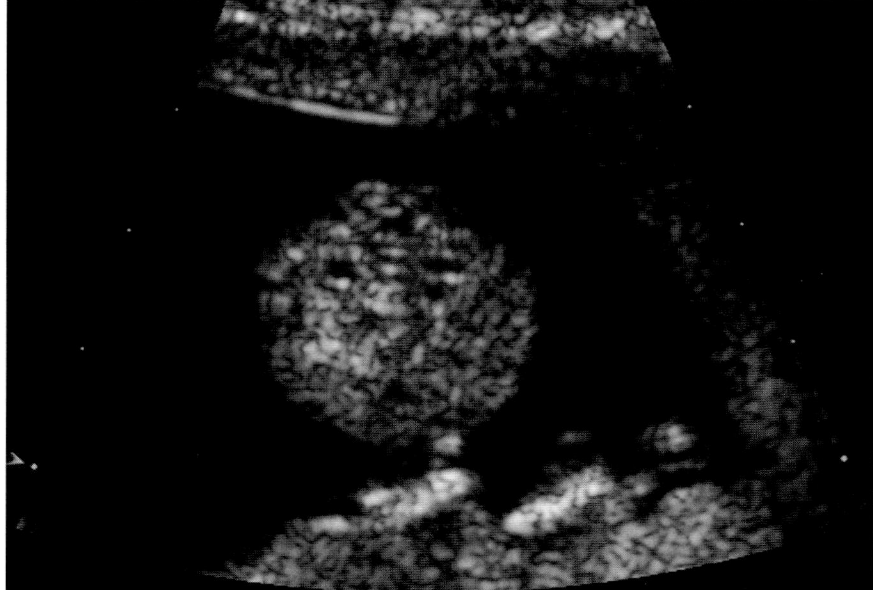

Fig. 1.**11** **First screening: early pregnancy, 8–11 weeks.** Cross-section of the fetal abdomen in a dorsoanterior fetal position at 13 + 0 weeks, showing the kidneys and the calyces of the renal pelvis on both sides.

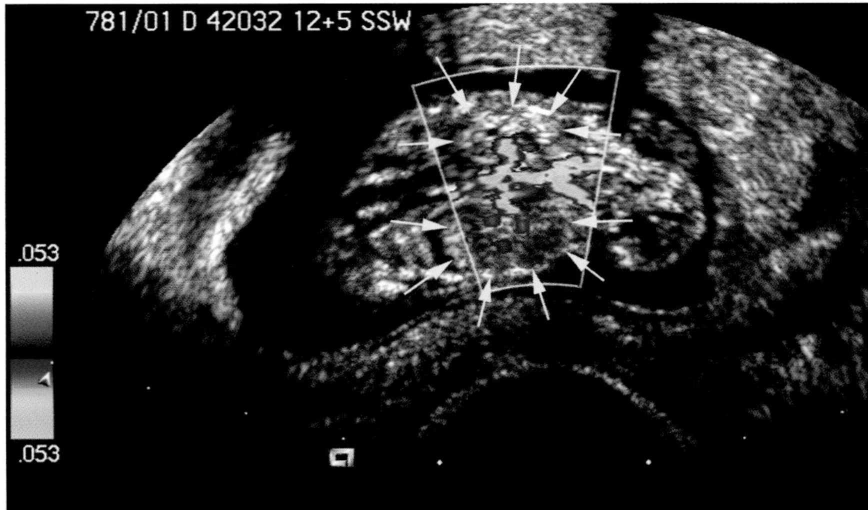

Fig. 1.**12** **First screening: early pregnancy, 8–11 weeks.** A section of the anterior region at 12 + 5 weeks, showing the fetal aorta up to its bifurcation, as well as both the renal arteries and the kidneys (arrows).

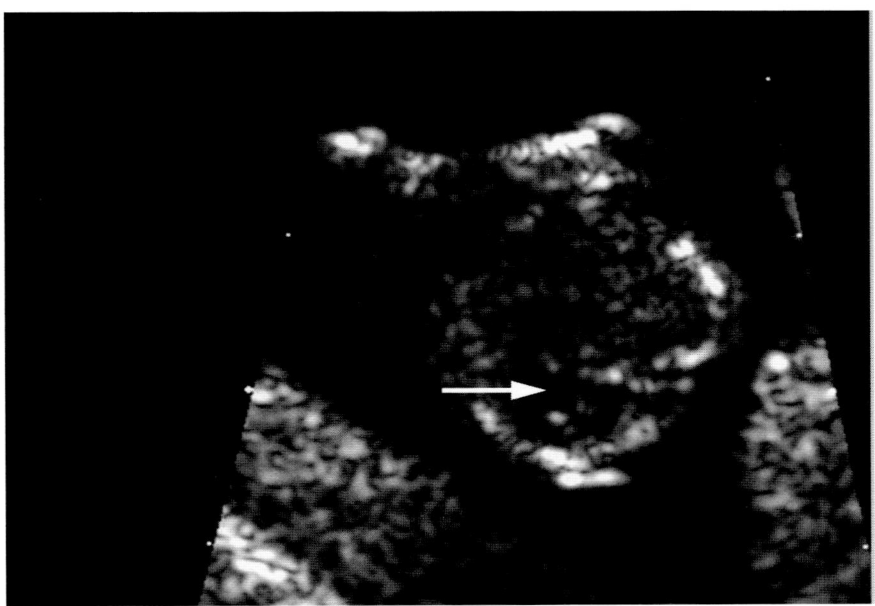

Fig. 1.**13** **First screening: early pregnancy, 8–11 weeks.** Cross-section of the fetal abdomen at 12 + 5 weeks, demonstrating the fetal stomach as an echo-free area.

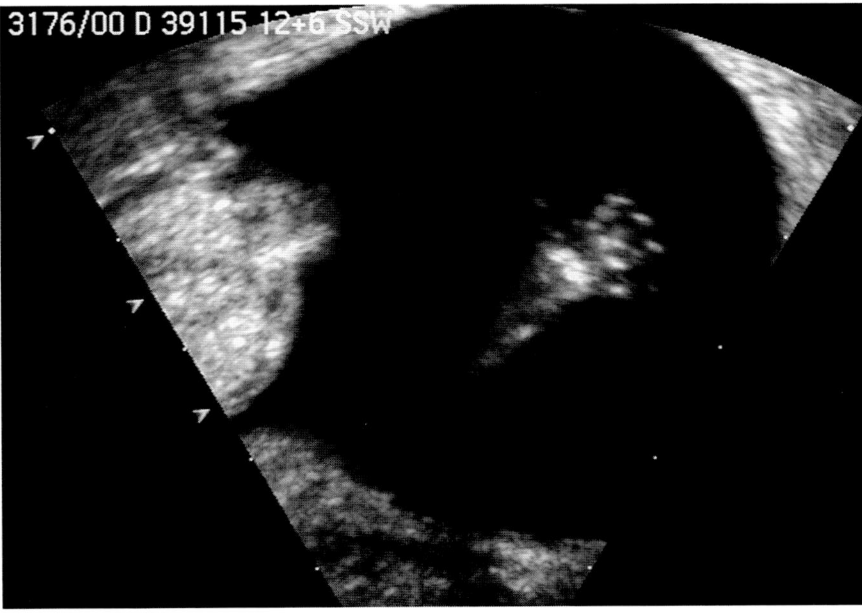

Fig. 1.**14** **First screening: early pregnancy, 8–11 weeks.** Fetal hand at 12 + 6 weeks. The phalanges of all the fingers are clearly seen.

1

Second Screening (18–21 Weeks)

In addition to confirming a viable pregnancy, the aim of this screening is to evaluate the number of fetuses, placental location, and—most importantly—*disturbances in fetal development and anomalies,* as well as assessment of the fetal heart and amniotic fluid.

For biometric assessment, biparietal and fronto-occipital diameters, abdominal circumference and femur length are measured. Measurements of other long bones may also prove useful.

For an effective survey of fetal anatomy, ultrasonography should be performed systematically. This is reported as follows.

Head: Important structures here are the middle echo, thalamus, lateral ventricles (normal width of the posterior horn up to 8–10 mm), size and form of the cerebellum, and the septum pellucidum. Eyes, nose, and lips should also be visualized.

Neck: Measurement of nuchal translucency in second-trimester screening is less predictive and cannot be analyzed statistically (Snijders and Nicolaides), but it should still be visualized as an extra parameter.

Thorax: The axis and location of the heart and lungs in the thorax should be identified. To exclude cardiac situs abnormalities, it is important to understand the fetal position within the uterus as well as the orientation of fetal heart within the thorax. Echocardiography is performed as an extra examination. The diaphragm is seen most easily in the longitudinal plane. For diagnosis of diaphragmatic hernia, a knowledge of the topography of the thoracic and abdominal organs is essential (mediastinal shift, displacement of the heart and stomach).

Abdomen: The stomach, liver, and gallbladder are readily detected in the upper abdomen, the kidneys lying caudally and dorsally. To visualize the kidney lying furthest from the transducer overshadowed by the vertebral column, the position of the transducer has to be changed often according to the fetal position. Doppler flow evaluation of renal arteries can also be useful in detecting renal anomalies such as double kidney, renal agenesis, and pelvic kidney. The insertion of the umbilical cord into the fetal abdomen, the bladder, and the genitals are localized more caudally. The umbilical arteries can be readily detected lateral to the bladder using Doppler flow, much more easily than in an umbilical cord floating free in amniotic fluid.

Spine: It is essential to examine the spine along its entire length, starting from the cervical region, and in a transverse plane. It is important to note that the three hyperechoic centers seen on ultrasonography represent the vertebral body and the laminae, but that the vertebral spines are not visualized. *Neural tube defects* are often detected as widening of the ossification centers of the laminae. In addition, soft tissue and skin overlying the spine should be viewed carefully. Examination of the head with regard to shape and form, as well as the configuration of the cerebellum and the ventricles, is important in detecting neural tube defects secondary to "head signs." Most neural tube defects are located in the lumbosacral region; lesions in the cervical and thoracic areas are an exception.

Extremities: Evaluation of the extremities in second-trimester screening can be difficult and time-consuming depending on the fetal position and maternal condition for sonography. Nevertheless, to detect *anomalies of the extremities,* all long bones, including bones of both the lower arm and lower leg, as well as fingers and toes, should be demonstrated. Measurement of the middle phalanx of the fifth finger as a method of screening for Down syndrome is neither practicable nor relevant, as the differences between normal and abnormal findings are too small to provide reasonable sensitivity and specificity.

Fetal echocardiography: A four-chamber view of the heart is obtained, and the location of the heart is confirmed (dextrocardia?). To measure the atria and ventricles, biometric assessment in B-mode is helpful. The four-chamber view makes it possible to monitor the *function of the atrioventricular (AV) valves (stenosis or insufficiency)* using CFM. To exclude a *ventricular septal defect (VSD),* the interventricular septum has to be demonstrated, especially below the level of the atrioventricular valves. For this, it is essential to visualize the heart from the side, as the apical view alone can easily produce a VSD artefact as a result of "echo dropout."

The transducer is turned slightly from the apical plane in the cranial direction of the fetus to observe the outflow tracts. The aortic stem with the aortic valve can be functionally demonstrated using CFM and Doppler sonography. The highest velocity over the aortic valve lies under 1 m/s. Turning the transducer further cranially, the crossing of the pulmonary artery over the aorta and the pulmonary valve are observed. The diameters of the aorta and pulmonary artery can be measured using B-mode sonography. Normally, the pulmonary artery is wider than the aorta, but if the aorta appears wider, this may suggest *pulmonary stenosis (Fallot's tetralogy?).* The ductus arteriosus (Botallo's duct) can be seen connecting the pulmonary artery and aorta. In the three-vessel view, the superior vena cava, aorta, and pulmonary artery can be demonstrated. The aortic arch can be seen in longitudinal axis, but the cranial outflow tracts have to be demonstrated to avoid confusion between the aortic arch, pulmonary trunk, and ductus arteriosus. When the pulse repetition frequency (PRF) function of CFM is selected for lower velocities, flow from the pulmonary vein into the left atrium and the junction of the superior and inferior vena cava into the right atrium can be visualized.

Placenta: Current data suggest that during second-trimester screening, it is worth measuring the velocity wave forms in both uterine arteries in order to help identify women who are at a higher risk of developing *placental dysfunction and placental abruption.* It is important here to measure the blood flow in the main uterine artery lying medial to the external iliac vein and not a small branch of the artery, which may show lower resistance values, misleading the examiner.

In addition, in certain cases, Doppler sonography of the umbilical arteries may help detect *early placental dysfunction.*

In case of pathological velocity wave forms, ultrasonography and Doppler examinations have to be repeated in the third trimester.

A one-sided "notch" and unilateral increased resistance in uterine artery flow are often associated with lateral location of the placenta and can also be a sign of possible development of placental dysfunction.

Multiple gestations: Zygosity in multiple gestations has to be confirmed if this has not been possible during the first screening. The wall separating the chorionic cavities is thinner in monochorionic twins (approx. 1 mm) than in dichorionic twins (> 1.5 mm). In addition, the "lambda sign" can be seen in dichorionic gestation. Visualizing the sex is also helpful (when there is a fetus of the opposite sex, the twins are dizygotic and therefore dichorionic and diamniotic).

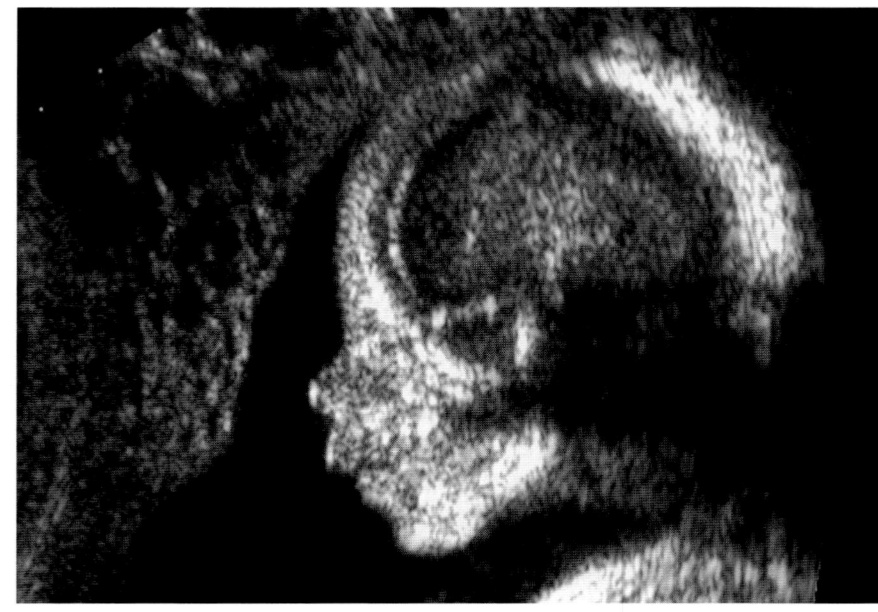

Fig. 1.**15** **Second screening, 18–21 weeks.** Fetal profile at 21 + 6 weeks

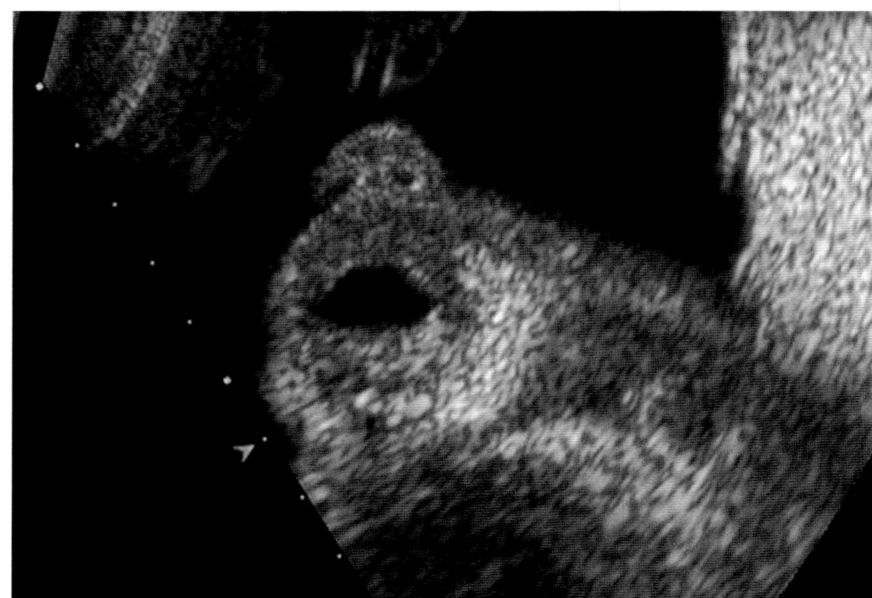

Fig. 1.**16** **Second screening, 18–21 weeks.** Frontal view of the fetal face, showing the lips and nostrils.

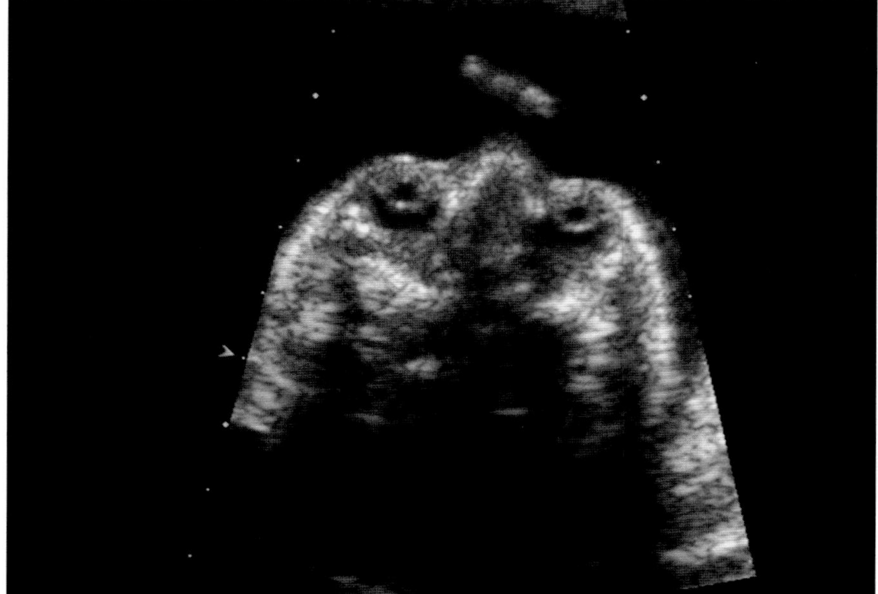

Fig. 1.**17** **Second screening, 18–21 weeks.** Cross-sectional view of the eye region, showing the fetal orbits and the lenses of the eyes.

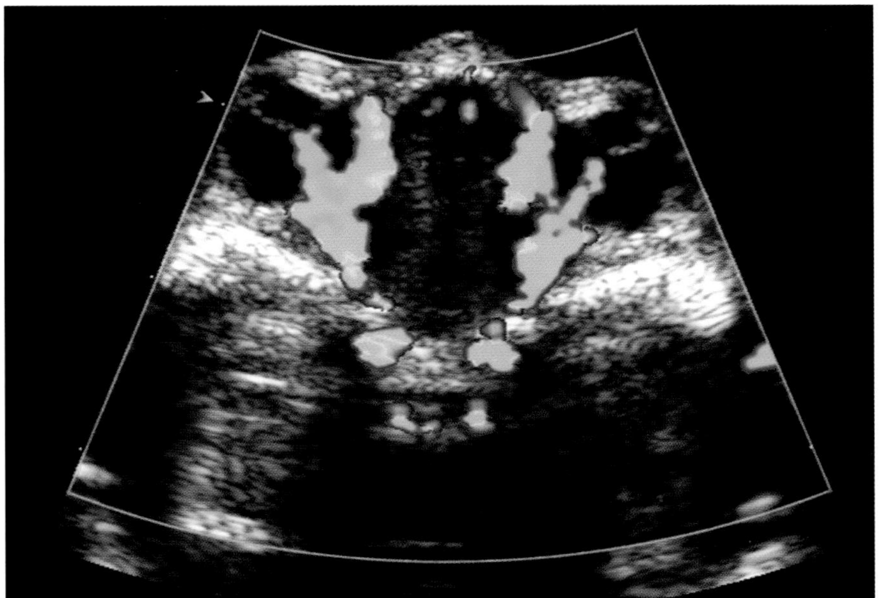

Fig. 1.**18** **Second screening, 18–21 weeks.** Cross-sectional view of the fetal eye region, demonstrating the hyaloid arteries supplying the lenses.

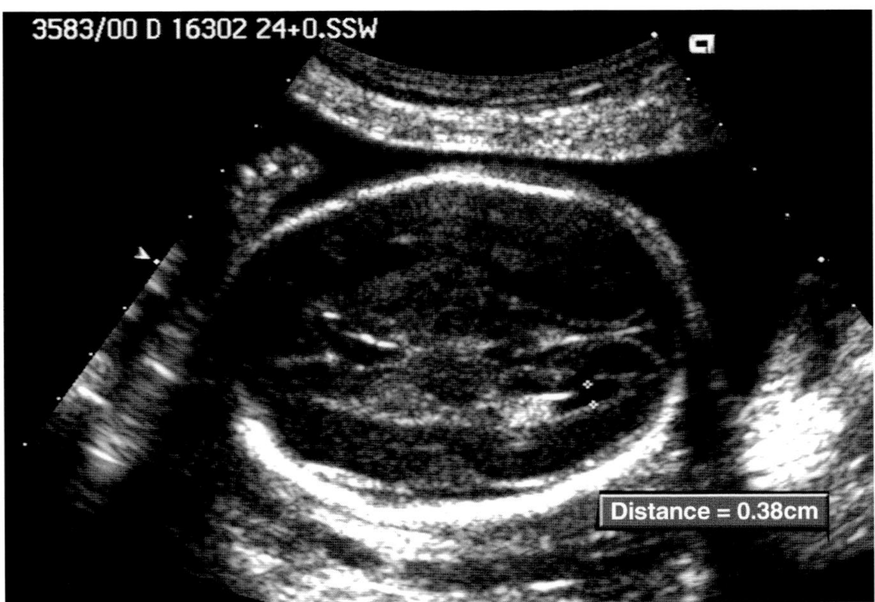

Fig. 1.**19** **Second screening, 18–21 weeks.** The posterior horn of the left lateral ventricle is seen, with a normal width measurement of 3.8 mm.

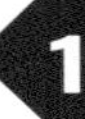

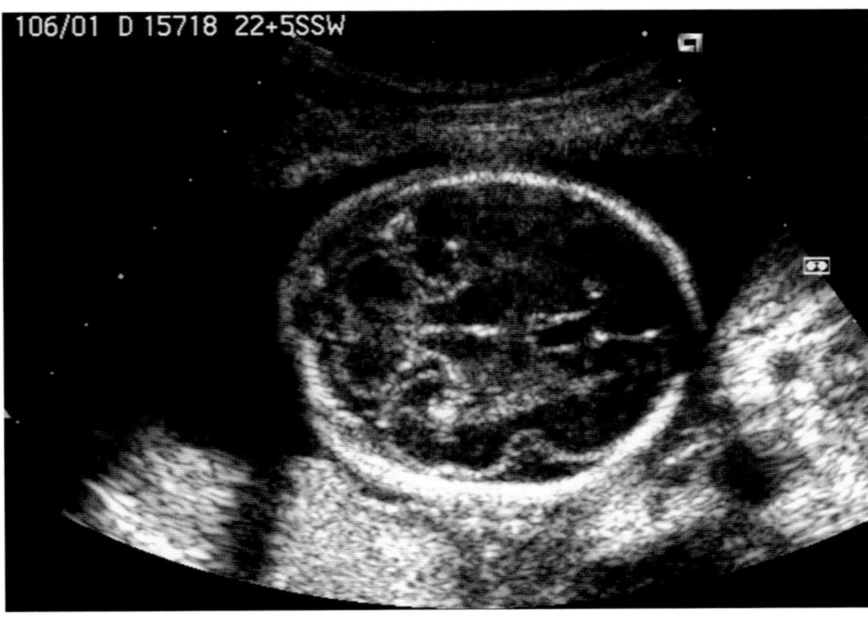

Fig. 1.**20** **Second screening, 18–21 weeks.** The normal cerebellum is recognized as a dumbbell shape. Between 20 and 23 weeks, its diameter in millimeters corresponds approximately to the gestational age (here 23 mm at 22 weeks).

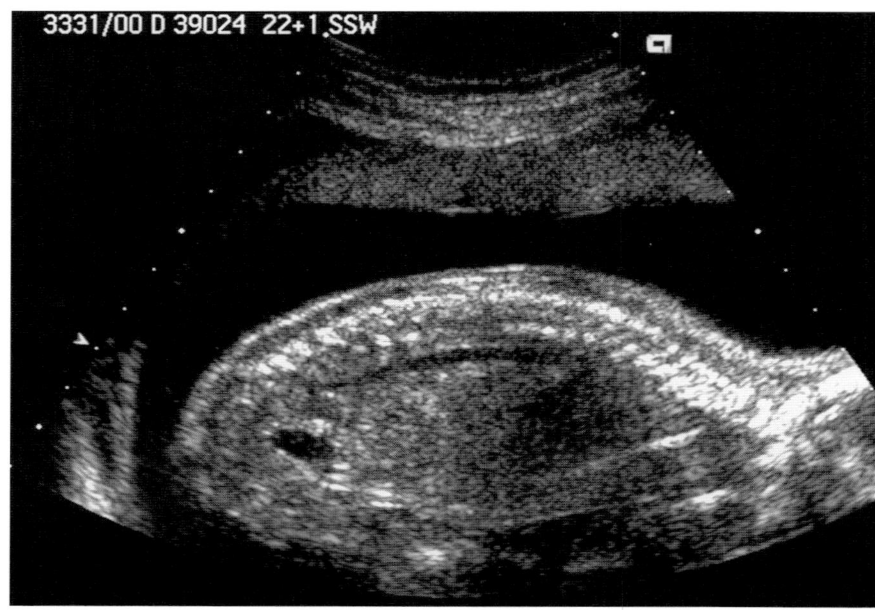

Fig. 1.**21** **Second screening, 18–21 weeks.** Longitudinal section of the fetal spinal column at 22 + 1 weeks, with the fetus lying dorsoanteriorly. The continuity of the main profile of the vertebral column is not interrupted. A section of the fetal aorta is seen at the front, and the urinary bladder is located in the pelvis. The neck region is normal.

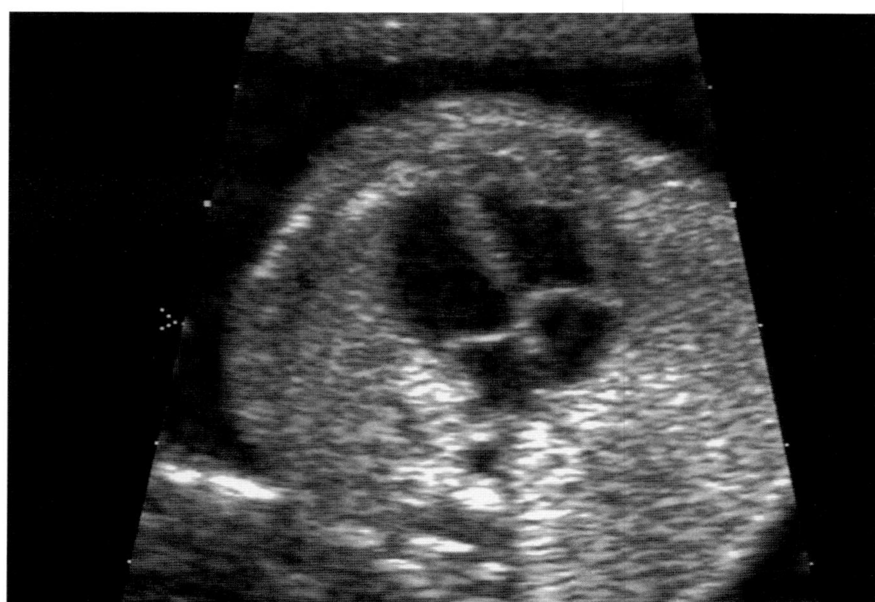

Fig. 1.**22** **Second screening, 18–21 weeks.** Cross-section of the fetal thorax at 22 + 0 weeks, showing an apical view of the four heart chambers in the early systolic phase. Both atrioventricular valves are closed, the tricuspid valve being slightly higher than the mitral valve. The septum primum, septum secundum, and foramen ovale are seen.

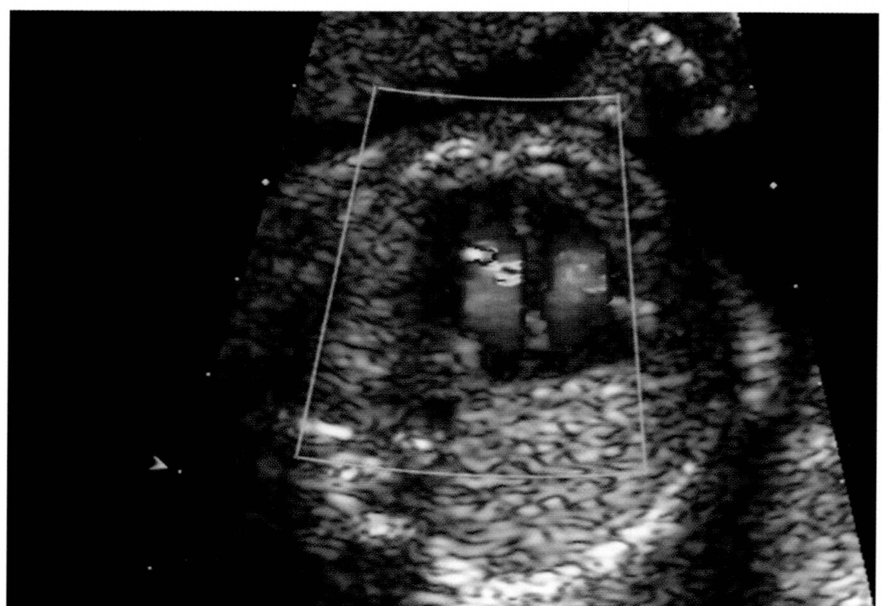

Fig. 1.**23** **Second screening, 18–21 weeks.** Apical view of the four chambers with color Doppler sonography in the diastolic phase. Blood flowing through both the valves into the ventricles can be well recognized.

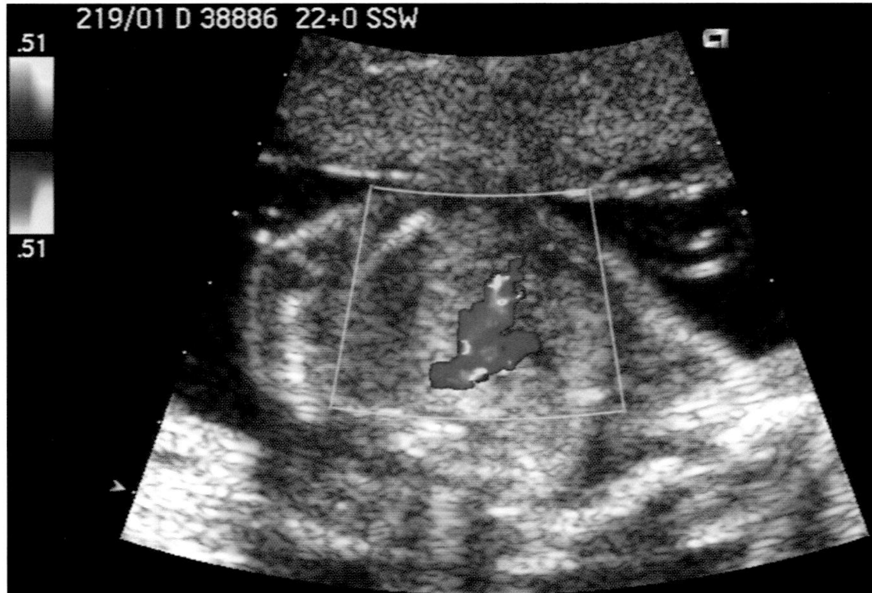

Fig. 1.**24** **Second screening, 18–21 weeks.** Color Doppler sonography of the outgoing vessels of the heart in the systolic phase, depicting the pulmonary trunk, the ductus arteriosus (Botallo's duct), and the fetal aorta.

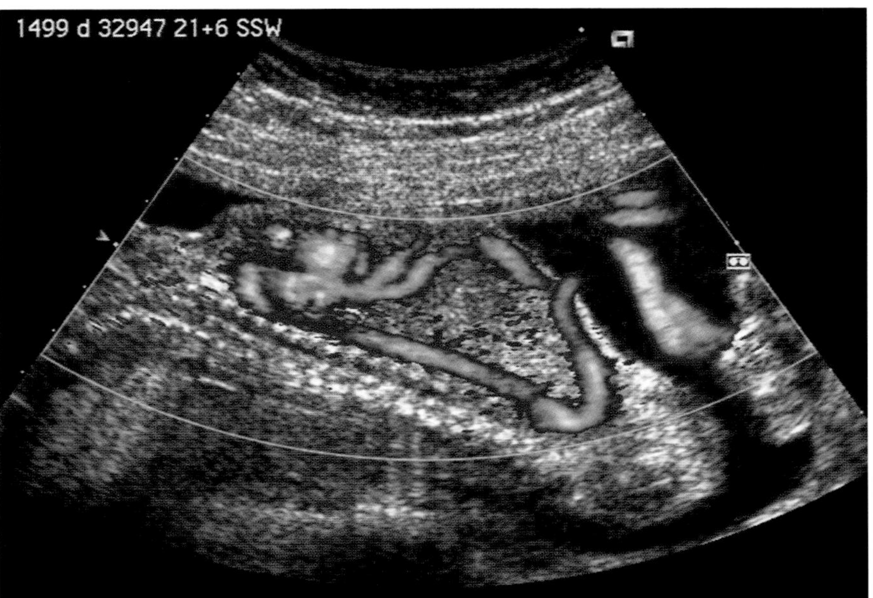

Fig. 1.**25** **Second screening, 18–21 weeks.** Fetal circulation at 21 weeks, depicted using the color Doppler energy mode. Visible here are the aortic arch leaving the heart, the thoracic and abdominal aorta, one of the two umbilical arteries and its course through the abdomen, as well as the intra-abdominal umbilical vein.

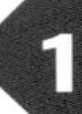

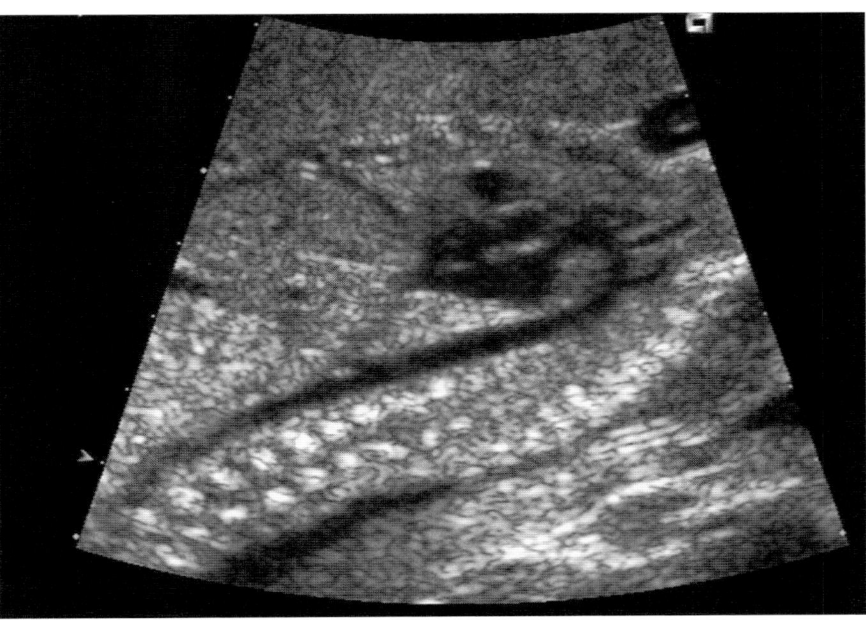

Fig. 1.**26** **Second screening, 18–21 weeks.** The fetal aorta (aortic arch with its three vessels arising from the cranial part, thoracic and abdominal aorta) as seen at 21 weeks, with the fetus lying dorsoposteriorly.

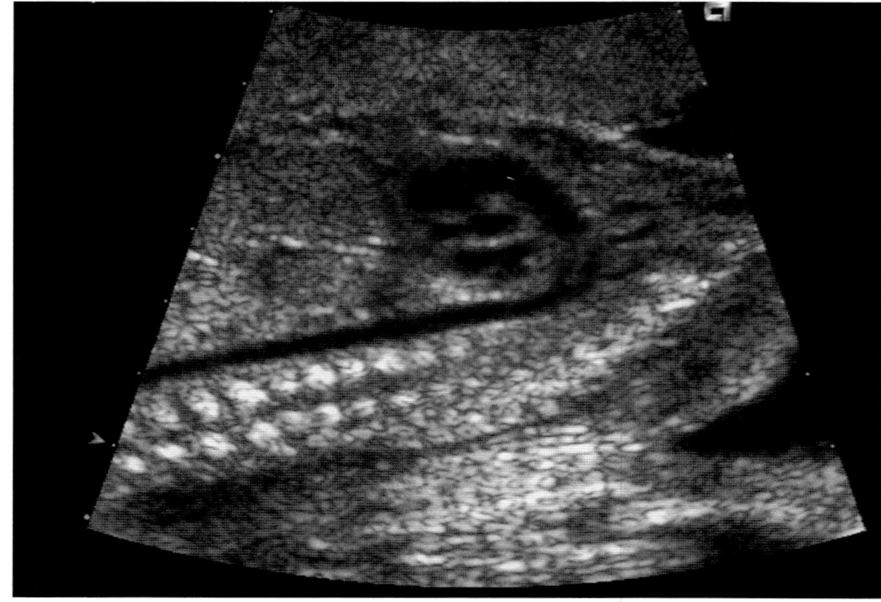

Fig. 1.27 **Second screening, 18–21 weeks.** The same view as in the previous figure, with the transducer slightly rotated. Flow from the ductus arteriosus (Botallo's duct) and aortic arch into the descending aorta can be seen.

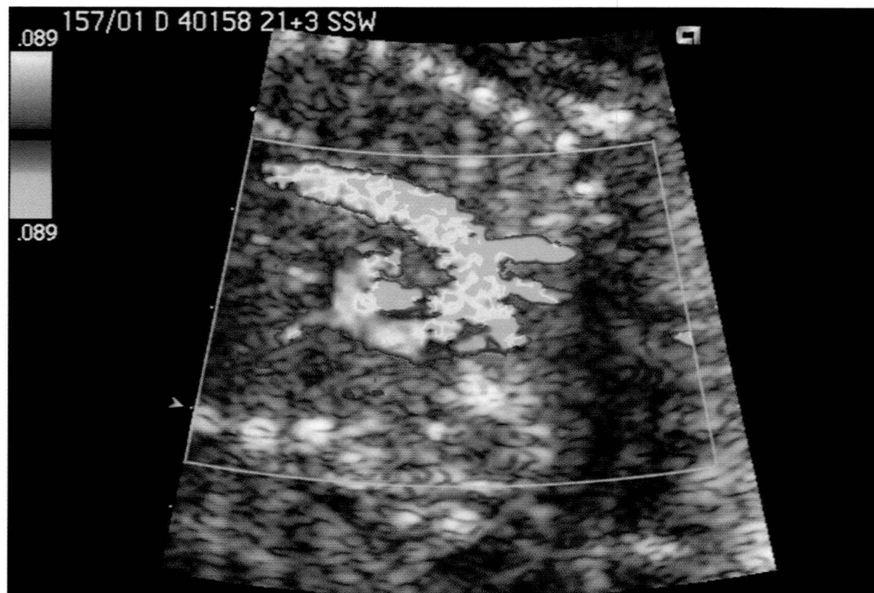

Fig. 1.28 **Second screening, 18–21 weeks.** The aortic arch and its branches are demonstrated using the color Doppler mode in a fetus lying dorsoanterior 21 weeks of gestation. This is a paramedian longitudinal section left of the vertebral column.

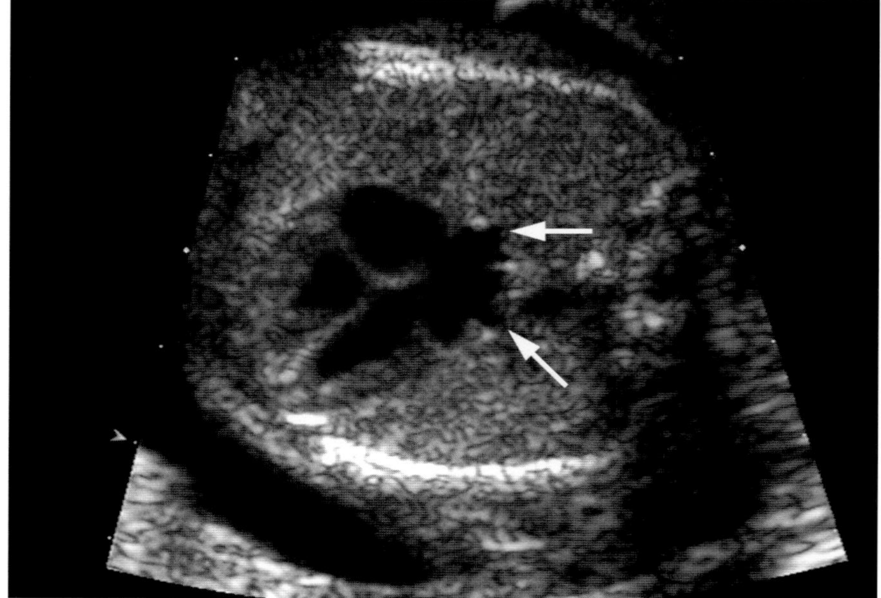

Fig. 1.29 **Second screening, 18–21 weeks.** Four-chamber view of the heart, showing the confluence of the pulmonary vein (arrows) into the left atrium at 21 + 4 weeks.

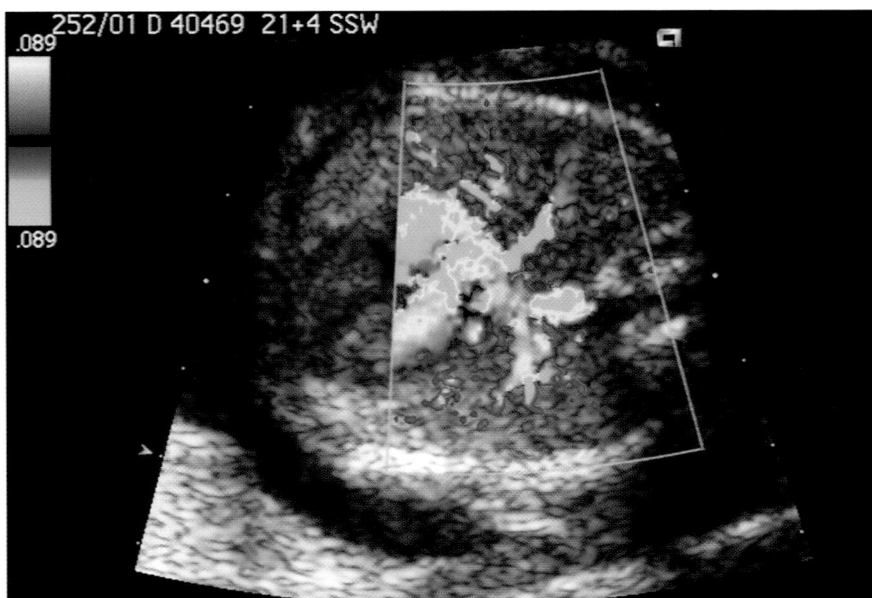

Fig. 1.**30** **Second screening, 18–21 weeks.** Same location as the previous view, with color Doppler mode.

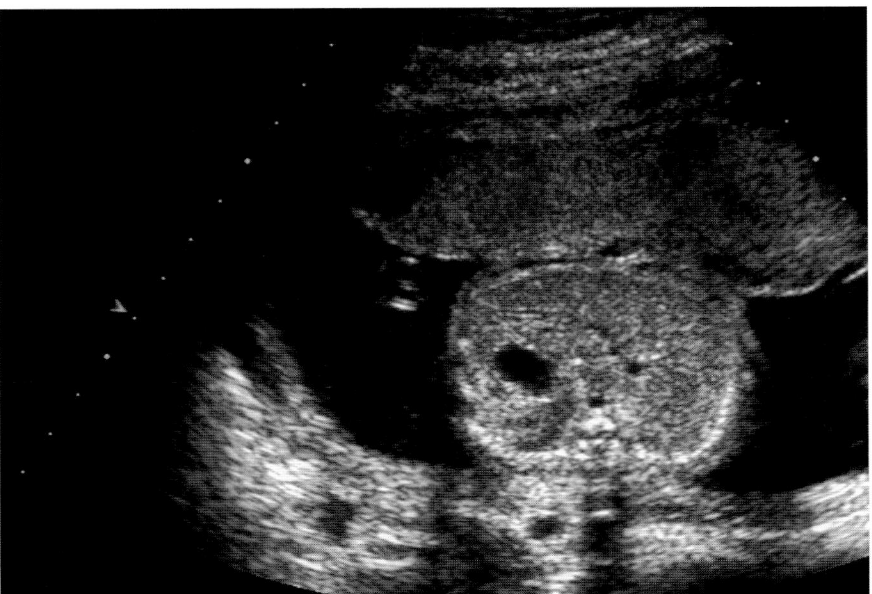

Fig. 1.**31** **Second screening, 18–21 weeks.** Cross-section of a fetal abdomen in the dorsoposterior position, showing the stomach at 22 + 0 weeks.

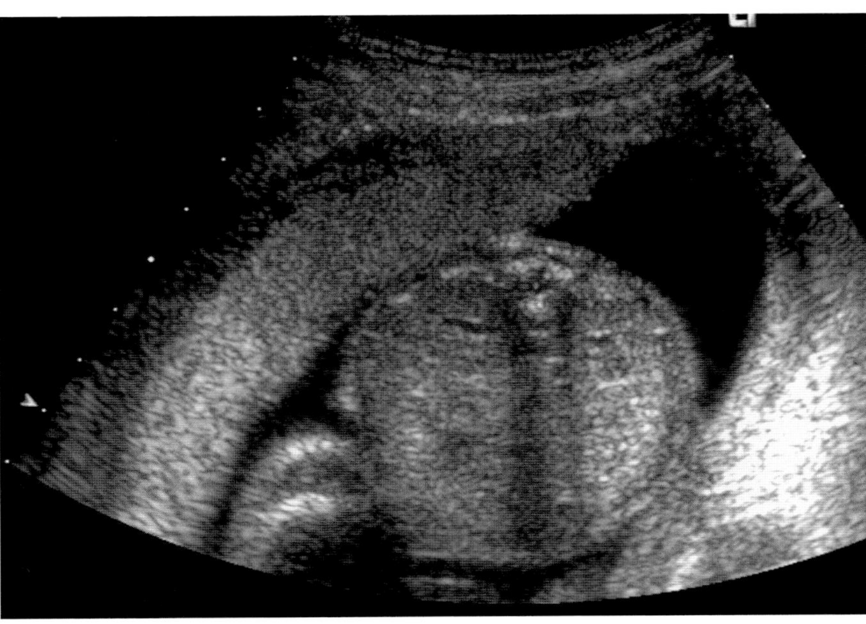

Fig. 1.**32** **Second screening, 18–21 weeks.** Cross-section of the fetal abdomen at 22 + 2 weeks in the dorsoanterior fetal position, showing the kidneys and undilated renal pelvis.

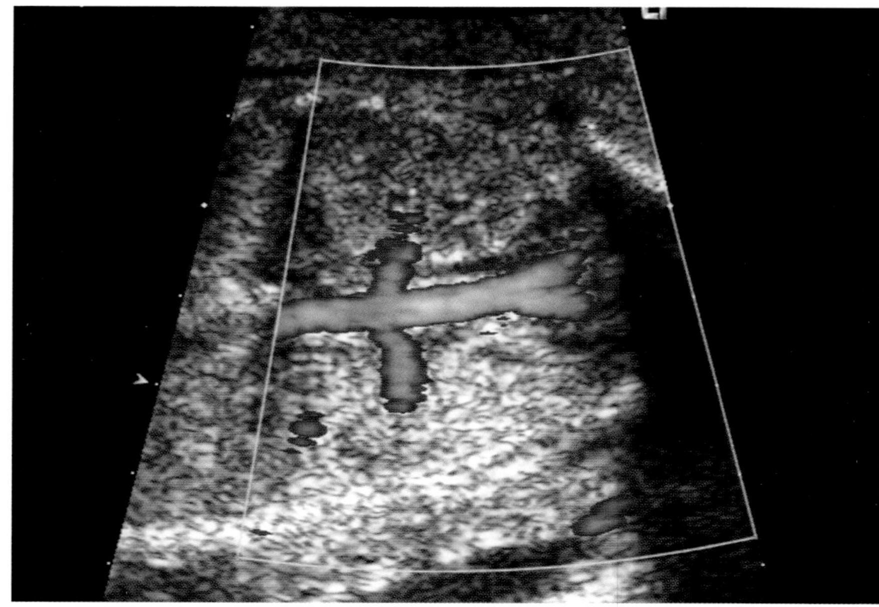

Fig. 1.**33** **Second screening, 18–21 weeks.** Frontal view of the fetal retroperitoneum at 21 + 4 weeks, showing the fetal aorta up to its bifurcation and the branching renal arteries (color Doppler energy mode).

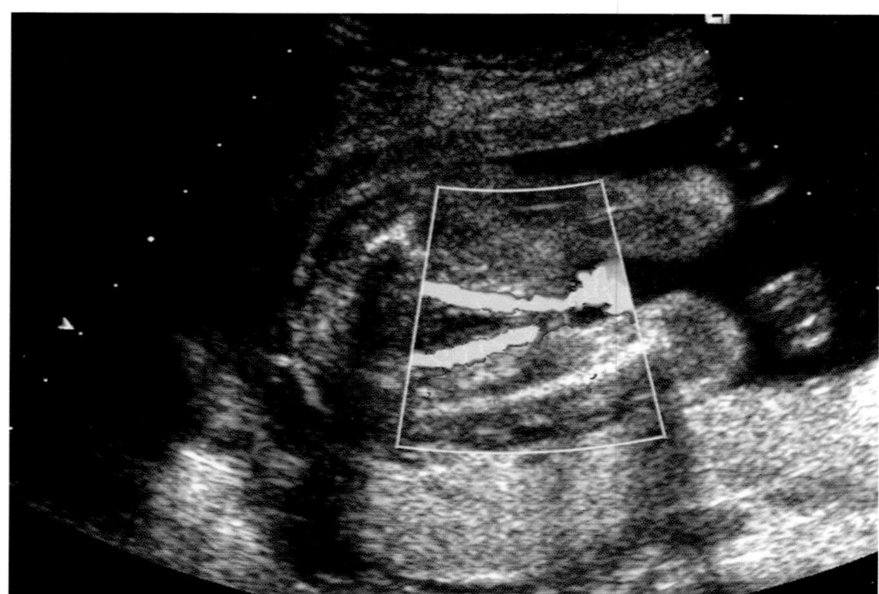

Fig. 1.**34** **Second screening, 18–21 weeks.** Cross-section of the fetal abdomen with tilted transducer at 23 + 3 weeks, showing both femurs, the urinary bladder, and both umbilical arteries running up to the navel (color Doppler sonography).

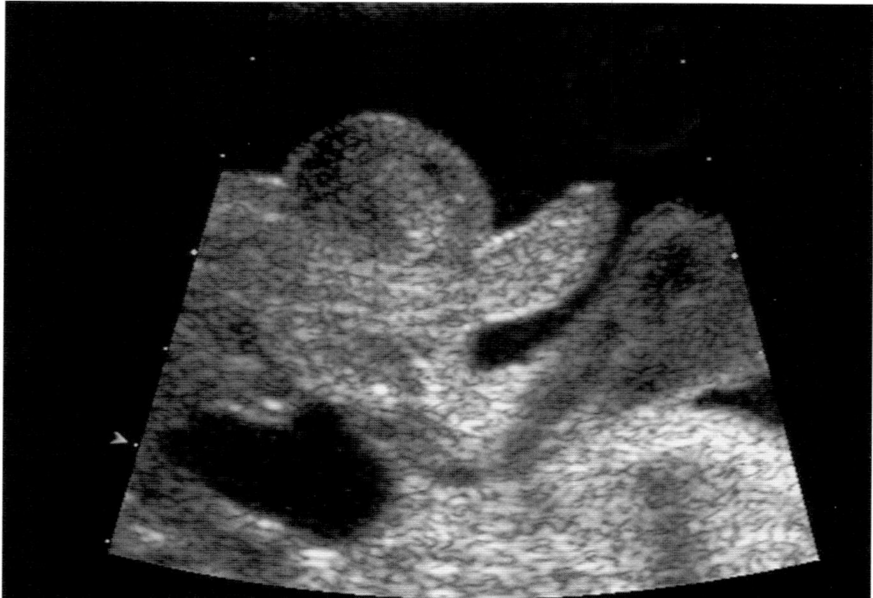

Fig. 1.**35** **Second screening, 18–21 weeks.** Longitudinal section of the lower fetal abdomen at 28 + 4 weeks with the fetus in the dorsoposterior position, demonstrating male genitals, urinary bladder, and navel.

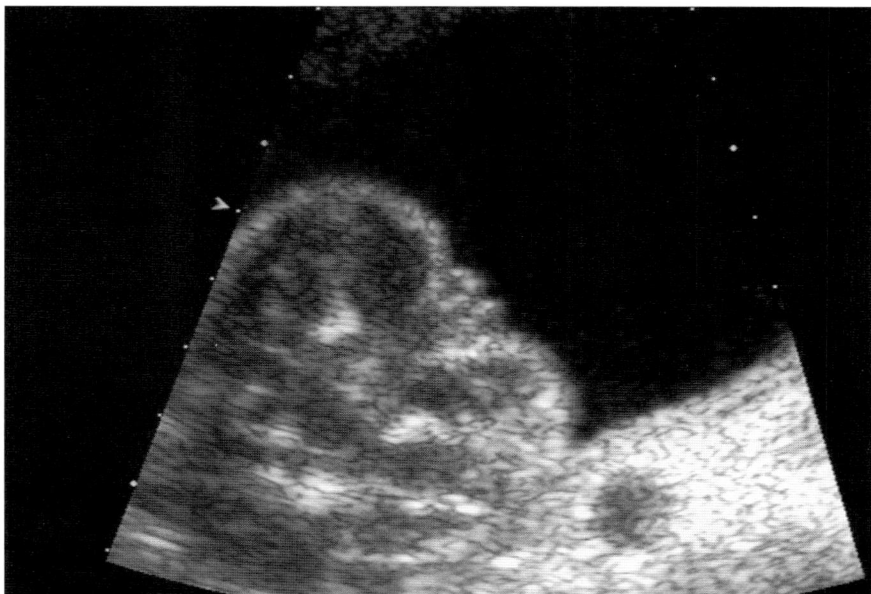

Fig. 1.**36** **Second screening, 18–21 weeks.** Cross-section of the fetal abdomen at 23 + 6 weeks, showing female genitals (labial folds).

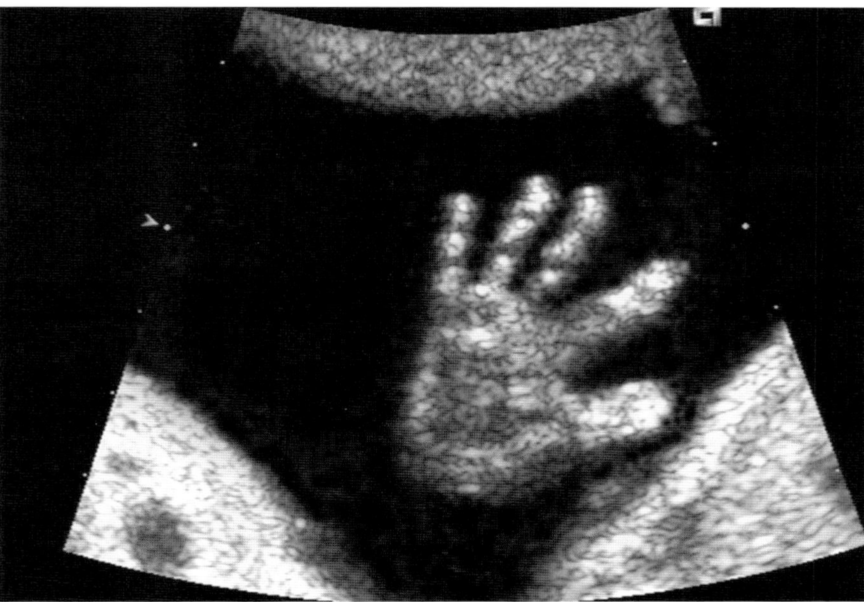

Fig. 1.**37** **Second screening, 18–21 weeks.** Fetal hand at 22 + 2 weeks. The phalanges are well demonstrated.

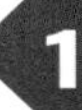

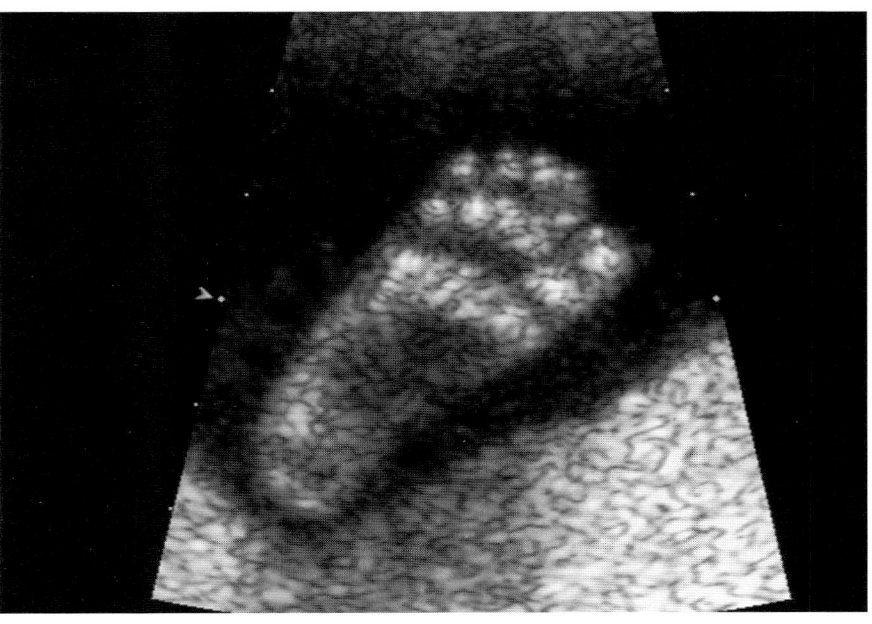

Fig. 1.**38** **Second screening, 18–21 weeks.** Fetal foot at 22 + 3 weeks.

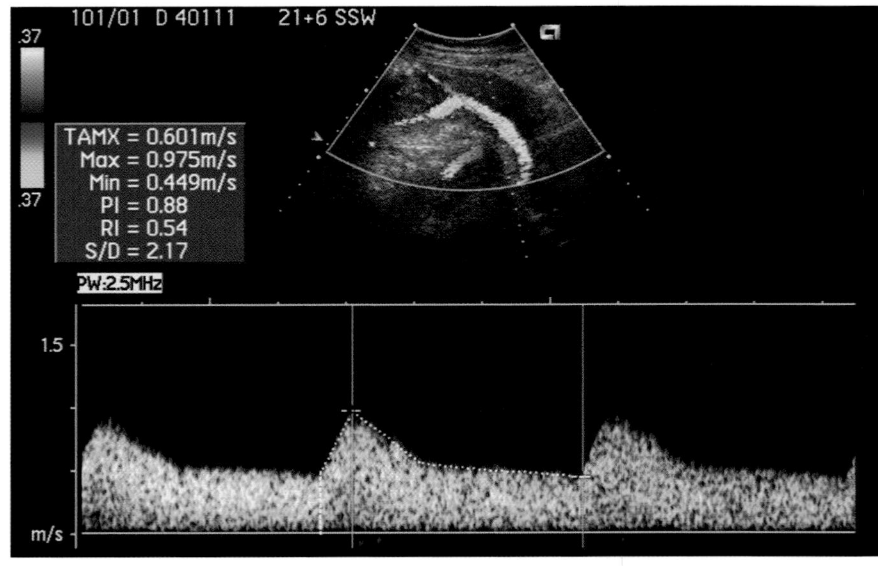

Fig. 1.**39** **Second screening, 18–21 weeks.** Uterine artery 21 + 6 weeks. *Top:* color Doppler sonography, showing the artery crossing the iliac artery. *Bottom:* Blood flow velocity curve using the pulsed Doppler mode. Normal findings.

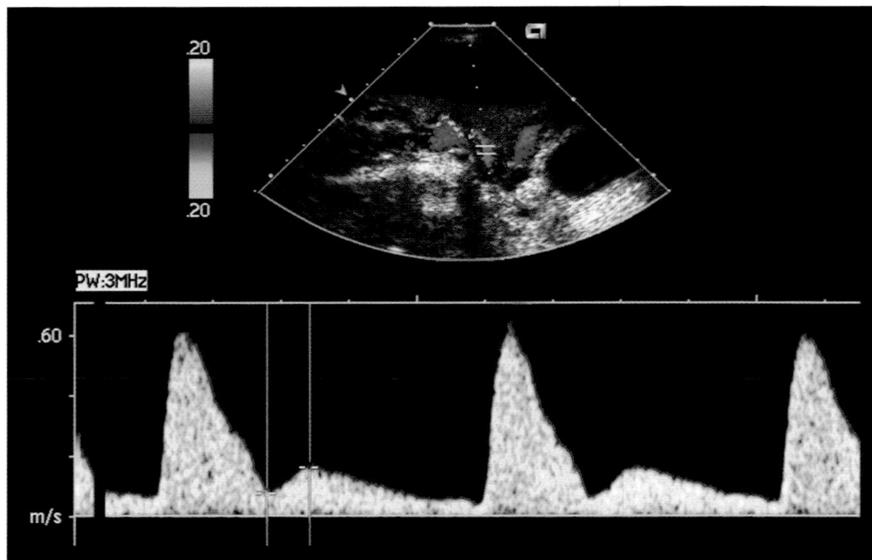

Fig. 1.**40** **Second screening, 18–21 weeks.** Color-coded Doppler sonography of the uterine artery, showing increased resistance and a significant "notch."

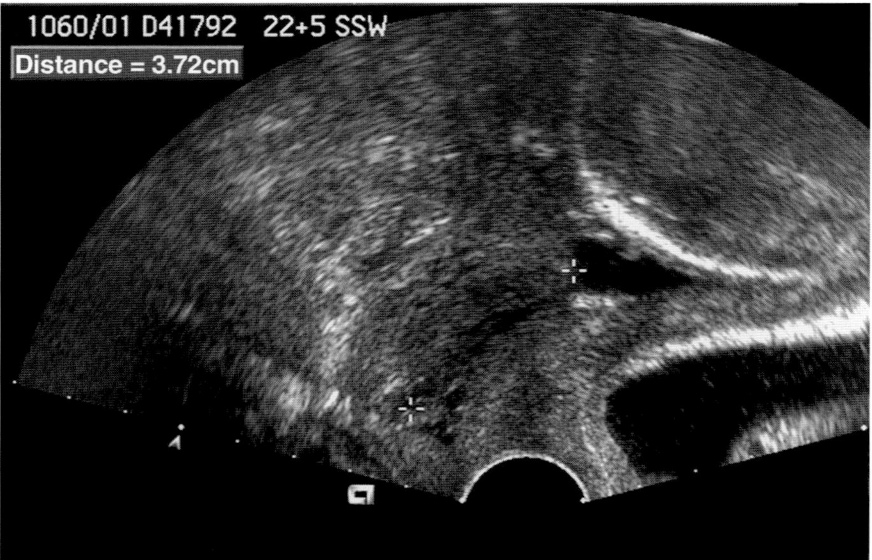

Fig. 1.**41** **Second screening, 18–21 weeks.** Cervix 22 + 5 weeks. Transvaginal sonography; the length of the cervix measures 37 mm. Apparently normal findings.

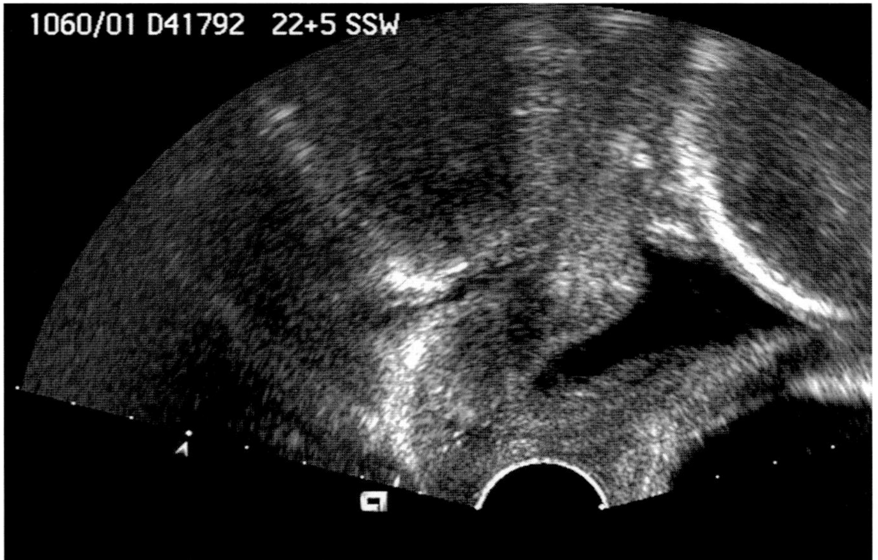

Fig. 1.**42** **Second screening, 18–21 weeks.** The same situation as before, but the patient is bearing down; the amniotic sac descends through the internal cervical os into the cervical canal.

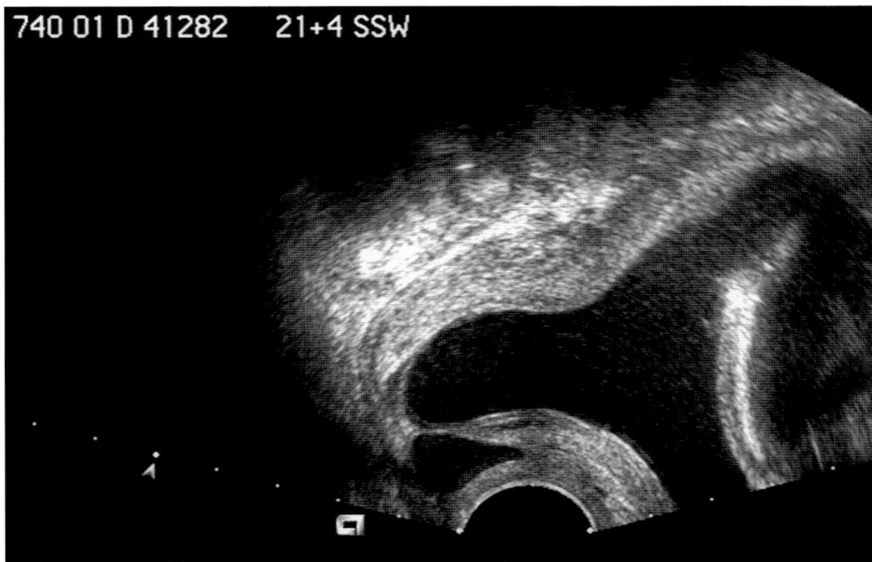

Fig. 1.**43** **Second screening, 18–21 weeks.** Vaginal sonography demonstrating the cervix at 21 + 4 weeks; the amniotic sac has prolapsed into the cervical canal, reaching the external cervical os. There is a Nabothian cyst as a concomitant finding.

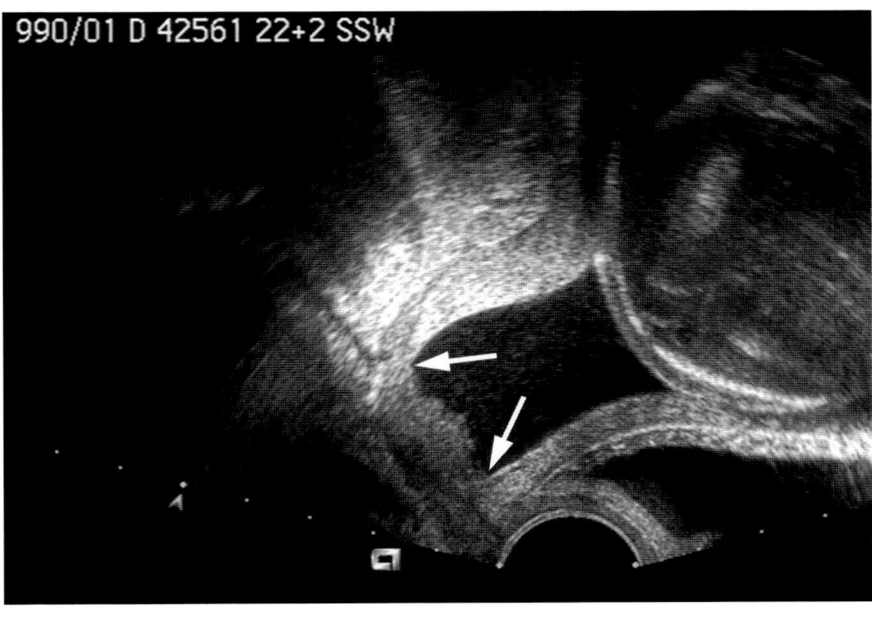

Fig. 1.**44** **Second screening, 18–21 weeks.** Vaginal sonography demonstrating the cervix at 22 + 2 weeks. Severe cervical insufficiency, with cervical dilation of 2 cm.

Table 1.1 Checklist of sonographic screening.

Fetomaternal unit		
	Number of fetuses Fetal position Localization of placenta (placenta previa?)	Is amount of amniotic fluid normal? (Oligohydramnios, anhydramnios, hydramnios) Cervical length (below 3 cm?), funneling of the cervical canal?
Biometric fetal assessment (correct due date, early growth restriction?)		
	Measurement of biparietal head diameter Fronto-occipital diameter Anteroposterior and transverse diameters of thorax Length of femur Measurement of other long bones—e.g., humerus, ulna, tibia (disproportion between long bones and body length?) Biometry of intracranial ventricles (e.g. width of the posterior horn of the lateral ventricle, hydrocephalus, asymmetry of the ventricular system?)	Diameter of cerebellum (hypoplasia? Banana sign? Correction of due date) Cisterna magna dilation? (Dandy–Walker malformation?) Cardiac biometry—ventricles, great vessels; disproportionate ventricular size? Narrowing of the great vessels? Is the pulmonary vessel smaller than the aorta (Fallot's tetralogy?)
Doppler sonography		
	Resistance index of umbilical artery (increased? Zero flow?)	Resistance index of the uterine artery at its crossing of external iliac artery. Notching?
Screening of fetal organs		
	Head	
	Normal shape? (Brachycephaly, lemon sign, strawberry sign?) Width and symmetry of the ventricles Choroid plexus cysts? Normal midline echo? (Holoprosencephaly?) Normal shape of cerebellum (banana sign, Dandy–Walker malformation	Demonstration of corpus callosum? (Agenesis?) Demonstration of septum pellucidum? (Agenesis of corpus callosum?) Widening of cisterna magna? (Dandy–Walker cysts?)
	Face	
	Are eyes in the right position? Is the nose visible? Mouth and palate normal? (Cleft lip and palate?)	Normal chin profile? (Retrognathia? Pierre-Robin sequence?).

Continue ▶

Table 1.1 (Continue)

Screening of fetal organs		
	Vertebral column	
	Normal? (Scoliosis? Spina bifida?)	
	Neck	
	Cystic hygroma? Encephalocele?	Goiter?
	Thorax	
	Normal cardiac location? (Situs inversus, cardiac displacement?)	Normal lung structure? (Cystic lesions, adenomatosis?)
	Heart	
	Cardiac rhythm normal? (Extrasystole, bradycardia, tachycardia?) Normal size, shape and axis of the heart? Presence of cardiac effusion? Is the four-chamber view normal? Is the ventricular septum normal, with normal flow? Are the atrial septum and oval foramen normal?	Are the AV valves and cardiac perfusion normal? Is there any evidence of heart defect? Are the great vessels, valves, and the crossing normal? Is the upper pulmonary vein visible, with flow into the left atrium? Are the aortic arch and its cranial branches visible?
	Abdomen	
	Is the stomach filled normally? Normal location of the liver? Are the intestines normal? (Echogenicity? Cysts? Obstruction?) Normal appearance of the kidneys without congestion?	Is the umbilicus visible (without hernia)? Is the urinary bladder filled normally? Are the genitals clearly visible and normal?
	Extremities	
	Normal lengths? Symmetrical? Radius aplasia?	Are the hands and fingers visible? Are the feet and toes visible?

Third Screening (28–31 Weeks)

The aim of this screening is to detect *placental dysfunction* (intrauterine growth restriction, oligohydramnios, pathological Doppler velocity forms). Some three-quarters of perinatal mortality are due to intrauterine deaths that could have been prevented by early delivery. In addition to biometric assessment, fetal organs should also be viewed to detect *anomalies* in later gestational weeks—for example, hydrocephalus may have developed after 21 weeks, and sonographic abnormalities are often first found after 24 weeks in cases of stenosis of the gastrointestinal tract.

Systematic Scanning of Fetal Anomalies

2 The Central Nervous System and the Eye

Anencephaly

Definition: Anencephaly, and in particular the exencephaly–anencephaly sequence, belongs to the group of cranial neural tube defects and is a condition in which the cranial vault, overlying skin, the meninges and brain are absent.

Incidence: Geographical differences are marked; in Germany and the United States, the figure is one in 1000, while in certain parts of the United Kingdom it is as high as one in 100 births.

Sex ratio: M : F = 1.0 : 3.7

Clinical history/genetics: Family history of neural tube defect; multifactorial transmission, with varying penetrance and influence of environmental factors, is assumed. Risk of recurrence 2–3%. In certain cases, X-chromosomal transmission has also been described.

Teratogens: Valproic acid, folic acid antagonists, diabetes mellitus, hyperthermia, folic acid deficiency.

Embryology: The neural tube closes between the 20th and 28th day after conception. In case of anencephaly, the cranial vault is absent. The developing brain seen in the early embryonic stage degenerates as the pregnancy progresses—mainly in the second trimester, apparently due to unprotected contact with the amniotic fluid.

Associated malformations: Spina bifida, facial clefts, omphalocele, renal anomalies, amniotic banding, Cantrell pentalogy.

Ultrasound findings: The cranial vault, usually fully formed at 9 weeks of pregnancy, is absent. At 9–11 weeks, the *cerebrovascular area* can be identified, but this degenerates up to 15 weeks. *Basal vessels* may even be seen later. Even at the end of first trimester, the form of the head appears unusual, and the cerebrovascular area and in particular the brain float freely, as seen on vaginal sonography. Biometric assessment at the beginning of the second trimester fails to demonstrate the biparietal diameter, thus confirming the diagnosis.

The lower part of the facial vault up to the level of the orbits is not affected, and even the brain stem remains intact. The fetal face often

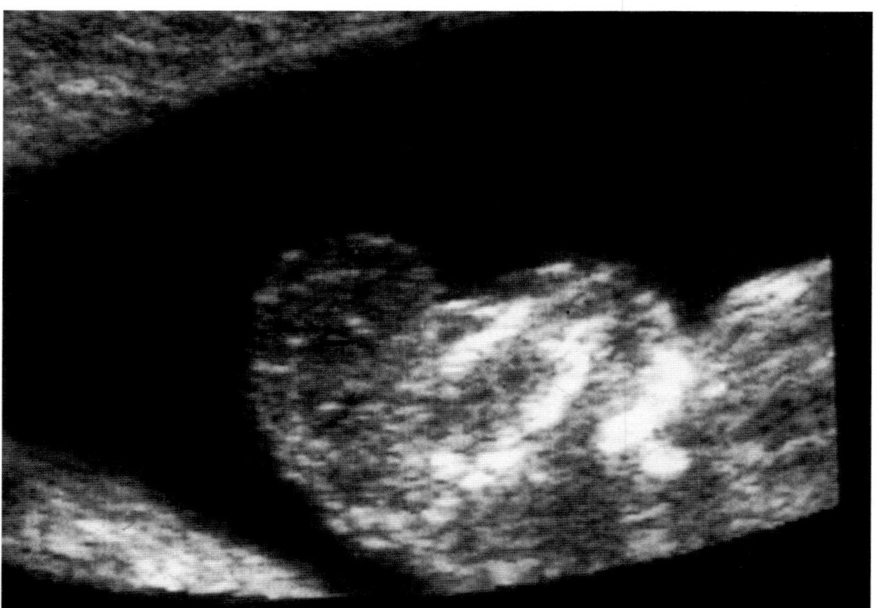

Fig. 2.1 **Exencephaly.** Floating brain in the absence of the cranial vault. Exencephaly, 16 + 6 weeks.

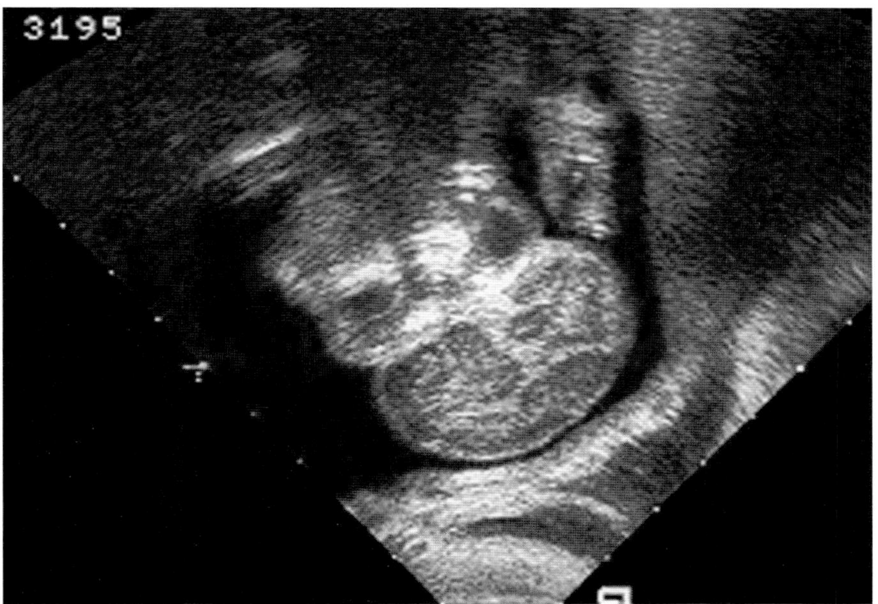

Fig. 2.**2** **Exencephaly.** Vaginal sonography, demonstrating the fetal head at 19 + 6 weeks. Aplasia of the cranial vault; brain tissue covered with meninges is floating in the amniotic fluid. Unusually late form of exencephaly without progression to anencephaly.

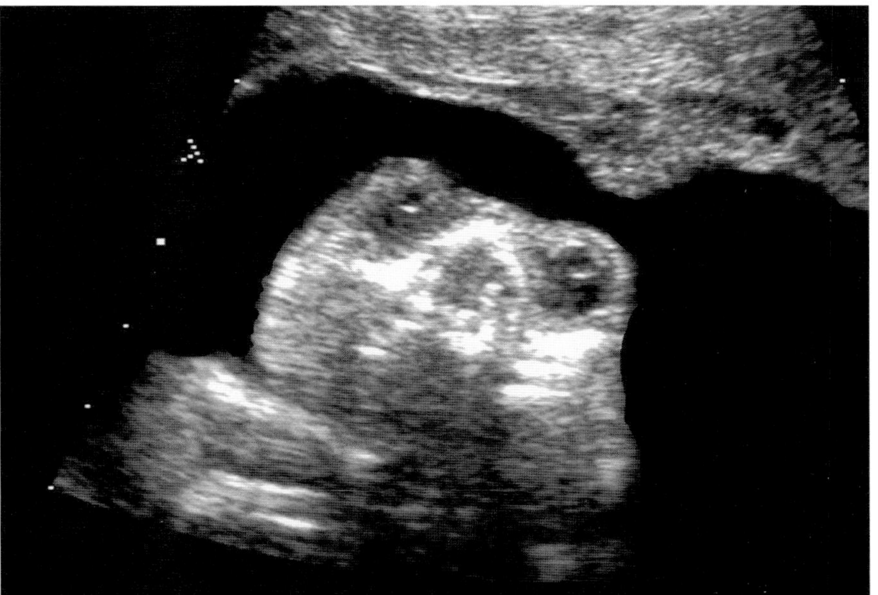

Fig. 2.**3** **Anencephaly.** Ultrasound showing the frontal view. The lenses of the eye are well recognized above the orbits, where the bony skull ends ("frog head").

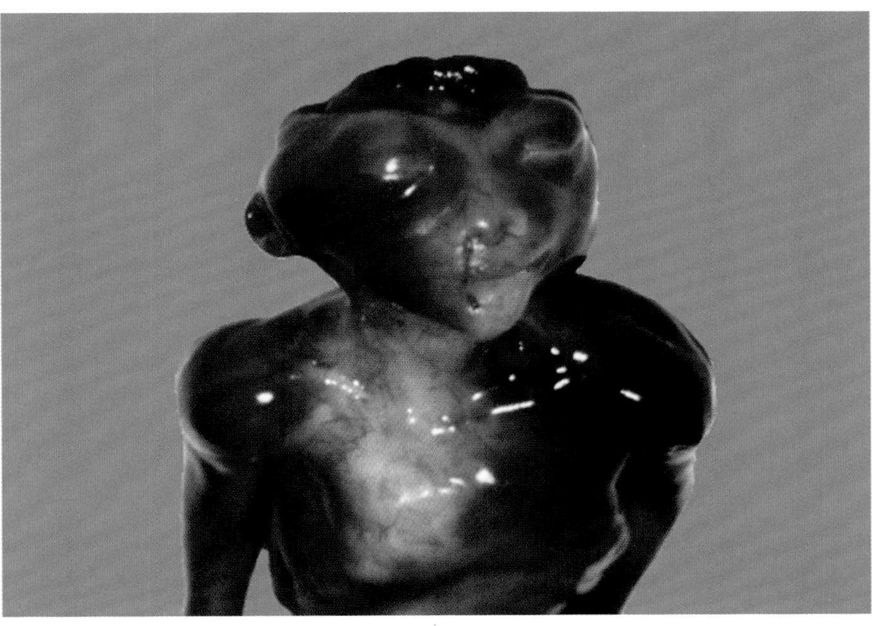

Fig. 2.**4** **Anencephaly.** Frontal view, showing the fetus after termination of pregnancy.

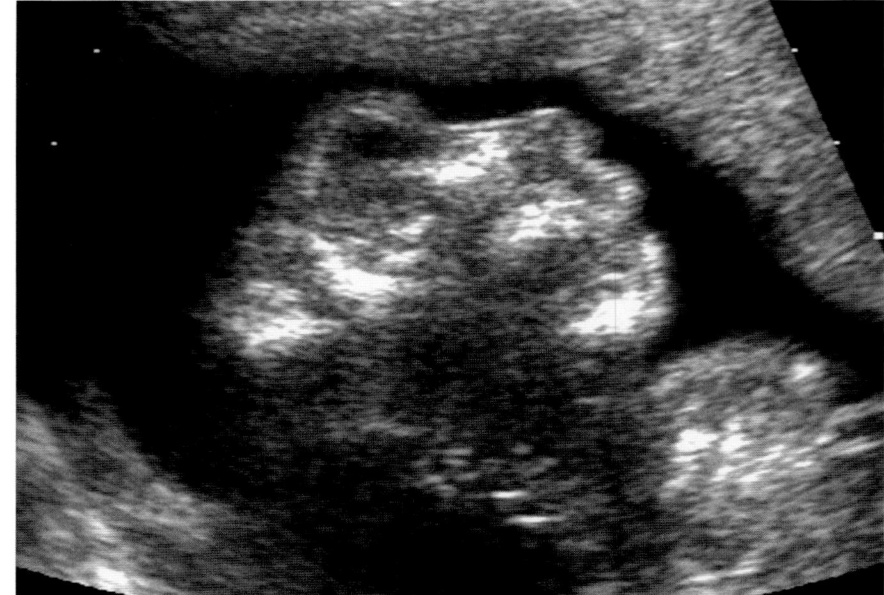

Fig. 2.5 **Anencephaly.** Ultrasound view in the sagittal plane.

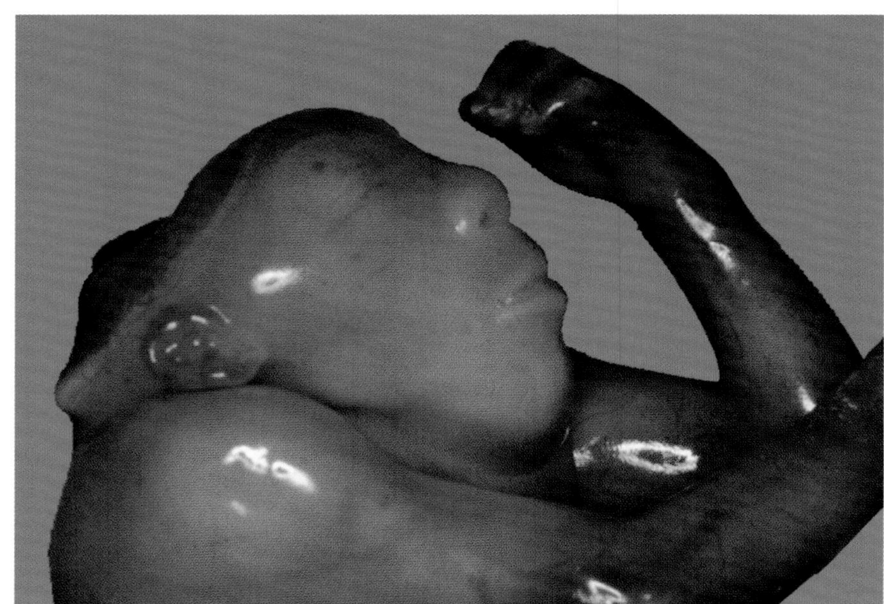

Fig. 2.6 **Anencephaly.** Sagittal view of the fetus after termination of pregnancy.

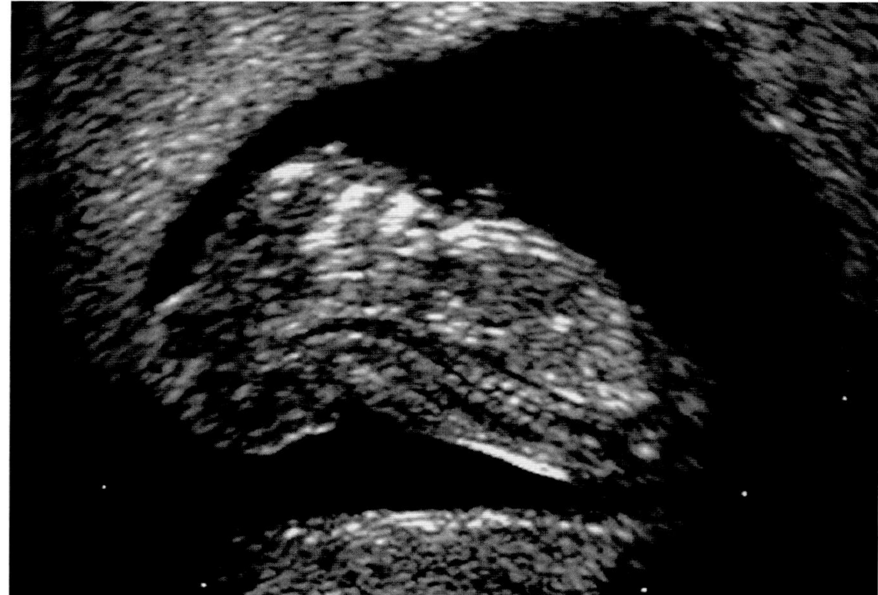

Fig. 2.7 **Exencephaly—anencephaly sequence.** 12 weeks. The cranial vault has not been formed. The brain tissue is floating in the amniotic fluid above the base of the skull.

has a "frog-like" appearance, with prominent orbits. *Myelomeningocele* in the cervical or lumbosacral region may accompany this anomaly. In late pregnancy, the absence of a swallowing reflex leads to *hydramnios*.

Clinical management: After the diagnosis is made, most women opt for termination of pregnancy. In the remaining cases, treatment for hydramnios is indicated to relieve maternal symptoms.

Procedure after birth: Therapy is not possible. Some of the affected neonates survive as much as a few days after birth.

Prognosis: This is considered to be a fatal malformation, resulting in intrauterine death in 50% of the affected fetuses, with the remaining 50% dying at the neonatal stage.

Recommendation for the patient: Before planning the next pregnancy, a regular daily intake of folic acid (4 mg/d) considerably reduces the risk of recurrence.

Self-Help Organization

Title: Anencephaly Support Foundation

Description: Provides support for parents who are continuing a pregnancy after being diagnosed with an anencephalic infant. Information and resources for parents and professionals. Phone support, pen pals, literature, pictures.

Scope: International network

Founded: 1992

Address: 20311 Sienna Pines Court, Spring, TX 77379, United States

Telephone: 1-888-206-7526

E-mail: asf@asfhelp.com

Web: http://www.asfhelp.com

References

Anon. Prevalence of neural tube defects in 20 regions of Europe and the impact of prenatal diagnosis, 1980–1986. EUROCAT Working Group. J Epidemiol Community Health 1991; 45: 52–8.

Becker R, Mende B, Stiemer B, Entezami M. Sonographic markers of exencephaly–anencephaly sequence at 9 + 3 gestational weeks. Ultrasound Obstet Gynecol 2000; 16: 582–4.

Boyd PA, Wellesley DG, De Walle HE, et al. Evaluation of the prenatal diagnosis of neural tube defects by fetal ultrasonographic examination in different centres across Europe. J Med Screen 2000; 7: 169–74.

Cuiller F. [Prenatal diagnosis of exencephaly at 10 weeks' gestation, confirmed at 13 weeks gestation; in French.] J Gynecol Obstet Biol Reprod (Paris) 2001; 30: 706–7.

Drugan A, Weissman A, Evans MI. Screening for neural tube defects. Clin Perinatol 2001; 28: 279–87.

Goldstein RB, Filly RA, Callen PW. Sonography of anencephaly: pitfalls in early diagnosis. JCU J Clin Ultrasound 1989; 17: 397–402.

Hardt W, Entezami M, Vogel M, Becker R. Die fetale Exenzephalie—Vorstadium der Anenzephalie? Ein kasuistischer Beitrag. Geburtshilfe Frauenheilkd 1999; 59: 135–8.

Wilkins HL, Freedman W. Progression of exencephaly to anencephaly in the human fetus: an ultrasound perspective. Prenat Diagn 1991; 11: 227–33.

Worthen NJ, Lawrence D, Bustillo M. Amniotic band syndrome: antepartum ultrasonic diagnosis of discordant anencephaly. JCU J Clin Ultrasound 1980; 8: 453–455.

Aqueduct Stenosis

Definition: Displacement or congenital malformation of the aqueduct of Sylvius resulting in a congenital obstructive hydrocephalus.

Incidence: One in 2000 births.

Sex ratio: M : F = 1.8 : 1

Clinical history/genetics: Most cases are sporadic; 2–5% of hydrocephalus cases unrelated to a neural tube defect are inherited recessively through an X-chromosome-linked gene. The cause seems to be mutations of the *L1 CAM* gene (gene locus Xq28).

Teratogens: Congenital infections (cytomegalovirus, rubella, toxoplasmosis).

Embryology: The sylvian aqueduct connects the third and fourth ventricles and develops in the 6th week after conception. In 50% of cases, local infection such as gliosis can be detected histologically.

Associated malformations: In X-linked aqueduct stenosis, 20% of the affected boys show deformities of the thumb. Additional malformations are present in 16% of cases. However, in cases of obstructive hydrocephalus, associated malformations are seen in 80%.

Ultrasound findings: The *third ventricle* and *lateral ventricles* are widened, but not the fourth ventricle. The cerebellum and cisterna magna are normal, except in severely affected cases. Measurement of the remaining cortex does not allow accurate prediction of the prognosis, the rim of cortex being thinnest in the occipital region. *Obstructive hydrocephalus* may also develop in the third trimester of pregnancy. Obstructive hydrocephalus does not always cause enlargement of the head, so that intrauterine head circumference measurements are not predictive.

Clinical management: Karyotyping procedure, possibly molecular-genetic diagnosis, and screening for intrauterine infections (TORCH). Intrauterine interventions such as placement of ventriculoamniotic shunt were attempted in the 1980 s, without adequate benefits. Regular sonographic assessments every 2–3 weeks as hydrocephalus may increase considerably. After 30 weeks of gestation, the benefit of early delivery and placement of a shunt has to be weighed up against the possible risks of a premature birth. In case of cephalic presentation and normal head circumference, cesarean section does not offer any advantage over vaginal delivery.

Procedure after birth: The postnatal management depends on the presence of associated anomalies. The placement of ventriculoperitoneal or ventriculoatrial shunts will depend on the enlarging head circumference and the protein content of the cerebrospinal fluid. Shunts have to be replaced frequently in repeated operations, due to obstruction or as the child grows. Fenestration of the third ventricle into the basal cisterns is an alternative to shunt therapy.

Prognosis: The neonatal mortality is in the range of 10–30%, depending on the accompanying malformations. Only 10% of survivors have an intelligence quotient (IQ) of over 70.

References

See section 2.9 (hydrocephalus).

Arachnoid Cysts

Definition: Echo-free structures arising from the arachnoid and located intracranially or in the spinal cord.

Incidence: Rare.

Clinical history/genetics: Mostly sporadic. Isolated cysts have been described, with autosomal-recessive inheritance.

Teratogens: Congenital infections.

Embryology: The etiology of congenital arachnoid cysts is uncertain. Maldevelopment of the leptomeninges may be responsible. After birth, these cysts may be acquired through infection or trauma.

Associated malformations: Obstructive hydrocephalus due to displacement of cerebrospinal fluid circulation.

Ultrasound findings: These cysts appear as echo-free single structures connected in places to the meninges and causing damage due to *compression* of brain tissue or cerebrospinal fluid circulation. This may cause obstructive hydrocephalus.

Clinical management: Repeated observations at short intervals. In cases of severe hydrocephalus and fetal maturity, premature delivery should be considered. Bleeding within the cysts may occur during labor.

Procedure after birth: Small cysts can be monitored at regular intervals. Surgical intervention such as placement of a shunt or fenestration of the cyst may be necessary for large cysts causing symptoms (seizures, hydrocephalus).

Prognosis: Generally good, depending on the location of the cyst and possible complications of surgical treatment.

Recommendation for the mother: The prognosis is very good, as this is one of the few cases in which the cause of hydrocephalus can be treated successfully.

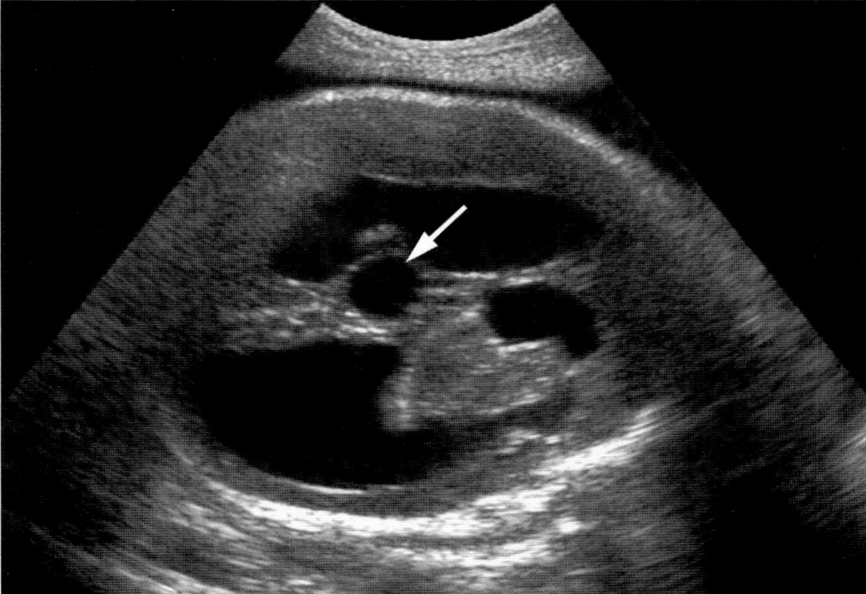

Fig. 2.8 **Central arachnoid cyst** (arrow). Seen at term, with consequent widening of both lateral ventricles.

References

Bannister CM, Russell SA, Rimmer S, Mowle DH. Fetal arachnoid cysts: their site, progress, prognosis and differential diagnosis. Eur J Pediatr Surg 1999; 9 (Suppl 1): 27–8.

Blaicher W, Prayer D, Kuhle S, Deutinger J, Bernaschek G. Combined prenatal ultrasound and magnetic resonance imaging in two fetuses with suspected arachnoid cysts. Ultrasound Obstet Gynecol 2001; 18: 166–8.

Caldarelli M, Di Rocco C. Surgical options in the treatment of interhemispheric arachnoid cysts. Surg Neurol 1996; 46: 212–21.

D'Addario V, Pinto V, Meo F, Resta M. The specificity of ultrasound in the detection of fetal intracranial tumors. J Perinat Med 1998; 26: 480–5.

Diakoumakis EE, Weinberg B, Mollin J. Prenatal sonographic diagnosis of a suprasellar arachnoid cyst. J Ultrasound Med 1986; 5: 529–30.

Elbers SE, Furness ME. Resolution of presumed arachnoid cyst in utero [review]. Ultrasound Obstet Gynecol 1999; 14: 353–5.

Limacher F, Kaiser G, Da Silva V. Fetal intracranial invasive cysts: diagnosis, procedure and therapy using the example of a case report (arachnoid cyst). Geburtshilfe Frauenheilkd 1984; 44: 444–50.

Meizner I, Barki Y, Tadmor R, Katz M. In utero ultrasonic detection of fetal arachnoid cyst. JCU J Clin Ultrasound 1988; 16: 506–9.

Pilu G, Falco P, Perolo A, et al. Differential diagnosis and outcome of fetal intracranial hypoechoic lesions: report of 21 cases. Ultrasound Obstet Gynecol 1997; 9: 229–36.

Rafferty PG, Britton J, Penna L, Ville Y. Prenatal diagnosis of a large fetal arachnoid cyst. Ultrasound Obstet Gynecol 1998; 12: 358–61.

Revel MP, Pons JC, Lelaidier C, et al. Magnetic resonance imaging of the fetus: a study of 20 cases performed without curarization. Prenat Diagn 1993; 13: 775–99.

Sandler MA, Madrazo BL, Riga PM, et al. Ultrasound case of the day: bilateral arachnoid cysts, diagnosed in utero. RadioGraphics 1988; 8: 358–61.

2

Agenesis of the Corpus Callosum

Definition: Complete or partial absence of the corpus callosum, a bundle of white matter connecting the cerebral hemispheres.

Incidence: One in 300–1500 births; however, when other anomalies of the central nervous system are present, it is detected in 50%. Mostly asymptomatic.

Clinical history/genetics: Mostly sporadic; inherited cases with autosomal-dominant, autosomal-recessive, and X-linked transmission have been reported.

Teratogens: Alcohol, rubella infection.

Embryology: The corpus callosum develops between 11 and 16 gestational weeks. Failure of development may be partial or complete.

Associated malformations: Hydrocephalus, microcephalus, pachygyria, lissencephaly. Dandy–Walker syndrome is the most frequently associated anomaly. Anomalies of the kidneys, heart, lungs, and diaphragm are frequently seen.

Associated syndromes: Over 240 syndromes have been described in association with corpus callosum depletion—for example, Gorlin syndrome, Meckel–Gruber syndrome, Miller–Dieker syndrome, Neu–Laxova syndrome, Walker–Warburg syndrome, Fanconi anemia, Apert syndrome, Crouzon syndrome, 4 p deletion, triploidy, trisomy 13, trisomy 18, arthrogryposis, and Fryns syndrome.

Ultrasound findings: In the absence of the corpus callosum, the third ventricle lies between the lateral ventricles. The posterior horns of the lateral ventricles are widened and are stretched ventrally (*teardrop sign*), and the medial borders run more parallel to the central echo than usual. The third ventricle may be connected to the lateral ventricles by a *cystic communication*. The septum pellucidum does not appear normal. The gyri of the hemispheres, which normally lie horizontally, tend to lie more ventrally in the absence of the corpus callosum. *N.b.:* a sagittal view through the midline is the best plane for diagnosing this condition. The diagnosis can be difficult and is often missed. Absence of the corpus callosum is rarely diagnosed before 16 weeks of gestation.

Clinical management: Karyotyping. Detailed sonographic screening of the fetus and vaginal sonography may help further in cephalic presentation. Sonographic exclusion of other anomalies and fetal echocardiography. Magnetic resonance imaging may be indicated in uncertain cases.

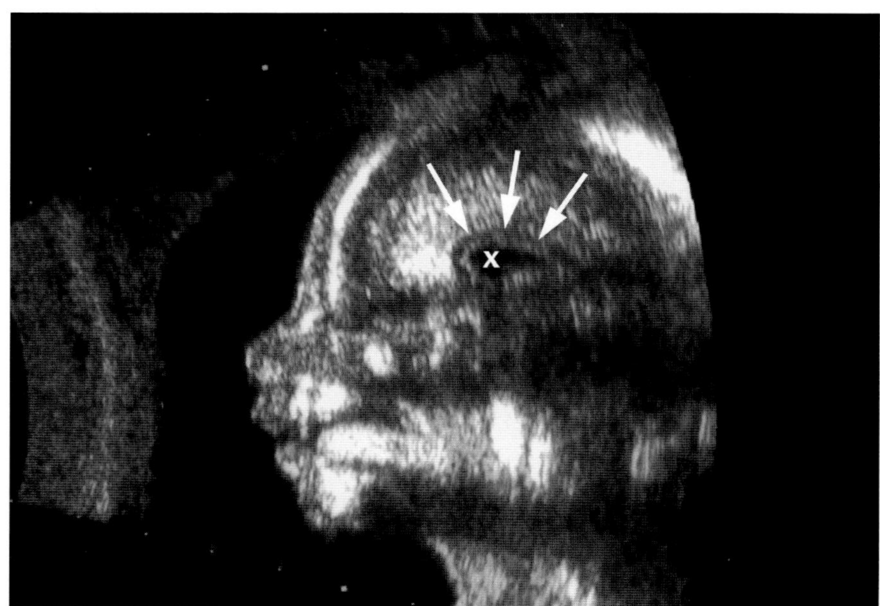

Fig. 2.**9** **Corpus callosum.** Midline sagittal section at 22 + 0 weeks, showing the septum pellucidum (x) and the corpus callosum (arrows).

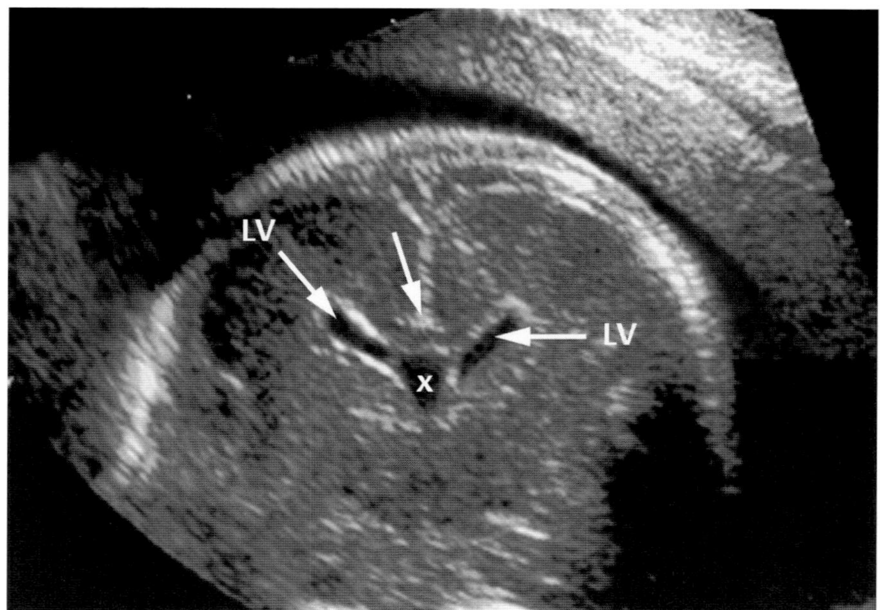

Fig. 2.**10** **Corpus callosum.** Frontal view through the forebrain. The anterior horns of both lateral ventricles (LV), septum pellucidum (x), and the cross-section of the corpus callosum (arrow) are well recognized.

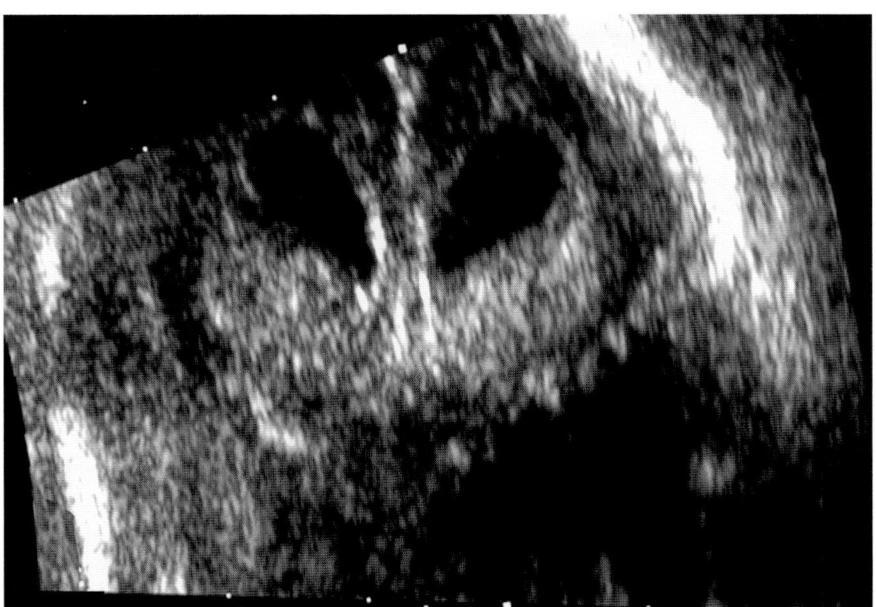

Fig. 2.**11** **Agenesis of the corpus callosum.** Frontal view of the anterior part of the brain in agenesis of corpus callosum at 22 weeks. The anterior horns of the lateral ventricles are seen, with widening of the structures separating them.

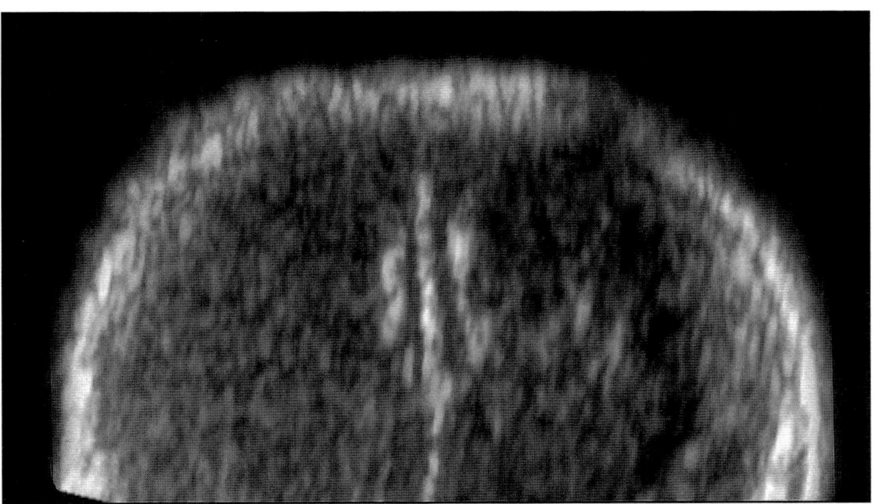

Fig. 2.**12** **Agenesis of the corpus callosum.** Frontal view of the anterior part of the brain in agenesis of corpus callosum: "three lines sign." The longitudinal fissure separating the cerebral hemispheres is widened.

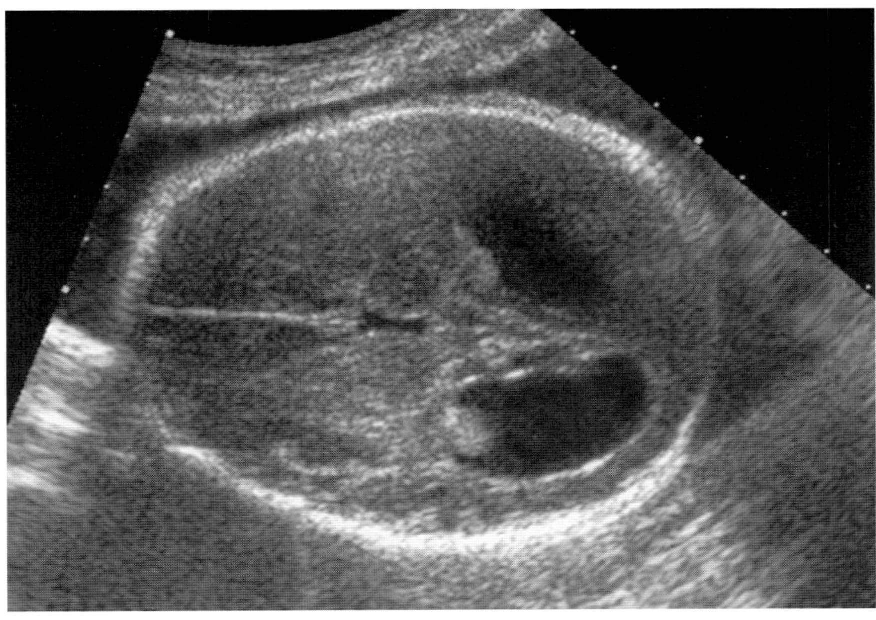

Fig. 2.**13** **Agenesis of the corpus callosum.** Transverse section of the fetal head in agenesis of corpus callosum. The septum pellucidum cannot be demonstrated at 30 weeks of gestation. The lateral ventricles are enlarged.

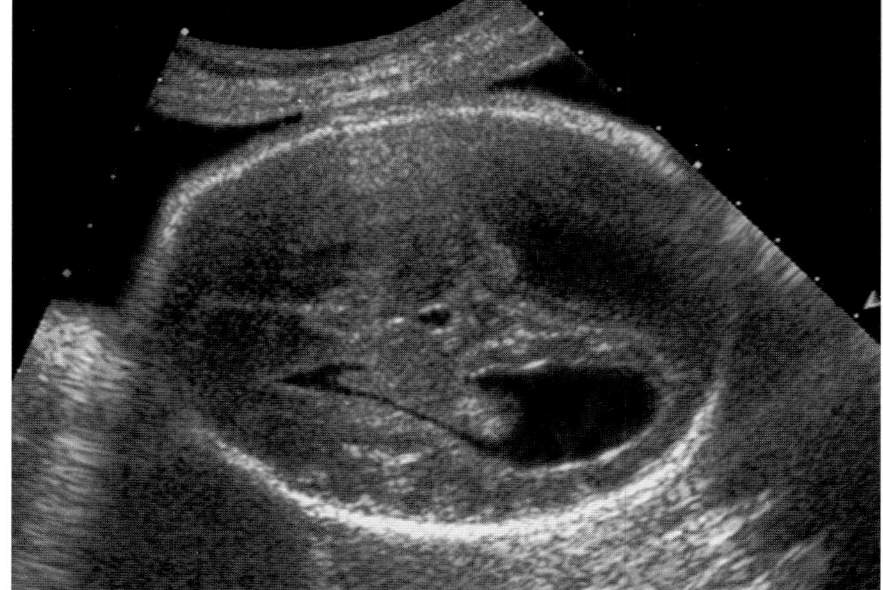

Fig. 2.**14** **Agenesis of corpus callosum.** Lateral ventricle in the case of agenesis of corpus callosum, with the "teardrop sign." The distance between the medial border of the lateral ventricle and the falx cerebri is larger in the part of the sharply pointed anterior horn than that from the posterior horn. The third ventricle is seen centrally; the septum pellucidum cannot be seen.

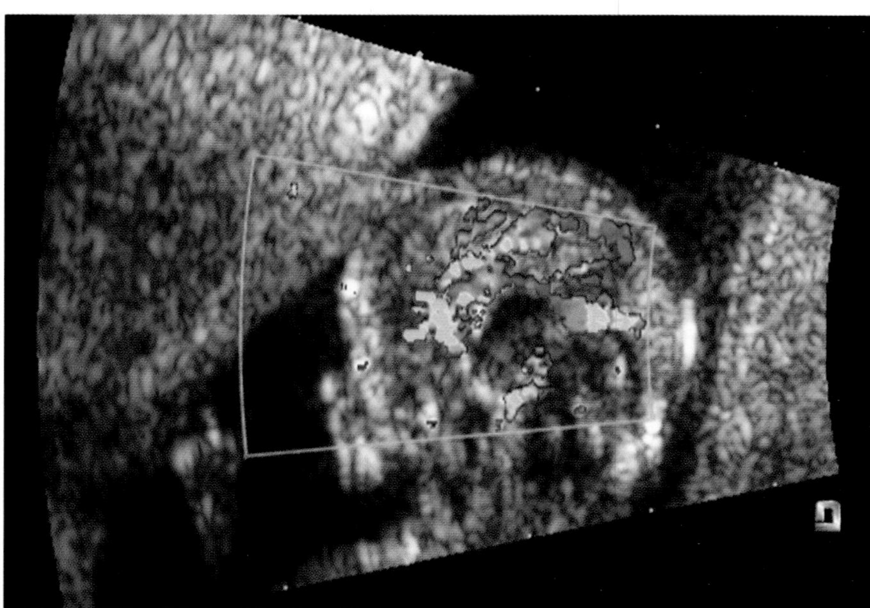

Fig. 2.**15** **Pericallosal artery.** Midline sagittal section at 13 + 4 weeks. The pericallosal artery is depicted using the color Doppler mode.

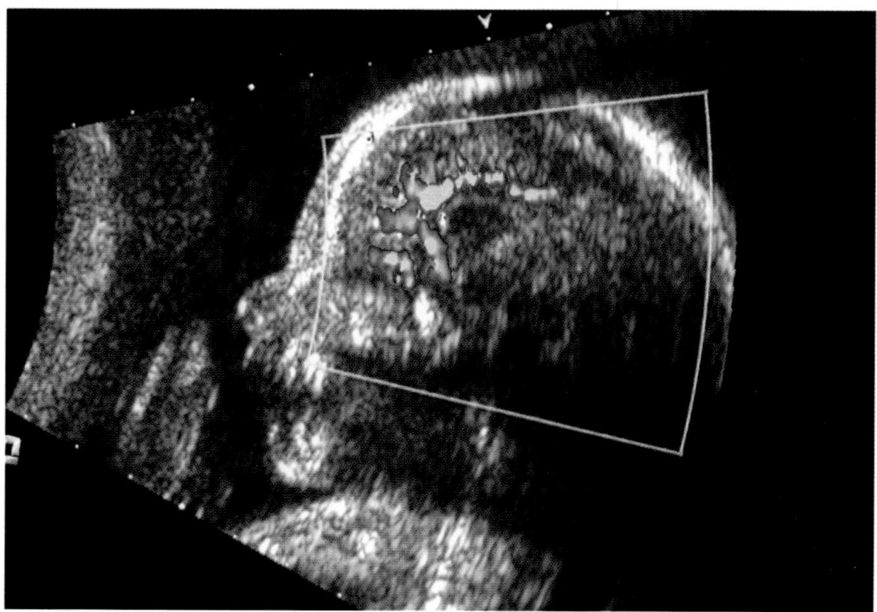

Fig. 2.**16** **Pericallosal artery.** Midline sagittal section at 22 + 2 weeks. The normal course of the artery is seen.

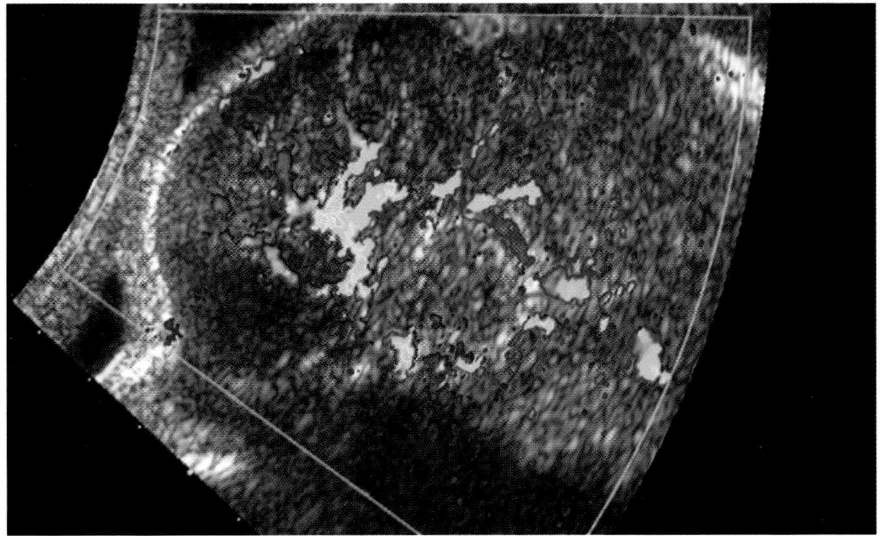

Fig. 2.17 **Agenesis of the corpus callosum.** Atypical course of the pericallosal artery due to agenesis of corpus callosum at 30 + 1 weeks.

Achieving a reliable prognosis and definitely excluding other central nervous system anomalies are difficult tasks. In counseling the parents, expert advice from neuropediatrician and a neuropathologist should be taken. Diseases with autosomal-dominant inheritance in the parents, such as tuberous sclerosis and basal-cell nevus syndrome, should be excluded. It is important to search for fetal infection (TORCH). Regular sonographic checks do not per se show any changes in the findings, but the associated ventriculomegaly may develop later in pregnancy.

Procedure after birth: There are no neurological deficits when agenesis of the corpus callosum is an isolated finding. Magnetic resonance imaging is considered the best method of confirming the diagnosis and excluding other central nervous system anomalies.

Prognosis: The isolated condition remains mainly asymptomatic, but seizures may occur. The prognosis in some syndromes—for example, Dandy–Walker syndrome—is poor when associated with absence of the corpus callosum; otherwise a good prognosis is expected.

Information for the patient: Up to 1 % of adults have congenital agenesis of the corpus callosum, without their knowledge and without symptoms. In the absence of associated anomalies, mental development is normal.

Self-Help Organization

Title: The ACC Network

Description: Helps individuals with agenesis, or other anomaly, of the corpus callosum, their families, and professionals. Helps identify others who are experiencing similar issues to share information and support. Phone support, information, newsletter and referrals. Coordinates an electronic discussion group on the internet.

Scope: International network

Founded: 1990

Address: University of Maine; 5749 Merrill Hall, Room 118, Orono, Maine 04469–5749, United States

Telephone: 207–581–3119

Fax: 207–581–3120

E-mail: UM-ACC@maine.maine.edu

References

Achiron R, Achiron A. Development of the human fetal corpus callosum: a high-resolution, cross-sectional sonographic study. Ultrasound Obstet Gynecol 2001; 18: 343–7.

Comstock CH, Culp D, Gonzalez J, Boal DB. Agenesis of the corpus callosum in the fetus: its evolution and significance. J Ultrasound Med 1985; 4: 613–6.

D'Ercole C, Girard N, Cravello L, et al. Prenatal diagnosis of fetal corpus callosum agenesis by ultrasonography and magnetic resonance imaging. Prenat Diagn 1998; 18: 247–53.

Greco P, Vimercati A, De Cosmo L, Laforgia N, Mautone A, Selvaggi L. Mild ventriculomegaly as a counselling challenge. Fetal Diagn Ther 2001; 16: 398–401.

Hilpert PL, Kurtz AB. Prenatal diagnosis of agenesis of the corpus callosum using endovaginal ultrasound. J Ultrasound Med 1990; 9: 363–5.
Maheut Le, Paillet C. Prenatal diagnosis of anomalies of the corpus callosum with ultrasound: the echographist's point of view. Neurochirurgie 1998; 44: 85–92.
Rapp B, Perrotin F, Marret H, Sembely-Taveau C, Lansac J, Body G. [Value of fetal cerebral magnetic resonance imaging for the prenatal diagnosis and prognosis of corpus callosum agenesis; in French.] J Gynecol Obstet Biol Reprod (Paris) 2002; 31: 173–82.
Sandri F, Pilu G, Cerisoli M, Bovicelli L, Alvisi C, Salvioli GP. Sonographic diagnosis of agenesis of the corpus callosum in the fetus and newborn infant. Am J Perinatol 1988; 5: 226–31.
Timor-Tritsch TI, Monteagudo A, Haratz-Rubinstein RN, Levine RU. Transvaginal sonographic detection of adducted thumbs, hydrocephalus, and agenesis of the corpus callosum at 22 postmenstrual weeks: the masa spectrum or L1 spectrum: a case report and review of the literature. Prenat Diagn 1996; 16: 543–8.
Valat AS, Dehouck MB, Dufour P, et al. Fetal cerebral ventriculomegaly: etiology and outcome—report of 141 cases. J Gynecol Obstet Biol Reprod (Paris) 1998; 27: 782–9.
Vergani P, Ghidini A, Mariam S, Greppi P, Negri R. Antenatal sonographic findings of agenesis of corpus callosum. Am J Perinatol 1988; 5: 105–8.

Dandy–Walker Syndrome

Definition: The Dandy–Walker syndrome is characterized by a cyst in the posterior fossa that communicates with the fourth ventricle, a defect in the cerebellar vermis, and varying degrees of hydrocephalus.

Incidence: One in 25 000–1 : 30 000 births, representing about 4% of hydrocephalic cases.

Clinical history/genetics: May appear sporadically, or may show autosomal-recessive or X-linked inheritance.

Teratogens: Congenital infections.

Embryology: The Dandy–Walker syndrome develops in the 5th to 6th week after conception.

Associated malformations: In 50% of the cases, other intracranial malformations are detected, especially agenesis of the corpus callosum. In 35%, other extracranial anomalies are evident such as those affecting the face (cleft lip and palate) or the heart (ventricular septal defects). Chromosomal aberrations are found in 15–30%. Dandy–Walker cysts are found often in the presence of encephalocele and neural tube defects.

Associated syndromes: These include Smith–Lemli–Opitz syndrome, Jubert syndrome, Meckel–Gruber syndrome, triploidy, trisomy 18, arthrogryposis, CHARGE association, Fryns syndrome, MURCS association.

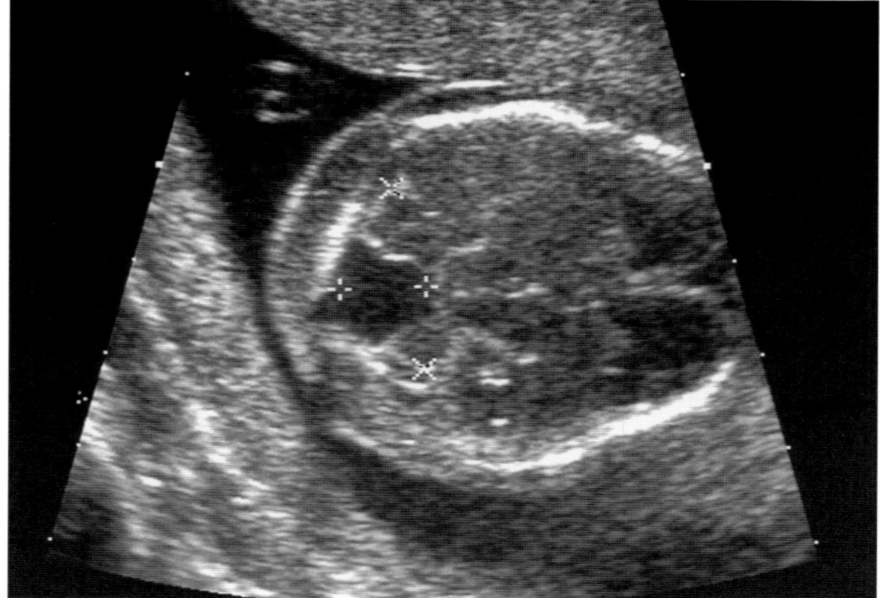

Fig. 2.**18** **Dandy–Walker syndrome.** Demonstration of the posterior cranial fossa in a case of Dandy–Walker syndrome. Cystic widening of the region below the cerebellar hemispheres is seen.

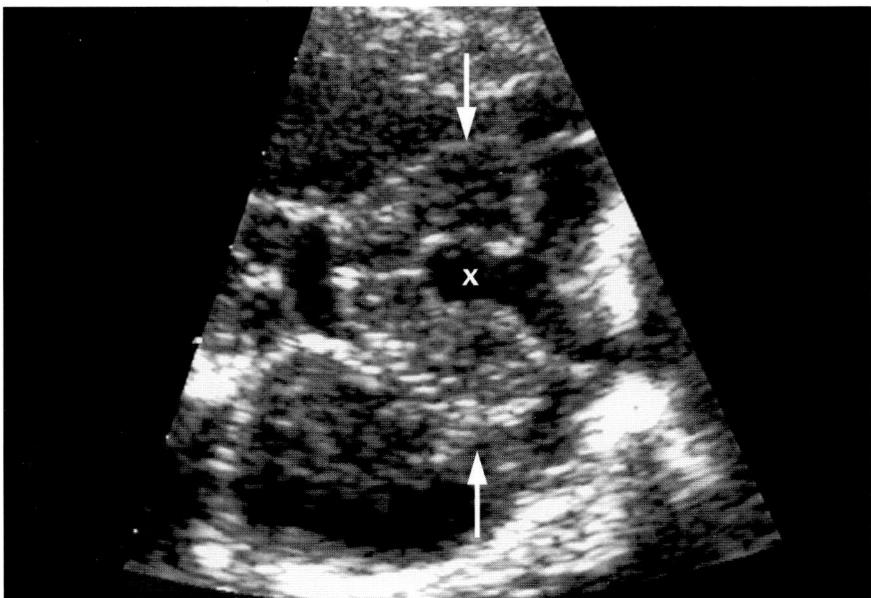

Fig. 2.**19** **Dandy–Walker variant.** Demonstration of the posterior cranial fossa in a case of Dandy–Walker variant. Widening of the space (x) lying between the two cerebellar hemispheres (arrows) is seen.

Ultrasound findings: Dandy–Walker cyst, seen as an echo-free structure, separates the cerebellar hemispheres. The cyst communicates with the fourth ventricle. The cerebellar vermis may be partially or totally absent. Hypoplasia of the cerebellum may also be present. The third ventricle and the lateral ventricles are widened in the presence of larger cysts.

Caution: The frequent finding of small cysts under the cerebellum may not be pathologic. A connection between the fourth ventricle and the cisterna magna is evident until 15–17 weeks.

Clinical management: Further sonographic screening, including fetal echocardiography. Karyotyping and search for infections (TORCH). Counseling with a neurosurgeon, neuropediatrician, or neuropathologist. If the mother decides to continue with the pregnancy, regular sonographic monitoring. Premature delivery should be considered if the hydrocephalus enlarges rapidly. This option is disputed because of bad prognosis. Prognosis is worsened if agenesis of the corpus callosum is also detected. If the diagnosis is uncertain, magnetic resonance imaging during the pregnancy can be useful in deciding the clinical management. Bleeding within the cysts may occur, and this should be borne in mind when choosing the mode of delivery.

Procedure after birth: Normal postnatal care for the newborn. In most infants with absence of intrauterine hydrocephalus, development of hydrocephalus occurs within 2 months after birth. Treatment for the Dandy–Walker cyst is only then indicated if the child develops symptoms (difficulty in swallowing, aspiration, a weak cry, underdeveloped sucking reflex). The usual management is placement of a cystoperitoneal shunt.

Prognosis: The overall postnatal mortality is about 35% and depends on the accompanying malformations. A third of the survivors have an IQ of over 80. Placement of a shunt is often necessary due to the presence of hydrocephalus.

Recommendation for the mother: The child should be investigated thoroughly, including genetic counseling. The parents should be advised regarding the risk for the next pregnancy.

Self-Help Organization

Title: Dandy–Walker Syndrome Network

Description: Provides mutual support, information and networking for families affected by Dandy–Walker syndrome. Phone support.

Scope: International network

Founded: 1993

Telephone: 612–423–4008

References

Achiron R, Achiron A, Yagel S. First trimester transvaginal sonographic diagnosis of Dandy–Walker malformation. J Clin Ultrasound 1993; 21: 62–4.

Bernard JP, Moscoso G, Renier D, Ville Y. Cystic malformations of the posterior fossa [review]. Prenat Diagn 2001; 21: 1064–9.

Blaicher W, Ulm B, Ulm MR, Hengstschlager M, Deutinger J, Bernaschek G. Dandy–Walker malformation as sonographic marker for fetal triploidy. Ultraschall Med 2002; 23: 129–33.
Dempsey PJ, Koch HJ. In utero diagnosis of the Dandy–Walker syndrome: differentiation from extra-axial posterior fossa cyst. JCU J Clin Ultrasound 1981; 9: 403–5.
Nyberg DA, Cyr DR, Mack LA, Fitzsimmons J, Hickok D, Mahony BS. The Dandy–Walker malformation: prenatal sonographic diagnosis and its clinical significance. J Ultrasound Med 1988; 7: 65–71.
Pilu G, Romero R, De Palma L, et al. Antenatal diagnosis and obstetric management of Dandy–Walker syndrome. J Reprod Med 1986; 31: 1017–22.
Serlo W, Kirkinen P, Heikkinen E, Jouppila P. Ante- and postnatal evaluation of the Dandy–Walker syndrome. Childs Nerv Syst 1985; 1: 148–51.
Ulm B, Ulm MR, Deutinger J, Bernaschek G. Dandy–Walker malformation diagnosed before 21 weeks of gestation: associated malformations and chromosomal abnormalities. Ultrasound Obstet Gynecol 1997; 10: 167–70.
Yuh WT, Nguyen HD, Fisher DJ, et al. MR of fetal central nervous system abnormalities. AJNR Am J Neuroradiol 1994; 15: 459–64.
Zimmermann R, Biedermann K, Wildhaber J, Huch A. Early recognition of fetal abnormalities by transvaginal ultrasonography. Ultraschall Med 1993; 14: 35–9.

Encephalocele

Definition: Encephalocele is herniation of some of the cranial contents through a midline defect in the bony skull, and belongs to the group of neural tube defects. Seventy-five percent of the defects are occipital, the remainder being frontal, parietal, and nasopharyngeal.

Incidence: One in 2000 births.

Sex ratio: M : F = 1 : 1

Clinical history/genetics: Mostly sporadic; the risk of recurrence is 2–5%. Encephalocele may constitute part of a syndrome.

Teratogens: Cocaine, rubella infection, hyperthermia, warfarin.

Embryology: The lesion is thought to occur due to failed closure of the rostral end of the neural tube in the 6th week of fetal life.

Associated malformations: Other central nervous system (CNS) malformations are often present, such as hydrocephalus, iniencephaly, and facial clefts and heart anomalies. Lumbosacral spina bifida is found in 7–15%.

Associated syndromes: Encephalocele has been described in over 30 syndromes. In Meckel–Gruber syndrome (autosomal-recessive transmission), encephalocele is accompanied by polycystic kidneys and polydactyly.

Ultrasound findings: Seventy-five percent of encephaloceles are located in the occipital region, 12% in the frontal, and 13% in the parietal region. It can be seen as a *purely cystic mass*, or may contain echoes from the *herniated brain tissue*. The larger the herniation of the brain tissue, the less remains intracranially, leading to *microcephaly*. In spite of an accompanying hydrocephalus, the head circumference remains small. *Hydramnios* develops secondary to these changes.

Clinical management: Further sonographic screening, including fetal echocardiography. Karyotyping and search for infections (TORCH). Counseling with a neuropediatrician. If the pregnancy continues, sonographic monitoring at regular intervals is advisable. In cases of severe microcephaly, the prognosis is poor, so that cesarean section for fetal distress during labor is a questionable option. Infants with a normal head circumference appear to have a better prognosis. A more gentle, atraumatic mode of delivery for the head and the encephalocele is achieved with cesarean section, avoiding intracranial bleeding.

Procedure after birth: In view of the overall prognosis and after parental consent, intensive medical intervention may not be considered. If vitally important brain structures are protruding into the herniation sac, neurosurgical intervention is not possible, as total resection of the herniated sac is required. In these cases, the prognosis is extremely poor.

Prognosis: This depends on the amount of affected brain tissue and the associated anomalies. If an isolated encephalocele without protrusion of brain tissue is the only finding, then normal mental development is possible in 50% of cases. Encephalocele located in the frontal region usually has a better prognosis.

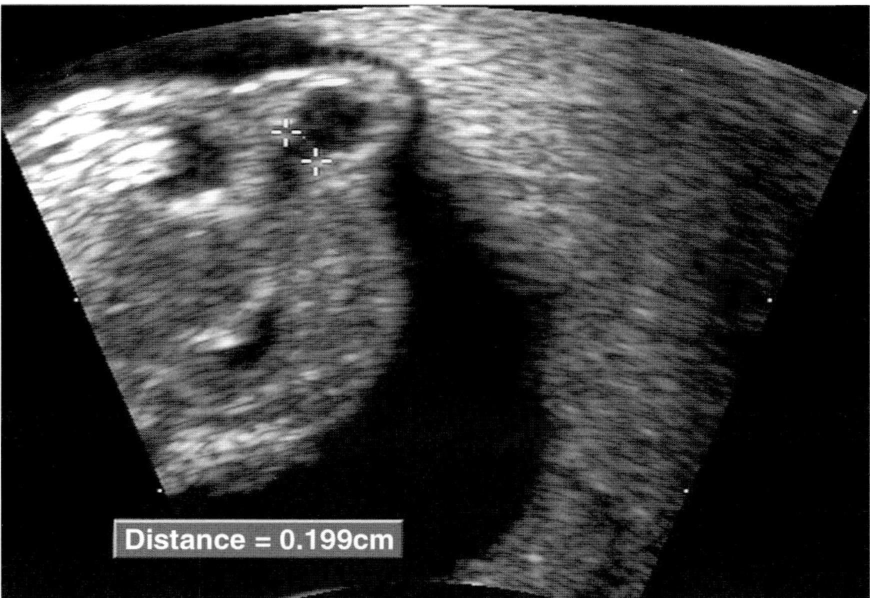

Fig. 2.**20** **Encephalocele.** Cross-section of the fetal head at 11 + 6 weeks, showing a small occipital encephalocele.

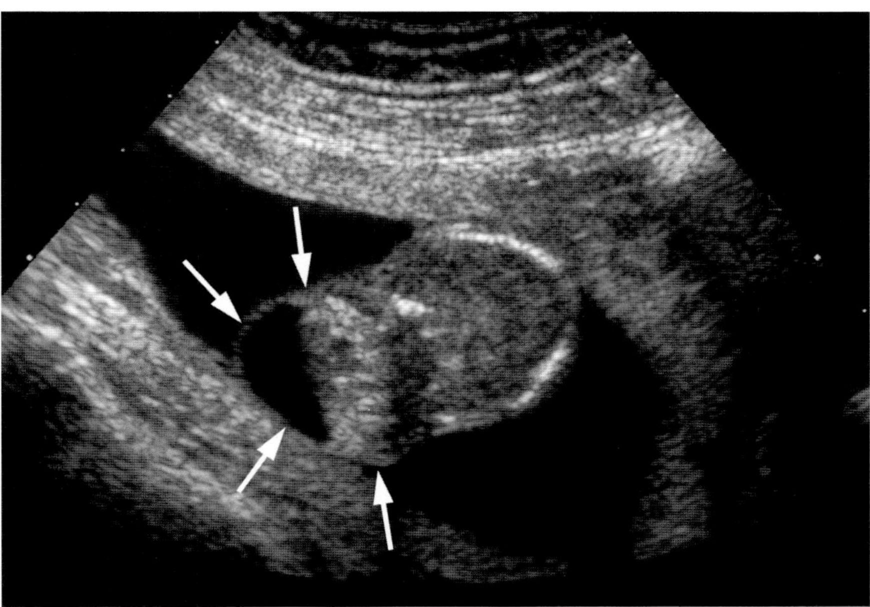

Fig. 2.**21** **Encephalocele.** Cross-section of the fetal head, showing a large occipital encephalocele (arrows) at 15 + 4 weeks.

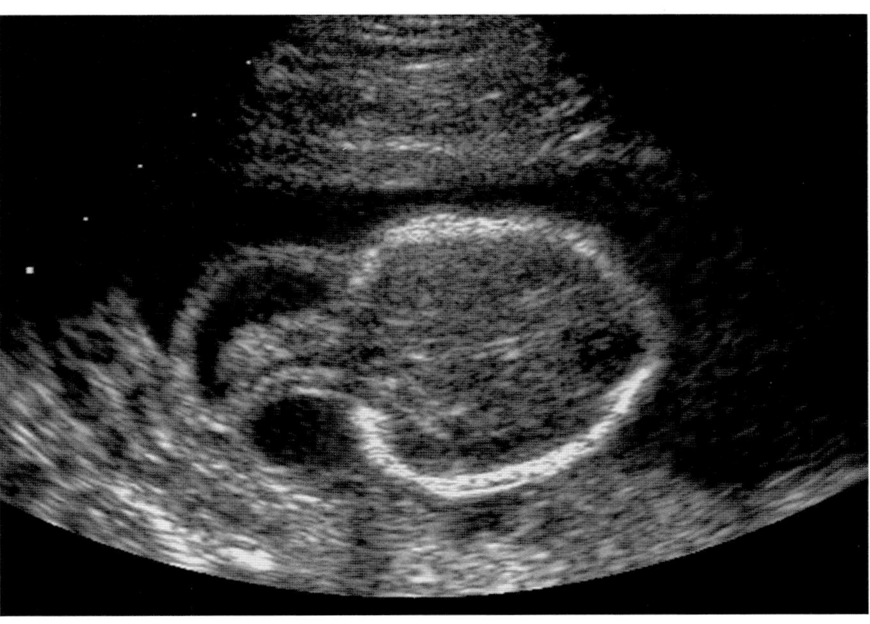

Fig. 2.**22** **Encephalocele.** Cross-section of the fetal head, showing a large occipital encephalocele at 18 + 2 weeks. Prolapse of brain tissue and consequent microcephaly are observed (see also under microcephaly).

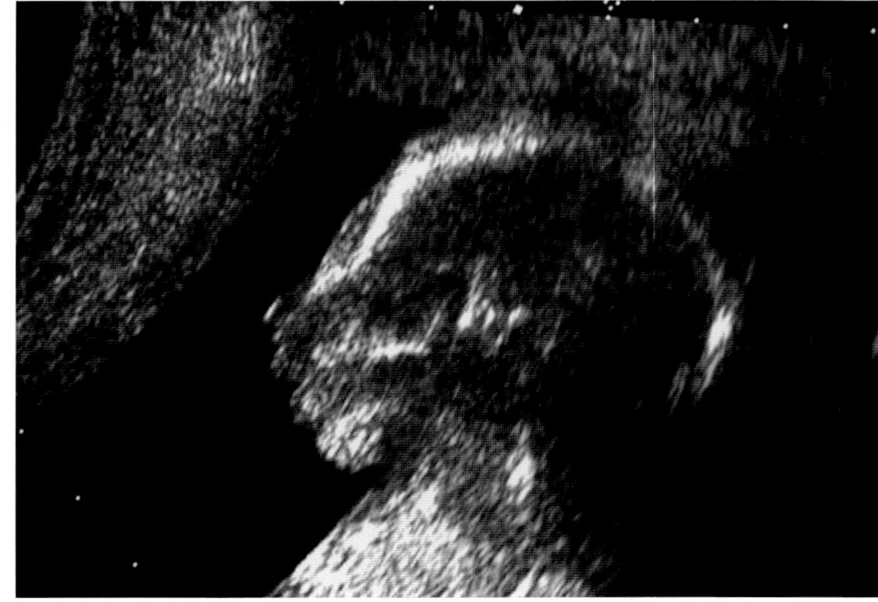

Fig. 2.**23** **Encephalocele.** The same fetus. The profile shows a flat forehead and consequent microcephaly due to displacement of intracranial contents into the occipital encephalocele.

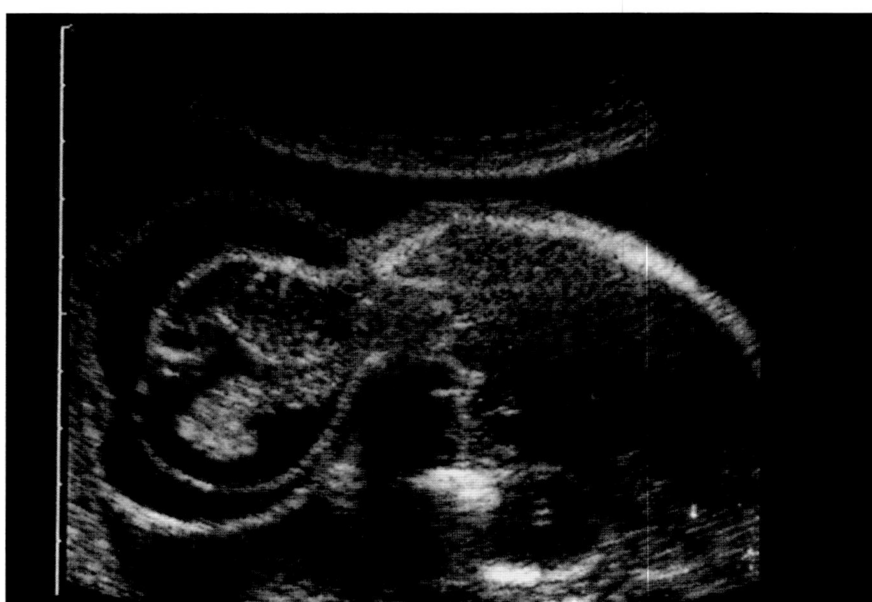

Fig. 2.**24** **Encephalocele.** Tilted sagittal section of the fetal head in a case of a severe fetal encephalocele, seen in one twin at 23 weeks.

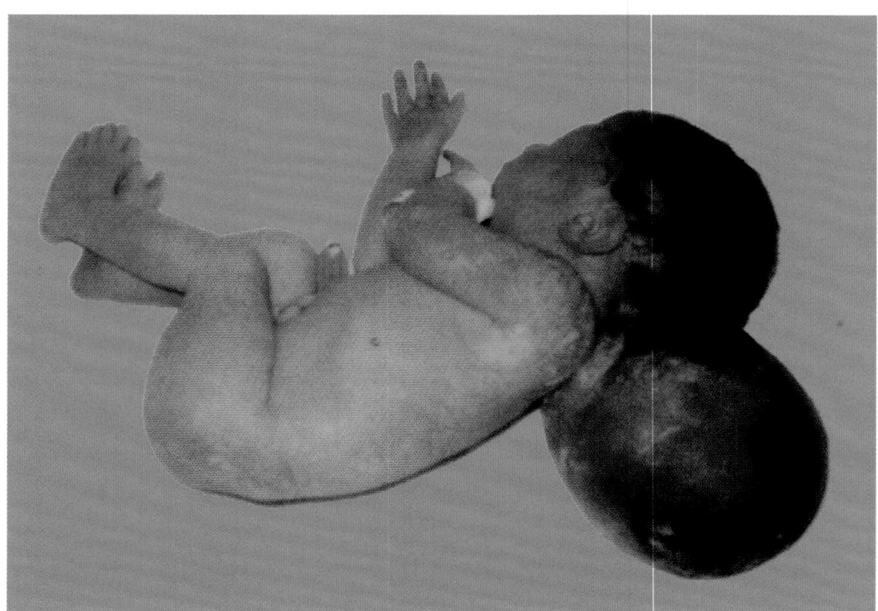

Fig. 2.**25** **Encephalocele.** The same twin after birth (spontaneous delivery as a second twin).

References

Becker R, Novak A, Rudolph KH. A case of occipital encephalocele combined with right lung aplasia in twin pregnancy: prenatal diagnosis, perinatal management, clinical outcome and review of the literature. J Perinat Med 1993; 21: 253–8.

Braithwaite JM, Economides DL. First-trimester diagnosis of Meckel–Gruber syndrome by transabdominal sonography in a low-risk case. Prenat Diagn 1995; 15: 1168–70.

Fink IJ, Chinn DH, Callen PW. A potential pitfall in the ultrasonographic diagnosis of fetal encephalocele. J Ultrasound Med 1983; 2: 313–4.

Fleming AD, Vintzileos AM, Scorza WE. Prenatal diagnosis of occipital encephalocele with transvaginal sonography. J Ultrasound Med 1991; 10: 285–6.

Flessa A, Rempen A, Schmausser B, Marx A. Meckel–Gruber syndrome. Z Geburtshilfe Neonatol 1996; 200: 66–8.

Noriega CA, Fleming AD, Bonebrake RG. A false-positive diagnosis of a prenatal encephalocele on transvaginal ultrasonography. J Ultrasound Med 2001; 20: 925–7.

Pachi A, Giancotti A, Torcia F, de Prosperi V, Maggi E. Meckel–Gruber syndrome: ultrasonographic diagnosis at 73 weeks' gestational age in an at-risk case. Prenat Diagn 1989; 9: 187–90.

Tanriverdi HA, Hendrik HJ, Ertan K, Schmidt W. Meckel–Gruber syndrome: a first-trimester diagnosis of a recurrent case. Eur J Ultrasound 2002; 15: 69–72.

Holoprosencephaly

Definition: Holoprosencephaly is characterized by an abnormal separation of the cerebral hemispheres due to absent or incomplete cleavage of the brain hemispheres. This results in fusion of lateral and third ventricles. Depending on the degree of severity, alobar, semilobar and lobar forms are identified (see below).

Incidence: One in 5000–10 000 births, but one in 250 embryos.

Sex ratio: M : F = 1 : 3 (alobar); M : F = 1 : 1 (lobar).

Clinical history/genetics: In multifactorial inheritance, the rate of recurrence is 6%. Autosomal-dominant and autosomal-recessive forms of inheritance have also been reported. Various syndromes have been described in addition to chromosomal abnormalities—for example, structural anomalies such as 7 q and 2 q deletion.

Teratogens: Alcohol, phenytoin, excessive vitamin A, diabetes mellitus, congenital infections, exposure to radiation.

Embryology: Separation of the hemispheres in the early embryonic stage is absent.

Associated malformations: Heart anomalies (especially double-outlet ventricle), omphalocele, Dandy–Walker syndrome, maldevelopment of the extremities, microcephaly and macrocephaly, and singular umbilical artery are often associated.

Associated syndromes: Shprintzen syndrome; ectrodactyly–ectodermal dysplasia–clefting (EEC) syndrome; chromosomal abnormality in up to 70%: trisomy 13, trisomy 18, triploidy, and various structural aberrations such as 7 q deletion.

Ultrasound findings: Early diagnosis is possible even before 12 weeks (single ventricular cavity and facial anomalies). In the *alobar and semilobar forms,* fusion of the thalami, absence of the third ventricle, and a single horseshoe-shaped intracranial ventricle are observed.

The common ventricle flows into a dorsal sac. The corpus callosum, falx cerebri and interhemispheric fissure are absent. Facial malformations are always present—such as hypotelorism, cyclopia, median facial clefts, and a flat nose with only one nasal opening. In the *lobar form,* the ventricle is fused with the falx in the frontal region, and the posterior horns of the lateral ventricle are separated. Hydranencephaly resembles alobar holoprosencephaly, except for the presence of the third ventricle and unfused thalami.

Clinical management: Karyotyping, exclusion of diabetes mellitus. If the mother continues the pregnancy, she should be informed about the poor prognosis so that she can decide about any interventions that may be necessary during labor. Vaginal delivery may be impossible due to the large fetal head. In such cases, cephalocentesis is indicated. In late pregnancy, development of hydramnios may cause premature labor and birth.

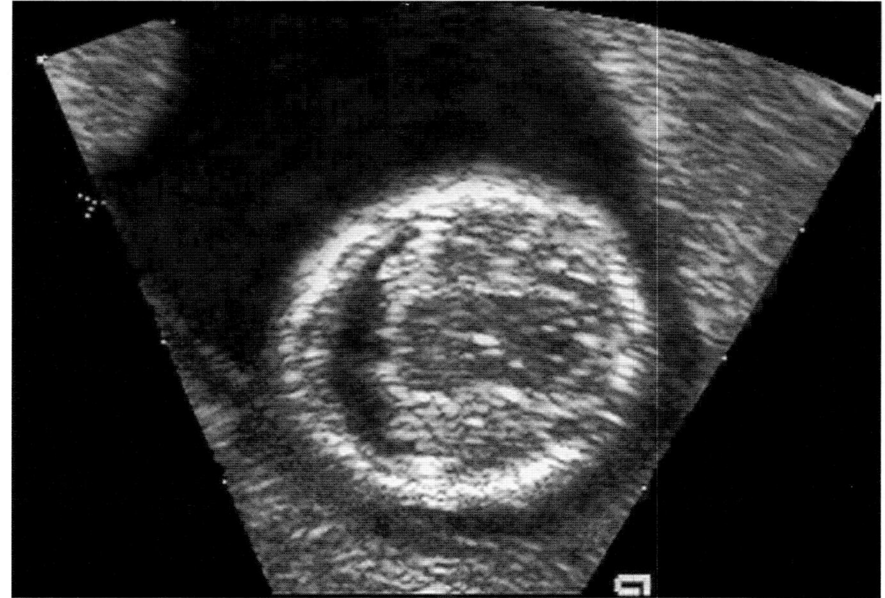

Fig. 2.**26** **Holoprosencephaly.** 12 + 5 weeks. In a case of trisomy 13, there is absent cleavage of the cerebral hemispheres in the frontal region.

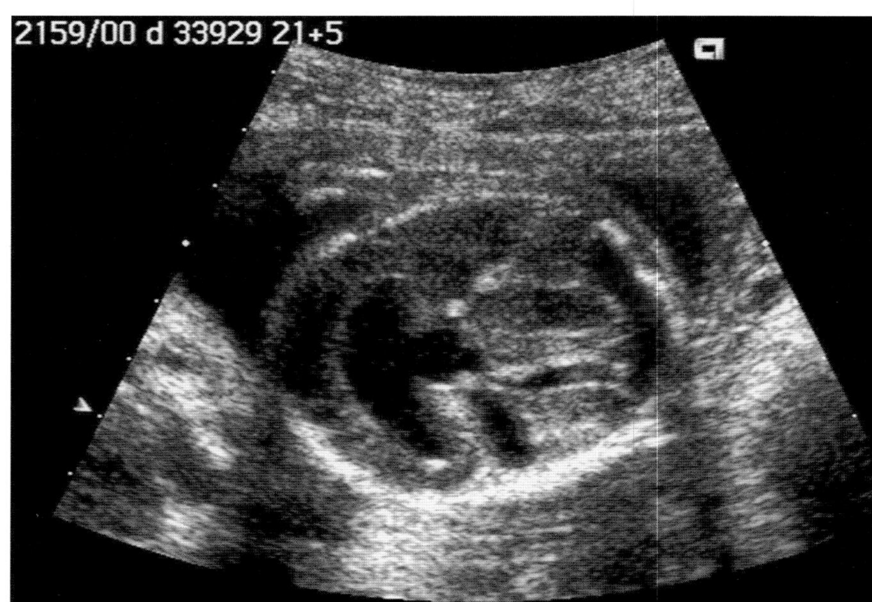

Fig. 2.**27** **Holoprosencephaly.** 21 + 5 weeks. Absent cleavage of the frontal lobes, causing confluent lateral ventricles combined with arrhinencephaly and proboscis. A cross-sectional view is seen here. No other malformations. Normal karyotype.

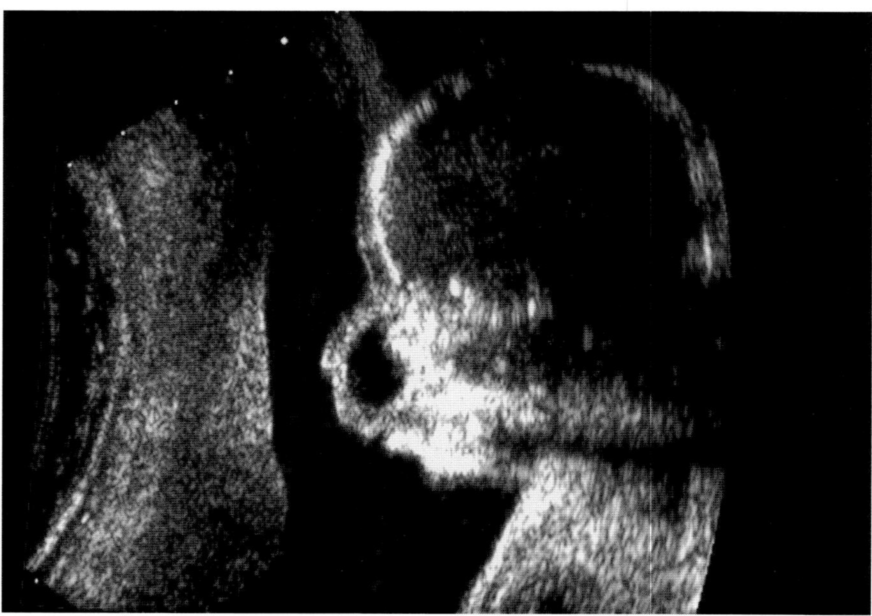

Fig. 2.**28** **Holoprosencephaly.** 21 + 5 weeks. Combined with arrhinencephaly and proboscis.

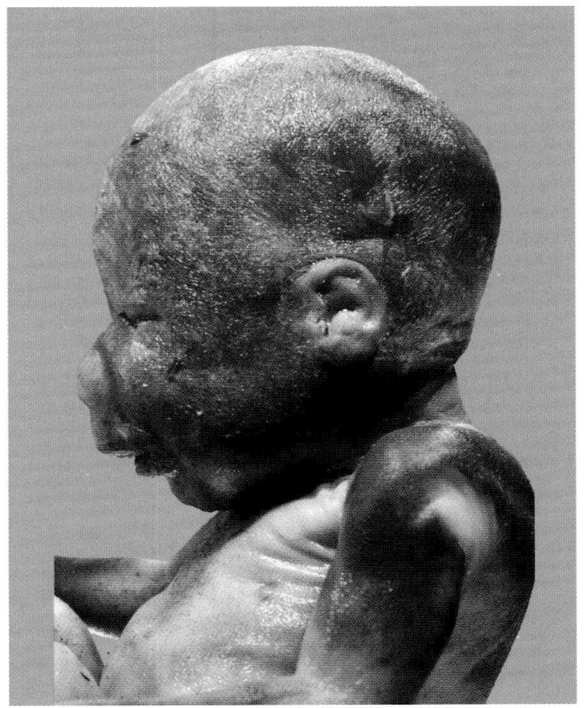

Fig. 2.**29** **Holoprosencephaly.** Facial profile. Termination of pregnancy.

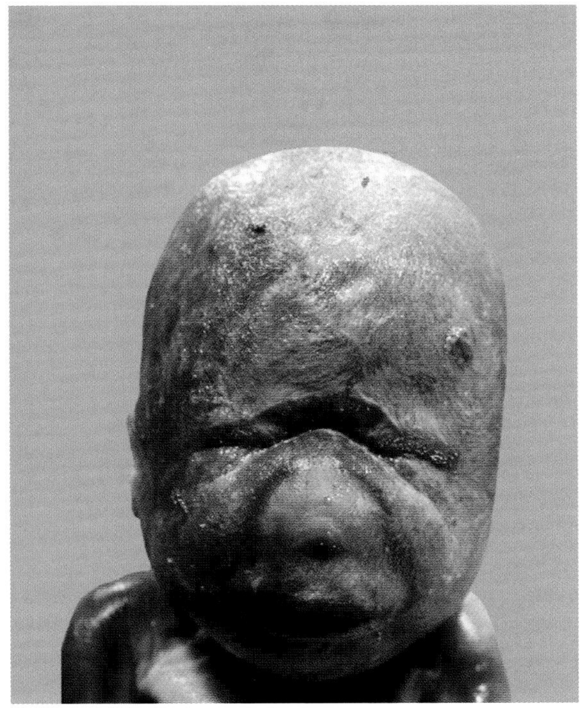

Fig. 2.**30** **Holoprosencephaly.** Frontal aspect. Termination of pregnancy.

Procedure after birth: Intensive life-saving measures are not indicated, due to the very poor prognosis.

Prognosis: Severely affected infants die within 6 months after birth. Less severely affected children may survive with various degree of mental impairment.

Self-Help Organization

Title: Holoprosencephaly Self-Help Group, Berliner Strasse 61 a, 63 110 Rodgau, Germany

Telephone: + 49–6106–18888

References

Bernard JP, Drummond CL, Zaarour P, Molho M, Ville Y. A new clue to the prenatal diagnosis of lobar holoprosencephaly: the abnormal pathway of the anterior cerebral artery crawling under the skull. Ultrasound Obstet Gynecol 2002; 19: 605–7.

Blaas HG, Eriksson AG, Salvesen KA, et al. Brains and faces in holoprosencephaly: pre- and postnatal description of 30 cases. Ultrasound Obstet Gynecol 2002; 19: 24–38.

Filly RA, Chinn DH, Callen PW. Alobar holoprosencephaly: ultrasonographic prenatal diagnosis. Radiology 1984; 151: 455–9.

Gembruch U, Baschat AA, Reusche E, Wallner SJ, Greiwe M. First-trimester diagnosis of holoprosencephaly with a Dandy-Walker malformation by transvaginal ultrasonography. J Ultrasound Med 1995; 14: 619–22.

Hoffman TJ, Horoupian DS, Koenigsberg M, Schnur MJ, Llena JF. Lobar holoprosencephaly with hydrocephalus: antenatal demonstration and differential diagnosis. J Ultrasound Med 1986; 5: 691–7.

Holzgreve W, Miny P, Gullotta F. Sonographic diagnosis of holoprosencephaly in the 2nd trimester. Geburtshilfe Frauenheilkd 1985; 45: 813–4.

Moog U, De Die-Smulders CE, Schrander-Stumpel CT, et al. Holoprosencephaly: the Maastricht experience. Genet Couns 2001; 12: 287–98.

Nelson LH, King M. Early diagnosis of holoprosencephaly. J Ultrasound Med 1992; 11: 57–9.

Tomd P, Costa A, Magnano GM, Cariati M, Lituania M. Holoprosencephaly: prenatal diagnosis by sonography and magnetic resonance imaging. Prenat Diagn 1990; 10: 429–36.

Turner CD, Silva S, Jeanty P. Prenatal diagnosis of alobar holoprosencephaly at 10 weeks of gestation. Ultrasound Obstet Gynecol 1999; 13: 360–2.

Wong HS, Lam YH, Tang MH, Cheung LW, Ng LK, Yan KW. First-trimester ultrasound diagnosis of holoprosencephaly: three case reports. Ultrasound Obstet Gynecol 1999; 13: 356–9.

Hydranencephaly

Definition: Extreme form of porencephaly where the cerebral cortex is either absent or only minimally preserved. Besides, severe hydrocephalus is present.

Incidence: Rare.

Sex ratio: M : F = 1 : 1.

Clinical history/genetics: Sporadic, occasionally familial inheritance. Described in over 20 syndromes.

Teratogens: Congenital infections, cocaine.

Embryology: Destruction of the cerebral tissue due to vascular occlusion or infection. Possibly resulting from an early stenosis of both internal carotid arteries. Hydrocephalus ex vacuo.

Associated malformations: None.

Ultrasound findings: There is practically *no evidence of cerebral tissue above the brain stem and diencephalon*. Even the falx cerebri is mostly absent. Infarction of the brain tissue may occur in the later part of pregnancy (30 weeks).

Clinical management: Karyotyping and search for infections (TORCH). The accompanying hydrocephalus does not progressively enlarge, as opposed to obstructive hydrocephalus (fluid-filled cavity ex vacuo). Termination of pregnancy is justified due to the unfavorable prognosis.

Prognosis: Fatal. Very few survive with severe mental retardation. Some may survive the immediate neonatal period.

References

Aguirre VC, Dominguez R. Intrauterine diagnosis of hydranencephaly by magnetic resonance. Magn Reson Imaging 1989; 7: 105–7.

Belfar HL, Kuller JA, Hill LM, Kislak S. Evolving fetal hydranencephaly mimicking intracranial neoplasm. J Ultrasound Med 1991; 10: 231–3.

Castro-Gago M, Pintos-Martinez E, Forteza-Vila J, et al. Congenital hydranencephalic–hydrocephalic syndrome with proliferative vasculopathy: a possible relation with mitochondrial dysfunction. J Child Neurol 2001; 16: 858–62.

Witters I, Moerman P, Devriendt K, et al. Two siblings with early-onset fetal akinesia deformation sequence and hydranencephaly: further evidence for autosomal-recessive inheritance of hydranencephaly, Fowler type. Am J Med Genet 2002; 108: 41–4.

Hadi HA, Mashini IS, Devoe LD, Holzman GB, Fadel HE. Ultrasonographic prenatal diagnosis of hydranencephaly: a case report. J Reprod Med 1986; 31: 254–6.

Lam YH, Tang MH. Serial sonographic features of a fetus with hydranencephaly from 11 weeks to term. Ultrasound Obstet Gynecol 2000; 16: 77–9.

McGahan JP, Ellis W, Lindfors KK, Lee BC, Arnold JP. Congenital cerebrospinal fluid-containing intracranial abnormalities: a sonographic classification. JCU J Clin Ultrasound 1988; 16: 531–44.

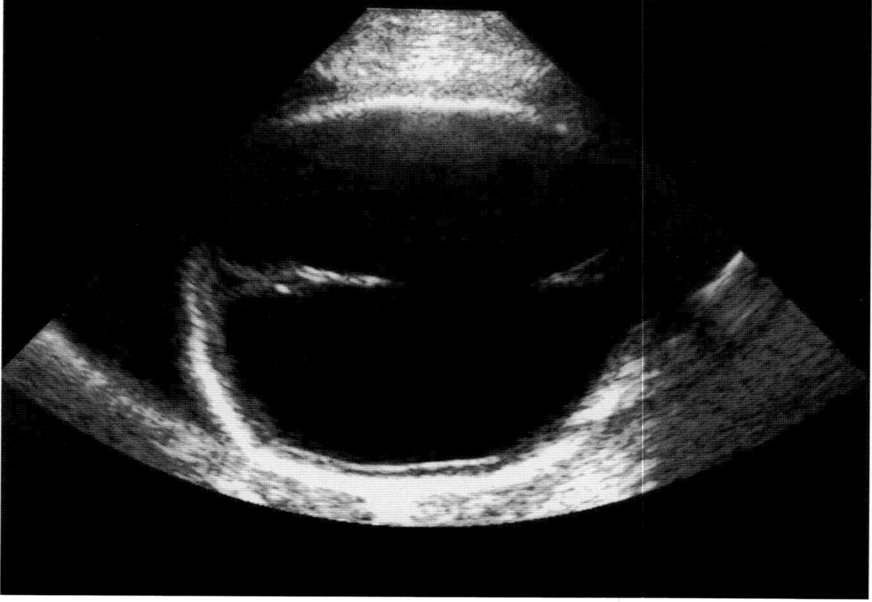

Fig. 2.**31** **Hydranencephaly.** 30 + 5 weeks. Severe dilation of the lateral ventricles. The rim of cortex measures 3 mm.

Stevenson DA, Hart BL, Clericuzio CL. Hydranencephaly in an infant with vascular malformations. Am J Med Genet 2001; 104: 295–8.

Vaughan JE, Parkes JR, Larsen P. Hydranencephaly: antenatal diagnosis using ultrasound [letter]. S Afr Med J 1984; 66: 675–6.

Hydrocephalus Internus

Definition: Widening of the lateral ventricles, as well as the third and the fourth ventricle. Alteration in the relationship between the rim of the cortex and the width of the ventricles. It is characterized by an abnormal accumulation of cerebrospinal fluid, due either to increased production or disturbed circulation and resorption. Prenatally, hydrocephalus is a consequence of obstruction or stenosis of the cerebral aqueduct. Hydrocephalus ex vacuo results from the destruction of brain tissue. It does not necessarily imply a large head, as this is a late and inconsistent sign.

Incidence: One in 1700–2000 births (hydrocephalus without neural tube defect).

Sex ratio: M : F = 0.7 : 1

Associated malformations: Associated malformations are expected in 80% of the cases. A neural tube defect may be the cause of hydrocephalus in 45–65%. In these cases, the characteristic “lemon sign” and “banana sign” are observed. In isolated cases, it may be difficult to detect the neural tube defect, especially if it is a simple spina bifida without a meningomyelocele. There is an increased occurrence of renal malformations. Chromosomal aberrations are evident in 20% of cases. Particularly in cases of trisomy 13, 18, and 21, an accompanying hydrocephalus is often present. Familial incidence through X-linked recessive inheritance is known to affect 50% of male infants, with hydrocephalus with stenosis of the aqueduct; 50% of females are asymptomatic carriers. Antenatal infections such as toxoplasmosis, cytomegalovirus, syphilis, and listeriosis are causative factors. In addition, hydrocephalus appears in association with other syndromes, for example, Meckel–Gruber syndrome, hydrolethalus, Peters anomaly, Miller–Diecker syndrome, osteogenesis imperfecta, and Apert syndrome.

Ultrasound findings: Assessment of ventricles is carried out routinely in the ultrasound screening of fetal anomalies. Under normal conditions, the width of the posterior horns of the lateral ventricles remains relatively constant from the end of the first trimester, with an upper limit of 8–10 mm. This means that the relationship of the ventricular width to the surrounding brain tissue changes in favor of the developing brain as the head circumference increases. In case of ventriculomegaly, it is most important to locate the defect (lateral ventricle, third or fourth ventricles). In addition, a very careful search for other anomalies is mandatory (for example, agenesis of corpus callosum, Dandy–Walker cyst).

Clinical management: Search for infections (TORCH), karyotyping, molecular-genetic diagnosis if necessary. Magnetic resonance imaging may be useful in the differential diagnosis. Repeated ultrasound at short intervals. Delivery should be planned in a center with a pediatric intensive-care unit with neuropediatric and neurosurgical experience. Intrauterine placement of a feto-amniotic shunt—a method propagated in the 1980s without the promised success—has been abandoned. There are no studies showing benefit of premature delivery for the sake of surgical intervention. In individual cases, delivery may be appropriate at 33 or 34 weeks. The benefit of a primary cesarean section is questionable. If the large fetal head poses a mechanical obstacle cephalocentesis may be an option in rare cases to enable a vaginal delivery. Even in severe cases of hydrocephalus, with only a tiny rim of cortex, decompression of the brain tissue may allow surprisingly good development of the brain.

Postnatally, intracranial pressure possibly may be estimated using Doppler sonography of the medial cerebral artery. Increased intracranial pressure is diagnosed when the diastolic flow velocity decreases, even showing reverse flow, and the resistance index increases. It is not yet clear whether these parameters are accurate for prenatal assessment of intracranial pressure.

Procedure after birth: Detailed diagnostic intervention, including molecular genetics, in the presence of aqueduct stenosis and “hitchhiker

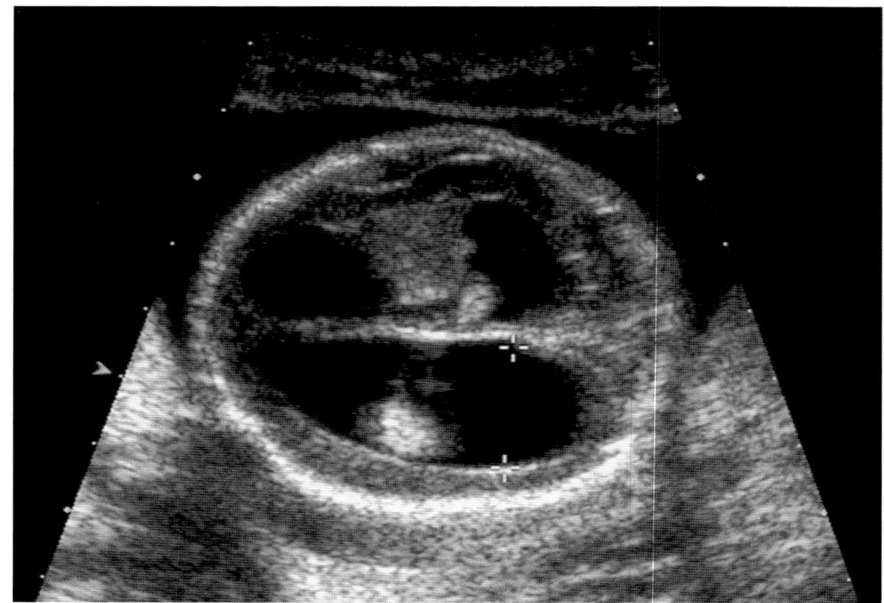

Fig. 2.**32** **Hydrocephalus.** 21 + 1 weeks. Widening of the lateral ventricles up to 17 mm.

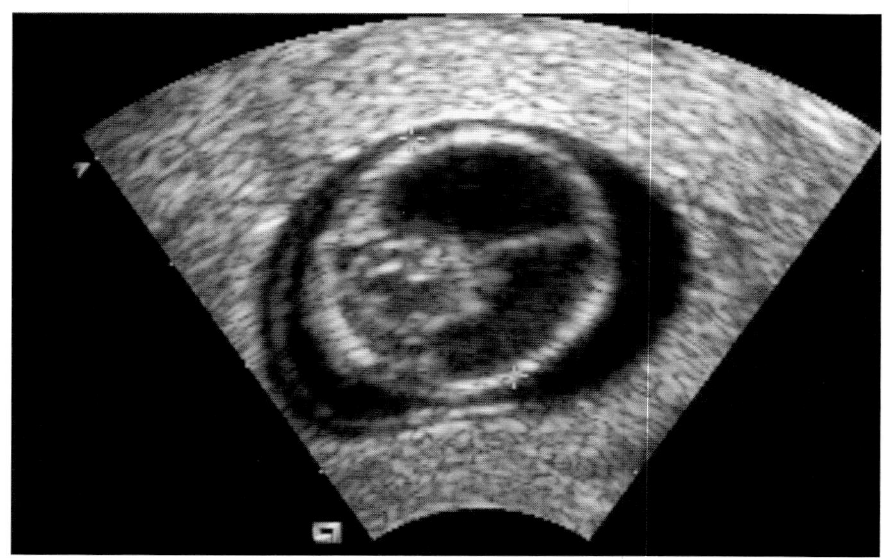

Fig. 2.**33** **Hydrocephalus.** A very early case of hydrocephalus, at 11 + 0 weeks.

thumb." Spinal tap to evaluate cerebrospinal fluid pressure and protein content. Considering the whole clinical situation, other forms of surgical intervention such as shunts should be considered.

Prognosis: The prognosis depends on associated malformations involving the CNS and other organs. Adequate therapy may lead to reasonable development of the brain, even when the initial findings are severe. Mental development in children with neural tube defect is usually good, even in cases of early hydrocephalus. Thinning of the cortical tissue due to increased intracranial pressure primarily affects the white matter, whereas the grey cells are not initially destroyed. For a good prognosis, it is important to achieve a sufficient decrease in intracranial pressure within the first 6 months of life.

Advice for the mother: The brain tissue of the neonate recovers amazingly well, so that in severe cases of hydrocephalus the prognosis may even be better than first expected. Here it is of utmost importance to evaluate the associated CNS and other anomalies for an accurate prognosis.

Self-Help Organizations

Title: Hydrocephalus Association

Description: Provides support, education and advocacy for people with hydrocephalus and their families. Provides a wealth of resource materials on hydrocephalus for all age groups, a quarterly newsletter, directory of neurosurgeons, biannual national conference, and scholarships for young adults.

Scope: National network

Founded: 1984.

Address: 870 Market St., Suite 705, San Francisco, CA 94102, United States

Telephone: 415–732–7040

Fax: 415–732–7044

E-mail: hydroassoc@aol.com

Web: http://www.hydroassoc.org

Title: Guardians of Hydrocephalus Research Foundation

Description: Information and referral service to persons affected by hydrocephalus. Phone networking for parents of children with hydrocephalus. Referrals to doctors, newsletter, literature and book for children and adults with hydrocephalus (in English and Spanish), video.

Scope: National network (bilingual)

Founded: 1977

Address: 2618 Ave. Z, Brooklyn, New York, NY 11235, United States

Telephone: 718–743–4473 or 1–800–458–8655.

Fax: 718–743–1171

E-mail: ghrf2618@aol.com

References

Clewell WH. Congenital hydrocephalus: treatment in utero. Fetal Ther 1988; 3: 89–97.

Clewell WH. Intra-uterine shunting procedures. Br J Hosp Med 1985; 34: 149–53.

Dreazen E, Tessier F, Sarti D, Crandall BF. Spontaneous resolution of fetal hydrocephalus. J Ultrasound Med 1989; 8: 155–157.

Goldstein I, Reece EA, Pilu GL, Hobbins JC, Bovicelli L. Sonographic evaluation of the normal developmental anatomy of fetal cerebral ventricles, 1: the frontal horn. Obstet Gynecol 1988; 72: 588–92.

Gupta JK, Bryce FC, Lilford RJ. Management of apparently isolated fetal ventriculomegaly. Obstet Gynecol Surv 1994; 49: 716–21.

Harrod MJ, Friedman JM, Santos RR, Rutledge J, Weinberg A. Etiologic heterogeneity of fetal hydrocephalus diagnosed by ultrasound. Am J Obstet Gynecol 1984; 150: 38–40.

Kirkinen P, Muller R, Baumann H, et al. Cerebral blood flow velocity waveforms in hydrocephalic fetuses. JCU J Clin Ultrasound 1988; 16: 493–8.

Mahony BS, Nyberg DA, Hirsch JH, Petty CN, Hendricks SK, Mack LA. Mild idiopathic lateral cerebral ventricular dilatation in utero: sonographic evaluation. Radiology 1988; 169: 715–21.

Reece EA, Goldstein I. Early prenatal diagnosis of hydrocephalus. Am J Perinatol 1997; 14: 69–73.

Schindelmann S, Sandner G, Harbeck N, Debus G. [Prenatal manifestation of a congenital glioblastoma: case report; in German]. Z Geburtshilfe Neonatol 2002; 206: 19–21.

Schrander SC, Fryns JP. Congenital hydrocephalus: posology and guidelines for clinical approach and genetic counselling. Eur J Pediatr 1998; 157: 355–62.

Seidman DS, Nass D, Mendelson E, Shehtman I, Mashiach S, Achiron R. Prenatal ultrasonographic diagnosis of fetal hydrocephalus due to infection with parainfluenza virus type 3. Ultrasound Obstet Gynecol 1996; 7: 52–4.

Senat MV, Bernard JP, Delezoide A, et al. Prenatal diagnosis of hydrocephalus-stenosis of the aqueduct of Sylvius by ultrasound in the first trimester of pregnancy: report of two cases. Prenat Diagn 2001; 21: 1129–32.

Siebert JR, Nyberg DA, Kapur RP. Cerebral mantle thickness: a measurement useful in anatomic diagnosis of fetal ventriculomegaly. Pediatr Dev Pathol 1999; 2: 168–75.

Weiner Z, Bronshtein M. Transient unilateral ventriculomegaly: sonographic diagnosis during the second trimester of pregnancy. J Clin Ultrasound 1994; 22: 59–61.

Iniencephaly

Definition: Defect of the cervical vertebrae causing exaggerated spinal lordosis and neural tube defect in the cervical region.

Incidence: Uncommon.

Sex ratio: M : F = 1 : 1

Clinical history/genetics: sporadic occurrence.

Teratogens: Not known.

Embryology: The pathogenesis is not known. It seems possible that the primary anomaly is a defective cervical column causing a secondary neural tube defect. It may even be the other way round, with the neural tube defect being the primary anomaly, as association with other neural tube defects has been described.

Associated malformations: Myelomeningocele and anencephaly.

Ultrasound findings: very short cervical spine with *absence of vertebrae and overextension of the fetal head*. A common finding is *dysraphism* of the cervical spine with an associated *meningomyelocele*.

Clinical management: Sonographic diagnosis is usually accurate enough for other diagnostic tools to be unnecessary. If the pregnancy continues, development of hydrocephalus is possible (caution: delivery obstacle). Difficulties are anticipated during labor and delivery due to overextension of the fetal head. In case of severe hydrocephalus, cephalocentesis is an option to allow a vaginal delivery. Rarely, embryotomy may be needed to avoid a cesarean section.

Procedure after birth: Intensive medical interventions should be avoided.

Prognosis: Mostly fatal.

Advice for the mother: This is a very rare anomaly with no increased risk of recurrence.

References

Foderaro AE, Abu YM, Benda JA, Williamson RA, Smit WL. Antenatal ultrasound diagnosis of iniencephaly. JCU J Clin Ultrasound 1987; 15: 550–4.

Guilleux MH, Serville F, Gaillac D, et al. Prenatal echographic diagnosis of iniencephaly: apropos of a case. J Gynecol Obstet Biol Reprod (Paris) 1987; 16: 85–8.

Hammer F, Scherrer C, Baumann H, Briner J, Schinzel F. Iniencephaly: prenatal and postnatal findings. Geburtshilfe Frauenheilkd 1990; 50: 491–4.

Jeanne-Pasquier C, Carles D, Alberti EM, Jacob B. [Iniencephaly: four cases and a review of the literature; in French; review.] J Gynecol Obstet Biol Reprod (Paris) 2002; 31: 276–82.

Marton T, Tanko A, Mezei G, Papp Z. Diagnosis of an unusual form of iniencephaly in the first trimester of pregnancy. Ultrasound Obstet Gynecol 2001; 18: 549–51.

Meizner I, Levi A, Katz M, Maor E. Iniencephaly: a case report. J Reprod Med 1992; 37: 885–8.

Morocz I, Szeifert GT, Molnar P, Toth Z, Csecsei K, Papp Z. Prenatal diagnosis and pathoanatomy of iniencephaly. Clin Genet 1986; 30: 81–6.

Sherer DM, Hearn SB, Harvey W, Metlay LA, Abramowicz JS. Endovaginal sonographic diagnosis of iniencephaly apertus and craniorachischisis at 13 weeks' menstrual age. J Clin Ultrasound 1993; 21: 124–7.

Shoham Z, Caspi B, Chemke J, Dgani R, Lancet M. Iniencephaly: prenatal ultrasonographic diagnosis case report. J Perinat Med 1988; 16: 139–43.

Intracranial Bleeding

Definition: Bleeding occurring within the parenchyma, in the ventricles, or in the intracranial space around the brain tissue.

Incidence: Rare.

Clinical history/genetics: Severe preeclampsia, twin–twin transfusion syndrome or intrauterine death of a monochorionic twin can lead to intracranial bleeding. Other causes can be congenital infections, vessel anomalies, autoantibodies, platelet antibodies (fetal alloimmune thrombocytopenia, FAIT) and trauma.

Teratogens: Congenital infections and cocaine.

Associated conditions: Bleeding into the lungs and liver are evident secondary to a hemorrhagic episode. Severe anemia resulting from the bleeding may cause hydrops fetalis.

Ultrasound findings: At first an *echogenic area* is seen intracranially, which may later turn *cystic*. *Echogenic blood clots* may be seen within the ventricles. *Subdural hematomas* appear between the skull and the brain tissue. The lateral or third ventricles may be widened, depending on the location of the bleeding. Intracranial bleeding is first recognized, if at all, in the third trimester. Often it is the resulting *hydrocephalus* and possibly the *differing widths of the lateral ventricles* that are detected sonographically.

Clinical management: Umbilical venous sampling to determine fetal hemoglobin and platelet count (caution: risk of bleeding in thrombocytopenia). Search for infections (TORCH). The delivery should proceed in a perinatal unit. If alloimmune thrombocytopenia is the cause, then platelet transfusion is given and cesarean section is preferred. The time of delivery is influenced by the development of the hydrocephalus.

Procedure after birth: In the case of fresh and severe bleeding, a transfusion of erythrocytes and platelets should be kept ready. Intensive medical intervention may be withheld in the most severely affected newborns. Magnetic resonance imaging is the best method for detecting associated vessel malformations.

Prognosis: This depends on the severity of brain damage and the cause of the bleeding, such as infection. As a result, hydrocephalus or porencephaly may develop.

References

Achiron R, Pinchas OH, Reichman B, et al. Fetal intracranial haemorrhage: clinical significance of in utero ultrasonographic diagnosis. Br J Obstet Gynaecol 1993; 100: 995–9.

Batukan C, Holzgreve W, Bubl R, Visca E, Radu EW, Tercanli S. Prenatal diagnosis of an infratentorial subdural hemorrhage: case report. Ultrasound Obstet Gynecol 2002; 19: 407–9.

Bondurant S, Boehm FH, Fleischer AC, Machin JE. Antepartum diagnosis of fetal intracranial hemorrhage by ultrasound. Obstet Gynecol 1984; 63: 25–27.

Burrows RF, Caco CC, Kelton JG. Neonatal alloimmune thrombocytopenia: spontaneous in utero intracranial hemorrhage. Am J Hematol 1988; 28: 98–102.

Fogarty K, Cohen HL, Haller JO. Sonography of fetal intracranial hemorrhage: unusual causes and a review of the literature. JCU J Clin Ultrasound 1989; 17: 366–70.

Guerriero S, Ajossa S, Mais V, et al. Color Doppler energy imaging in the diagnosis of fetal intracranial hemorrhage in the second trimester. Ultrasound Obstet Gynecol 1997; 10: 205–8.

Kirkinen P, Partanen K, Ryynanen M, Orden MR. Fetal intracranial hemorrhage: imaging by ultrasound and magnetic resonance imaging. J Reprod Med 1997; 42: 467–72.

Kirkinen P, Ordén MR, Partanen K. Cerebral blood flow changes associated with fetal intracranial hemorrhages. Acta Obstet Gynecol Scand 1997; 76: 308–12.

Kuhn MJ, Couch SM, Binstadt DH, et al. Prenatal recognition of central nervous system complications of alloimmune thrombocytopenia. Comput Med Imaging Graph 1992; 16: 137–42.

Sasidharan CK, Kutty PM, Ajithkumar, Sajith N. Fetal intracranial hemorrhage due to antenatal low dose aspirin intake. Indian J Pediatr 2001; 68: 1071–2.

Stirling HF, Hendry M, Brown JK. Prenatal intracranial haemorrhage. Dev Med Child Neurol 1989; 31: 807–11.

Strigini FA, Cioni G, Canapicchi R, Nardini V, Capriello P, Carmignani A. Fetal intracranial hemorrhage: is minor maternal trauma a possible pathogenetic factor? Ultrasound Obstet Gynecol 2001; 18: 335–42.

Cataract

Definition: Echogenic lenses of the eye, which can be seen with high-frequency ultrasound (e.g., 7 MHz transvaginal sonography).

Incidence: Rare.

Clinical history/genetics: Family history, isolated finding resulting from autosomal-recessive or autosomal-dominant transmission.

Teratogens: Unknown.

Ultrasound findings: The earliest diagnosis was made at 15 weeks with a positive family history. Otherwise, prenatal diagnosis is unlikely.

Differential diagnosis: Infections (cytomegalovirus, rubella, toxoplasmosis, varicella), coloboma, congenital aniridia, microphthalmia, glucose-6-phosphate dehydrogenase deficiency, homocysteinuria, arthrogryposis, chondroplasia punctata, Hallermann–Streiff syndrome, hypochondroplasia, Kniest syndrome, Marfan syndrome, Roberts syndrome, Smith–Lemli–Opitz syndrome, Walker–Warburg syndrome.

Clinical management: Genetic counseling, TORCH serology.

Procedure after birth: Early ophthalmic treatment can prevent the development of severe amblyopia.

Prognosis: Variable, depending on the associated anomalies. Surgical treatment of isolated cataracts is very successful.

References

Bornemann A, Pfeiffer R, Beinder E, et al. Three siblings with Walker–Warburg syndrome. Gen Diagn Pathol 1996; 141: 371–5.

Cengiz B, Baxi L. Congenital cataract in triplet pregnancy after IVF with frozen embryos: prenatal diagnosis and management. Fetal Diagn Ther 2001; 16: 234–6.

Drysdale K, Kyle PM, Sepulveda W. Prenatal detection of congenital inherited cataracts. Ultrasound Obstet Gynecol 1997; 9: 62–3.

Monteagudo A, Timor TI, Friedman AH, Santos R. Autosomal-dominant cataracts of the fetus: early detection by transvaginal ultrasound. Ultrasound Obstet Gynecol 1996; 8: 104–8.

Pedreira DA, Diniz EM, Schultz R, Faro LB, Zugaib M. Fetal cataract in congenital toxoplasmosis. Ultrasound Obstet Gynecol 1999; 13: 266–7.

Rahi JS, Dezateux C. Congenital and infantile cataract in the United Kingdom: underlying or associated factors. British Congenital Cataract Interest Group. Invest Ophthalmol Vis Sci 2000; 41: 2108–14.

Romain M, Awoust J, Dugauquier C, Van Maldergem L. Prenatal ultrasound detection of congenital cataract in trisomy 21. Prenat Diagn 1999; 19: 780–2.

Zimmer EZ, Bronshtein M, Ophir E, et al. Sonographic diagnosis of fetal congenital cataracts. Prenat Diagn 1993; 13: 503–11.

Microcephaly

Definition: Microcephaly is defined as severely reduced head circumference (lower limit < 2 or < 3 SD) in otherwise normal body measurements, resulting in thoracocephalic disproportion. The small head circumference is caused mostly due to insufficient development of the brain tissue, leading to reduction in brain volume. A premature synostosis of fetal skull is a rare cause of microcephaly.

Incidence: One in 6000–10 000 births.

Sex ratio: M : F = 1 : 1.

Clinical history/genetics: It may be inherited as an autosomal-recessive or dominant trait. Over 300 syndromes have been described in which microcephaly is an accompanying feature.

Teratogens: Congenital infections, radiation, various drugs, and alcohol have been implicated as causal factors. In addition, maternal phenylketonuria may also cause fetal microcephaly.

Embryology: Microcephaly results from underdevelopment of the brain tissue. The first prenatal manifestation of this may be late in the third trimester, or even after birth.

Associated malformations: Meningoceles and porencephalic cysts are associated with microcephaly. Others include holoprosencephaly, intracranial calcifications, ventricular distension, lissencephaly.

Depending on the presence of other syndromes, heart and other anomalies are evident.

Associated syndromes: Cornelia de Lange syndrome, Seckel syndrome, Smith–Lemli–Opitz syndrome, Meckel–Gruber syndrome, Miller–Diecker syndrome, Neu–Laxova syndrome, Shprintzen syndrome, Walker–Warburg syndrome, Fancini anemia, Freeman syndrome, multiple pterygium syndrome, Roberts syndrome, Wolf–Hirschhorn syndrome (4 p deletion), cri-du-chat syndrome (5 p deletion), Jacobsen syndrome (11 q deletion), trisomy 9 mosaic, trisomy 13, arthrogryposis.

Ultrasound findings: The head circumference is small, whereas the facial structures are normal. In order to minimize false-positive findings, microcephaly should only be diagnosed when the head circumference measures less than three standard deviations below average. Measurement of the frontal lobes may help in diagnosis. Microcephaly cannot always be diagnosed with certainty before 23 weeks. Repeated controls maybe helpful. False-positive findings are seen in up to 70% of cases; this means that in these cases, there is no evidence of microcephaly postnatally.

Caution: Small head may be a familial condition and may not be a pathological finding.

Clinical management: Detailed clinical and family history and exclusion of phenylketonuria is important. TORCH serology, further sonographic screening including fetal echocardiography, karyotyping, possibly magnetic resonance imaging.

Procedure after birth: Magnetic resonance imaging may detect associated neural malformations.

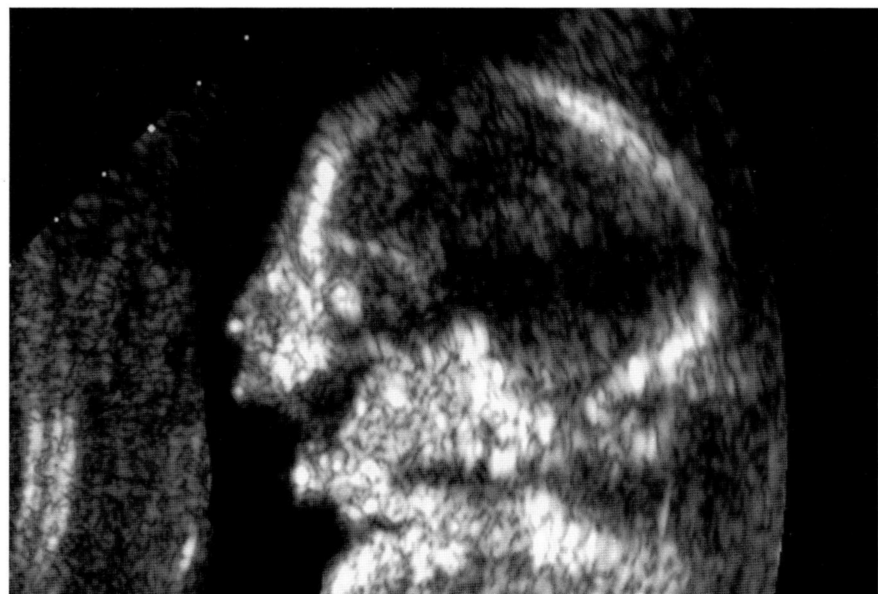

Fig. 2.**34** **Microcephaly.** Fetal profile at 21 + 6 weeks in a case of familial microcephaly.

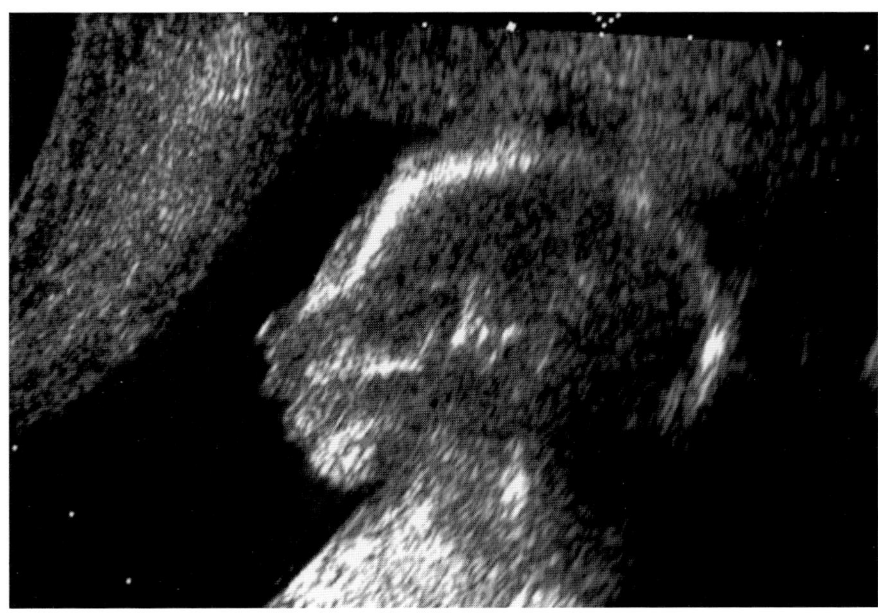

Fig. 2.**35** **Microcephaly.** At 18 + 2 weeks, as a result of an encephalocele displacing the brain tissue dorsally.

Prognosis: This depends on the extent of the brain anomaly, but severe mental retardation is expected. Normal intelligence is rarely found.

Self-Help Organization

Title: Brain Talk MGH Neurology Web Forum

Description: Provides both unmoderated message boards and chat rooms for various neurological disorders, such as: aneurysms, atrioventricular malformations (AVMs), Bell's palsy, central pain syndrome, cauda equina syndrome, PANDAS, premenstrual dysphoric disorder, thoracic outlet syndrome, and over a hundred others—including rare neurological conditions—and workers' compensation, both under the "General Subjects" category.

Scope: Online

Web: http://www.BrainTalk.org

References

Bromley B, Benacerraf BR. Difficulties in the prenatal diagnosis of microcephaly. J Ultrasound Med 1995; 14: 303–6.

Chervenak FA, Rosenberg J, Brightman RC, Chitkara U, Jeanty P. A prospective study of the accuracy of ultrasound in predicting fetal microcephaly. Obstet Gynecol 1987; 69: 908–10.

Dahlgren L, Wilson RD. Prenatally diagnosed microcephaly: a review of etiologies. Fetal Diagn Ther 2001; 16: 323–6.

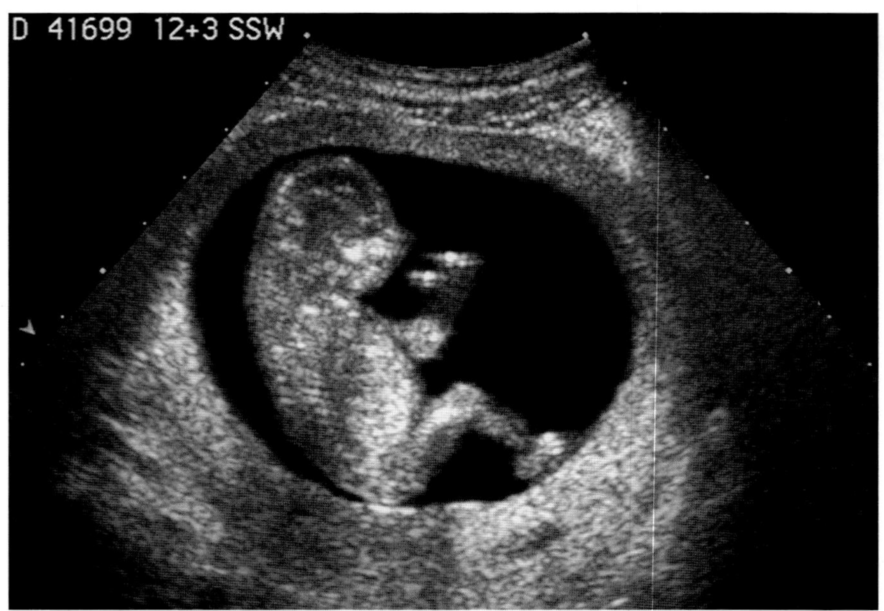

Fig. 2.**36** **Microcephaly.** An unusually early detection of microcephaly at 12 + 3 weeks.

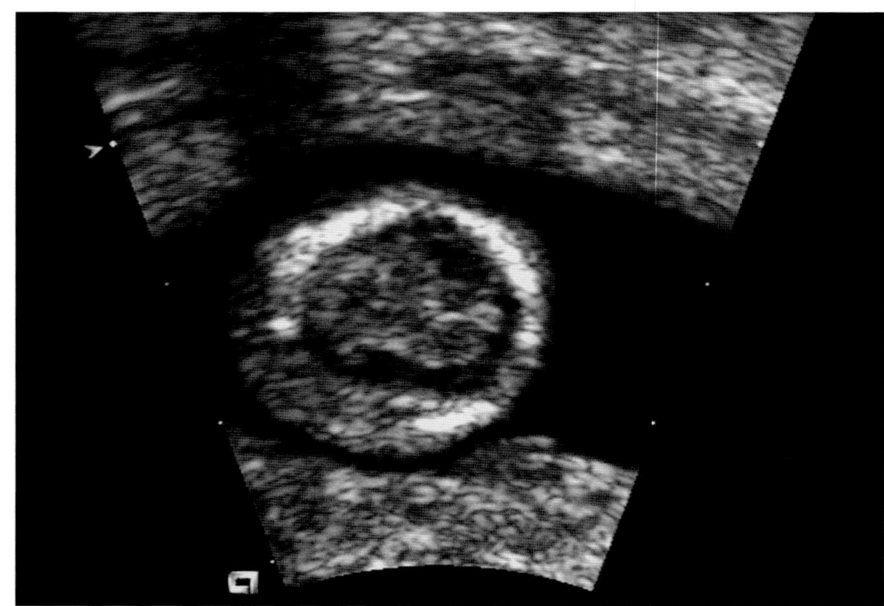

Fig. 2.**37** **Microcephaly.** Same case as before. Cross-sectional view of the microcephalic fetal head at 12 + 3 weeks.

Durr-e-Sabih, Khan AN, Sabih Z. Prenatal sonographic diagnosis of Neu–Laxova syndrome. J Clin Ultrasound 2001; 29: 531–4.

Kurtz AB, Wapner RJ, Rubin CS, Cole BC, Ross RD, Goldberg BB. Ultrasound criteria for in utero diagnosis of microcephaly. JCU J Clin Ultrasound 1980; 8: 11–6.

Lenke RR, Platt LD, Koch R. Ultrasonographic failure of early detection of fetal microcephaly in maternal phenylketonuria. J Ultrasound Med 1983; 2: 177–9.

Majoor KD, Wladimiroff JW, Stewart PA, van de Harten JJ, Niermeijer ME. Microcephaly, micrognathia and bird-headed dwarfism: prenatal diagnosis of a Seckel-like syndrome. Am J Med Genet 1987; 27: 183–8.

Pilu G, Falco P, Milano V, Perolo A, Bovicelli L. Prenatal diagnosis of microcephaly assisted by vaginal sonography and power Doppler. Ultrasound Obstet Gynecol 1998; 11: 357–60.

Rees AE, Bates A, Clarke H. Cerebellar hypoplasia in the second trimester associated with microcephaly at birth. Ultrasound Obstet Gynecol 1995; 5: 206–8.

The HN, Pescia G, Deonna T, Bakaric O. Early prenatal diagnosis of genetic microcephaly. Prenat Diagn 1985; 5: 345–347.

Tolmie JL, McNay M, Stephenson JB, Doyle D, Connor JM. Microcephaly: genetic counselling and antenatal diagnosis after the birth of an affected child. Am J Med Genet 1987; 27: 583–94.

Wilson RD, Hitchman D, Wittman BK. Clinical follow-up of prenatally diagnosed isolated ventriculomegaly, microcephaly and encephalocele. Fetal Ther 1989; 4: 49–57.

Spina Bifida Aperta, (Myelo-)Meningocele

Definition: Midline defect of the vertebra combined with a neural tube defect, leading to herniation and exposure of neural tissue and the meninges. This results in a considerable loss of neurological function. The defect is located in the lumbosacral region in 90% of cases, in the thoracic region in 6–8%, and in the cervical vertebrae in 2–4%. In 75%, the herniated sac shows a myelomeningocele and in 25% a meningocele.

Incidence: Varies geographically; in Germany one in 1000, in the USA between one in 500 and one in 2000 births.

Sex ratio: M : F = 1 : > 1

Clinical history/genetics: Alpha fetoprotein in serum is elevated in 80% of mothers. The recurrence rate after one affected child is 2–3%, and after two affected children 10%.

Teratogens: Valproic acid, folic acid antagonists, high doses of vitamin A, thalidomide, diabetes mellitus, hyperthermia, folic acid deficiency.

Embryology: A defect in the posterior arch of the vertebra, which develops up to the 6th week. The usual location is lumbosacral, with hydrocephalus resulting from the Arnold–Chiari malformation present in 90% of the cases.

Associated malformations: Arnold–Chiari malformation ("banana sign") and hydrocephalus, deformation of the head with overlapping of the frontal bones ("lemon sign"), club feet, occasionally hydronephrosis and heart defect.

Associated syndromes: Over 90 chromosomal and nonchromosomal syndromes have been described.

Ultrasound findings: *Widening of the vertebral column* in the affected region appears as a *U shape* in transverse section. Frequently, a *cystic elevation* is found *dorsal to the vertebral column*. Most commonly located in the lumbosacral region. (The upper edge of the iliac bone represents the 5th lumbar vertebra). Sometimes a *bulge* is seen in the affected area. The vertebral column should be viewed in the horizontal and longitudinal axis. In small defects, *Arnold–Chiari malformation* ("banana sign") and "lemon sign" are more easily recognized than the defect in the vertebra. Widening of the lateral ventricles is often present, the head circumference however may still be small. Ninety-eight percent of the myelomeningoceles are detected through ultrasound screening of the head and the vertebral column. Club feet and absence of movement in the lower extremities predicts a poor prognosis. On the other hand, spontaneous movement of the lower extremities does not assure normal neurological function postnatally or after surgery.

Clinical management: Karyotyping (chromosomal aberrations in 10%), measurement of amniotic fluid alpha fetoprotein and acetylcholinesterase. Progression of hydrocephalus should be monitored regularly. Premature delivery after 31 weeks of gestation may be advised if hydrocephalus progresses. Recommendations regarding the mode of delivery are inconsistent. Recent reports have shown that primary cesarean section prior to onset of labor allows the greatest preservation of motor skills.

Procedure after birth: The delivery should take place in a perinatal unit. Gentle handling of the defect without causing trauma is essential; the defect should be covered using aseptic measures. Hydrocephalus may develop even after the defect has been surgically repaired. It is often necessary to place a ventriculoperitoneal shunt prior to surgery. Recurrent urogenital infections and orthopedic dysfunction are treated symptomatically.

Prognosis: This depends on the size and location of the meningomyelocele. There is a 10% risk of mental retardation. A certain degree of neurological deficit in the lower extremities and urinary bladder dysfunction are expected.

Recommendation for the mother: Intake of folic acid (4 mg/d) prior to conception reduces the risk of recurrence significantly.

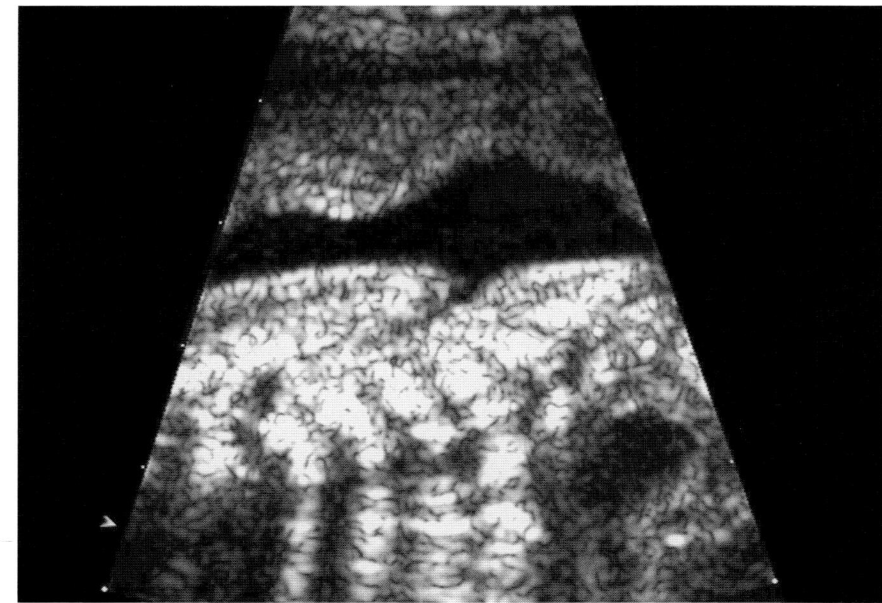

Fig. 2.**38** **Spina bifida aperta.** 21 + 1 weeks, dorsoanterior longitudinal section. There is an interruption in the continuity of the skin fold.

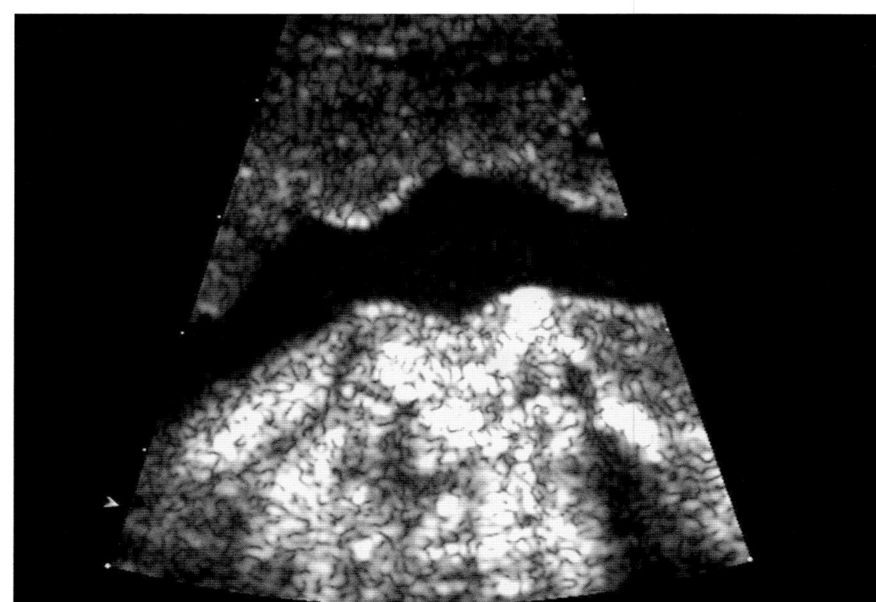

Fig. 2.**39** **Spina bifida aperta.** 21 + 1 weeks, the same case in cross-section. Absence of closure of the posterior vertebral arch.

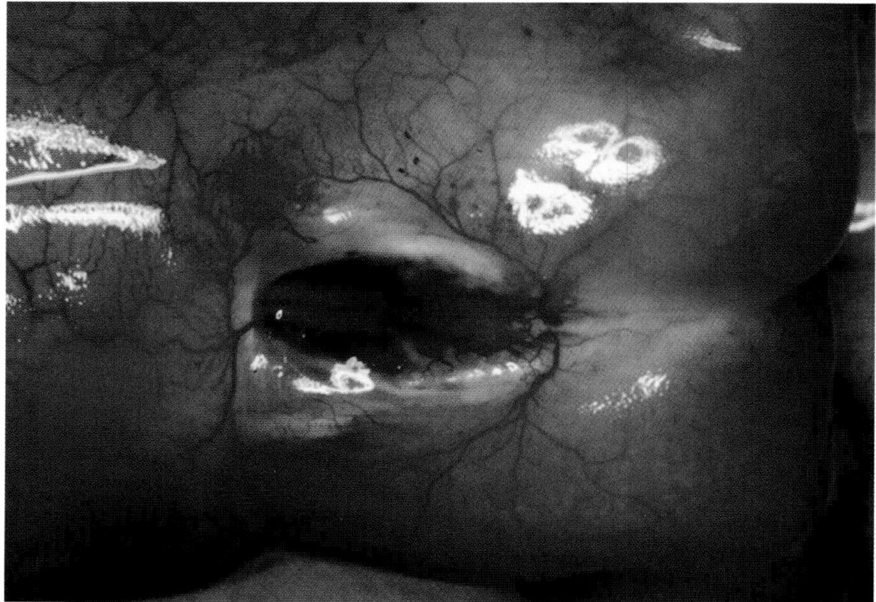

Fig. 2.**40** **Spina bifida aperta.** Absence of any herniation. Termination of pregnancy.

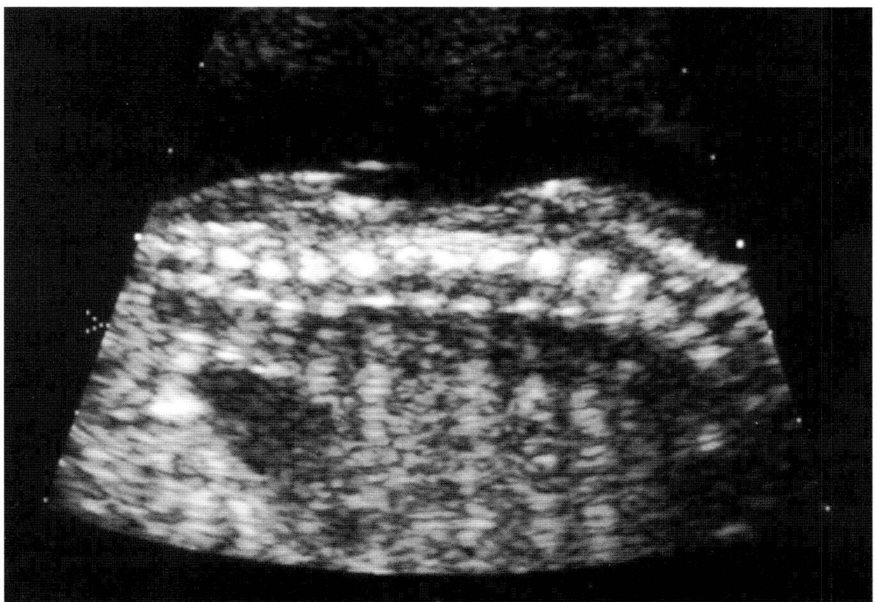

Fig. 2.41 **Spina bifida aperta.** Severe finding in the lumbosacral region extending over several vertebrae at 21 + 3 weeks.

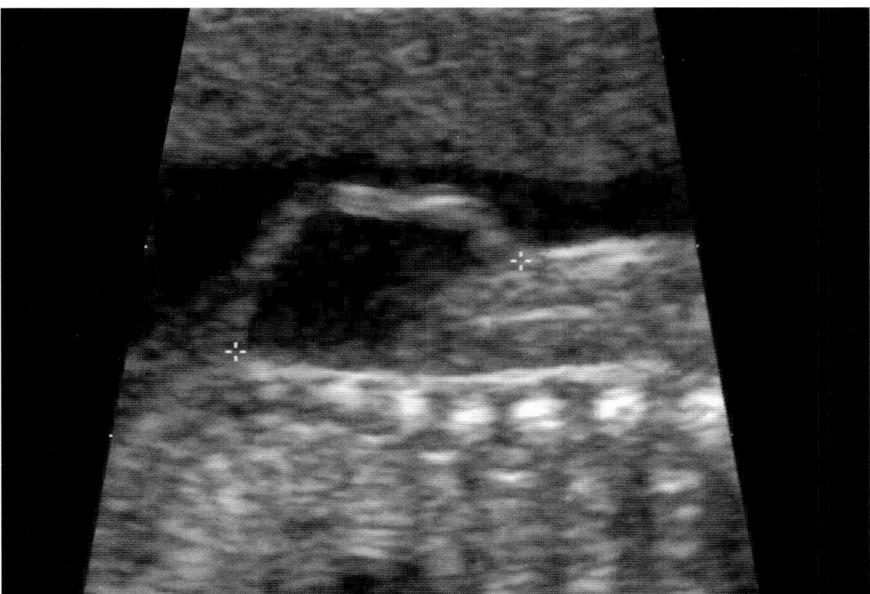

Fig. 2.42 **Spina bifida aperta.** Here in the region of the sacrum with a meningomyelocele at 19 + 6 weeks. Longitudinal section, with the fetus in a dorsoanterior position.

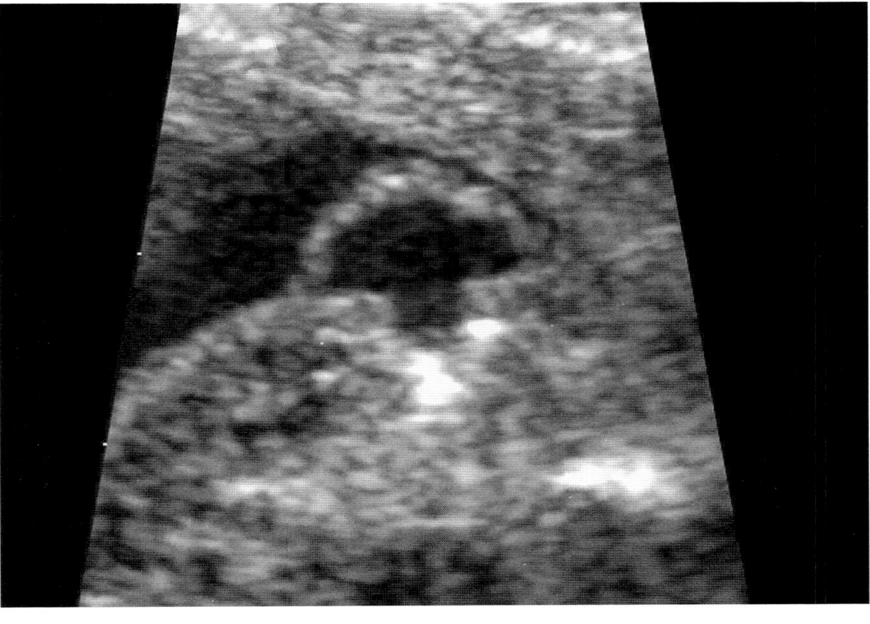

Fig. 2.43 **Spina bifida aperta.** Same as the previous case, in cross-section.

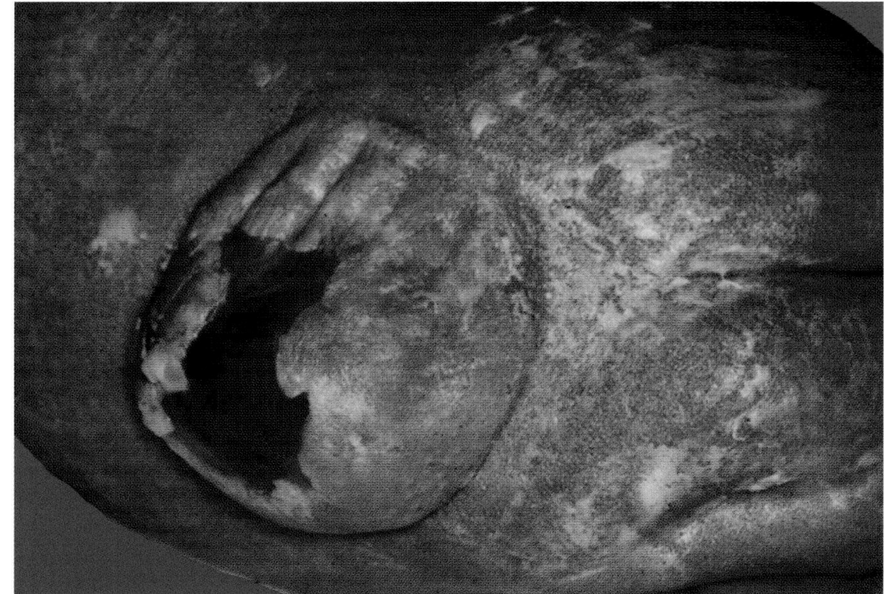

Fig. 2.**44** **Spina bifida aperta.** Seen here with a meningocele of the lower vertebral column, after termination of the pregnancy.

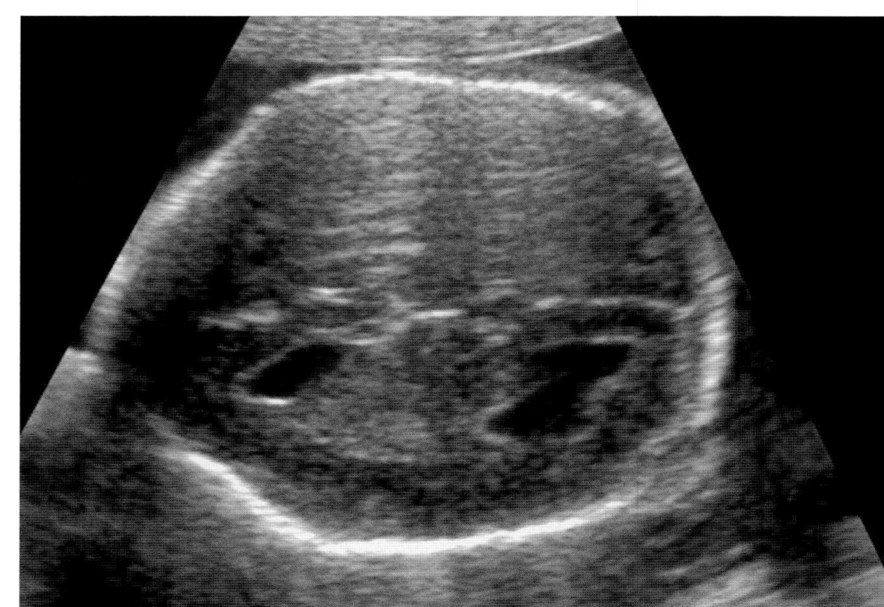

Fig. 2.**45** **Spina bifida aperta.** Fetal head at 21 + 1 weeks in a case of spina bifida aperta of the lower vertebrae, showing widening of the cerebrospinal fluid space and indentation of the frontal bone ("lemon sign").

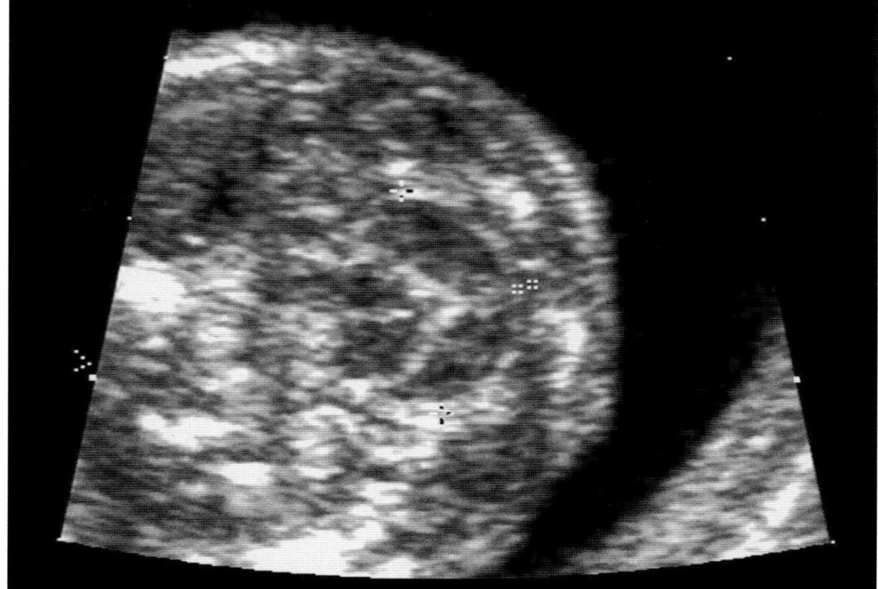

Fig. 2.**46** **Spina bifida aperta.** Depiction of cerebellum in a fetus with spina bifida aperta at 17 + 4 weeks. Due to the descent of some brain tissue into the upper vertebral column (Arnold–Chiari malformation), the appearance of the cerebellum is more like a banana in shape than the normal dumbbell form—the "banana sign."

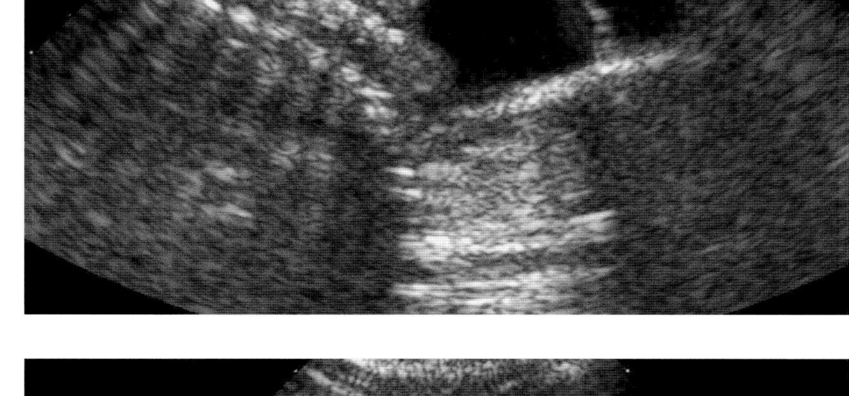

Fig. 2.**47** **Cervical spina bifida.** With a meningocele at 32 + 2 weeks. Longitudinal view, with the fetus in the dorsoanterior position.

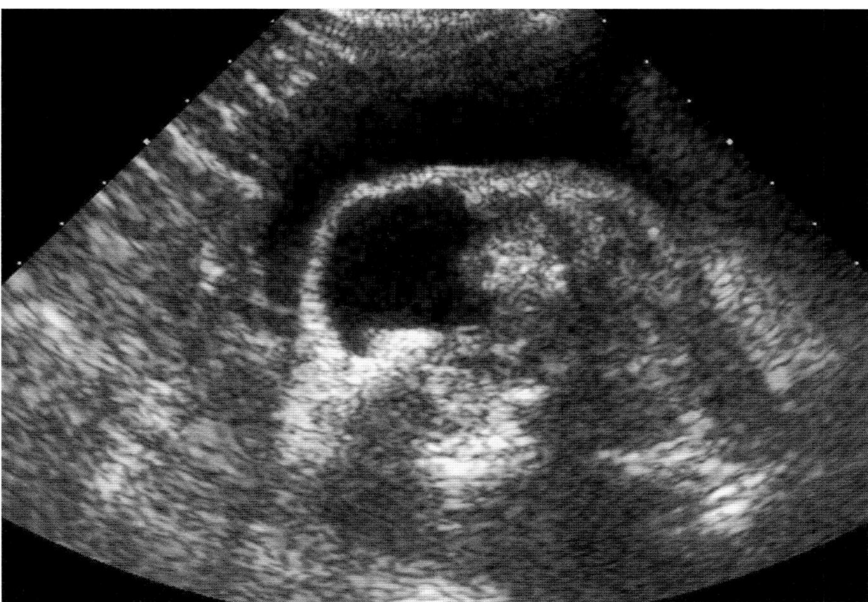

Fig. 2.**48** **Cervical spina bifida.** With a meningocele at 32 + 2 weeks. Cross-section, showing clearly the absence of closure of the vertebral arch.

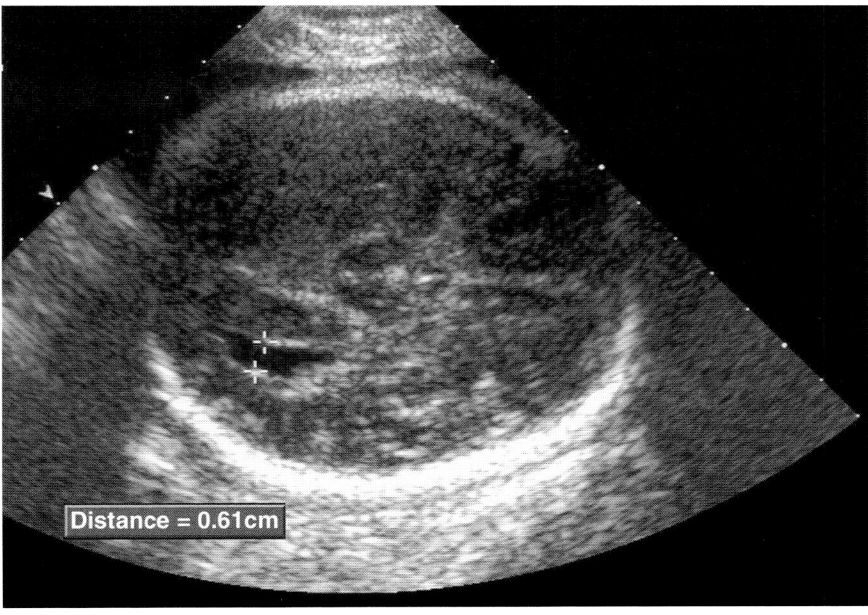

Fig. 2.**49** **Lateral ventricle and cervical spina bifida.** 32 + 2 weeks. There is no dilation of the cerebrospinal fluid space.

Self-Help Organization

Title: Spina Bifida Association of America

Description: Encourages educational and vocational development of patients. Promotes public awareness, advocacy and research. Newsletter, chapter development guidelines, national resource center, scholarships, film/videotapes.

Scope: National

Number of groups: 75 chapters

Founded: 1972

Address: 4590 MacArthur Blvd. NW, Suite 250, Washington, DC 20007, United States

Telephone: 1-800-621-3141 or 202-944-3285

Fax: 202-944-3295

E-mail: sbaa@sbaa.org

Web: http://www.sba.org

References

Babcock CJ. Ultrasound evaluation of prenatal and neonatal spina bifida. Neurosurg Clin N Am 1995; 6: 203–18.

Bernard JP, Suarez B, Rambaud C, Muller F, Ville Y. Prenatal diagnosis of neural tube defect before 12 weeks' gestation: direct and indirect ultrasonographic semeiology. Ultrasound Obstet Gynecol 1997; 10: 406–9

Buisson O, De Keersmaecker B, Senat MV, Bernard JP, Moscoso G, Ville Y. Sonographic diagnosis of spina bifida at 12 weeks: heading towards indirect signs. Ultrasound Obstet Gynecol 2002; 19: 290–2.

Chan A, Robertson EF, Haan EA, Ranieri E, Keane RJ. The sensitivity of ultrasound and serum alpha-fetoprotein in population-based antenatal screening for neural tube defects, South Australia 1986–1991. Br J Obstet Gynaecol 1995; 102: 370–6.

Gremm B, Sohn C, Beldermann F Bastert G. Increased AFP in maternal serum as an indication for invasive diagnosis. Zentralbl Gynäkol 1997; 119: 560–6.

Lee W, Chaiworapongsa T, Romero R, et al. A diagnostic approach for the evaluation of spina bifida by three-dimensional ultrasonography. J Ultrasound Med 2002; 21: 619–26.

Lindhout D, Omtzigt JG. Teratogenic effects of antiepileptic drugs: implications for the management of epilepsy in women of childbearing age. Epilepsia 1994; 35 (Suppl 4): S19 -S28.

Nadel AS, Green JK, Holmes LB, Frigoletto FDJ, Benacerraf BR. Absence of need for amniocentesis in patients with elevated levels of maternal serum alpha-fetoprotein and normal ultrasonographic examinations. N Engl J Med 1990; 323: 557–61.

Petrikovsky BM. Predicting ambulation by checking leg withdrawal in fetuses with spina bifida. Am J Obstet Gynecol 2002; 187: 256; discussion 256.

Reece EA, Homko CJ, Wiznitzer A Goldstein I. Needle embryofetoscopy and early prenatal diagnosis. Fetal Diagn Ther 1995; 10: 81–2.

Sebire NJ, Noble PL, Thorpe BJ, Snijders, RJ, Nicolaides KH. Presence of the "lemon" sign in fetuses with spina bifida at the 10–14-week scan. Ultrasound Obstet Gynecol 1997; 10: 403–5.

Williams LJ, Mai CT, Edmonds LD, et al. Prevalence of spina bifida and anencephaly during the transition to mandatory folic acid fortification in the United States. Teratology 2002; 66: 33–9.

Williamson P, Alberman E, Rodeck C, Fiddler M, Church S, Harris R. Antecedent circumstances surrounding neural tube defect births in 1990–1991. The Steering Committee of the National Confidential Enquiry into Counselling for Genetic Disorders. Br J Obstet Gynaecol 1997; 104: 51–6.

Teratoma (Intracranial)

Definition: Teratomas are germ-cell tumors arising from omnipotent stem cells. They consist of ectoderm, endoderm, and mesoderm.

Incidence: Rare.

Sex ratio: M : F = 5 : 1

Teratogens: Unknown.

Embryology: Only 3% of teratomas are located intracranially, but 50% of intrauterine brain tumors are teratomas.

Ultrasound findings: Intracranial *tumor* with solid and cystic areas. *Calcification* may be found. Only large tumors are mostly detected prenatally. The resulting disturbance of swallowing reflex also causes *hydramnios* .

Differential diagnosis: Other primary brain tumors, lipomas, and intracranial bleeding have to be considered.

Clinical management: To clarify the findings further, umbilical venous sampling (alloimmune thrombocytopenia, bleeding?) and TORCH serology are indicated. Magnetic resonance imaging may also help. Changes in head circumference should be monitored regularly using ultrasound.

Procedure after birth: Resection of the tumor is possible, depending on its size and extent. Mature teratomas are often completely resectable, whereas immature ones can only be partly excised and thus tend to have a high recurrence rate.

Prognosis: This depends on the size and extent of the tumor. In severe forms, the prognosis is fatal.

References

Broeke ED, Verdonk GW, Roumen FJ. Prenatal ultrasound diagnosis of an intracranial teratoma influencing management: case report and review of the literature. Eur J Obstet Gynecol Reprod B 45: 210–4.

Chan KL, Tang MH, Tse HY, et al. Factors affecting outcomes of prenatally diagnosed tumours. Prenat Diagn 2002; 22: 437–43.

D'Addario V, Pinto V, Meo F, Resta M. The specificity of ultrasound in the detection of fetal intracranial tumors. J Perinat Med 1998; 26: 480–5.

DiGiovanni LM, Sheikh Z. Prenatal diagnosis, clinical significance and management of fetal intracranial teratoma: a case report and literature review. Am J Perinatol 1994; 11: 420–2.

Eckmann C, Huneke B, Schlotfeldt TC, Carstensen MH, Reinhold S. Prenatal diagnosis of malignant intracranial teratoma in the fetus. Geburtshilfe Frauenheilkd 1991; 51: 859–60.

Ferreira J, Eviatar L, Schneider S, Grossman R. Prenatal diagnosis of intracranial teratoma: prolonged survival after resection of a malignant teratoma diagnosed prenatally by ultrasound: a case report and literature review. Pediatr Neurosurg 1993; 19: 84–8.

Hoff NR, Mackay IM. Prenatal ultrasound diagnosis of intracranial teratoma. JCU J Clin Ultrasound 1980; 8: 247–9.

Horton D, Pilling DW. Early antenatal ultrasound diagnosis of fetal intracranial teratoma. Br J Radiol 1997; 70: 1299–1301.

Rodriguez-Mojica W, Goni M, Correa MS, Colon LE, Volnikh V. Prenatal sonographic evaluation of two intracranial teratomas. P R Health Sci J 2002; 21: 43–5.

Shipp TD, Bromley B, Benacerraf B. The ultrasonographic appearance and outcome for fetuses with masses distorting the fetal face. J Ultrasound Med 1995; 14: 673–8.

Aneurysm of the Vein of Galen

Definition: Aneurysmal dilation of the vein of Galen may be an isolated or a multiple finding. It results from arteriovenous malformations connecting the arteries and the veins of the brain.

Incidence: Rare.

Sex ratio: M : F = 2 : 1.

Clinical history/genetics: Sporadic occurrence.

Teratogens: Unknown.

Associated malformations: Heart defect, cystic hygroma, hydrops fetalis.

Ultrasound findings: In the posterior part of the skull, an echo-free region is observed lying in the midline above the third ventricle. The arteries leading to the aneurysm can be demonstrated using the Doppler sonography. The *flow within the aneurysm* can also be detected using Doppler. This may result in widening of the intracranial ventricles. Cardiac insufficiency may follow, showing signs of *cardiomegaly* and *hepatosplenomegaly*. *Hydrops fetalis* develops in severe cases.

Differential diagnosis: Arachnoid cysts (differentiated using Doppler sonography).

Clinical management: Cardiac insufficiency is the limiting factor, and early detection of it is important. In case of severe cardiac insufficiency and hydrops, early delivery is indicated. The benefit of primary cesarean section has not been proven.

Procedure after birth: If the newborn is asymptomatic, intervention is not needed and regular follow-up is sufficient. In cases of hydrocephalus or cardiac insufficiency, endovascular or even neurosurgical interventions may be needed. These interventions are associated with high morbidity and mortality rates.

Prognosis: In the presence of cardiac insufficiency and hydrops, the prognosis is very poor; otherwise, a perioperative mortality of 20% is expected. Survivors rarely show symptoms in later life.

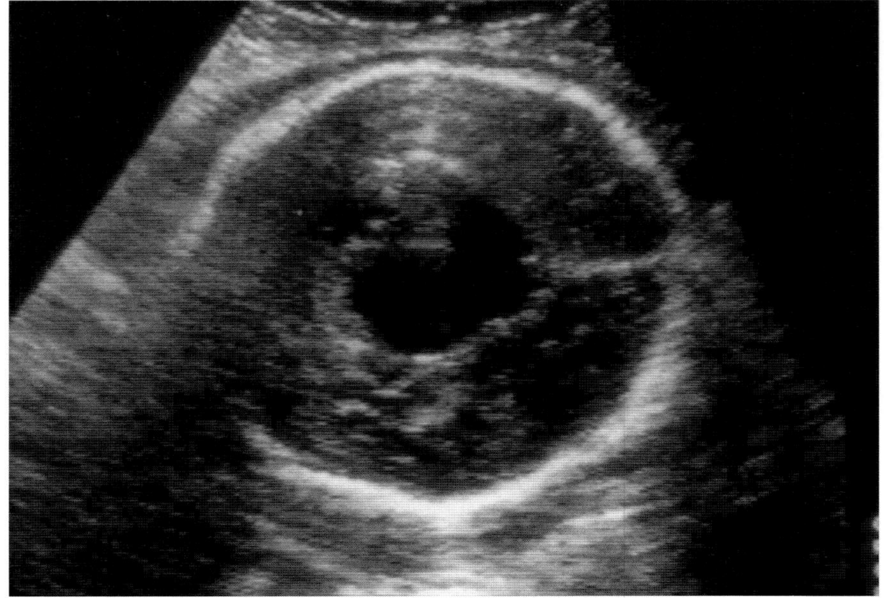

Fig. 2.**50** **Aneurysm of the vein of Galen,** showing a cystic lesion in the brain situated centrally. After spontaneous delivery, the neonate died due to decompensated heart failure.

Self-Help Organization

Title: BrainTalk MGH Neurology WebForums

Description: Provides both unmoderated message boards and chat rooms for various neurological disorders such as: aneurysms, AVMs, Bell's palsy, central pain syndrome, cauda equina syndrome, PANDAS, premenstrual dysphoric disorder, thoracic outlet syndrome, and over a hundred others, including rare neurological conditions, and workers' compensation, both under the "General Subjects" category.

Scope: Online

Web: http://www.BrainTalk.org

References

Alden TD, Ojemann JG, Lytle RA Jr, Park TS. Vein of Galen aneurysmal malformation. Pediatr Neurosurg 2001; 35: 51.

Ballester MJ, Raga F, Serra SV, Bonilla MF. Early prenatal diagnosis of an ominous aneurysm of the vein of Galen by color Doppler ultrasound. Acta Obstet Gynecol Scand 1994; 73: 592–5.

Chisholm CA, Kuller JA, Katz VL, McCoy MC. Aneurysm of the vein of Galen: prenatal diagnosis and perinatal management. Am J Perinatol 1996; 13: 503–6.

Doren M, Tercanli S, Holzgreve W. Prenatal sonographic diagnosis of a vein of Galen aneurysm: relevance of associated malformations for timing and mode of delivery. Ultrasound Obstet Gynecol 1995; 6: 287–9.

Evans AJ, Twining P. Case report: in utero diagnosis of a vein of Galen aneurysm using colour flow Doppler. Clin Radiol 1991; 44: 281–2.

Kurihara N, Tokieda K, Ikeda K, et al. Prenatal MR findings in a case of aneurysm of the vein of Galen. Pediatr Radiol 2001; 31: 160–2.

Mai R, Rempen A, Kristen P. Prenatal diagnosis and prognosis of a vein of Galen aneurysm assessed by pulsed and color Doppler sonography [letter]. Ultrasound Obstet Gynecol 1996; 7: 228–30.

Mizejewski GJ, Polansky S, Mondragon TF, Ellman AM. Combined use of alpha-fetoprotein and ultrasound in the prenatal diagnosis of arteriovenous fistula in the brain. Obstet Gynecol 1987; 70: 452–3.

Paladini D, Palmieri S, DAngelo A, Martinelli P. Prenatal ultrasound diagnosis of cerebral arteriovenous fistula. Obstet Gynecol 1996; 88: 678–81.

Pilu G, Falco P, Perolo A, et al. Differential diagnosis and outcome of fetal intracranial hypoechoic lesions: report of 21 cases. Ultrasound Obstet Gynecol 1997; 9: 229–36.

3 Face and Neck

Facial Clefts (Cleft Lip and Cleft Palate)

Definition: Clefts are defects involving the upper lip and/or the upper jaw and palate; most defects are lateral; they are located medially in less than 1%.

Incidence: One in 700–1000 for cleft lip and/or cleft palate and jaw; one in 1000 for cleft palate alone.

Sex ratio: M > F.

Clinical history/genetics: Mostly sporadic, but may occur often in families due to autosomal-dominant, recessive, and X-linked inheritance. If one sibling is affected, the recurrence rate is 4%, with two affected siblings it is 10%. If one parent and one child have this condition, then the rate of recurrence is 14%.

Teratogens: Alcohol, maternal phenylketonuria, hyperthermia, hydantoin, aminopterin, methotrexate, metronidazole, carbamazepine, cortisone, radiation, valproic acid.

Embryology: Incomplete fusion of the frontonasal process 5–6 weeks after conception. Unilateral or bilateral defects are possible.

Associated malformations: If detected prenatally, associated malformations are seen in almost 50%. Over 300 syndromes have been described in association with facial clefts. If the defect lies in the midline, neural tube defects are to be expected, especially holoprosencephaly.

Associated syndromes: Van der Woude syndrome seen in 2%, amnion band sequence, arthrogryposis, chromosomal anomalies (especially trisomy 13), holoprosencephaly, Meckel–Gruber syndrome, MURCS association, Nager syndrome, Pierre Robin sequence, Roberts syndrome, short rib–polydactyly syndrome and others.

Ultrasound findings: *Clefting of the upper lip* is seen, and this can be followed up to the palate and the jaw when these are affected. *Hydramnios* may develop due to an inadequate swallowing reflex. As the fusion of the maxillary bone is completed at 17 weeks, detection of cleft lip may

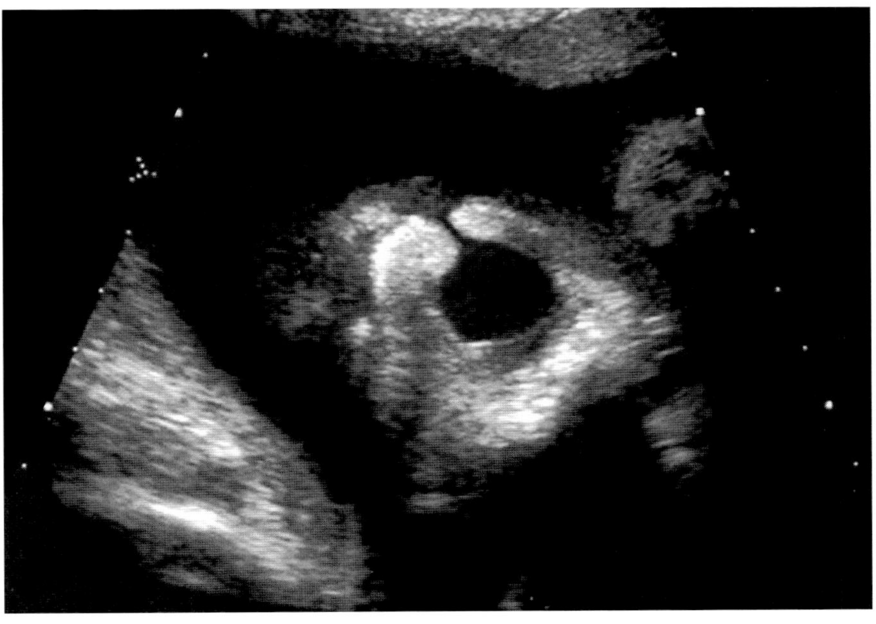

Fig. 3.1 **Cleft lip and palate.** Frontal view of the open mouth at 27 + 2 weeks. The continuity of the upper lip is interrupted: one-sided cleft lip.

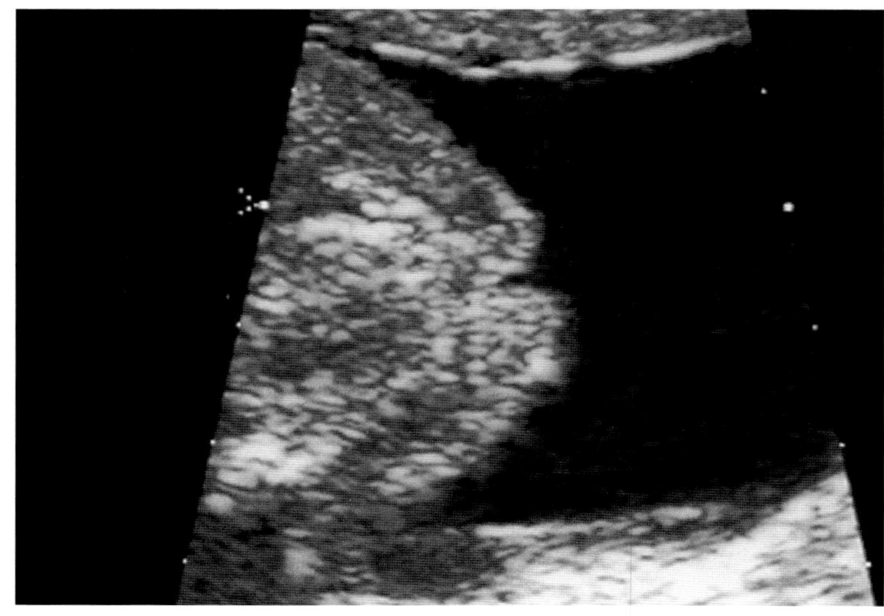

Fig. 3.2 **Cleft lip and palate.** Cross-section of the upper lip region and the upper jaw at 22 + 2 weeks. Whereas the contour of the upper lip is interrupted, the upper jaw is not affected: isolated one-sided cleft lip.

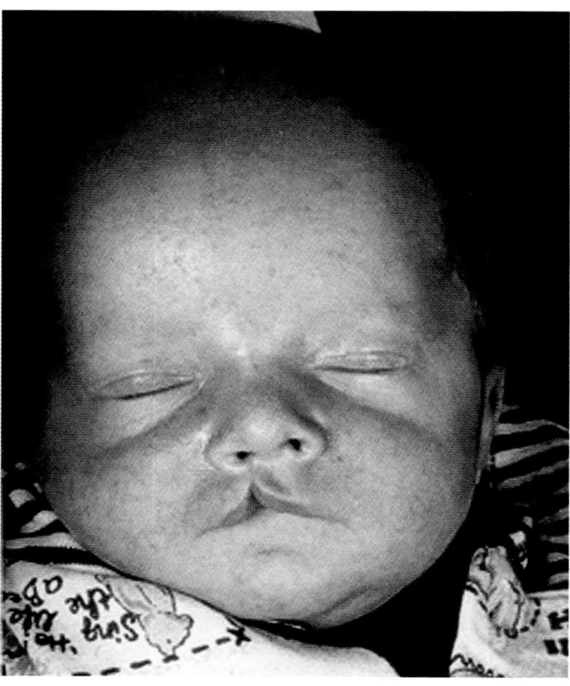

Fig. 3.3 **Cleft lip and palate.** Same case; small one-sided cleft lip post partum.

not necessarily mean involvement of the palate and the jaw. Diagnosis of cleft lip can be made as early as 12 weeks of gestation.

Clinical management: Screening for other defects and fetal echocardiography. In the presence of other anomalies, karyotyping, parental counseling by an oromaxillary surgeon. Normal antenatal checks, more frequent if hydramnios is present (premature labor). Normal delivery.

Procedure after birth: Specific measures are not indicated. Assistance may be required for feeding, depending on individual assessment. Repeated surgical interventions are necessary; correction of the cleft lip is usually carried out during the first 6 months of life.

Prognosis: If the finding is isolated, the prognosis is very good; otherwise, it depends on the accompanying anomalies. Midline defects have a poor prognosis, as they are more often associated with other brain anomalies.

Self-Help Organizations

Title: Prescription Parents, Inc.

Description: Support group for families of children with cleft lip and palate. Education for parents of newborns, presentations by professionals. Family social events, phone support network, group development guidelines.

Scope: Model

Founded: 1973

Address: P.O. Box 920554, Needham, MA 02492, United States

Telephone: 781-431-1398

Web: http://www.samizdat.com/pp1.html

Title: Cleft Palate Foundation

Description: Provides information and referrals to individuals with cleft lip and palate or other craniofacial anomalies. Referrals are made to local cleft palate/craniofacial teams

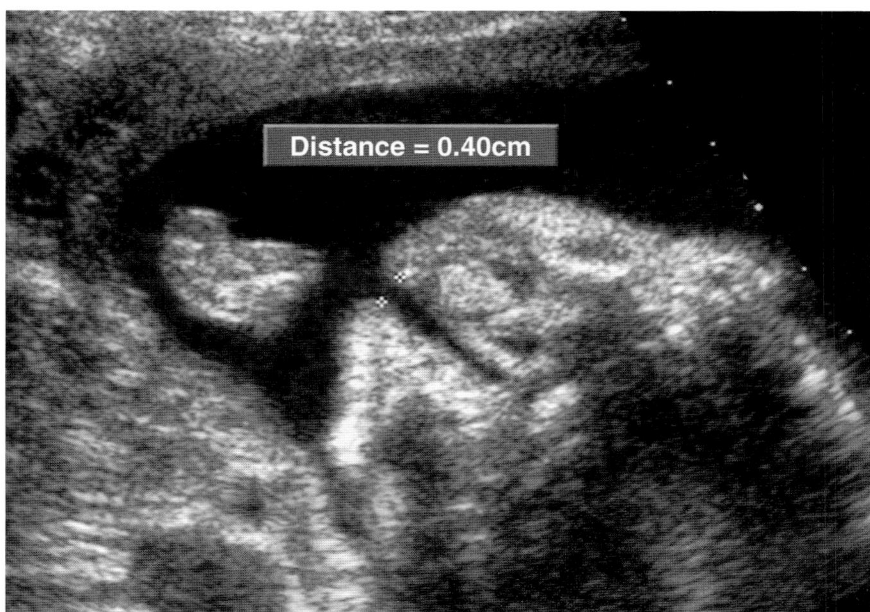

Fig. 3.4 **Cleft lip and palate.** Cross-section of the upper lip and upper jaw at 22 + 1 weeks. One-sided cleft lip and palate.

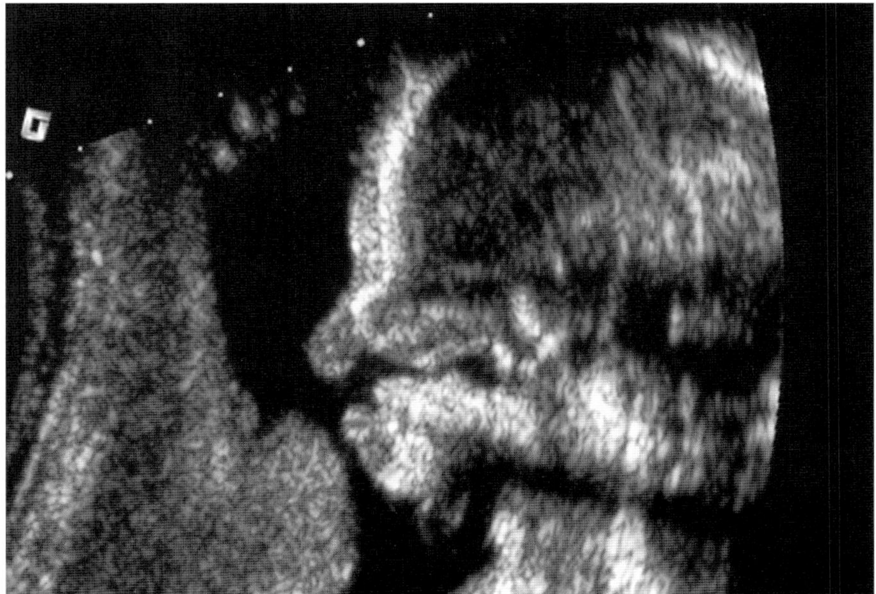

Fig. 3.5 **Cleft lip and palate.** Same case at 22 + 1 weeks; lateral longitudinal view in a case of one-sided cleft lip and palate.

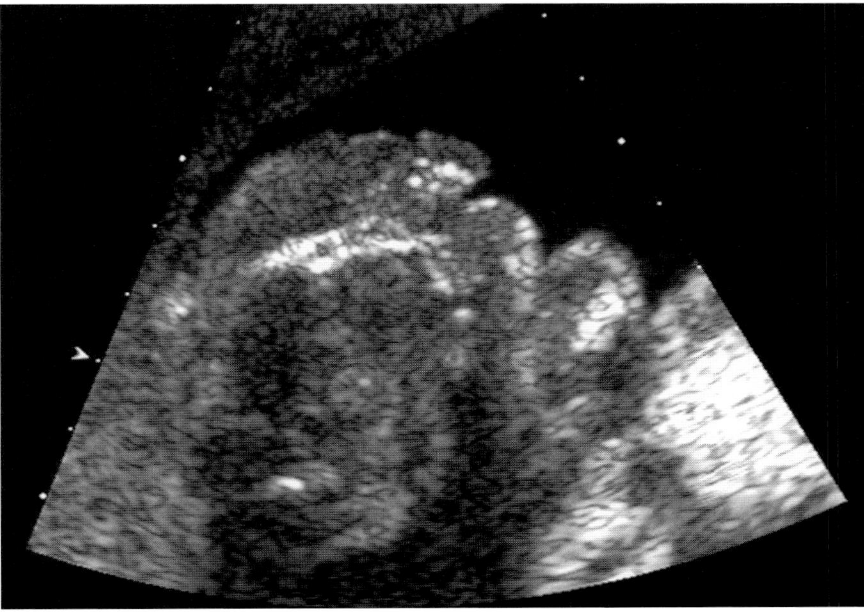

Fig. 3.6 **Cleft lip and palate.** Cross-section of a double-sided facial cleft at 21 + 3 weeks. Outcome: intrauterine fetal death at 36 weeks.

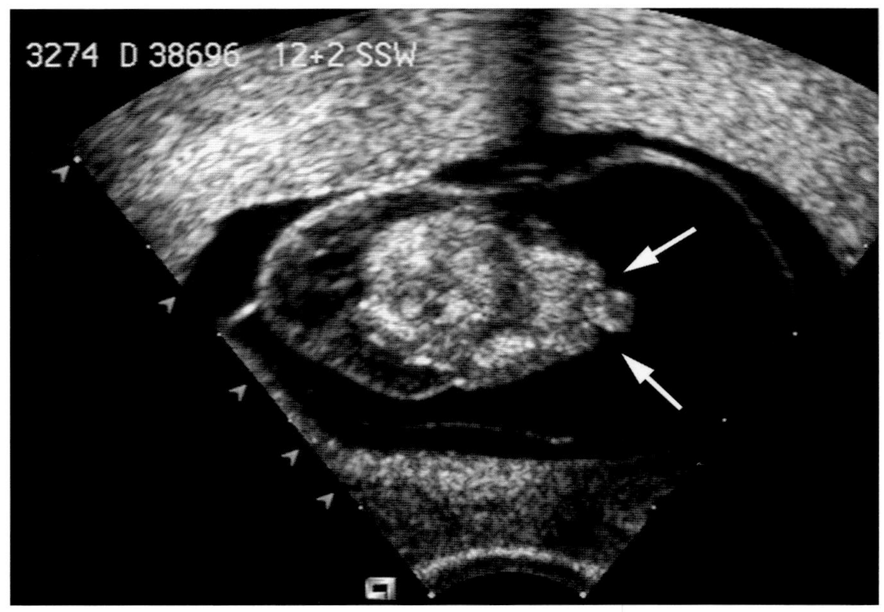

Fig. 3.**7** **Cleft lip and palate.** Cross-section of the fetal head at 12 + 2 weeks; double-sided cleft lip and cleft palate. Severe hygroma colli is seen in the neck region.

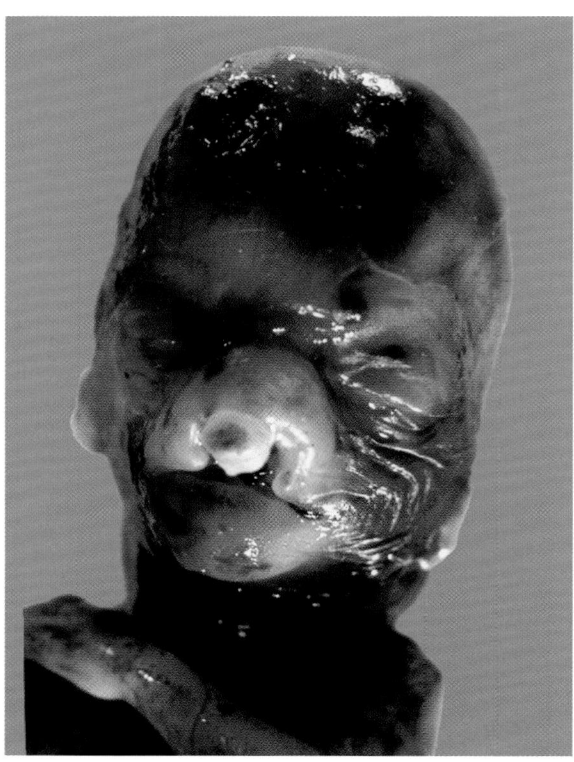

Fig. 3.**8** **Cleft lip and palate.** Finding after termination of pregnancy for trisomy 13, confirmed by chorionic villus sampling.

for treatment and to parent support groups. Free information on various aspects of clefting for parents and individuals.

Scope: National network

Founded: 1973

Address: 104 S. Estes Dr., Suite 204, Chapel Hill, NC 27514, United States

Telephone: 1-800-24-CLEFT or 919-933-9044

Fax: 919-933-9604

E-mail: cleftline@aol.com

Web: http://www.cleftline.org

Title: Forward Face

Description: Mutual support for people with craniofacial disfigurement and their families. Strongly advocates educating members and the public in the quest for understanding and acceptance. Liaison with medical personnel. Newsletter. Videotapes. Teen/young adult support group The Inner Faces.

Scope: Model

Founded: 1978

Address: 317 E. 34th St., New York, NY 10016, United States

Telephone: 1-800-393-3223 or 212-684-5

Fax: 212-684-5864

References

Aspinall CL. Dealing with the prenatal diagnosis of clefting: a parent's perspective. Cleft Palate Craniofac J 2002; 39: 183–7.

Babcook CJ, McGahan JP. Axial ultrasonographic imaging of the fetal maxilla for accurate characterization of facial clefts. J Ultrasound Med 1997; 16: 619–25.

Berge SJ, Plath H, Von Lindern JJ, et al. Natural history of 70 fetuses with a prenatally diagnosed orofacial cleft. Fetal Diagn Ther 2002; 17: 247–51.
Hafner E, Sterniste W, Scholler J, Schuchter K, Philipp K. Prenatal diagnosis of facial malformations. Prenat Diagn 1997; 17: 51–8.
Küffer E, Asseryanis E, Eppel W Schurz B, Reinold E. A case of Patau syndrome: fetal heart defect and lip–jaw–palate cleft as indicators. Ultraschall Med 1994; 15: 217–8.
Lee A, Deutinger J, Bernaschek G. Three dimensional ultrasound: abnormalities of the fetal face in surface and volume rendering mode. Br J Obstet Gynaecol 1995; 102: 302–6.
Matthews MS, Cohen M, Viglione M, Brown AS. Prenatal counseling for cleft lip and palate. Plast Reconstr Surg 1998; 101: 1–5.
Monni G, Ibba RM, Olla G, Cao A, Crisponi G. Color Doppler ultrasound and prenatal diagnosis of cleft palate. J Clin Ultrasound 1995; 23: 189–91.
Nyberg DA, Mahony BS, Kramer D. Paranasal echogenic mass: sonographic sign of bilateral complete cleft lip and palate before 20 menstrual weeks. Radiology 1992; 184: 757–9.
Raposio E, Panarese P, Sand P. Fetal unilateral cleft lip and palate: detection of enzymic anomalies in the amniotic fluid. Plast Reconstr Surg 1999; 103: 391–4.
Shipp TD, Mulliken JB, Bromley B, Benacerraf B. Three-dimensional prenatal diagnosis of frontonasal malformation and unilateral cleft lip/palate. Ultrasound Obstet Gynecol 2002; 20: 290–3.
Strauss RP, Davis JU. Prenatal detection and fetal surgery of clefts and craniofacial abnormalities in humans: social and ethical issues. Cleft Palate J 1990; 27: 176–82.
Wayne C, Cook K, Sairam S, Hollis B, Thilaganathan B. Sensitivity and accuracy of routine antenatal ultrasound screening for isolated facial clefts. Br J Radiol 2002; 75: 584–9.

Hygroma Colli (Cystic Hygroma of the Neck)

Definition: Collection of fluid in the soft tissue of the neck caused by local lymphedema. It must be differentiated from nuchal translucency, which has been given a lot of attention recently in prediction of the risk of chromosomal anomalies at 11–13 weeks. Nuchal translucency is detected in each embryo, the upper limit being 2.5 mm.

Incidence: One in 875 spontaneous abortions, about one in 1000 births.

Sex ratio: M = F.

Teratogens: Alcohol.

Embryology: Delayed development of the lymphatic drainage system in the neck. The connection between the lymphatic vessels and the venous system forms later (jugular lymphatic obstruction sequence).

Associated malformations: Chromosomal anomalies are found in 60% of cases (triploidy, Turner syndrome, trisomy 13, 18, and 21).Other malformation syndromes are: multiple pterygium syndrome, Pena–Shokeir syndrome, Roberts syndrome, Cornelia de Lange syndrome, Noonan syndrome, Smith–Lemli–Opitz syndrome, Fryns syndrome, Joubert syndrome, achondrogenesis, EEC syndrome, Apert syndrome, Pallister–Killian syndrome.

Ultrasound findings: Huge *cystic lesions* are seen bilaterally in the neck region. *Hydrops fetalis* may accompany. The cysts may be simple or may contain septa. Spontaneous remission of the lesion has been described. *Oligohydramnios* is frequent.

Clinical management: Further screening for other anomalies, karyotyping, fetal echocardiography. Spontaneous remission has been reported in course of the pregnancy. Severe forms detected in the third trimester show poor prognosis. Spontaneous remission does not necessarily exclude an abnormal karyotype. Most frequent outcome is intrauterine death (at least in 75%). Decompression or drainage of severe findings is indicated only to ease vaginal delivery. Regular screening for hydrops fetalis. Normal delivery should be attempted.

Procedure after birth: This depends on the clinical condition after birth. Respiratory obstruction caused by pharyngeal edema may cause breathing problems.

Prognosis: Severe forms lead to intrauterine death. Complete or partial remission in uterus is possible (pterygium colli post partum).

Self-Help Organization

Title: CALM (Children Anguished with Lymphatic Malformations)

Description: Networking of families of children with cystic hygroma and lymphangioma. Sharing of experiences and coping skills. Research into alternative treatment op-

2

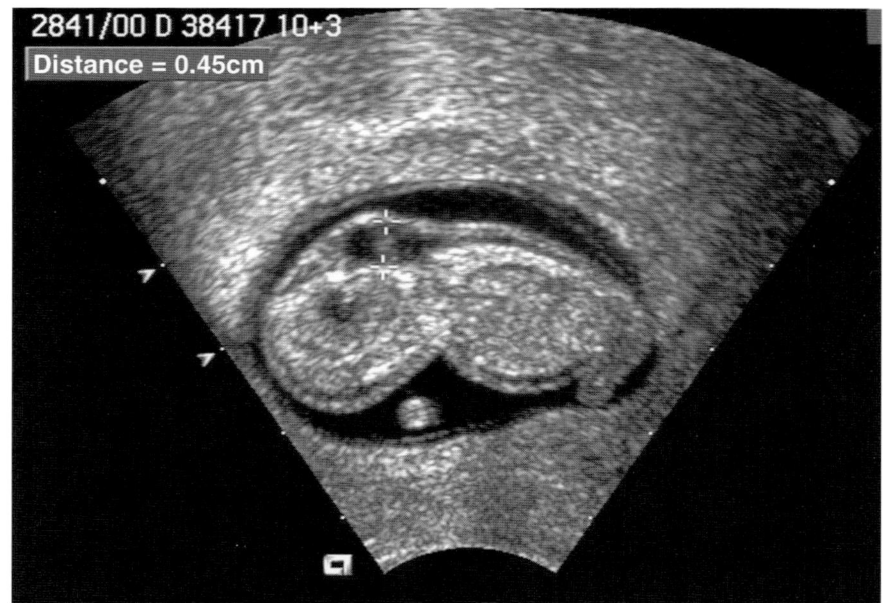

Fig. 3.9 **Hygroma colli.** A lesion measuring 4.5 mm at 10 + 3 weeks in a fetus with Turner syndrome. Early development of nonimmunological hydrops, subcutaneous edema of the whole fetus.

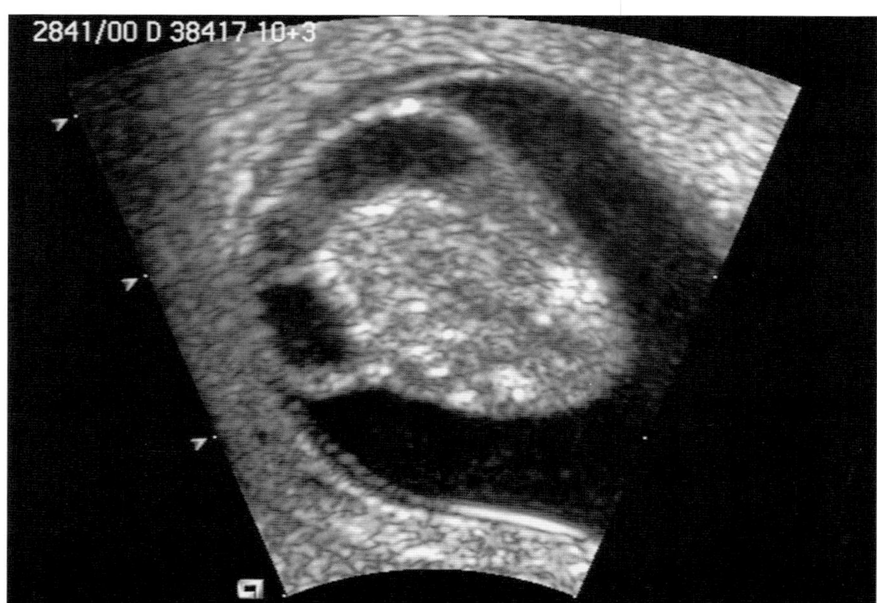

Fig. 3.10 **Hygroma colli.** Same case. Cross-section of the neck region, showing a septum. Termination of pregnancy followed.

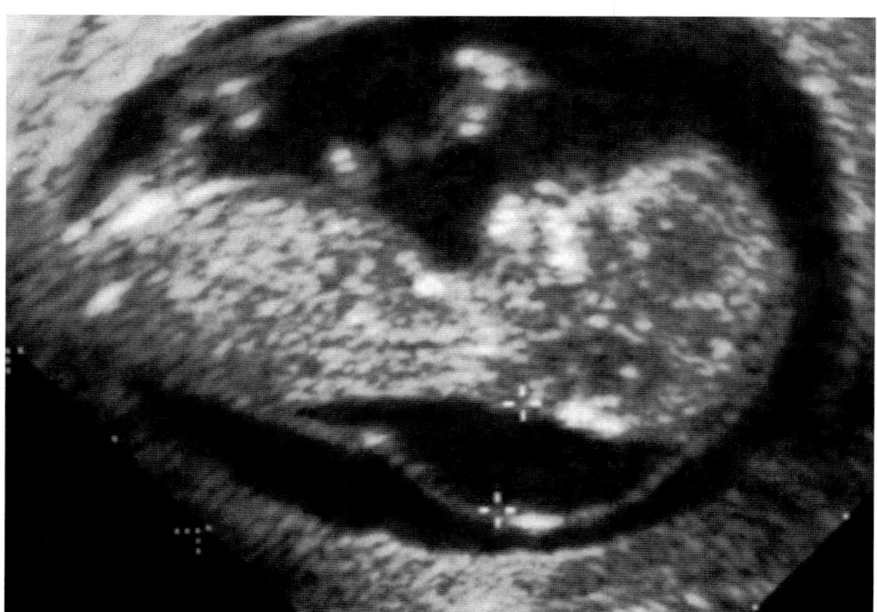

Fig. 3.11 **Hygroma colli.** A very large echo-free hygroma measuring 11 mm (CRL 55 mm, 11 + 3 weeks) by normal karyotype. A fetal cardiac anomaly (AV channel) was suspected.

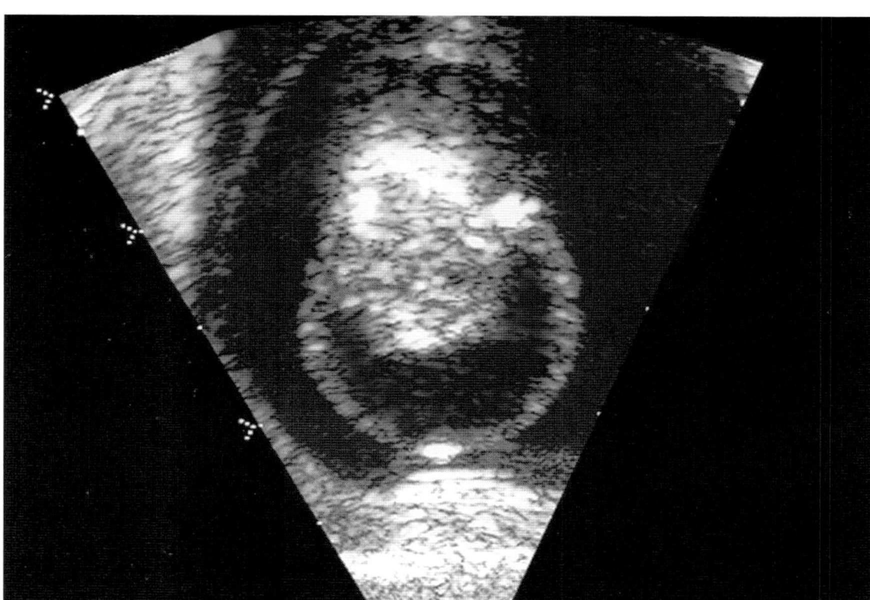

Fig. 3.**12** **Hygroma colli.** Same case as before. Cross-section of the fetal neck.

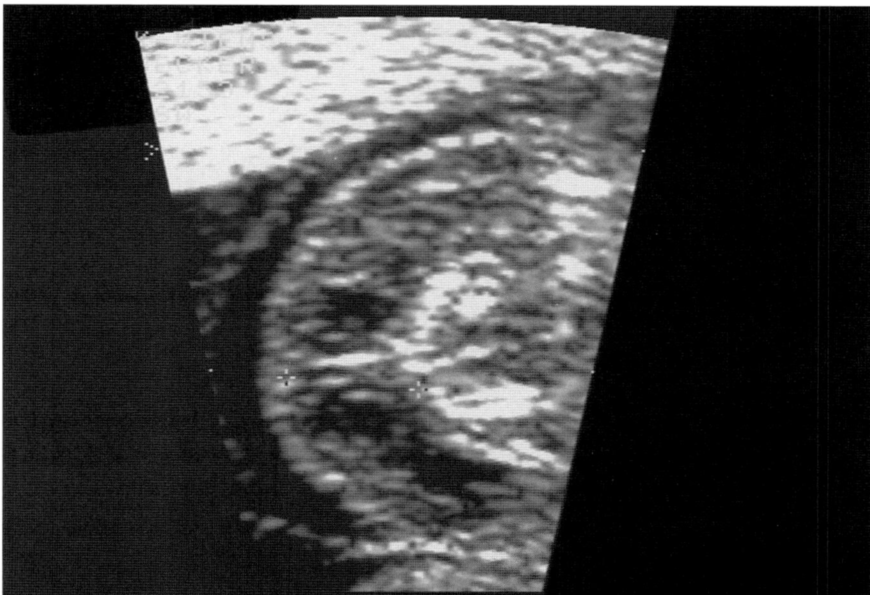

Fig. 3.**13** **Hygroma colli.** This finding measures 5.6 mm in a fetus with Down syndrome.

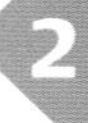

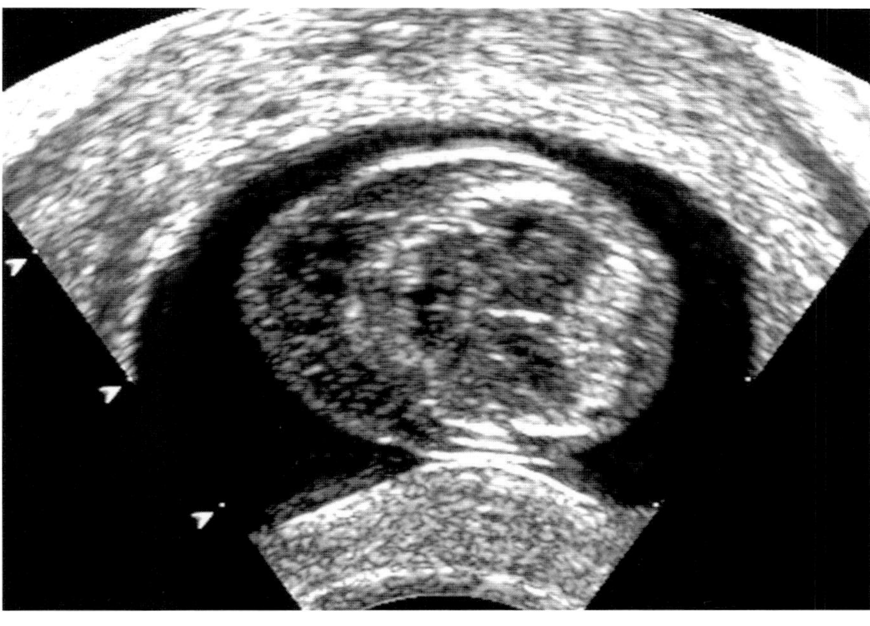

Fig. 3.**14** **Hygroma colli.** A finding of 4.7 mm in the 11 + 1 weeks in a fetus with nonbalanced Robertson translocation trisomy 21.

tions, literature, phone support, pen pals, information and referrals, newsletter, family reunion, symposiums for medical community.

Scope: National network

Founded: 1993

Address: 1141 Prestige, Frisco, TX 75034, United States

Telephone: 972-377-4326 (voice/fax)

Fax: 972-377-4326

E-mail: stayCALM93@aol.com or j1m1@airmail.net

Web: http://web2.airmail.net/j1m1/

References

Boyd PA, Anthony MY, Manning N, Rodriguez CL, Wellesley DG, Chamberlain P. Antenatal diagnosis of cystic hygroma or nuchal pad: report of 92 cases with follow up of survivors. Arch Dis Child Fetal Neonatal Ed 1996; 74: F38–F42.

Droste S, Hendricks SK, Von Alfrey H, Mack LA. Cystic hygroma colli: perinatal outcome after prenatal diagnosis. J Perinat Med 1991; 19: 449–54.

Fisher R, Partington A, Dykes E. Cystic hygroma: comparison between prenatal and postnatal diagnosis. J Pediatr Surg 1996; 31: 473–6.

Gilbert B, Yardin C, Briault S, et al. Prenatal diagnosis of female monozygotic twins discordant for Turner syndrome: implications for prenatal genetic counselling. Prenat Diagn 2002; 22: 697–702.

Hösli IM, Tercanli S, Rehder H, Holzgreve W. Cystic hygroma as an early first-trimester ultrasound marker for recurrent Fryns syndrome. Ultrasound Obstet Gynecol 1997; 10: 422–4.

Nadel A, Bromley B, Benacerraf BR. Nuchal thickening or cystic hygromas in first- and early second-trimester fetuses: prognosis and outcome. Obstet Gynecol 1993; 82: 43–8.

Ozeren S, Yüksel A, Tükel T. Prenatal sonographic diagnosis of type I achondrogenesis with a large cystic hygroma [letter]. Ultrasound Obstet Gynecol 1999; 13: 75–6.

Rosati P, Guariglia L. Transvaginal ultrasound detection of septated and non-septated cystic hygroma in early pregnancy. Fetal Diagn Ther 1997; 12: 132–5.

Sepúlveda WH, Ciuffardi I. Early sonographic diagnosis of fetal cystic hygroma colli. J Perinat Med 1992; 20: 149–52.

Tanriverdi HA, Hendrik HJ, Ertan AK, Axt R, Schmidt W. Hygroma colli cysticum: prenatal diagnosis and prognosis. Am J Perinatol 2001; 18: 415–20.

Goiter (Fetal)

Definition: Enlargement of the thyroid.

Incidence: Rare.

Clinical history/genetics: Sporadic. Pendred syndrome consists of goiter and neurosensory deafness (autosomal-recessive).

Teratogens: Propylthiouracil, iodine, lithium.

Embryology: Hypothyroidism is the main cause of development of goiter. This may be due to iodine deficiency, iodine toxication, medication given to the mother for thyroid disease and disturbance in production of thyroid hormones. Hyperthyroidism results from antibodies responsible for the stimulation of maternal thyroid, acting on fetal thyroid. Fetal goiter develops in one in 70 cases of mothers suffering from Basedow disease.

Ultrasound findings: *Enlargement of fetal thyroid* can be seen in sagittal and horizontal axis. The neck may be over extended if large lesion is present. Fetal growth restriction is a frequent feature. Earliest prenatal diagnosis has been reported at 25 weeks of gestation. Development of hydramnios leads to premature labor. In addition to cardiac insufficiency, AV block or tachycardia may follow.

Clinical management: Amniotic fluid alpha fetoprotein and thyroid-stimulating hormone (TSH) determination. Successful treatment of hyperthyroidism after intra-amniotic injection of thyroid hormones has been reported. Regular sonographic controls of hydramnios and cardiac failure are advised. Monstrous enlargement may cause obstruction of labor. In addition, overextension of the head may be a hindrance for vaginal delivery.

Procedure after birth: Huge thyroid masses can cause respiratory distress. Emergency tracheostomy may be required. Other therapeutic possibilities depend on accompanying symptoms.

Prognosis: Depends on the cause for the goiter.

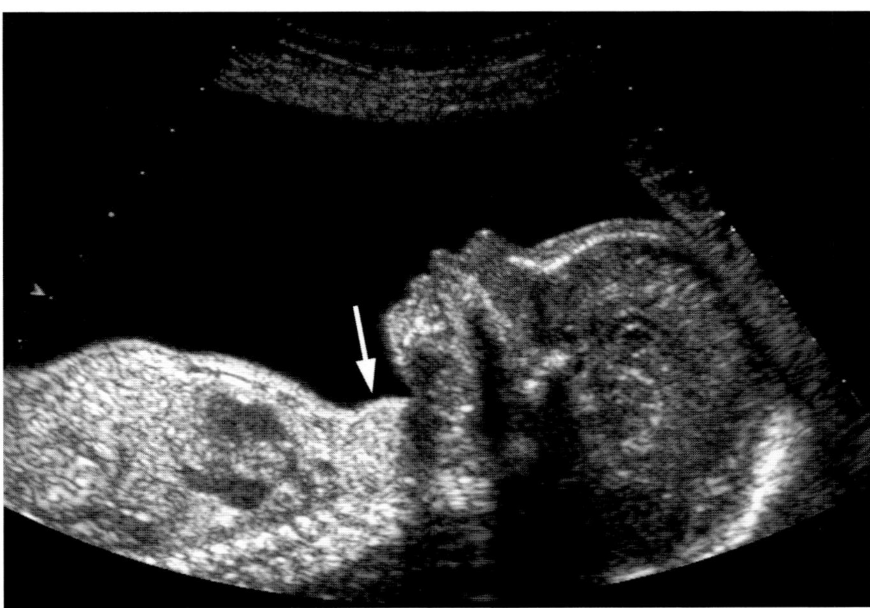

Fig. 3.**15** **Fetal goiter.** Fetal profile at 21 + 5 weeks, thickening of the neck due to fetal goiter.

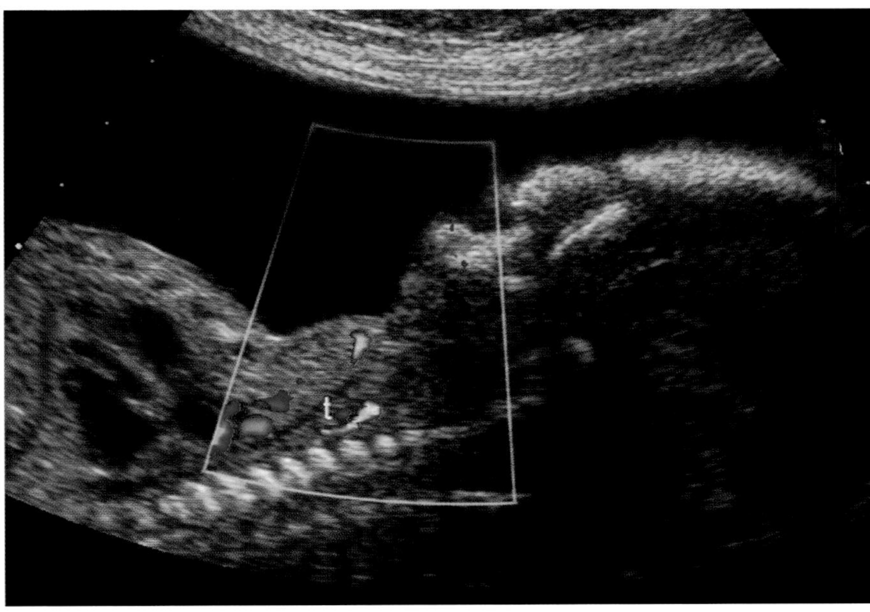

Fig. 3.**16** **Fetal goiter.** Same case. Color Doppler sonography, demonstrating the goiter and the supplying vessels.

Self-Help Organization

Title: American Foundation of Thyroid Patients

Description: Mutual support and education for thyroid disease patients. "Sharing Network" matches patients together for support and exchange of information. Newsletter, physician referrals, speakers bureau. Online patient chat room. Offers low-cost thyroid screening. Assistance in starting chapters.

Scope: National

Number of groups: Six affiliated groups

Founded: 1993

Address: 18534 N. Lyford, Katy, TX 77 449, United States

Telephone: 1–888–996–4460; 281–855–6608 (in Houston)

E-mail: thyroid@flash.net

Web: http://www.thyroidfoundation.org

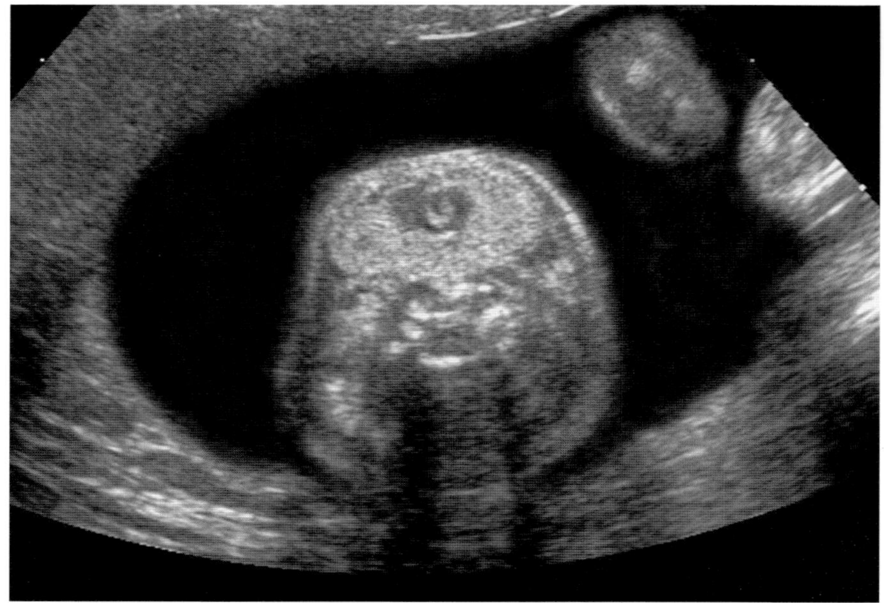

Fig. 3.**17** **Fetal goiter.** Cross-section of the fetal neck showing an echogenic lesion corresponding sonomorphologically to a fetal goiter. The fetal larynx is seen in the middle of it.

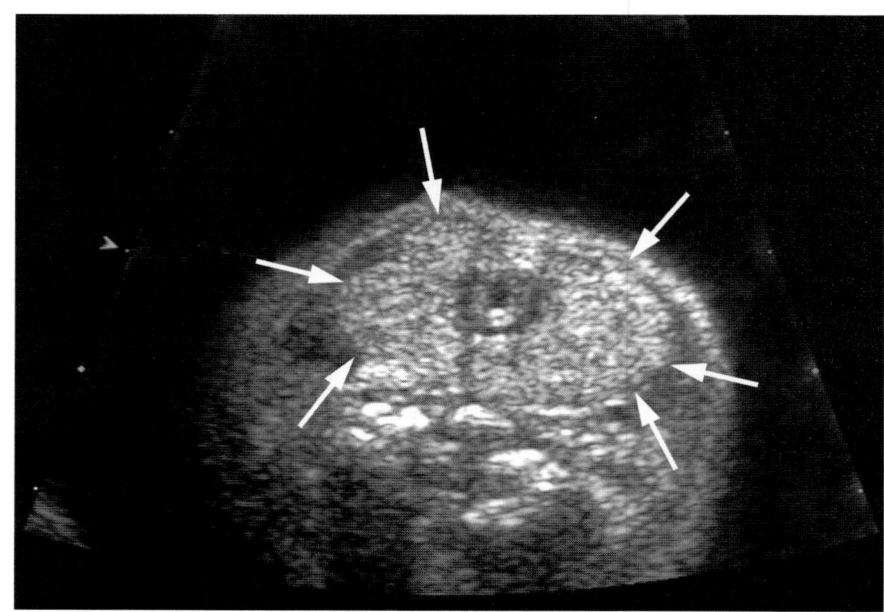

Fig. 3.**18** **Fetal goiter.** The same case, with magnification.

References

Abuhamad AZ, Fisher DA, Warsof SL, et al. Antenatal diagnosis and treatment of fetal goitrous hypothyroidism: case report and review of the literature. Ultrasound Obstet Gynecol 1995; 6: 368–71.

Agrawal P, Ogilvy-Stuart A, Lees C. Intrauterine diagnosis and management of congenital goitrous hypothyroidism. Ultrasound Obstet Gynecol 2002; 19: 501–5.

Bruner JP, Dellinger EH. Antenatal diagnosis and treatment of fetal hypothyroidism: a report of two cases. Fetal Diagn Ther 1997; 12: 200–4.

Hadi HA, Strickland D. Prenatal diagnosis and management of fetal goiter caused by maternal Graves disease. Am J Perinatol 1995; 12: 240–2.

Heckel S, Favre R, Schlienger JL, Soskin P. Diagnosis and successful in utero treatment of a fetal goitrous hyperthyroidism caused by maternal Graves' disease: a case report. Fetal Diagn Ther 1997; 12: 54–8.

Jackson IM. Inherited hypothyroidism. Clin Perinatol 1976; 3: 221–30.

Karabulut N, Martin DR, Yang M, Boyd BK. MR Imaging findings in fetal goiter caused by maternal Graves disease. J Comput Assist Tomogr 2002; 26: 538–40.

Morine M, Takeda T, Minekawa R, et al. Antenatal diagnosis and treatment of a case of fetal goitrous hypothyroidism associated with high-output cardiac failure. Ultrasound Obstet Gynecol 2002; 19: 506–9.

Noia G, De Santis M, Tocci A, et al. Early prenatal diagnosis and therapy of fetal hypothyroid goiter. Fetal Diagn Ther 1992; 7: 138–43.

Pradeep VM, Ramachandran K, Sasidharan K, Sulekha C. Fetal goiter: a case detected by ultrasonography. J Clin Ultrasound 1991; 19: 571–4.

Soliman S, McGrath F, Brennan B, Glazebrook K. Color Doppler imaging of the thyroid gland in a fetus with congenital goiter: a case report. Am J Perinatol 1994; 11: 21–3.

Vicens CE, Potau N, Carreras E, Bellart J, Albisu MA, Carrascosa A. Diagnosis and treatment in utero of goiter with hypothyroidism caused by iodide overload. J Pediatr 1998; 133: 147–8.

4 Thorax

Congenital Cystic Adenomatoid Malformation (CCAM) of the Lung

Definition: Congenital cystic adenomatoid malformation of the lung corresponds to a hamartoma with hyperplasia and dysplasia of the terminal bronchioli. Three forms are described (after Stocker): *macrocystic form* (type I), a *mixed form* (type II) and a *microcystic form* (type III).

Incidence: Rare.

Sex ratio: M : F = 1 : 1.

Clinical history/genetics: Sporadic occurrence.

Teratogens: Unknown.

Embryology: This malformation occurs in the first 6 weeks after conception due to dysplasia of the bronchioli (after conception).

Associated malformations: These are found in 26% of cases, and consist of chest malformation (pectus excavatum), renal agenesis and fetal hydrops.

Ultrasound findings: *Stocker type I:* Cysts measuring 2–10 cm in diameter; sometimes only one cyst is found. *Stocker type II*: Cysts smaller than 2 cm in diameter with echogenic tissue lying in between. *Stocker type III:* the echogenicity of the affected tissue is much stronger. In each case, displacement of the heart and the diaphragm is possible. Concomitant hydrops is found more often in type III. Up to sixty-five percent of cases develop hydramnios. Spontaneous regression of the lung anomaly has been known, such that the lesions may disappear completely. In addition, the echogenicity of the affected tissue may change during the course of pregnancy.

Differential diagnosis: Diaphragmatic hernia, bronchogenic or neuroenteric cysts.

Clinical management: Further ultrasound screening and regular monitoring, fetal echocardiography, if hydrops develops invasive treatment is necessary (cannulation of the cyst, drainage), or by reaching fetal maturity labor induction. Intrauterine surgery is still in experimental stages. Criteria for operative intervention (hydrops, size of the lesion, displacement of the heart) remain uncertain. Prophylactic treatment is disputed, as spontaneous resolution is possible.

Procedure after birth: In severe cases, respiratory distress immediately after birth is common. Mechanical ventilation may even worsen the condition due to expansion of the lesion (over ventilation of nonfunctioning areas). Selective intubation of the healthy lung is a possibility. The newborn is placed on the side of the lesion to prevent overexpansion of the affected lung. The severity of the condition can be assessed postnatally using the magnetic resonance imaging (planning for surgery). The affected part of the lung is resected. Perioperatively, extracorporeal membrane oxygenation (ECMO) can be lifesaving.

Prognosis: The *macrocystic form* rarely causes fetal hydrops and has an overall survival rate of more than 70%. The *microcystic form,* associated with hydrops, has a poorer prognosis. If symptoms such as dyspnea and tachypnea appear in the newborn, then the mortality is up to 78%. In older studies, fifty percent of patients have clinical symptoms later in life, and have a good survival rate. In severe cases, resection of a complete lobe may be necessary, causing deformation of the thoracic cage. This can be corrected with placement of expanders.

However, if part of the lung can be preserved, it expands, filling the hemithorax and resulting in improved functional capacity.

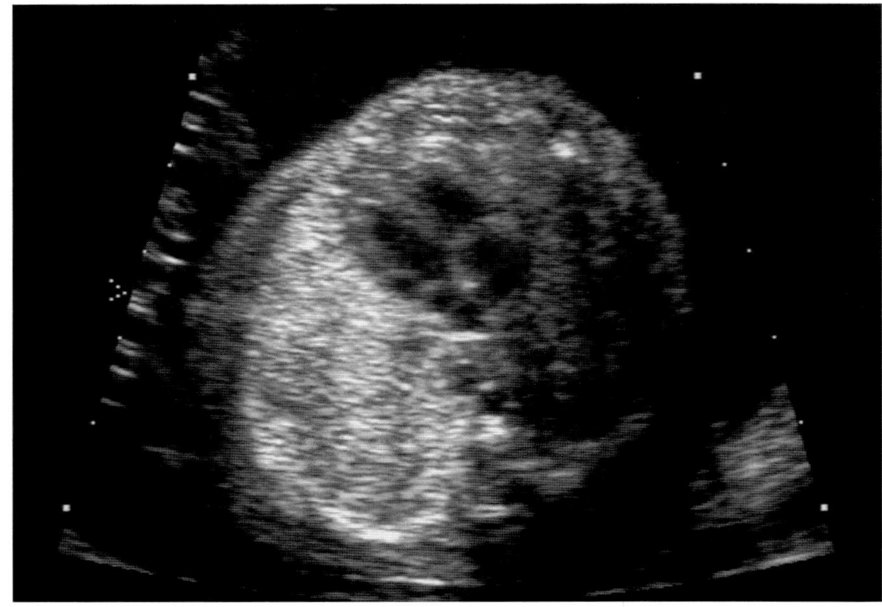

Fig. 4.**1** **Congenital cystic adenomatoid malformation of the lung.** Cross-section of a fetal thorax at 21 + 6 weeks. The left lung appears to be full of small cysts. Displacement of the heart to the right. The right lung is not affected.

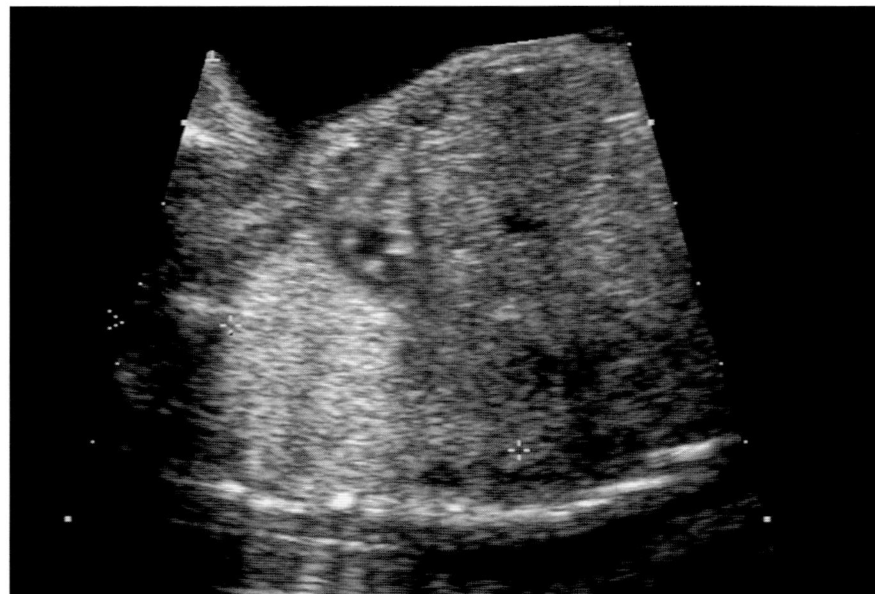

Fig. 4.**2** **Congenital cystic adenomatoid malformation of the lung.** Same patient as in the previous image, in a longitudinal section showing the liver and echogenic lung tissue.

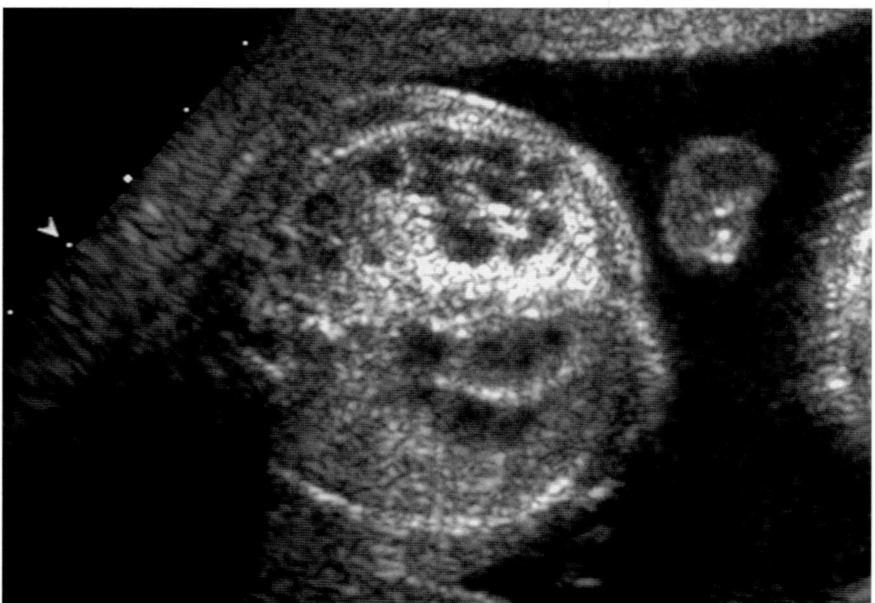

Fig. 4.**3** **Congenital cystic adenomatoid malformation of the lung.** Left-sided anomaly at 21 + 2 weeks consisting of large cystic lesions, displacing the heart to the right.

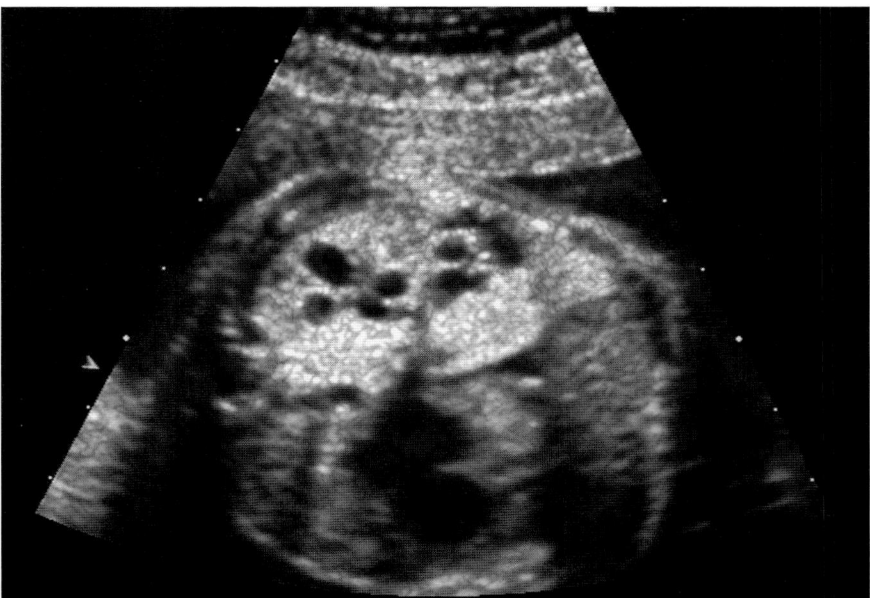

Fig. 4.**4** **Congenital cystic adenomatoid malformation of the lung.** Same case as in the previous image, at 23 + 5 weeks.

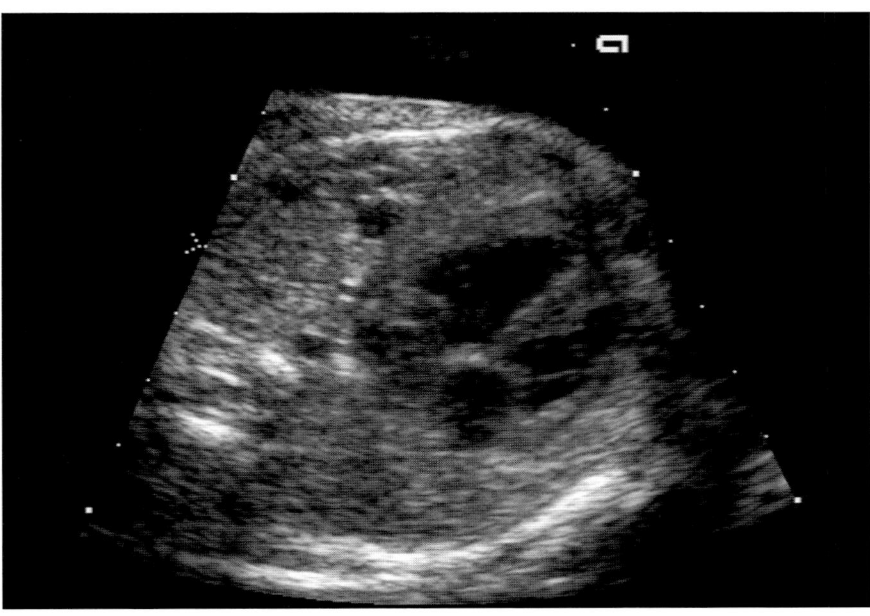

Fig. 4.**5** **Congenital cystic adenomatoid malformation of the lung.** The same patient seen at 28 + 3 weeks. The findings are now less severe, with partial resolution of the echogenicity of the affected lung and displacement of the heart.

References

Adzick NS, Harrison MR, Glick PL, et al. Fetal cystic adenomatoid malformation: prenatal diagnosis and natural history. J Pediatr Surg 1985; 20: 483–8.

Barret J, Chitayat D, Sermer M, et al. The prognostic factors in the prenatal diagnosis of the echogenic fetal lung. Prenat Diagn 1995; 15: 849–53.

Bouchard S, Johnson MP, Flake AW, et al. The EXIT procedure: experience and outcome in 31 cases. J Pediatr Surg 2002; 37: 418–26.

Entezami M, Halis G, Waldschmidt J, Opri F, Runkel S. Congenital cystic adenomatoid malformation of the lung and fetal hydrops: a case with favourable outcome. Eur J Obstet Gynecol Reprod Biol 1998; 79: 99–101.

Keidar S, Ben-Sira L, Weinberg M, Jaffa AJ, Silbiger A, Vinograd I. The postnatal management of congenital cystic adenomatoid malformation. Isr Med Assoc J 2001; 3: 258–61.

Laberge JM, Flageole H, Pugash D, et al. Outcome of the prenatally diagnosed congenital cystic adenomatoid lung malformation: a Canadian experience. Fetal Diagn Ther 2001; 16: 178–86.

Morris E, Constantine G, McHugo J. Cystic adenomatoid malformation of the lung: an obstetric and ultrasound perspective. Eur J Obstet Gynecol Reprod Biol 1991; 40: 11–5.

Pinson CW, Harrison MW, Thornburg KL, Campbell JR. Importance of fetal fluid imbalance in congenital cystic adenomatoid malformation of the lung. Am J Surg 1992; 163: 510–4.

Winters WD, Effmann EL, Nghiem HV, Nyberg DA. Congenital masses of the lung: changes in cross-sectional area during gestation. J Clin Ultrasound 1997; 25: 372–7.

Zangwill BC, Stocker JT. Congenital cystic adenomatoid malformation within an extralobar pulmonary sequestration. Pediatr Pathol 1993; 13: 309–15.

Esophageal Atresia

Definition: Esophageal atresia is a congenital disorder caused by closure of the esophagus with a blind end. In 90% of cases, there is an associated tracheo-esophageal fistula at the distal end.

Incidence: One in 800–5000 births.

Clinical history/genetics: sporadic occurrence.

Teratogens: Retinoic acid, alcohol.

Embryology: The anomaly arises due to defective division of the anterior intestines into trachea and esophagus during the 6th–7th week after menstruation (21–34 days after conception). In over 90% of cases, a tracheo-esophageal fistula is present, so that hydramnios—an important diagnostic clue—may be absent, as the amniotic fluid is diverted over the fistula into the stomach.

Associated malformations: Other anomalies are evident in 50%, cardiac anomalies in 20%—especially ventricular septal defects (VSDs) or atrial septal defects (ASDs), other gastrointestinal defects in 10%, anal atresia in a further 10%, and VACTERL association in about 6%. Twenty-five syndromes have been described in association with esophageal atresia, with Down syndrome in 2–3%.

Ultrasound findings: Esophageal atresia should be suspected when, in the presence of *hydramnios* (rare before 25 weeks), repeated screening examinations *fail to demonstrate the fetal stomach*. Due to the presence of tracheo-esophageal fistula in most cases, the stomach may be filled, but its small size is suspicious. In some cases, *the blind end* of the esophagus *filled with fluid* is detectable. Severe *hydramnios* may be present. In chromosomal anomaly or VACTERL association, fetal growth retardation may be evident. Failure to demonstrate the stomach in repeated examinations and concomitant hydramnios are suspicious signs for esophageal atresia.

Clinical management: Sonographic screening, fetal echocardiography. Karyotyping. High risk for premature labor due to hydramnios. If symptoms appear in the mother due to hydramnios (dyspnea, premature contractions), therapeutic drainage of the amniotic fluid is indicated. Vaginal delivery is allowed. Delivery should take place in a center with neonatal intensive care and pediatric surgical units.

Procedure after birth: In case of respiratory distress, primary intubation is preferred to ventilation using a mask. This prevents overextension of the stomach. To prevent aspiration, oral feeding is avoided and repeated emptying of the blind end through suction is advised.

Prognosis: The prognosis depends on the accompanying anomalies. In isolated esophageal atresia the overall survival is excellent with 95%, and a good functional outcome is expected. Cardiac anomalies and premature birth reduce the survival down to 50–70%.

Self-Help Organization

Title: EA/TEF Child and Family Support Connection, Inc.

Description: Dedicated to providing educational resources and emotional and practical support for families of children with esophageal atresia and tracheo-esophageal fistula. Offers a newsletter, a family directory for telephone networking, information, lending library, educational brochures, and literature. A "sunshine program" sends birthday greetings and gifts to hospitalized children.

Scope: International

Number of groups: More than 11 chapters

Address: 111 West Jackson Blvd., Suite 1145, Chicago, IL 60604–3502, United States

Telephone: 312–987–9085

Fax: 312–987–9086

E-mail: eatef2@aol.com

Web: http://eatef.org

1

2

3

4

5

References

Chitty LS, Goodman J, Seller MJ, Maxwell D. Esophageal and duodenal atresia in a fetus with Down's syndrome: prenatal sonographic features. Ultrasound Obstet Gynecol 1996; 7: 450–2.

D'Elia A, Pighetti M, Nappi C. Prenatal ultrasonographic appearance of esophageal atresia. Eur J Obstet Gynecol Reprod Biol 2002; 105: 77.

Eyheremendy E, Pfister M. Antenatal real-time diagnosis of esophageal atresias. JCU J Clin Ultrasound 1983; 11: 395–7.

Farrant P. The antenatal diagnosis of oesophageal atresia by ultrasound. Br J Radiol 1980; 53: 1202–3.

Kalache KD, Chaoui R, Mau H, Bollmann R. The upper neck pouch sign: a prenatal sonographic marker for esophageal atresia. Ultrasound Obstet Gynecol 1998; 11: 138–40.

Langer JC, Hussain H, Khan A, et al. Prenatal diagnosis of esophageal atresia using sonography and magnetic resonance imaging. J Pediatr Surg 2001; 36: 804–7.

Pretorius DH, Drose JA, Dennis MA, Manchester DK, Manco JM. Tracheoesophageal fistula in utero: twenty-two cases. J Ultrasound Med 1987; 6: 509–13.

Pretorius DH, Meier PR, Johnson ML. Diagnosis of esophageal atresia in utero. J Ultrasound Med 1983; 2: 475–6.

Rahmani MR, Zalev AH. Antenatal detection of esophageal atresia with distal tracheoesophageal fistula. JCU J Clin Ultrasound 1986; 14: 143–5.

Sase M, Asada H, Okuda M, Kato H. Fetal gastric size in normal and abnormal pregnancies. Ultrasound Obstet Gynecol 2002; 19: 467–70.

Stoll C, Alembik Y, Dott B, Roth MP. Evaluation of prenatal diagnosis of congenital gastro-intestinal atresias. Eur J Epidemiol 1996; 12: 611–6.

Tsukerman GL, Krapiva GA, Kirillova IA. First-trimester diagnosis of duodenal stenosis associated with oesophageal atresia. Prenat Diagn 1993; 13: 371–6.

Vijayaraghavan SB. Antenatal diagnosis of esophageal atresia with tracheoesophageal fistula. J Ultrasound Med 1996; 15: 417–9.

Zemlyn S. Prenatal detection of esophageal atresia. JCU J Clin Ultrasound 1981; 9: 453–4.

Primary Fetal Hydrothorax

Definition: Collection of fluid (mostly chyle) within the pleural cavity; the right side of the thorax is affected more frequently than the left.

Incidence: One in 10 000 births.

Sex ratio: M : F = 2 : 1.

Teratogens: Unknown.

Embryology: An overproduction or malresorption of lymph fluid may be the cause.

Associated malformations: In addition to sporadic appearance, in which the hydrothorax is caused by anomalies of the lymphatic vessels, combined forms have been described in over 50 different syndromes, especially Turner and Down syndrome. It may also appear in cases of fetal hydrops.

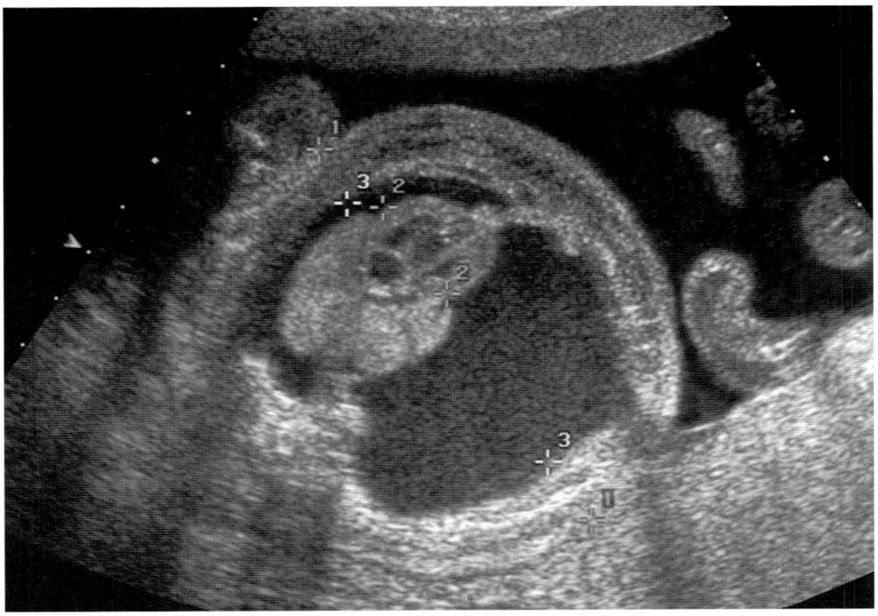

Fig. 4.6 **Primary fetal hydrothorax.** Findings affecting both sides at 24 + 5 weeks. The left-sided thorax is more compromised and the mediastinum and the heart are displaced to the right.

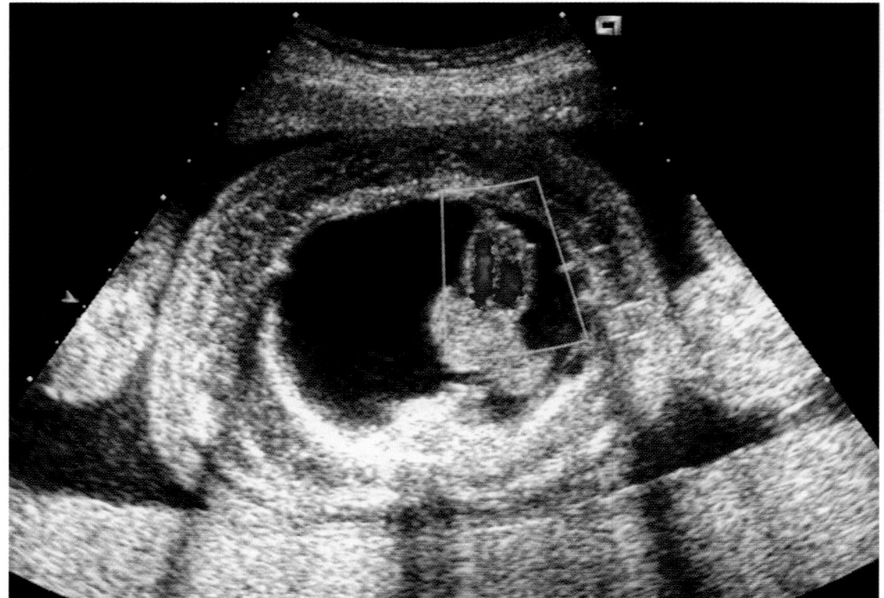

Fig. 4.7 **Primary fetal hydrothorax.** Same patient as in the previous image, at 27 + 1 weeks. Cross-section of the fetal thorax. Color Doppler sonography, demonstrating diastolic blood flow into the ventricles. Development of severe anasarca (hydrops).

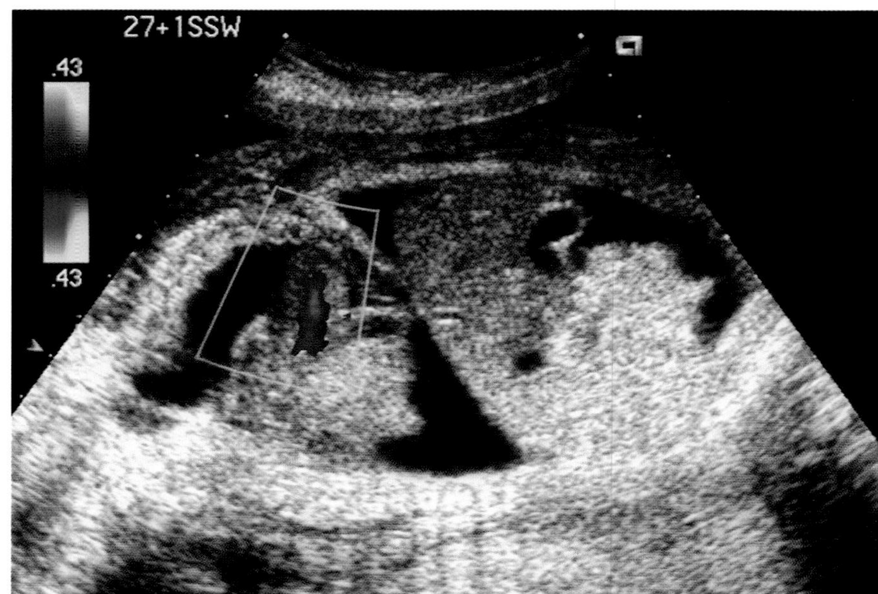

Fig. 4.8 **Primary fetal hydrothorax.** Same case. Longitudinal section: hydrothorax, anasarca, ascites.

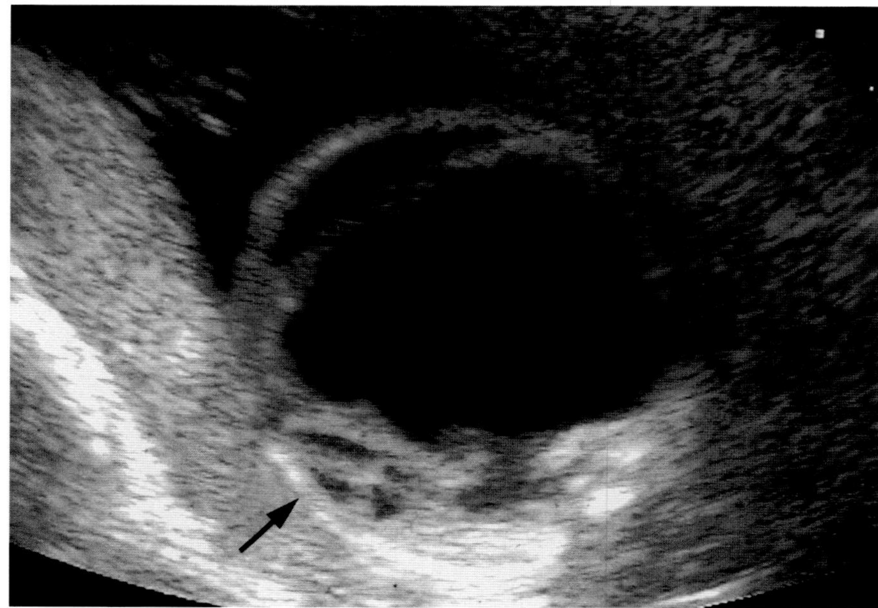

Fig. 4.9 **Primary left-sided fetal hydrothorax.** Severe displacement of the heart to the right at 21 weeks (black arrow) and subsequent hydrops; crescent-shaped appearance of the ascites.

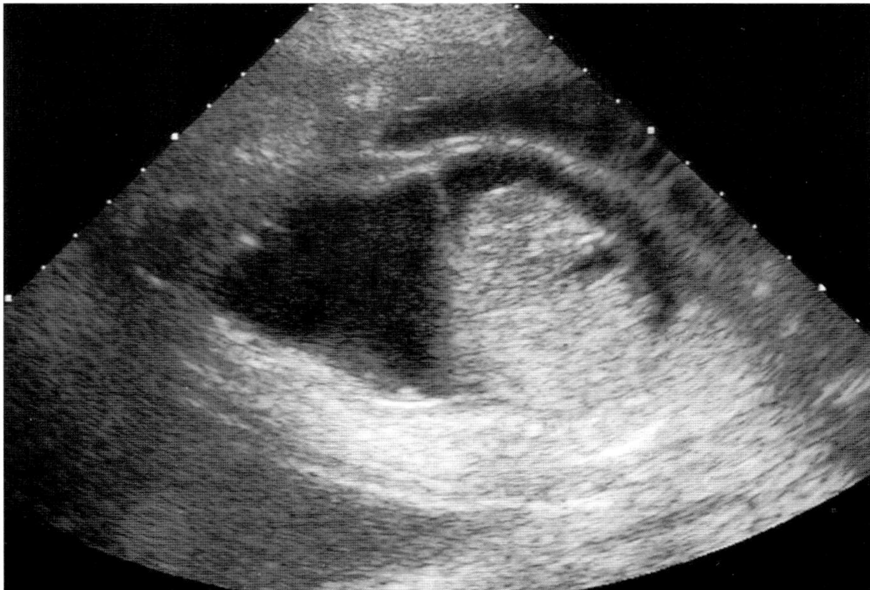

Fig. 4.**10** **Primary fetal hydrothorax.** The same fetus in longitudinal section, showing hydrothorax and ascites.

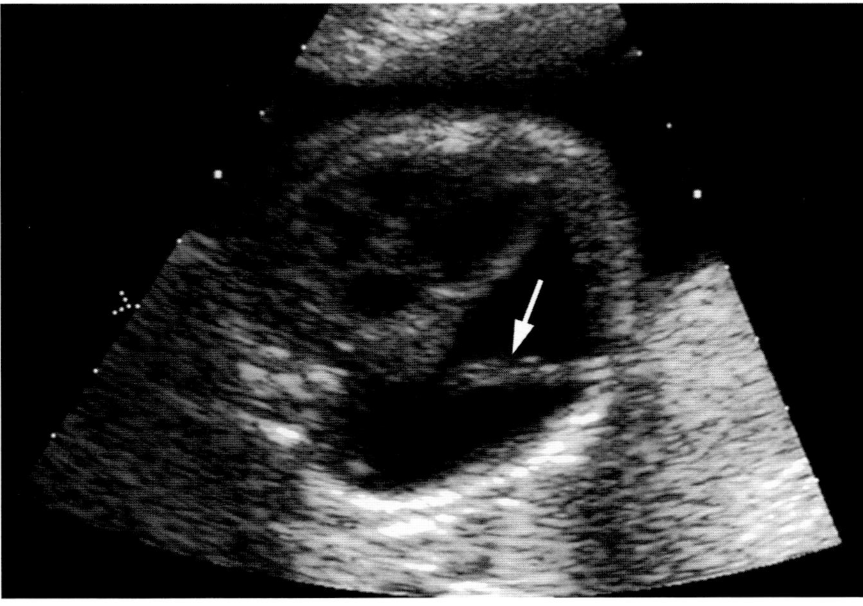

Fig. 4.**11** **Primary fetal hydrothorax.** The findings improved considerably after placement of a pleuroamniotic shunt (arrow). A healthy girl was born at 33 weeks.

Ultrasound findings: The lungs are surrounded by fluid. The finding can be unilateral or bilateral. Secondary development of hydrops is possible. Hydramnios is sometimes observed. Hypoplasia of the lung may further support the development of hydrothorax.

Caution: In severe forms of pericardial effusion, the lungs are displaced dorsally.

Clinical management: Sonographic screening, including fetal echocardiography. Karyotyping. TORCH serology. If the finding is persistent, decompression by thoracocentesis may be successful. Lymphocytes are the main component of the contents. Before birth, decompression of chylothorax may ease the management of the neonate after birth. Regular ultrasound checks are important. Often, a pleural–amniotic shunt is successful. Spontaneous resolution has also been reported. Induction of labor should be considered if hydrops develops after 32 weeks.

Procedure after birth: Preparation for intubation or thoracocentesis should be made. Repeated decompression or thorax drainage for a few days may be required.

Prognosis: A mortality rate of 50% is expected if the pleural effusions are diagnosed prenatally. The prognosis worsens if fetal prematurity, hypoplasia of the lungs, and hydrops are present.

References

Becker R, Arabin B, Entezami M, Novak A, Weitzel HK. Fetal hydrothorax: successful treatment by longtime drainage from week 23. Fetal Diagn Ther 1993; 8: 331–7.

Bernaschek G, Deutinger J, Hansmann M, Bald R, Holzgreve W, Bollmann R. Feto-amniotic shunting: report of the experience of four European centres. Prenat Diagn 1994; 14: 821–33.

Bovicelli L, Rizzo N, Orsini LF, Carderoni P. Ultrasonic real-time diagnosis of fetal hydrothorax and lung hypoplasia. JCU J Clin Ultrasound 1981; 9: 253–4.

Crombleholme TM, Dalton M, Cendron M, et al. Prenatal diagnosis and the pediatric surgeon: the impact of prenatal consultation on perinatal management. J Pediatr Surg 1996; 31: 156–62.

Kristoffersen SE, Ipsen L. Ultrasonic real time diagnosis of hydrothorax before delivery in an infant with extralobar lung sequestration. Acta Obstet Gynecol Scand 1984; 63: 723–5.

Meizner I, Levy A. A survey of non-cardiac fetal intrathoracic malformations diagnosed by ultrasound. Arch Gynecol Obstet 1994; 255: 31–6.

Merz E, Miric TD, Bahlmann F, Weber G, Hallermann C. Prenatal sonographic chest and lung measurements for predicting severe pulmonary hypoplasia. Prenat Diagn 1999; 19: 614–9.

Nyberg DA, Resta RG, Luthy DA, et al. Prenatal sonographic findings of Down syndrome: review of 94 cases. Obstet Gynecol 1990; 76: 370–7.

Diaphragmatic Hernia

Definition: Diaphragmatic hernia is a defect of varying size in the diaphragm resulting in displacement of abdominal content into the thoracic cavity. They occur most commonly in the posterolateral part of the diaphragm and are left sided (75–85 %). Retrosternal location is rare.

Incidence: One in 2000–5000 births.

Sex ratio: M : F = 2 : 1.

Clinical history/genetics: Mostly sporadic. Multifactorial inheritance: risk of recurrence in a sibling 2%. Rarely autosomal-dominant or X-linked transmission.

Teratogens: Unknown.

Embryology: Forms between 5 and 8 weeks.

Associated malformations: Associated anomalies are expected in almost 75% of cases. Cardiac anomalies in 20%, CNS anomalies in 30%. Chromosomal aberrations, particularly trisomy 18, are also observed. It is also associated with over 30 syndromes.

Associated syndromes: Wolf–Hirschhorn syndrome (deletion 4 p), Fryns syndrome, Multiple pterygium syndrome, Pallister–Killian syndrome (tetrasomy 12 p), partial trisomy 9, trisomy 18.

Ultrasound findings: A *left-sided diaphragmatic hernia* is the most common finding. Displacement of the heart to the right is obvious. Stomach, bowel, and parts of the liver may be detected next to the heart in the left hemithorax. In cases of the rare *right-sided diaphragmatic hernia,* the liver lies in the right hemithorax, displacing the heart to the left. Organ displacement and mediastinal shift can lead to obstruction of the intestines, resulting in hydramnios. This is prognostically unfavorable. The defect in the diaphragm is not always seen, so that it is often difficult to estimate its size (one-sided agenesis of the diaphragm?).

Clinical management: Sonographic screening, including fetal echocardiography. Karyotyping. Counseling of the parents by the pediatrician and pediatric surgeon concerning the findings and their possible prognostic significance. Fetal surgery (tracheal occlusion) is still at the experimental stage. Premature birth in association with diaphragmatic hernia has a poor prognosis. Delivery by cesarean section may be considered in order to organize intensive therapeutic measures (ECMO preparation).

Procedure after birth: Ventilation using a nasopharyngeal mask should be avoided (overventilation of the stomach). Immediate intubation and drainage of the stomach contents. High risk of pneumothorax. Possibly, high-frequency respiration and application of surfactant. Stabilizing the neonate for at least 12–24 h is important prior to surgery. The prognosis is very poor if the "honeymoon" stage (short-lived improvement of ventilation) has not been achieved. The role of ECMO (preoperative or postoperative) is at present still uncertain, but promising.

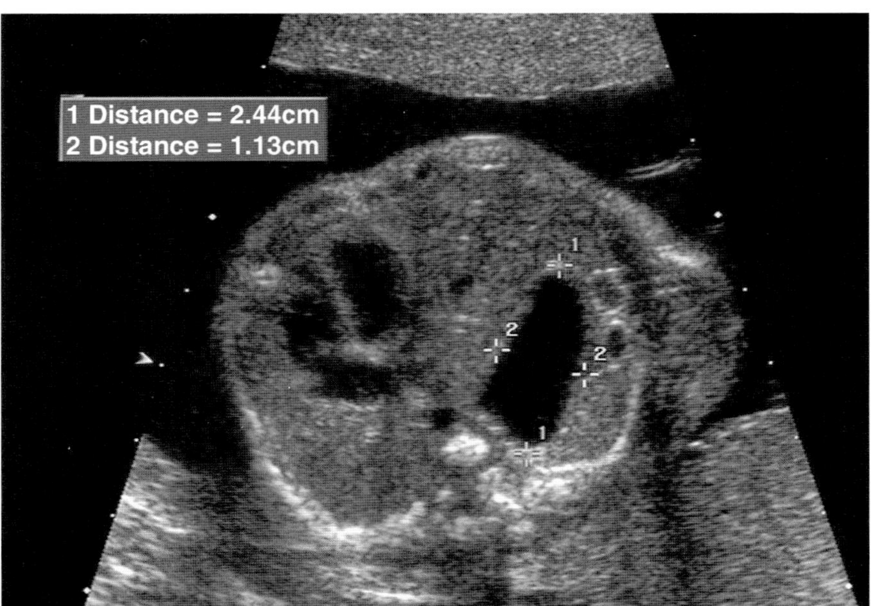

Fig. 4.**12** **Left-sided diaphragmatic hernia.** Fetus in breech presentation at 23 + 3 weeks. The fetal heart is shifted to the right due to prolapse of the stomach into the thoracic cavity. Loops of bowel are seen next to it.

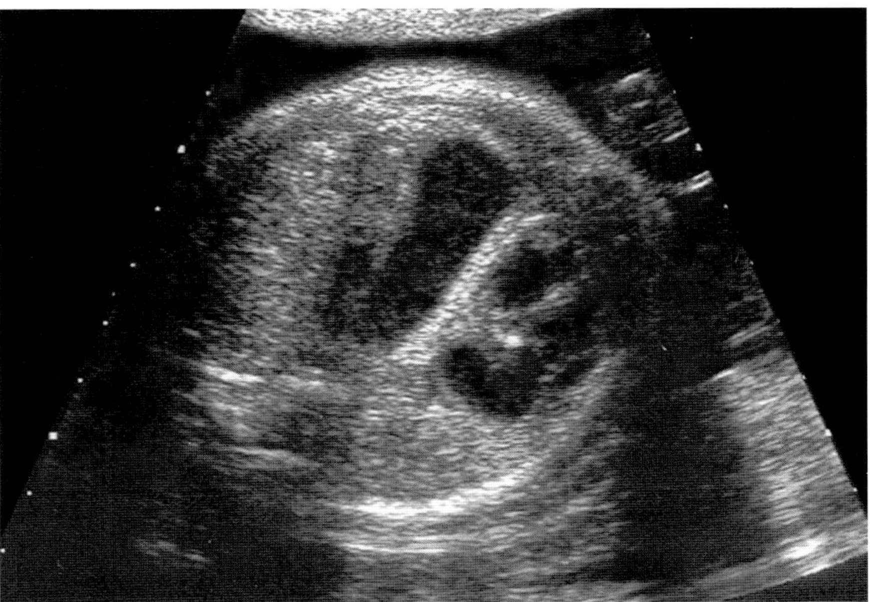

Fig. 4.**13** **Left-sided diaphragmatic hernia** at 29 weeks, showing herniation of the stomach and bowel into the thorax and displacing the heart to the right.

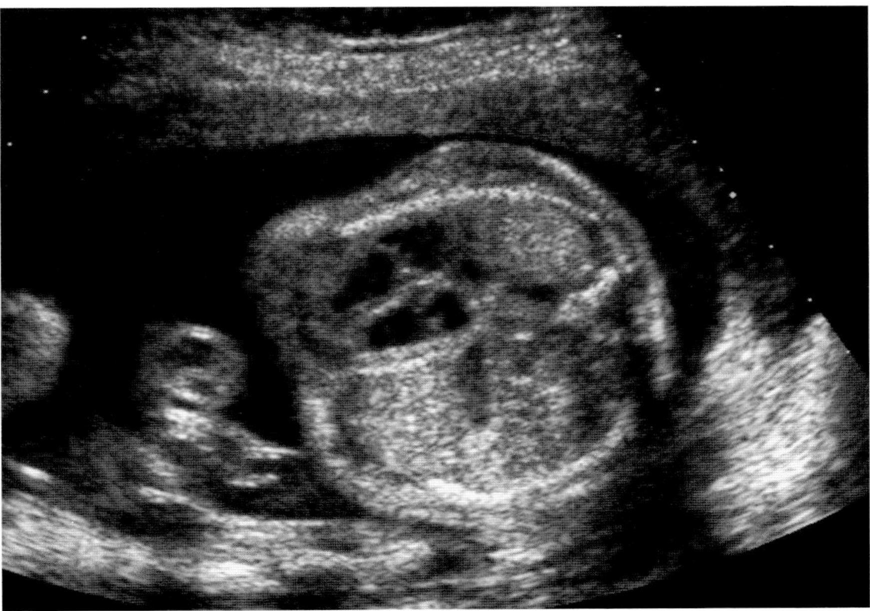

Fig. 4.**14** **Left-sided diaphragmatic hernia** at 23 + 2 weeks. Herniation of bowel into the thoracic cavity has caused cardiac displacement to the right.

Fig. 4.**15** **Left-sided diaphragmatic hernia.** The same case viewed longitudinally. The diaphragm is seen ventrally but not dorsally. The intestine is seen continuously up into the thorax.

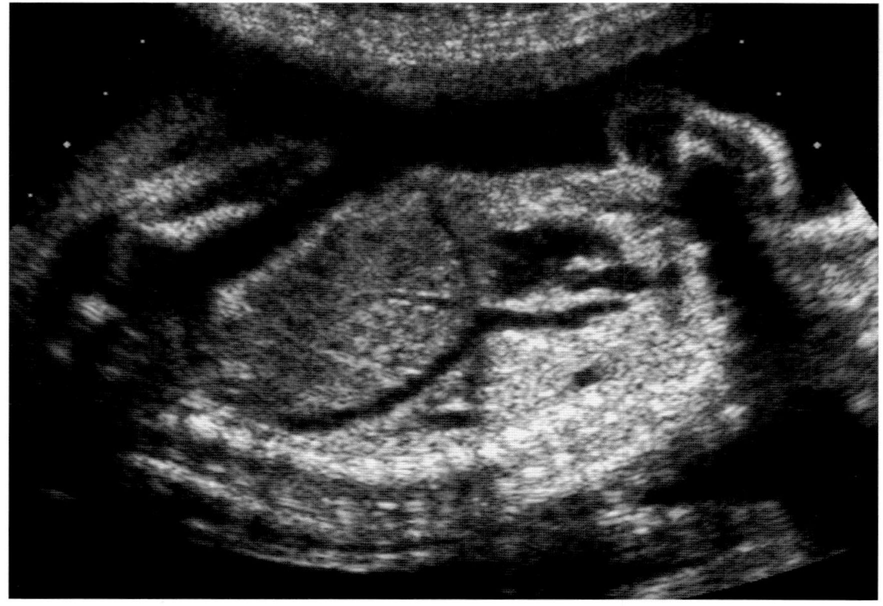

Prognosis: The prognosis depends on the severity of respiratory distress, especially hypoplasia of the lung and other concomitant anomalies. The earlier the diagnosis is made in prenatal screening, the poorer the prognosis (15–50% mortality). The prognosis worsens if the diagnosis is made prior to 24 weeks' gestation and hydramnios develops. Mortality is influenced by the neonatologist's experience and possibly also concurrent the use of extracorporeal membrane oxygenation (ECMO). The value of intrauterine prognostic factors for determining the extent of hypoplasia of the lungs (area of the lung, Doppler sonography of the pulmonary artery, and amniotic flow in the trachea) is uncertain. Intrauterine fetal surgery (e.g., tracheal blockage) is still in the experimental phase. Neonates who can be stabilized postnatally prior to surgery have about a 65–85% chance of survival. Some children develop a chronic respiratory distress syndrome.

Self-Help Organization

Title: CHERUBS Association for Congenital Diaphragmatic Hernia Research, Advocacy, and Support

Description: Support and information to families of children born with congenital diaphragmatic hernias. Phone support, online services, on-call volunteers, state and country representatives, pen pals, medical research, information and referrals, newsletter.

Scope: International network

Founded: 1995

Address: P.O. Box 1150, Creedmoor, NC 27 565, United States

Telephone: 1-888-834-8158 or 919-693-8158

Fax: 707-924-1114

E-mail: info @cherubs-cdh.org

Web: http://www.cherubs-cdh.org

References

Adzick NS, Vacanti JP, Lillehei CW, O'Rourke PP, Crone RK, Wilson JM. Fetal diaphragmatic hernia: ultrasound diagnosis and clinical outcome in 38 cases. J Pediatr Surg 1989; 24: 654–7.

Albanese CT, Lopoo J, Goldstein RB, et al. Fetal liver position and perinatal outcome for congenital diaphragmatic hernia. Prenat Diagn 1998; 18: 1138–42.

Al-Shanafey S, Giacomantonio M, Henteleff H. Congenital diaphragmatic hernia: experience without extracorporeal membrane oxygenation. Pediatr Surg Int 2002; 18: 28–31.

Kalache KD, Chaoui R, Hartung J, Wernecke KD, Bollmann R. Doppler assessment of tracheal fluid flow during fetal breathing movements in cases of congenital diaphragmatic hernia. Ultrasound Obstet Gynecol 1998; 12: 27–32.

Kasales CJ, Coulson CC, Meilstrup JW, Ambrose A, Botti JJ, Holley GP. Diagnosis and differentiation of congenital diaphragmatic hernia from other noncardiac thoracic fetal masses. Am J Perinatol 1998; 15: 623–8.

Lewis DA, Reickert C, Bowerman R, Hirschl RB. Prenatal ultrasonography frequently fails to diagnose congenital diaphragmatic hernia. J Pediatr Surg 1997; 32: 352–6.

Merz E, Miric TD, Bahlmann F, Weber G, Hallermann C. Prenatal sonographic chest and lung measurements for predicting severe pulmonary hypoplasia. Prenat Diagn 1999; 19: 614–9.

Milner R, Adzick NS. Perinatal management of fetal malformations amenable to surgical correction. Curr Opin Obstet Gynecol 1999; 11: 177–83.

Norio R, Kaariainen H, Rapola J, Herva R, Kekomaki M. Familial congenital diaphragmatic defects: aspects of etiology, prenatal diagnosis, and treatment. Am J Med Genet 1984; 17: 471–83.

Skari H, Bjornland K, Frenckner B, et al. Congenital diaphragmatic hernia in Scandinavia from 1995 to 1998: predictors of mortality. J Pediatr Surg 2002; 37: 1269–75.

Stevens TP, Chess PR, McConnochie KM, et al. Survival in early- and late-term infants with congenital diaphragmatic hernia treated with extracorporeal membrane oxygenation. Pediatrics 2002; 110: 590–6.

Witters I, Legius E, Moerman P, et al. Associated malformations and chromosomal anomalies in 42 cases of prenatally diagnosed diaphragmatic hernia. Am J Med Genet 2001; 103: 278–82.

5 The Heart

General Considerations

Congenital heart disease is relatively frequent, with an incidence of eight per 1000 live births (0.8%, or one affected child in 125 births). Half of these cases constitute severe cardiac anomalies, which require surgical intervention after birth. Not all malformations are detected prenatally, as some are due to the presence of the physiological fetal circulation between the heart and the great vessels (a normal state before birth) persisting even after birth; the malformations are therefore only detected after birth (e.g., open ductus arteriosus/Botallo duct). The *rate of detection* of cardiac anomalies during prenatal screening is extremely variable; according to the literature, it ranges from 5% to 85%, so that at best 17 of 20 cardiac anomalies may be detected prenatally, or at worst only one in 20. There are three reasons for this wide variation.

1 Time of Screening

On the one hand, the frequency of cardiac malformations depends on the age of the pregnancy (cardiac anomalies which lead to spontaneous demise in early pregnancy are rarely detected at a later gestational stage). On the other hand, the sensitivity of the method of examination depends on the gestational age—i.e., the percentage in which the anomaly is detected. In our experience, the best time for cardiac screening is around 21 weeks. In obese patients, a control screening examination may further be necessary at 23 to 24 weeks. The present trend is to detect cardiac anomalies as early as possible; in individual cases, this can mean as early as 12 weeks.

2 Personal Competence

"You can only detect what you know." An experienced examiner who has seen a large number of cardiac malformations in pregnancy and who only carries out ultrasound examinations obviously has more certainty in his or her diagnosis and thus has a better chance of detecting an anomaly than an examiner who provides basic care and only carries out ultrasound examinations in pregnancy occasionally.

3 Quality of the Equipment

The quality of ultrasound equipment varies considerably, with new equipment costing anything between $20 000 and $200 000. In addition to B-mode sonography, *color flow imaging Doppler sonography* is a must for detecting fetal cardiac anomalies, as it establishes the direction of blood flow and determines flow velocities in such a way that detailed hemodynamic evaluation is possible.

If cardiac anomaly is suspected after prenatal screening, then the following measures are taken:

1. In case of cardiac or any other anomalies, it is important to obtain a second opinion from another specialist in ultrasound screening to confirm the initially suspected diagnosis.
2. If the diagnosis of cardiac malformation is confirmed, then a detailed examination of the structures involved must be carried out. This is easier said than done, as it may take up to 2 hours in a physician's practice to confirm the diagnosis with certainty and to decide what sort of consequences the anomaly may have. It is useful to involve a pediatric cardiologist at this stage who can interpret this and who can also counsel the patient.
3. Cardiac anomalies may be an isolated finding, may appear in association with other malformations, or may constitute part of a syndrome. Thus, it is absolutely necessary to do a complete and detailed fetal screening for other malformations to confirm either an isolated finding or a complex syndrome with an accompanying cardiac anomaly.
4. Cardiac malformation may indicate a chromosomal anomaly—for example, an AV septal defect is associated with trisomy 21 in about 50% of cases. After an anomaly of this type has been diagnosed, the parents should be informed about further tests that are available for detecting genetic abnormalities (amniocentesis and the prenatal Quick test, especially the fluorescent in-situ hybridization (FISH) test, placental biopsy, or fetal blood sampling).

5. In cases of severe cardiac anomalies, the patient may opt for termination of the pregnancy. From our point of view, it is very important that after counseling, this decision comes solely from the patient (nondirective counseling) and that she should not be rushed into taking a decision because of lack of time (in Germany, there is no gestation limit for a medical indication for the termination of pregnancy at present). Psychotherapeutic sessions should also be offered to the parents.

6. Detecting a cardiac anomaly does not necessarily alter the plan of antenatal care or the method of delivery. Usually, a normal delivery can be expected at due date. However, the pregnancy must be monitored more often using ultrasonography.

7. The presence of a cardiac anomaly does not always mean delivery by cesarean section, but the delivery should take place in a center in which a pediatric intensive-care unit as well as an experienced pediatric cardiology team are available. After birth, the cardiologist performs an echocardiography and decides which other measures are immediately necessary. Anomalies such as ventricular septal defect or atrial septal defect do not always have to be treated, as many resolve spontaneously within the first year of life.

The advantages of fetal echocardiography can be summarized as follows:

1. The main advantage of routine fetal echocardiography during pregnancy is to dispel any fear of having cardiac anomalies when the fetal ultrasound screening is normal.

2. If a severe cardiac anomaly is diagnosed or cardiac malformation suggests genetic disease, the parents have the option of whether or not to carry on with the pregnancy.

3. If the mother decides to carry on with the pregnancy after diagnosis of a fetal cardiac anomaly, the prenatal diagnosis allows optimal monitoring of the pregnancy, labor, delivery, and neonatal care of the child, which otherwise might have had a very poor chance of surviving, if any.

Information for the Mother of an Affected Fetus

Title: CHASER (Congenital Heart Anomalies—Support, Education, Resources)

Description: Opportunity for parents of children born with heart defects to network with other parents with similar needs and concerns. Education on hospitalization, surgeries, medical treatments, etc. Newsletter, information and referral, phone support. Heart surgeons and facilities directory.

Scope: National

Founded: 1992

Address: 2112 N. Wilkins Rd., Swanton, OH 43558, United States

Telephone: 419–825–5575 (day)

Fax: 419–825–2880

E-mail: chaser@compuserve.com

Web: http://www.csun.edu/~hfmth006/chaser/

2

Coarctation of the Aorta

Definition: Narrowing of the aorta over a variable distance near the junction of ductus arteriosus (Botallo's duct).

Incidence: One in 1600 births.

Sex ratio: M : F = 1.5 : 1.

Clinical history/genetics: Multifactorial inheritance; risk of recurrence with one affected child 2%, with two affected children 6%; if the mother is affected, then the risk of recurrence rises to 18%, in case of an affected father it is 5%.

Teratogens: Diabetes mellitus, high doses of vitamin A.

Associated malformations: Other cardiac anomalies such as VSD, valvular aortic stenosis, transposition of the great arteries.

Associated syndromes: Turner syndrome (35% of affected children have coarctation of the aorta). This vessel anomaly has also been described in over 25 different syndromes.

Ultrasound findings: *Asymmetrical heart chambers with dilation of the right heart* (atrium, ventricle, and pulmonary trunk dilation) may be the first indication. *Narrowing of the aortic arch* itself is difficult to demonstrate, as this often appears secondary to constriction of Botallo's duct in the neonatal stage and is less obvious prior to this. Cross-sectional view of vena cava, aorta and pulmonary artery (*three-vessel view*) is the best method of demonstrating *the relative narrowing of the aorta*. In extreme cases, it resembles a *hypoplastic left heart*. In mild cases, intrauterine diagnosis is often very difficult.

Clinical management: Further sonographic screening. Karyotyping. Ultrasound monitoring at regular intervals to detect increasing asymmetry of the ventricles. Vaginal delivery is possible.

Procedure after birth: The decision on whether to undertake early therapeutic intervention depends on the severity of the existing lesion or of aortic stenosis appearing after the closure of Botallo's duct. In severe cases, prostaglandin can be given as a prophylactic measure (inadequate liver and kidney perfusion, severe dysfunction of the left ventricle). Early surgical therapy or balloon angioplasty is indicated if signs of heart failure or inadequate perfusion of the periphery develop. In children without symptoms, the operation can be delayed until the age of 3–5 years.

Prognosis: The prognosis is good after successful surgical treatment. When the lesion is isolated, the perioperative mortality is below 1%. In the presence of other anomalies, however, the mortality rate rises to 5–15%. Recurrence of stenosis is expected in 15–30% of patients.

References

Beekman RH. Coarctation of the aorta. In: Emmanouilides GC, Allen HD, Riemenschneider TA, Gutgesell HP, editors. Moss and Adams heart disease in infants, children, and adolescents, including the fetus and young adult. Baltimore: Williams & Wilkins, 1995: 1111–33.

Benacerraf BR, Saltzman DH, Sanders SP. Sonographic sign suggesting the prenatal diagnosis of coarctation of the aorta. J Ultrasound Med 1989; 8: 65–9.

Bronshtein M, Zimmer EZ. Early sonographic diagnosis of fetal small left heart ventricle with a normal proximal outlet tract: a medical dilemma. Prenat Diagn 1997; 17: 249–53.

Bronshtein M, Zimmer EZ. Sonographic diagnosis of fetal coarctation of the aorta at 14–16 weeks of gestation. Ultrasound Obstet Gynecol 1998; 11: 254–7.

Franklin O, Burch M, Manning N, Sleeman K, Gould S, Archer N. Prenatal diagnosis of coarctation of the aorta improves survival and reduces morbidity. Heart 2002; 87: 67–9.

Nomiyama M, Ueda Y, Toyota Y, Kawano H. Fetal aortic isthmus growth and morphology in late gestation. Ultrasound Obstet Gynecol 2002; 19: 153–7.

Wenstrom KD, Williamson RA, Hoover WW, Grant SS. Achondrogenesis type II (Langer–Saldino) in association with jugular lymphatic obstruction sequence. Prenat Diagn 1989; 9: 527–32.

Atrioventricular Septal Defect (AV Canal)

Definition: The most frequent form is *complete AV canal*, characterized by a large septal defect involving the atrial as well as the ventricular septa and the presence of a common atrioventricular valve. In the case of an *incomplete AV canal*, the AV valvular rims are separated and at least one anomaly of the AV valve is present (mostly a "cleft anterior mitral leaflet," combined with an atrial septal defect of the foramen primum type and/or an inlet VSD).

Incidence: 3.6 : 10 000; 2% of all congenital cardiac malformations.

Clinical history/genetics: Down syndrome is confirmed in 50% of cases; in a further 10%, there is Ivemark syndrome (agenesis of the spleen or polysplenia). The rate of recurrence is 2.5% if one sibling is affected and 8% with two affected siblings. In the case of an affected mother, the recurrence rate is 6%, and it is 1.5% if the father is affected.

Associated malformations: Fallot-type pulmonary stenosis, fibromuscular subaortic stenosis, coarctation of the aorta; AV valve stenosis; anomalies of the spleen (Ivemark syndrome). Hydrops develops only in association with fetal cardiac arrhythmia.

Associated syndromes: Down syndrome, Ivemark syndrome.

Ultrasound findings: A *combined atrial and ventricular septal defect* in the mid-region of the AV valve (inlet VSD). The anterior and posterior *AV valves are fused together*, or lie much closer together than is normally expected. Using color

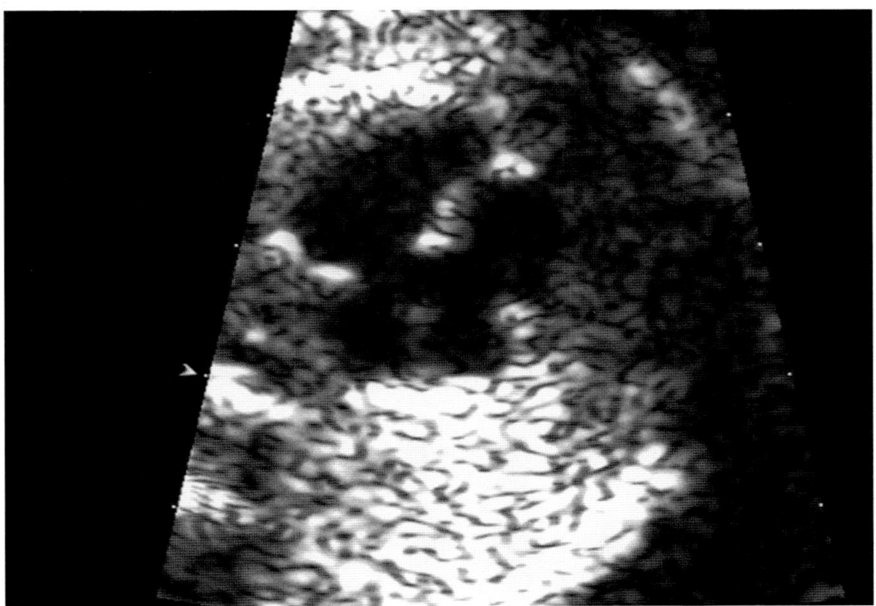

Fig. 5.**1** **Complete atrioventricular septal defect.** Apical view of the four chambers, at 21 + 6 weeks. The ventricular septum ends below the level of the valve, primary septum is missing, tricuspid and mitral valves are not separated: a complete atrioventricular septal defect.

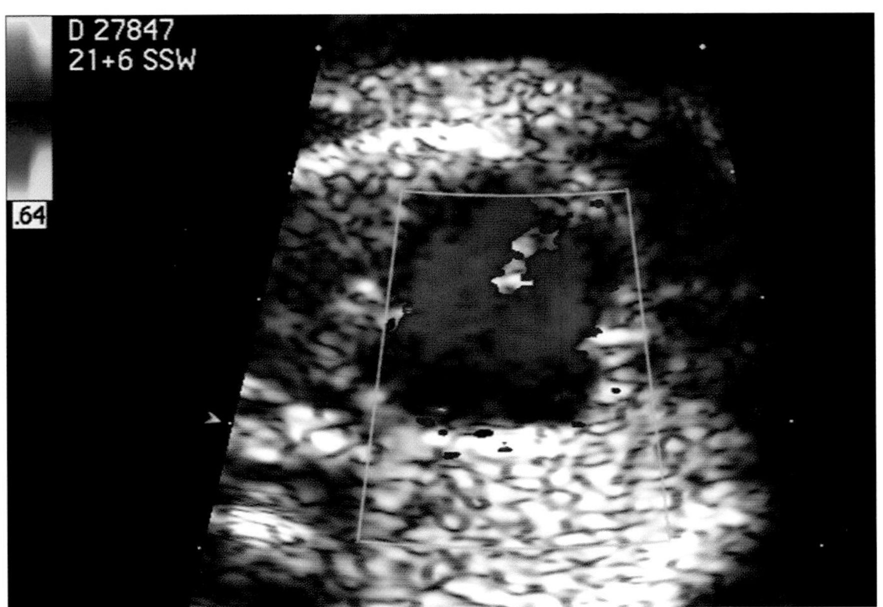

Fig. 5.**2** **Complete atrioventricular septal defect.** Same case, diastolic phase, using color flow mapping. Blood is streaming through a common valve into both chambers.

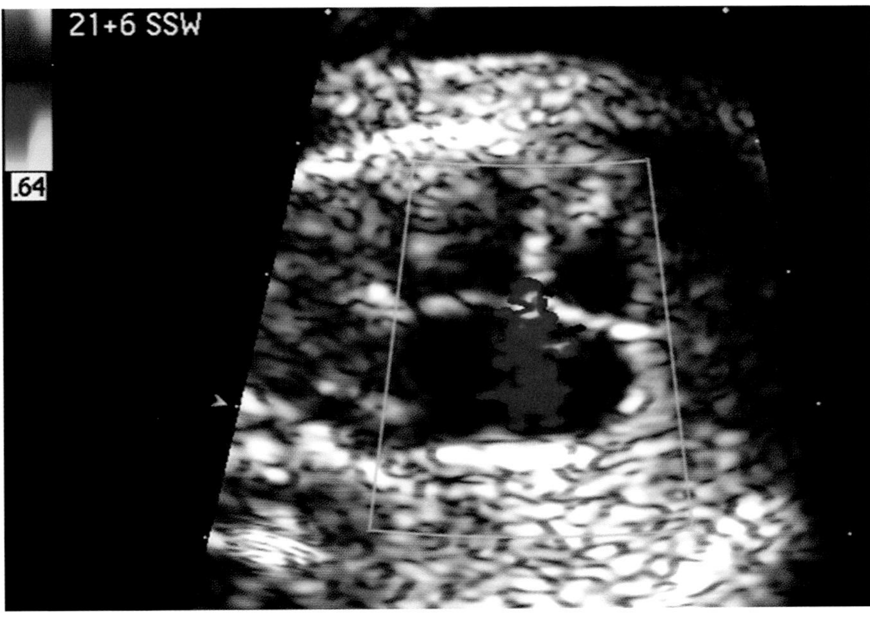

Fig. 5.**3** **Complete atrioventricular septal defect.** Same case, systolic phase. Incompetence of the communicating atrioventricular valve, with regurgitation.

2

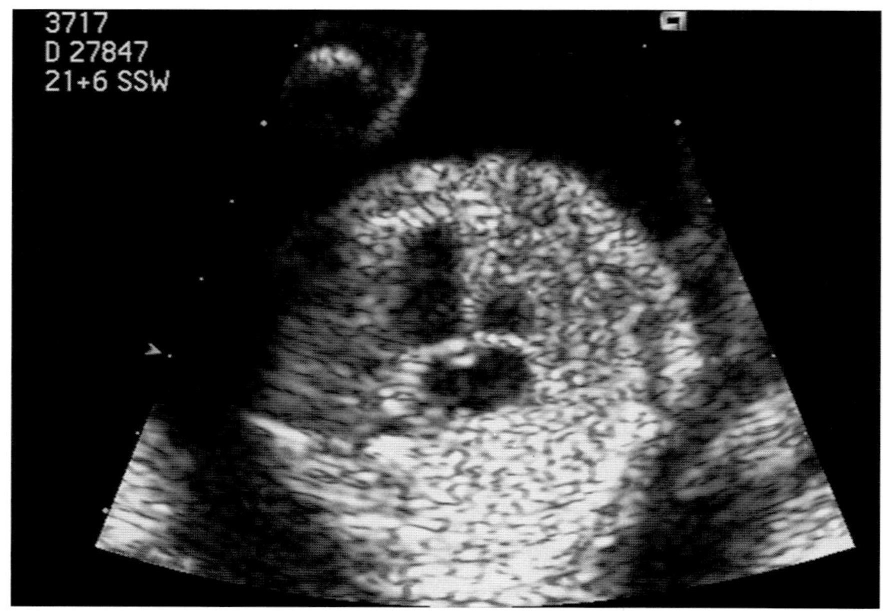

Fig. 5.**4** **Complete atrioventricular septal defect.** Same case. Slight tilting of the scanner produces almost a normal appearance.

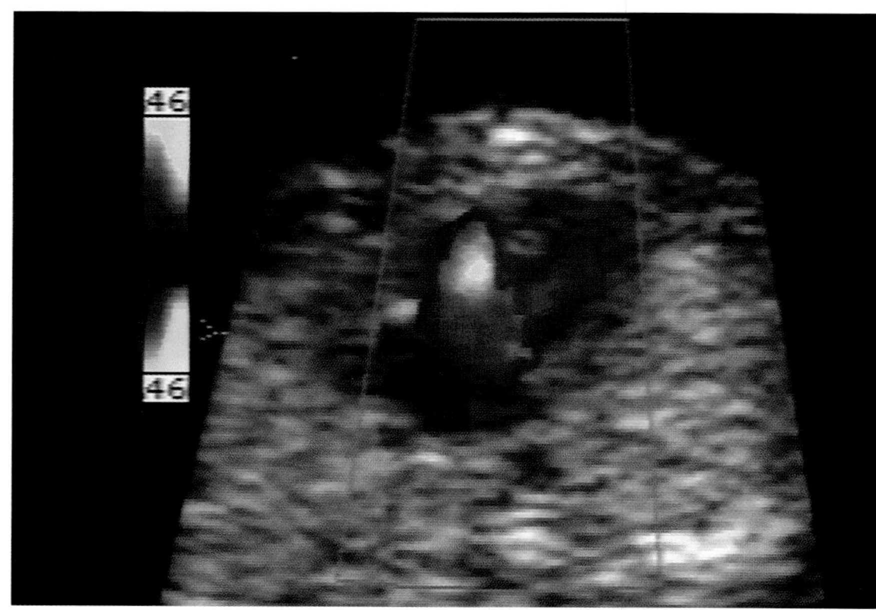

Fig. 5.**5** **Atrioventricular septal defect,** 14 + 5 weeks. Apical view of the four chambers using color flow mapping.

flow Doppler imaging, AV valvular incompetence can often be detected. Disturbances in stimulus conduction may lead to cardiac arrhythmia (AV block, extrasystoles).

Clinical management: Further fetal ultrasound screening. Karyotyping. Ultrasound monitoring at regular intervals for early detection of cardiac failure or fetal hydrops. Vaginal delivery is possible.

Procedure after birth: Immediate postnatal complications are not to be expected in the absence of stenosis of great vessels. However, all children require surgical correction, which is usually carried out during the first year of life. Initial symptoms develop at the age of 4–6 weeks after birth (tachypnea, tachycardia).

Prognosis: In most cases, it is possible to correct the defect surgically. The perioperative mortality is 5%. The prognosis becomes unfavorable if obstruction of the pulmonary artery is also present.

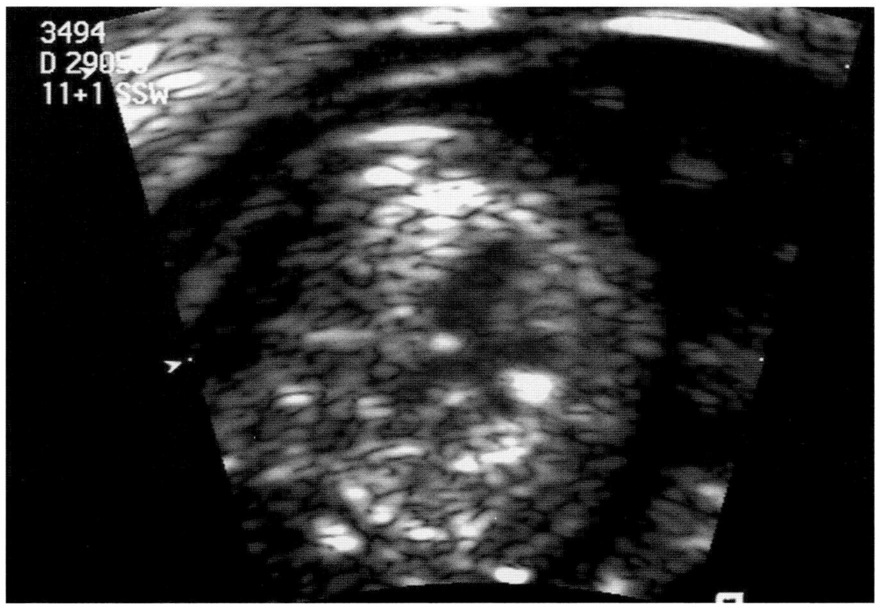

Fig. 5.6 **Atrioventricular septal defect.** Cross-section of fetal thorax, at 11 + 1 weeks. Apical four-chamber view with AV septal defect in a case of Down syndrome.

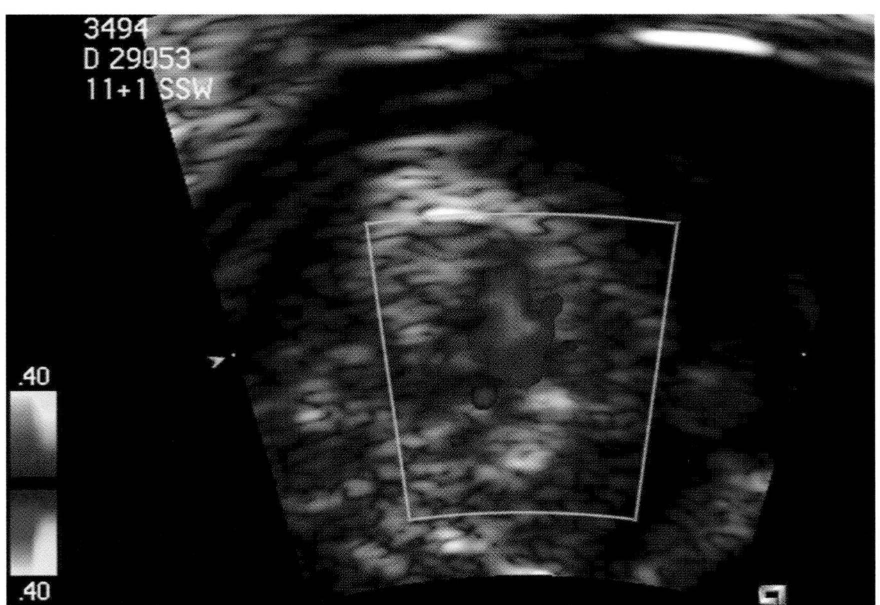

Fig. 5.7 **Atrioventricular septal defect.** Same case. Demonstration of blood flow over the AV valve using color flow mapping.

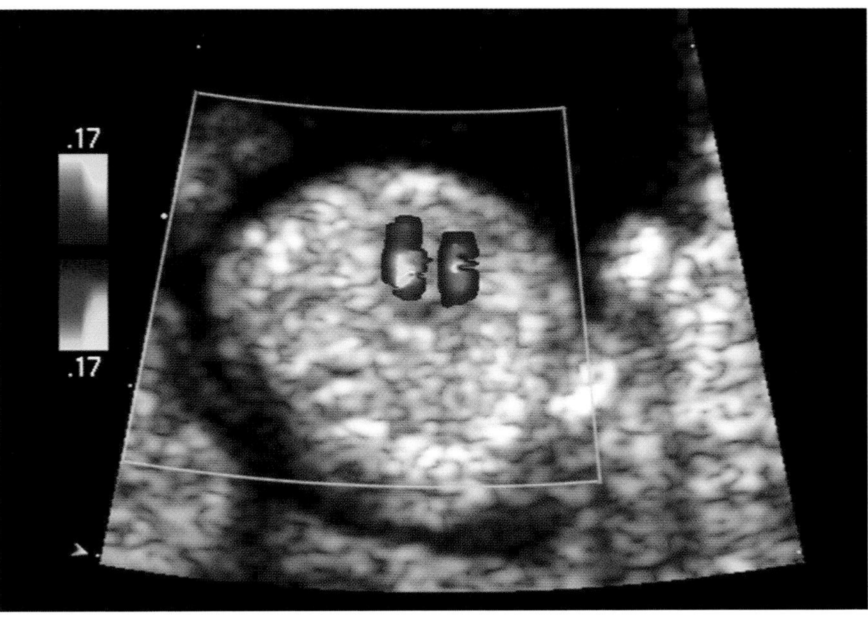

Fig. 5.8 **For comparison,** the flow pattern in a normal fetus at 12 weeks.

Fig. 5.9 **Atrioventricular septal defect.** Demonstration of blood flow over the defective AV valve using color flow mapping as well as pulsed Doppler sonography.

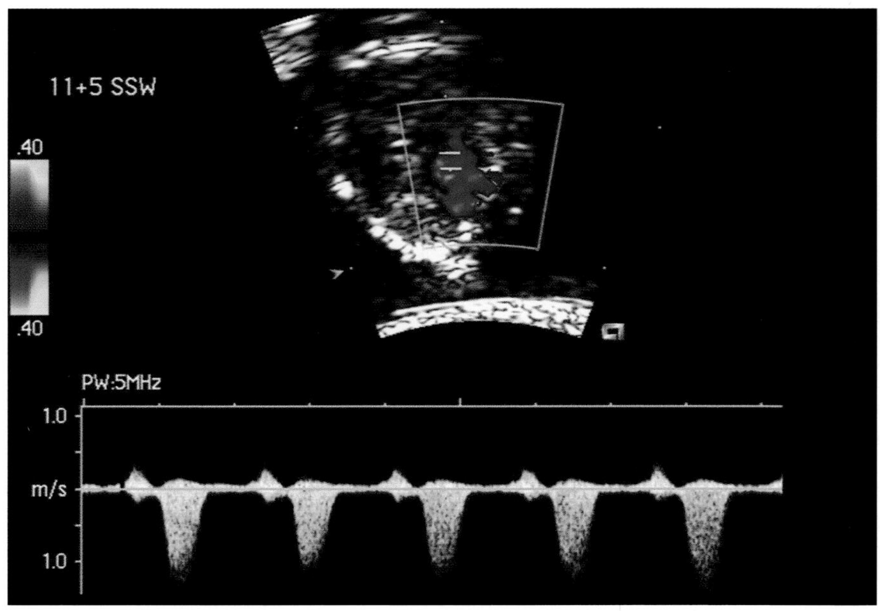

References

Achiron R, Rotstein Z, Lipitz S, Mashiach S, Hegesh J. First-trimester diagnosis of fetal congenital heart disease by transvaginal ultrasonography. Obstet Gynecol 1994; 84: 69–72.

Allan LD, Anderson RH, Cook AC. Atresia or absence of the left-sided atrioventricular connection in the fetus: echocardiographic diagnosis and outcome. Ultrasound Obstet Gynecol 1996; 8: 295–302.

Areias JC, Matias A, Montenegro N, Brandao O. Early antenatal diagnosis of cardiac defects using transvaginal Doppler ultrasound: new perspectives? Diagn Ther 1998; 13: 111–14.

Benacerraf BR, Gelman R, Frigoletto FDJ. Sonographic identification of second-trimester fetuses with Down's syndrome. N Engl J Med 1987; 1371–6.

Feldt RH, Porter CJ, Edwards WD, Puga FJ, Seward JB. Atrioventricular septal defects. In: In: Emmanouilides GC, Allen HD, Riemenschneider TA, Gutgesell HP, editors. Moss and Adams heart disease in infants, children, and adolescents, including the fetus and young adult. Baltimore: Williams & Wilkins, 1995: 704–24.

Murphy DJ Jr. Atrioventricular canal defects. Curr Treat Options Cardiovasc Med 1999; 1: 323–34.

Paladini D, Calabrb R, Palmieri S, Dandrea T. Prenatal diagnosis of congenital heart disease and fetal karyotyping. Obstet Gynecol 1993; 81: 679–82.

Park JK, Taylor DK, Skeels M, Towner DR. Dilated coronary sinus in the fetus: misinterpretation as an atrioventricular canal defect. Ultrasound Obstet Gynecol 1997; 10: 126–9.

Stoll C, Dott B, Alembik Y, Roth MP. Evaluation of routine prenatal ultrasound examination in detecting fetal chromosomal abnormalities in a low risk population. Hum Genet 1993; 91: 37–41.

Tennstedt C, Chaoui R, Korner H, Dietel M. Spectrum of congenital heart defects and extracardiac malformations associated with chromosomal abnormalities: results of a seven year necropsy study. Heart 1999; 82: 34–9.

Bradycardia

Definition: Heart frequency below 100 beats per minute.

Incidence: One in 20 000 births.

Clinical history/genetics: 50% of cases are due to a complete AV block resulting from an autoimmune disease. The rate of recurrence is 8% if one child is affected.

Teratogens: Not known.

Embryology: Autoantibodies can disturb the cardiac stimulus conduction system. If structural malformation is the cause, then the atrioventricular septum is mostly involved.

Associated malformations: In 50% of cases, complex cardiac anomalies are present such as AV canal, VSD, atrial isomerism, or abnormal venous flow. Fetal hydrops must be excluded. If there is sinus bradycardia, malformation of the central nervous system and fetal growth restriction should be looked for.

Ultrasound findings: A very slow heartbeat is the first sign detected in B-mode. M-mode echocardiography is needed for further differentiation.

In a *complete AV block,* the atria and ventricles beat regularly but are completely dissociated from one another. In *sinus bradycardia,* 1 : 1 conduction takes place from the atria to the ventricles. In case of atrial bigeminal rhythm, certain isolated beats are transferred to the ventricles and others are not. In *second-degree AV block,* 3 : 1 or 2 : 1 conduction to the ventricles is possible.

Clinical management: Further sonographic screening, anti-Rho, anti-La and antiphospholipid antibodies should be determined either to confirm or to exclude autoimmune disease. If there is structural malformation, karyotyping is advised. After 32 completed weeks, premature delivery is an option if cardiac insufficiency and hydrops develop. At earlier gestation, maternal therapy with steroids or plasmapheresis may be successfully administered. There is no consensus regarding the mode of delivery. "Fetal distress" is difficult to diagnose using cardiotocography during labor, and repeated fetal blood analysis is only valuable for a short period. Pulse oximetry may help in this situation. Cesarean section should be considered if hydrops develops and if the prognosis is not hopeless due to other cardiac anomalies.

Procedure after birth: Intensive cardiac care is needed in the neonatal stage. If there is a bigeminal pulse and sinus bradycardia, therapy is usually not needed. In the presence of a complete AV block with a bradycardia of under 55 bpm or generalized hydrops, pacemaker installation should be considered.

Prognosis: This depends on the cause of the bradycardia. Cases of bigeminal pulse have a good prognosis and the condition may disappear spontaneously. However, in 1% of cases, tachyarrhythmia may develop. A heart frequency of 80–100 bpm is found in sinus bradycardia; this may be sufficient for normal development of the child. The prognosis is poor if a complete AV block resulting from a complex malformation is diagnosed, or if the frequency is below 55 bpm. The fetus is not affected hemodynamically if there is a second-degree AV block.

References

Beinder E, Grancay T, Menendez T, Singer H, Hofbeck M. Fetal sinus bradycardia and the long QT syndrome. Am J Obstet Gynecol 2001; 185: 743–7.

Brucato A, Frassi M, Franceschini F, et al. Risk of congenital complete heart block in newborns of mothers with anti-Ro/SSA antibodies detected by counterimmunoelectrophoresis: a prospective study of 100 women. Arthritis Rheum 2001; 44: 1832–5.

Carpenter RJJ, Strasburger JF, Garson AJ, Smith RT, Deter RL, Engelhardt HTJ. Fetal ventricular pacing for hydrops secondary to complete atrioventricular block. J Am Coll Cardiol 1986; 8: 1434–6.

Fermont L, Batisse A, Le Bidois J. Prenatal cardiology: can we treat the fetal heart? Pediatrie (Bucur) 1992; 47: 339–45.

Friedman DM, Rupel A, Glickstein J, Buyon JP. Congenital heart block in neonatal lupus: the pediatric cardiologist's perspective [review]. Indian J Pediatr 2002; 69: 517–22.

Mendoza GJ, Almeida O, Steinfeld L. Intermittent fetal bradycardia induced by midpregnancy fetal ultrasonographic study. Am J Obstet Gynecol 1989; 160: 1038–40.

Nurnberg JH, Weng Y, Lange PE, Versmold H. [Transthoracic pacing in a very low birth weight infant with congenital complete atrioventricular block. Case report; in German.] Klin Pädiatr 2002; 214: 89–92.

Silverman NH, Enderlein MA, Stanger P, Teitel DF, Hamann MA, Golbus MS. Recognition of fetal arrhythmias by echocardiography. JCU J Clin Ultrasound 1985; 13: 255–63.

Wladimiroff JW, Stewart PA, Tonge HM. Fetal bradyarrhythmia: diagnosis and outcome. Prenat Dial 1988; 8: 53–7.

Yaman C, Tulzer G, Arzt W Tews G. Doppler ultrasound of the umbilical vein in fetal 3rd degree atrioventricular block. Ultraschall Med 1998; 19: 142–5.

Double-Outlet Right Ventricle (DORV)

Definition: This is a complex cardiac anomaly in which both great vessels arise from the right ventricle. The left ventricle is emptied through a VSD to the right ventricle.

Incidence: Rare; 1.5–2% of congenital heart disease.

Sex ratio: M : F = 1 : 1.

Clinical history/genetics: Sporadic occurrence. With one affected sibling, the rate of recurrence is 3–4%. Chromosomal aberration is found in 10–15% of cases.

Teratogens: Not known.

Associated malformations: Tracheo-esophageal fistula.

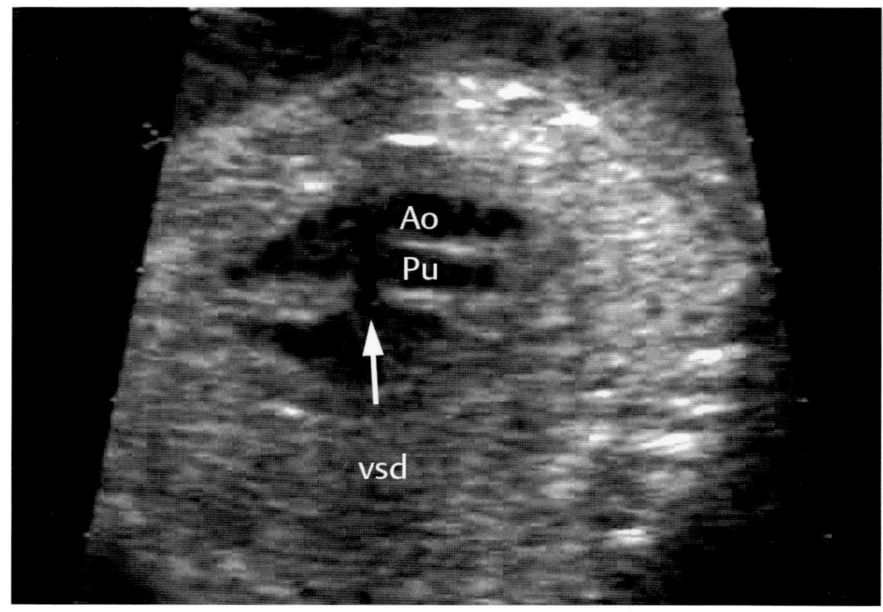

Fig. 5.**10** **Atypical four-chamber view,** 22 weeks. There is transposition of the great arteries, both arising from the right ventricle—double-outlet right ventricle. In addition, there is a ventricular septal defect (arrow). These findings were confirmed after termination of the pregnancy.

Associated syndromes: Trisomy 18.

Ultrasound findings: Three different forms of DORV are recognized:

1. *Side-by-side positioning of the great vessels.* The aorta lies to the right and the pulmonary artery to the left. Subaortic VSD (46% of all cases and thus the most frequent form). Subpulmonary VSD (also known as Taussig–Bing anomaly, 9%). Subaortic and subpulmonary VSD (3%). VSD away from the great vessels (7%).

2. *Right-sided malpositioning of great vessels.* The aorta lies in front to the right and the pulmonary artery behind it to the left. Here there are only two variations of VSD: subaortic (16%) and subpulmonary (10%).

3. *Left-sided malpositioning of the great vessels.* The aorta lies in the front to the left and the pulmonary artery behind to the right. Again, two VSD variations are known here—subaortic (3%) and subpulmonary (2%).

Echocardiography has to demonstrate whether both vessels arise from the right ventricle (trabecular and moderator band in the right ventricle) and their position relative to each other. The size of the left ventricle should be determined (hypoplasia?). Other cardiac anomalies should be looked for (pulmonary stenosis, coarctation of the aorta, AV valve defect).

Differential diagnosis: Tetralogy of Fallot (if the overriding of the aorta is less than 50% of its diameter over the VSD, then it is likely to be Fallot's tetralogy; in this case, the aorta and the narrowed pulmonary artery lie normally).

Clinical management: Further sonographic screening for other anomalies. Karyotyping including FISH diagnosis to exclude Di George syndrome. Cardiac insufficiency with development of hydrops is seen rarely in DORV. However, regular sonographic controls are necessary to detect such complications early. If there are no signs of cardiac insufficiency, then vaginal delivery is possible.

Procedure after birth: Complications are not expected immediately after delivery. In individual cases, infusion therapy with prostaglandin may be useful, especially if severe cyanosis is present.

Prognosis: Surgical intervention is necessary. The perioperative mortality depends on the type of DORV and on other associated anomalies, and lies between 10% and 20%. The long-term prognosis varies according to the primary finding. In favorable conditions, the child may survive without major impairment. For accurate prognosis, counseling with a pediatric cardiologist is advised.

References

Bollmann R, Schilling H, Abet L, Reinhold RL, Zienert A. Ultrasound diagnosis of severe fetal abnormalities. Zentralbl Gynäkol 1989; 111: 1185–8.

Greenberg F, Gresik MV, Carpenter RJ, Law SW, Hoffman LP, Ledbetter DH. The Gardner–Silengo–Wachtel or genito-palato-cardiac syndrome: male pseudohermaphroditism with micrognathia, cleft palate, and conotruncal cardiac defect. Am J Med Genet 1987; 26: 59–64.

Hagler DJ. Double-outlet right ventricle. In: Emmanouilides GC, Allen HD, Riemenschneider TA, Gutgesell HP, editors. Moss and Adams heart disease in infants, children, and adolescents, including the fetus and young adult. Baltimore: Williams & Wilkins, 1995: 1246–70.

Shenker L, Reed KL, Marx GR, Donnerstein RL, Allen HD, Anderson CF. Fetal cardiac Doppler flow studies in prenatal diagnosis of heart disease. Am J Obstet Gynecol 1988; 158: 1267–73.

Smith RS, Comstock CH, Kirk JS, Lee W, Riggs T, Weinhouse E. Double-outlet right ventricle: an antenatal diagnostic dilemma. Ultrasound Obstet Gynecol 1999; 14: 315–9.

Stewart PA, Wladimiroff JW, Essed CE. Prenatal ultrasound diagnosis of congenital heart disease associated with intrauterine growth retardation: a report of 2 cases. Prenat Diagn 1983; 3: 279–85.

Tennstedt C, Chaoui R, Korner H, Dietel M. Spectrum of congenital heart defects and extracardiac malformations associated with chromosomal abnormalities: results of a seven year necropsy study. Heart 1999; 82: 34–9.

Tometzki AJ, Suda K, Kohl T, Kovalchin JP, Silverman NH. Accuracy of prenatal echocardiographic diagnosis and prognosis of fetuses with conotruncal anomalies. J Am Coll Cardiol 1999; 33: 1696–701.

Wladimiroff JW, Stewart PA, Reuss A, Sachs ES. Cardiac and extra-cardiac anomalies as indicators for trisomies 13 and 18: a prenatal ultrasound study. Prenat Diagn 1989; 9: 515–20.

Ebstein Anomaly

Definition: Displacement of the free parts of the septal and posterior cusps of the tricuspid valve in the direction of the apex of the heart, such that the left atrium appears larger and the left ventricle smaller.

Incidence: One in 20 000 live births; less than 1% of congenital cardiac anomalies.

Sex ratio: M : F = 1 : 1.

Clinical history/genetics: Sporadic, multifactorial inheritance: recurrence rate of 1% if one sibling and 3% if two siblings are affected.

Teratogens: Lithium.

Associated malformations: Micrognathia, renal aplasia, megacolon, undescended testes, low-set ears.

Ultrasound findings: Due to adhesions of the septal and posterior cusps of the valve to the adjoining septum and the free wall of the right ventricle, *the tricuspid valve appears to be displaced towards the cardiac apex.* The right atrium is enlarged. Part of the right ventricle lies within the atrium. *Tricuspid valve incompetence* is a concomitant finding, and in severe cases *pulmonary stenosis* is present. From the physiological point of view, the tricuspid valve lies more apically than the mitral valve. However, if the tricuspid valve lies more than 15 mm lower towards the apex and tricuspid incompetence is diagnosed, it is more likely to be an Ebstein anomaly. The following intracardiac anomalies have to be excluded: VSD, inverted ventricle, Fallot's tetralogy, anomalies of the mitral valve, coarctation of the aorta, atrial septal defect, and anomaly of the pulmonary vein.

Clinical management: Further ultrasound screening is necessary. Karyotyping should be carried out, although chromosomal aberrations are rare in Ebstein anomaly. For prognostic evaluation, a pediatric cardiologist should be consulted. Regular monitoring is advised because of the risk of tachyarrhythmia (Wolff–Parkinson–White syndrome) developing during the course of pregnancy. Cardiac failure may result secondary to severe tricuspid incompetence. Vaginal delivery is possible as long as cardiac failure and hydrops are not diagnosed.

Procedure after birth: This is an anomaly causing cyanosis. In certain cases, administration of prostaglandin improves perfusion of the lungs. Severe cyanosis, decreasing physical performance and compression of the right lung due to an enlarged atrium may make surgical intervention necessary. Cardiac arrhythmia can be treated by ablation of additional atrioventricular conduction systems using cardiac catheterization.

Prognosis: This depends on the severity of pulmonary stenosis. If only the tricuspid valve is involved, then the prognosis is favorable. In these cases, cardiac surgery is not necessary. An unfavorable prognosis is expected if severe pulmonary stenosis or pulmonary atresia is present.

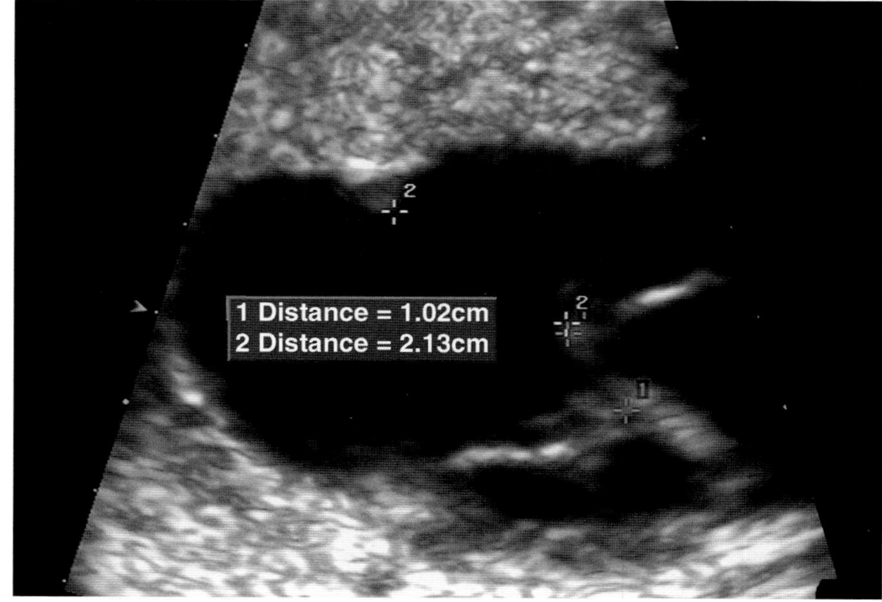

Fig. 5.**11** **Ebstein anomaly,** 38 weeks. The right ventricle is considerably smaller compared to the left, and the tricuspid valve is displaced about 10 mm in the direction of the cardiac apex. Both atria are significantly enlarged.

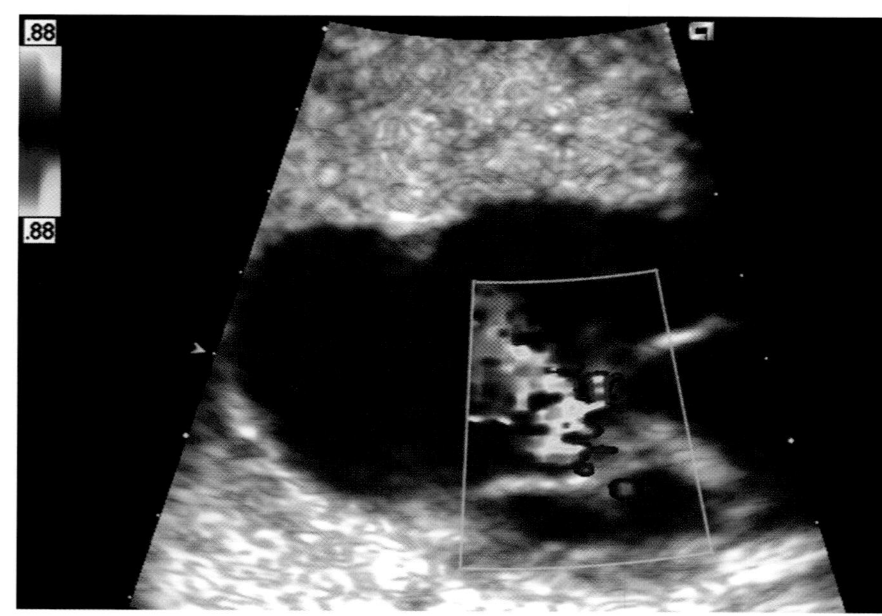

Fig. 5.**12** **Tricuspid valve insufficiency.** Depiction using color flow mapping.

1
2
3
4
5

References

Benson CB, Brown DL, Roberts DI. Uhl's anomaly of the heart mimicking Ebstein's anomaly in utero. J Ultrasound Med 1995; 14: 781–3.

Chaoui R, Bollmann R, Hoffmann H, Zienert A, Bartho S. Ebstein anomaly as a rare cause of a non-immunological fetal hydrops: prenatal diagnosis using Doppler echocardiography. Klin Pädiatr 1990; 202: 173–5.

Chiba Y, Kanzaki T, Kobayashi H, Murakami M, Yutani C. Evaluation of fetal structural heart disease using color flow mapping. Ultrasound Med Biol 1990; 16: 221–9.

DeLeon MA, Gidding SS, Gotteiner N, Backer CL, Mavroudis C. Successful palliation of Ebstein's malformation on the first day of life following fetal diagnosis. Cardiol Young 2000; 10: 384–7.

Durán M, Gómez I, Palacio A. Ebstein's anomaly with pulmonary hypoplasia: diagnosis with Doppler color echocardiography in the fetus. Rev Esp Cardiol 1992; 45: 541–2.

Epstein ML. Congenital stenosis and insufficiency of the tricuspid valve. In: Emmanouilides GC, Allen HD, Riemenschneider TA, Gutgesell HP, editors. Moss and Adams heart disease in infants, children, and adolescents, including the fetus and young adult. Baltimore: Williams & Wilkins, 1995: 919–29.

Faivre L, Morichon DN, Viot G, et al. Prenatal detection of a 1 p36 deletion in a fetus with multiple malformations and a review of the literature. Prenat Diagn 1999; 19: 49–53.

Silva SR, Bruner JP, Moore CA. Prenatal diagnosis of Down's syndrome in the presence of isolated Ebstein's anomaly. Fetal Diagn Ther 1999; 14: 149–51.

Song TB, Lee JY, Kim YH, Oh BS, Kim EK. Prenatal diagnosis of severe tricuspid insufficiency in Ebstein's anomaly with pulmonary atresia and intact ventricular septum: a case report. J Obstet Gynaecol Res 2000; 26: 223–6.

Ectopia Cordis/Cantrell Pentalogy

Definition: The pentalogy of Cantrell consists of five malformations: ectopia cordis, abdominal wall defect, sternoschisis, defect of the diaphragm and of the pericardium.

Incidence: Less than one in 100 000.

First description: Described by James R. Cantrell in 1958.

Sex ratio: M : F = 2 : 1.

Clinical history/genetics: Sporadic. Sometimes seen in trisomy 21.

Teratogens: Not known.

Embryology: The pentalogy of Cantrell is due to disturbance in development of the mesoderm in the early embryonic stage. This results in failure of closure of structures such as the diaphragm, sternum, pericardium, and abdominal wall and causes protrusion of the heart through this defect.

Associated malformations: Cardiac anomalies (especially VSD, ASD, pulmonary stenosis, tetralogy of Fallot), neural tube defects, omphalocele, gastroschisis, malformation of the extremities and caudal regression are the most frequently associated malformations.

Ultrasound findings: In the *thoracic form*, the sternum is split, the heart lying in front of the thorax and the cardiac apex pointing cranially. The thoracic cavity is small. In the *thoracico-abdominal form*, the defect lies further caudal and there is frequently also an omphalocele, which may even be ruptured. This is often accompanied by evisceration of the liver, stomach and intestines (laparoschisis).

Differential diagnosis: Amnion band sequence, chromosomal aberrations, "limb–body stalk" abnormality.

Clinical management: After the condition is confirmed, further diagnostic evaluation does not change the prognosis. If the mother decides to continue with the pregnancy, karyotyping should be advised.

Procedure after birth: If surgical correction is considered, then the findings should be evaluated by specialists already in the prenatal stage.

Prognosis: Surgical correction is possible only in very mild forms. The full-blown form of the pentalogy of Cantrell is fatal.

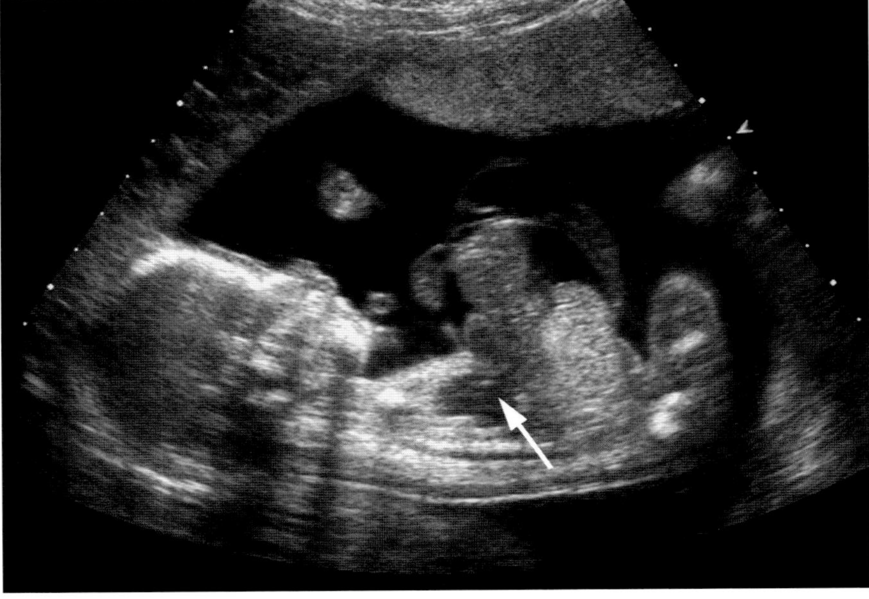

Fig. 5.**13** **Ectopia cordis.** Longitudinal section, 19 + 2 weeks. The liver and bowel have herniated through a defect in the anterior abdominal wall. The fetal heart (arrow) is partly displaced into the abdomen through a diaphragmatic hernia.

2

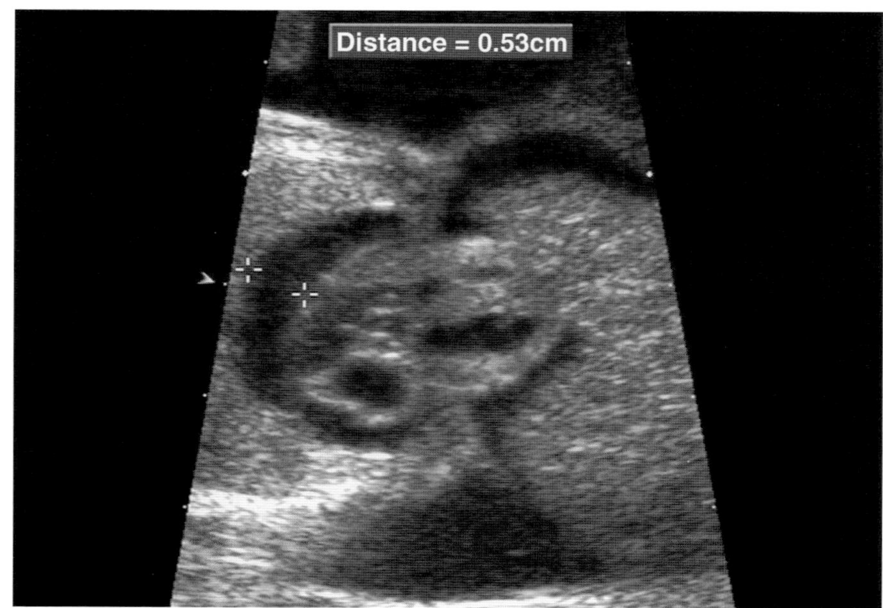

Fig. 5.**14** **Ectopia cordis.** Section at the level of upper abdomen showing herniation of fetal heart through the diaphragm.

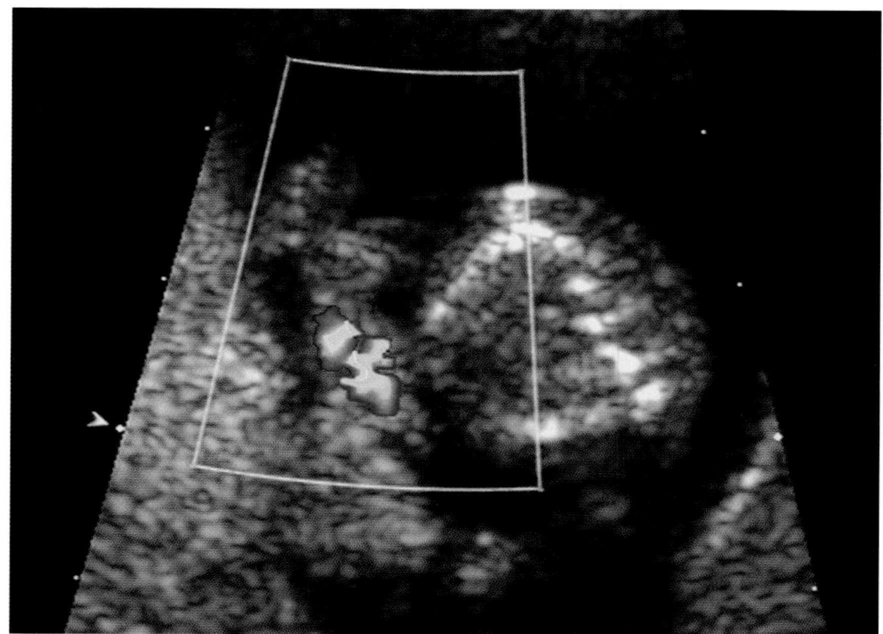
Fig. 5.**15** **Pentalogy of Cantrell,** 13 + 2 weeks. Color flow mapping, showing an ectopic fetal heart.

References

Abu YM, Wray AB, Williamson RA, Bonsib SM. Antenatal ultrasound diagnosis of variant of pentalogy of Cantrell. J Ultrasound Med 1987; 6: 535–8.

Baker ME, Rosenberg ER, Trofatter KF, Imber MJ, Bowie JD. The in utero findings in twin pentalogy of Cantrell. J Ultrasound Med 1984; 3: 525–7.

Bennett TL, Burlbaw J, Drake CK, Finley BE. Diagnosis of ectopia cordis at 12 weeks gestation using transabdominal ultrasonography with color flow Doppler. J Ultrasound Med 1991; 10: 695–6.

Bognoni V, Quartuccio A. First-trimester sonographic diagnosis of Cantrell's pentalogy with exencephaly. J Clin Ultrasound 1999; 27: 276–8.

Fleming AD, Vintzileos AM, Rodis JF, Scorza WE, Nardi D, Salafia C. Diagnosis of fetal ectopia cordis by transvaginal ultrasound. J Ultrasound Med 1991; 10: 413–5.

Ghidini A, Sirtori M, Romero R, Hobbins JC. Prenatal diagnosis of pentalogy of Cantrell. J Ultrasound Med 1988; 7: 567–72.

Haynor DR, Shuman WP, Brewer DK, Mack LA. Imaging of fetal ectopia cordis: roles of sonography and computed tomography. J Ultrasound Med 1984; 3: 25–7.

Leca F, Thibert M, Khoury W, Fermont L, Laborde F, Dumez Y. Extrathoracic heart (ectopia cordis). Report of two cases and review of the literature. Int J Cardiol 1989; 22: 221–8.

Liang RI, Huang SE, Chang FM. Prenatal diagnosis of ectopia cordis at 10 weeks of gestation using two-dimensional and three-dimensional ultrasonography. Ultrasound Obstet Gynecol 1997; 10: 137–9.

Extrasystoles (Supraventricular)

Definition: This is defined as heart beats occurring additionally to the sinus rhythm. The most frequent cause of extrasystoles is premature contractions of the atrium, which appear more than 8 ms prior to the expected atrial contractions. The stimulation arises mostly from an ectopic focus within the atrium and not from the sinoatrial node.

Incidence: Seen often in the early stage of the third trimester.

Clinical history/genetics: Caffeine intake by the mother has been described as a possible cause. Certain drugs may also be responsible (fenoterol and some vasoactive substances such as those in nasal sprays).

Associated malformations: Structural cardiac anomalies; 1 % of cases may be complicated by development of supraventricular tachycardia.

Ultrasound findings: The *arrhythmic contractions* are first diagnosed in B-mode. They can be differentiated further using M-mode.

Clinical management: Further sonographic screening, including fetal echocardiography, to exclude cardiac anomaly. Weekly control of the heart frequency is necessary for early detection and treatment of supraventricular tachycardia, before the development of cardiac failure with fetal hydrops. Abstinence from caffeine is advised and β-mimetics should be avoided.

Procedure after birth: If the arrhythmia is present until just before birth, then 24-h monitoring of the heart frequency of the newborn is recommended. ECG is useful.

Prognosis: Spontaneous remission in the late stages of pregnancy or just after birth is the usual course.

References

Bollmann R, Chaoui R, Schilling H, Hoffmann H, Reiche M, Pahl L. Prenatal diagnosis and management of fetal arrhythmias. Z Geburtshilfe Perinatol 1988; 192: 266–72.

Fyfe DA, Meyer KB, Case CL. Sonographic assessment of fetal cardiac arrhythmias. Semin Ultrasound CT MR 1993; 14: 286–97.

Goraya JS, Parmar VR. Fetal and neonatal extrasystoles. Indian Pediatr 2000; 37: 784–6.

Hata T, Takamori H, Hata K, Takamiya O, Murao F, Kitao M. Antenatal diagnosis of congenital heart disease and fetal arrhythmia by ultrasound: prospective study. Gynecol Obstet Invest 1988; 26: 118–25.

Kleinman CS, Hobbies JC, Jaffe CC, Lynch DC, Talner NS. Echocardiographic studies of the human fetus: prenatal diagnosis of congenital heart disease and cardiac dysrhythmias. Pediatrics 1980; 65: 1059–67.

Pál A, Gembruch U, Hansmann M. Practical importance of the exact diagnosis of fetal arrhythmias. Orv Hetil 1991; 132: 1359–62.

Southall DP, Richards J, Hardwick RA, et al. Prospective study of fetal heart rate and rhythm patterns. Arch Dis Child 1980; 55: 506–11.

Tsujimoto H, Takeshita S, Kawamura Y, Nakatani K, Sato M. Isolated congenital left ventricular diverticulum with perinatal dysrhythmia: a case report and review of the literature. Pediatr Cardiol 2000; 21: 175–9.

Tetralogy of Fallot

Definition: A combined cardiac malformation consisting of four anomalies: VSD, pulmonary stenosis, hypertrophy of the right heart (postnatal) and overriding of the aorta (over VSD).

Incidence: One in 2000 births, 6–10% of all congenital heart malformations.

Clinical history/genetics: Mostly a sporadic, multifactorial inheritance. Recurrence rate of 2.5% with one affected sibling and of 8% when two siblings are affected; in case of an affected mother the probability of recurrence is 2.5 %, and with an affected father it is 1.5%. Autosomal-dominant inheritance has also been reported in rare cases.

Teratogens: High doses of Vitamin A, thalidomide, trimethadione, sexual steroids and alcohol.

Associated malformations: Extracardiac malformations are seen in a total of 16%.

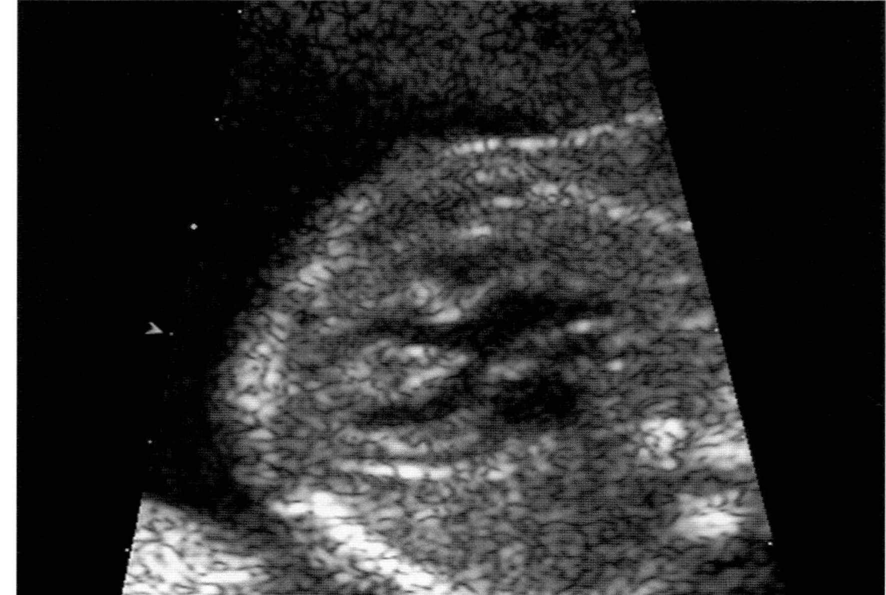

Fig. 5.**16** **Tetralogy of Fallot,** 22 weeks. A membranous ventricular septal defect is clearly seen. An overriding aorta is also diagnosed; it is wider than the pulmonary trunk.

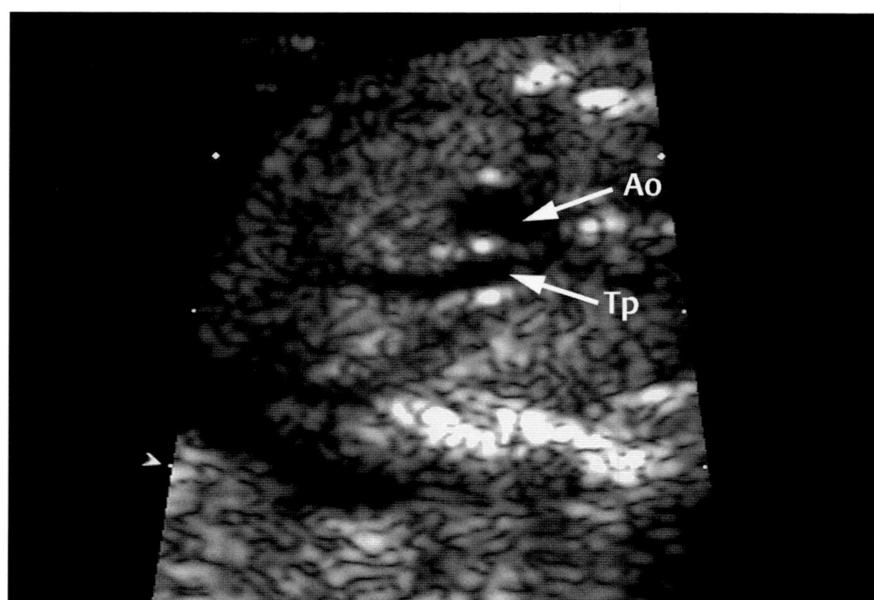

Fig. 5.**17** **Tetralogy of Fallot.** Outflow tract of the fetal heart, showing the aorta and pulmonary artery. This differs from the normal findings in that the diameter of the aorta (AO) is greater than that of the pulmonary trunk (Tp).

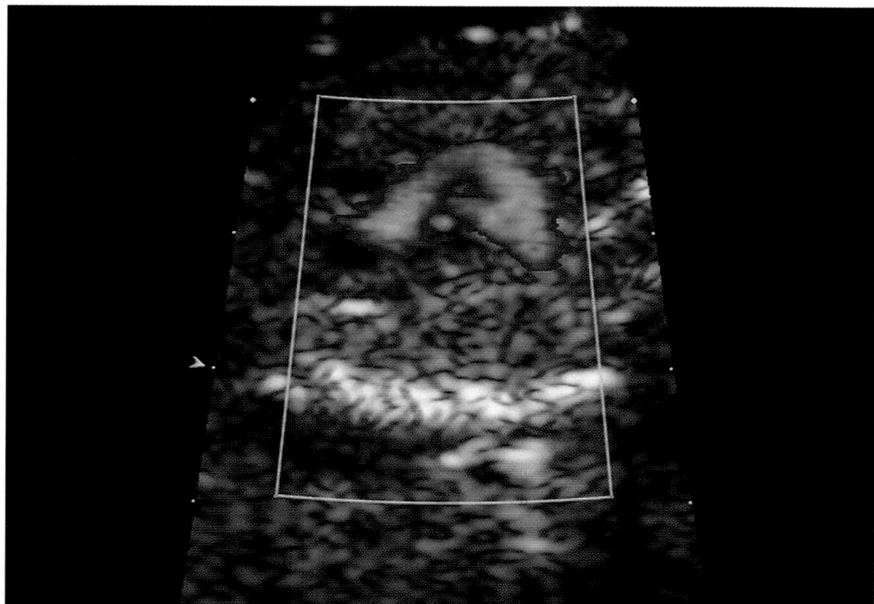

Fig. 5.**18** **Tetralogy of Fallot.** Color flow mapping (color Doppler energy), showing aortic widening and narrowing of the pulmonary trunk.

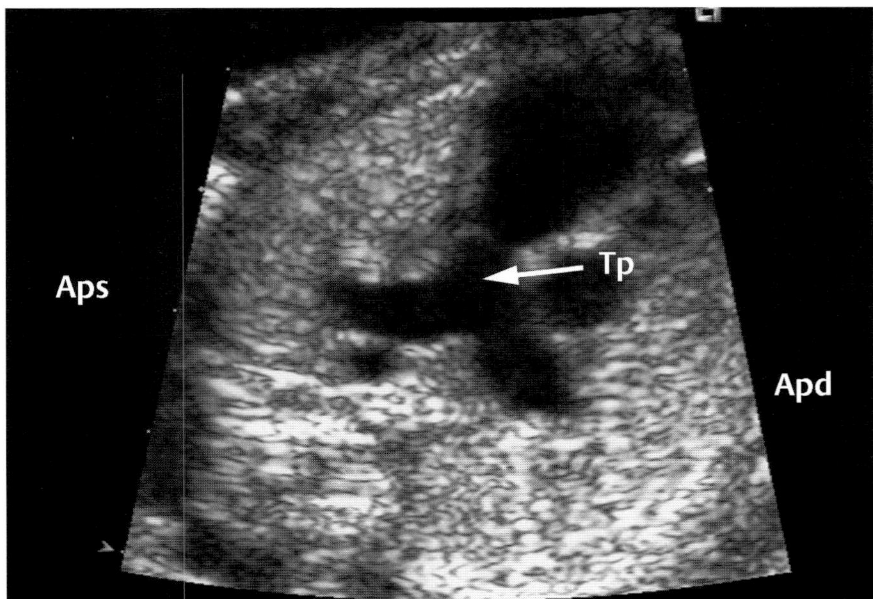

Fig. 5.**19** **Tetralogy of Fallot** with absent pulmonary valve: the pulmonary trunk (Tp) branches into the right (dextra, Apd) and left (sinistra, Aps) pulmonary arteries. Both are significantly dilated. The ductus arteriosus (Botallo's duct) is not seen.

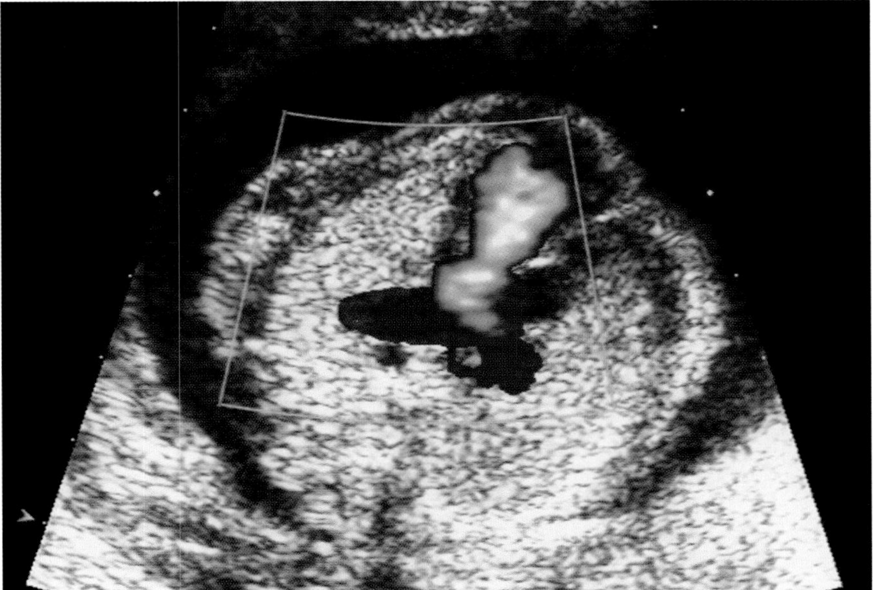

Fig. 5.**20** **Tetralogy of Fallot.** Color flow mapping of the same case. In the diastolic phase, a large amount of blood flows back into the right ventricle through the dysplastic pulmonary valve.

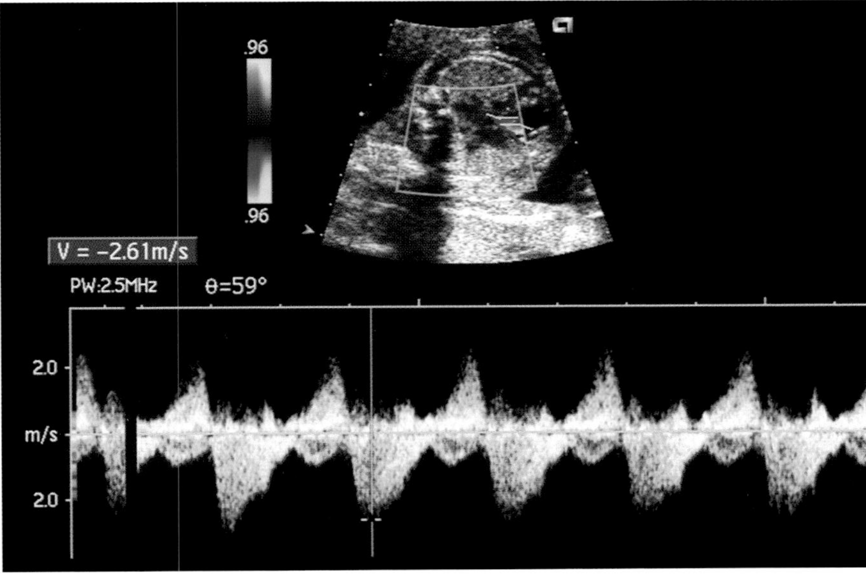

Fig. 5.**21** **Tetralogy of Fallot.** Pulsed Doppler ultrasound, showing blood flowing in both directions through a dysplastic pulmonary valve.

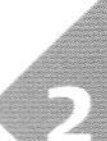

Associated syndromes: De Lange syndrome, Klippel–Feil syndrome, VACTERL association, CHARGE association, Goldenhar syndrome, hemifacial microsomy syndrome, chromosomal anomalies (especially trisomy 21 and 18, Di George syndrome, partial monosomy 22 q).

Ultrasound findings: *Subaortic ventricle septum defect, pulmonary stenosis and a relatively widened aorta overriding the VSD* are characteristic findings. Hypertrophy of the right ventricle develops actually after birth. The pulmonary stenosis may be located in the infundibular region. The pulmonary trunk is smaller than the aorta. Sometimes an ASD may also exist. Hydramnios is a frequent finding.

Clinical management: Further screening of the other organs. Karyotyping, counseling with pediatric cardiologist and advising the parents. In cases of complete pulmonary atresia, development of fetal hydrops is possible. Vaginal delivery is possible in almost all cases. If fetal hydrops is present, delivery by cesarean section may be indicated, but this is controversial because of the poor prognosis.

Procedure after birth: This is a cardiac anomaly causing cyanosis, so that intensive care of the neonate is necessary. Prostaglandin administration early on in therapy. Oxygen therapy above 40–60% is not given concomitantly with prostaglandin treatment. Surgical intervention is mostly during the first year of life.

Prognosis: The prognosis in tetralogy of Fallot is favorable in the absence of pulmonary atresia. Surgical correction is always necessary. The perioperative mortality lies between 2% and 7%. After correction, the quality of life is mostly good. Repeated surgical intervention is rarely needed.

References

Achiron R, Golan PN, Gabbay U, et al. In utero ultrasonographic measurements of fetal aortic and pulmonary artery diameters during the first half of gestation. Ultrasound Obstet Gynecol 1998; 11: 180–4.

Achiron R, Rotstein Z, Lipitz S, Mashiach S, Hegesh J. First-trimester diagnosis of fetal congenital heart disease by transvaginal ultrasonography. Obstet Gynecol 1994; 84: 69–72.

Anderson CF, McCurdy CMJ, McNamara MF, Reed KL. Diagnosis: color Doppler aided diagnosis of tetralogy of Fallot. J Ultrasound Med 1994; 13: 341–2.

Becker R, Schmitz L, Guschmann M, Wegner RD, Stiemer B, Entezami M. Prenatal diagnosis of familial absent pulmonary valve syndrome: case report and review of the literature. Ultrasound Obstet Gynecol 2001; 17: 263–7.

Benacerraf BR, Pober BR, Sanders SP. Accuracy of fetal echocardiography. Radiology 1987; 165: 847–9.

Lee W, Smith RS, Comstock CH, Kirk JS, Riggs T, Weinhouse E. Tetralogy of Fallot: prenatal diagnosis and postnatal survival. Obstet Gynecol 1995; 86: 583–8.

Moon-Grady AJ, Tacy TA, Brook MM, Hanley FL, Silverman NH. Value of clinical and echocardiographic features in predicting outcome in the fetus, infant, and child with tetralogy of Fallot with absent pulmonary valve complex. Am J Cardiol 2002; 89: 1280–5.

Hypoplasia of the Left Heart

Definition: This is defined as hypoplasia of the left ventricle associated with aortic stenosis or atresia and a severe mitral stenosis.

Incidence: One in 10 000 births.

Sex ratio: M : F = 2 : 1.

Clinical history/genetics: Multifactorial inheritance, recurrence rate with one affected sibling circa 3%, with two affected siblings 10%. Autosomal-recessive inheritance has also been occasionally described.

Teratogens: High doses of vitamin A, diabetes mellitus.

Associated malformations: Turner syndrome, trisomies, situs inversus, renal agenesis, omphalocele and diaphragmatic hernia. Twenty-nine percent of cases show anomalies of the central nervous system (microcephalus, holoprosencephaly, agenesis of the corpus callosum).

Ultrasound findings: *The left ventricle is very small* and the right ventricle comparatively large. The apex of the left ventricle ends more proximally than that of the right. *Mitral and aortic valves show hypoplasia* rarely showing atresia. Hypoplasia of the aorta is common and it is filled often through retrograde flow from the ductus arteriosus (Botallo's duct). The left atrium is small. In some cases, the full-blown form is

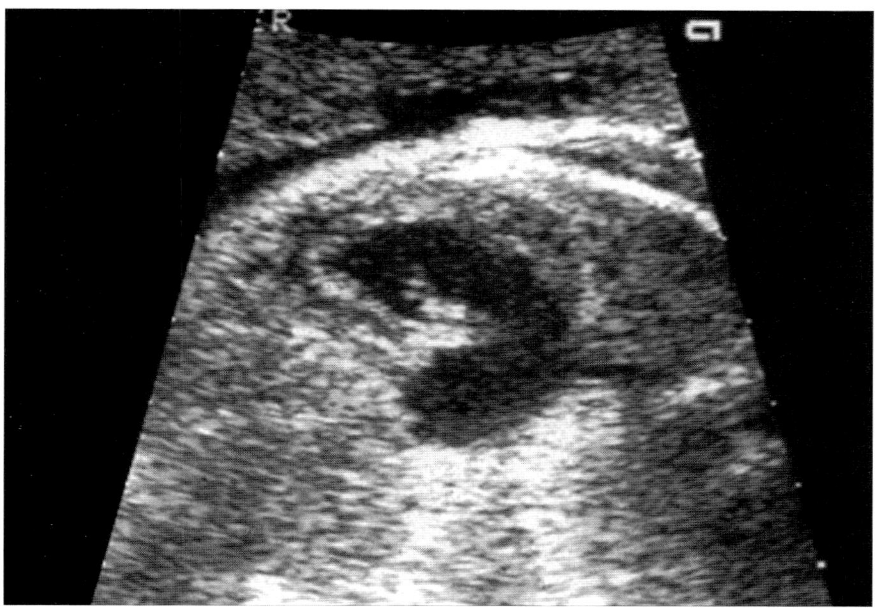

Fig. 5.**22** **Hypoplastic left heart syndrome,** 22 weeks. The left ventricle is seen as an echogenic structure, significantly smaller than normal, next to a large right ventricle (in the diastolic phase the tricuspid valve is open).

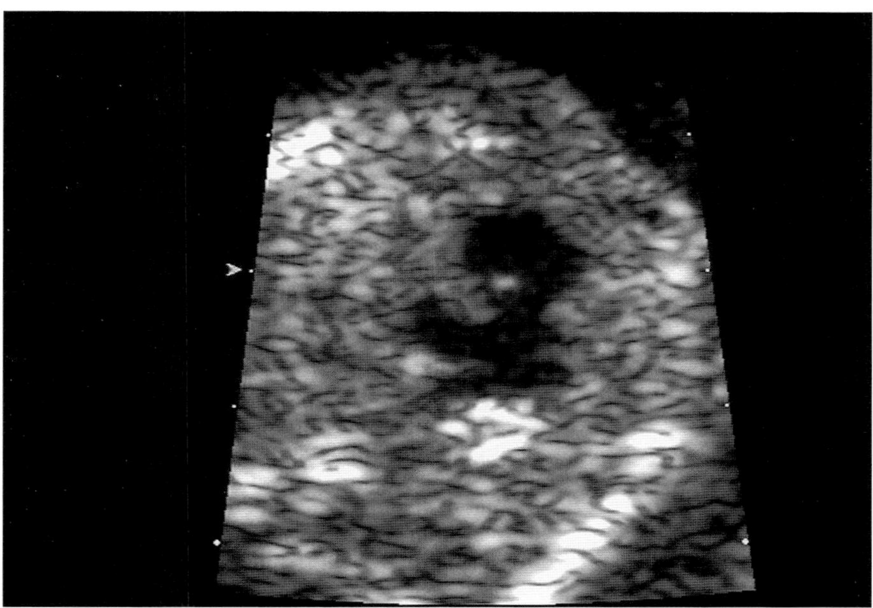

Fig. 5.**23** **Hypoplastic left heart syndrome.** Four-chamber view at 19 + 1 weeks, with a large right ventricle. The atria are seen, but not the left ventricle.

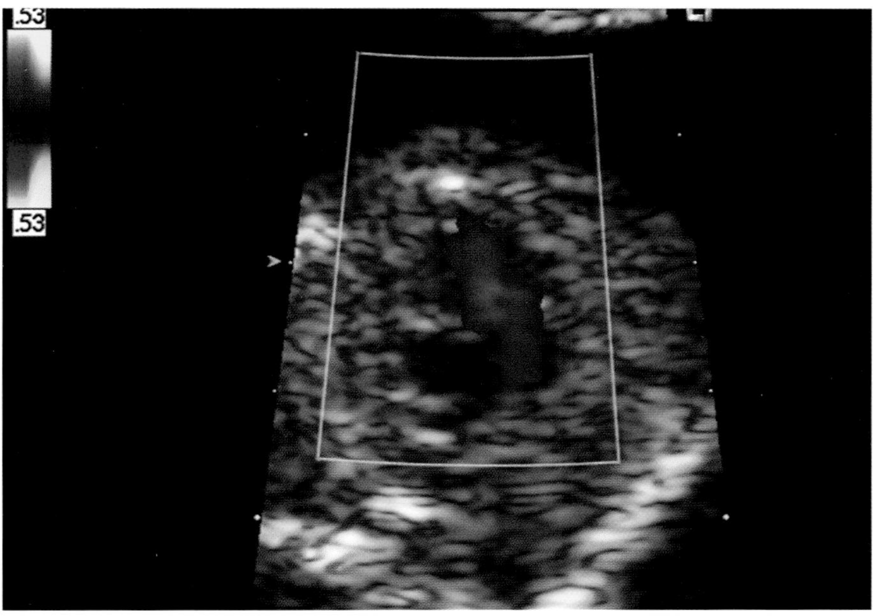

Fig. 5.**24** **Hypoplastic left heart syndrome.** Same situation as before; color flow mapping shows blood flowing into the right ventricle, but flow into the left ventricle is not evident.

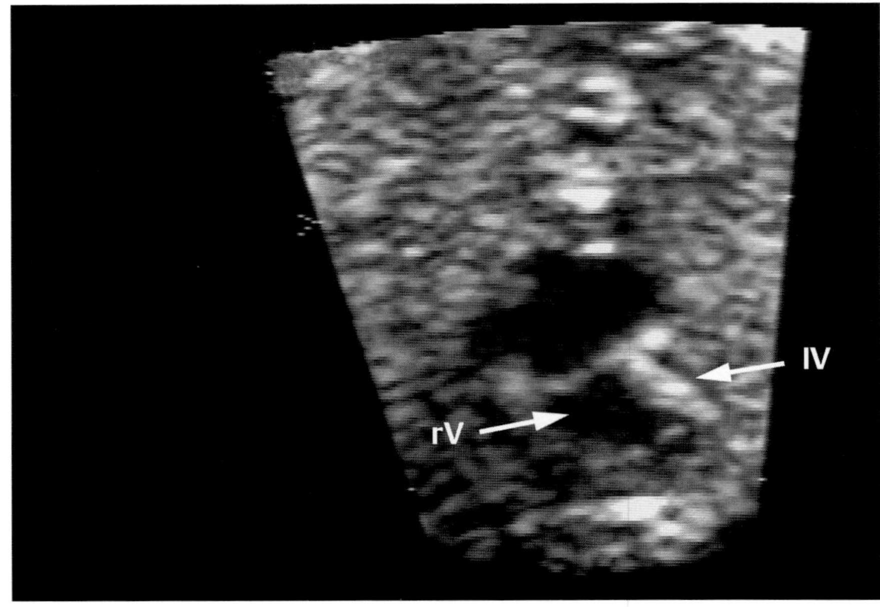

Fig. 5.**25** **Hypoplastic left heart syndrome,** 15 weeks, four-chamber view (apical), transvaginal sonography. The right ventricle (rV) appears large in comparison with the left ventricle (lV), which is barely visible.

seen for the first time as late as in the third trimester.

Clinical management: Further sonographic screening. Karyotyping, consultation with pediatric cardiologist. Vaginal delivery is possible.

Procedure after birth: As this anomaly is associated with and dependent on the Botallo's duct, oxygen administration should not exceed 40–60%. Therapy with prostaglandin should start immediately after birth.

Prognoses: This is a fatal condition without surgical intervention. Cardiac surgical procedures such as the Norwood operation (at least three surgical corrections) are performed, with survival rates of 20–70%. Heart transplantation has also been tried in these children recently; the success rate has been reported to be as high as 70%. In the long run, the quality of life after these interventions remains limited. After the Norwood operation, persistent neurological deficits have been described in up to 70% of the infants.

References

Allan LD. Fetal diagnosis of fatal congenital heart disease. J Heart Lung Transplant 1993; 12: S159–60.
Allan LD, Cook A, Sullivan I, Sharland GK. Hypoplastic left heart syndrome: effects of fetal echocardiography on birth prevalence. Lancet 1991; 337: 959–61.
Anderson NG, Brown J. Normal size left ventricle on antenatal scan in lethal hypoplastic left heart syndrome. Pediatr Radiol 1991; 21: 436–7.
Andrews R, Tulloh R, Sharland G, et al. Outcome of staged reconstructive surgery for hypoplastic left heart syndrome following antenatal diagnosis. Arch Dis Child 2001; 85: 474–7.
Bauer J, Thul J, Kramer U, et al. Heart transplantation in children and infants: short-term outcome and long-term follow-up. Pediatr Transplant 2001; 5: 457–62.
Byrne BM, Morrison JJ. Prenatal diagnosis of lethal fetal malformation in Irish obstetric practice. Ir Med J 1999; 92: 271–3.
Cartier MS, Emerson D, Plappert T, Sutton MS. Hypoplastic left heart with absence of the aortic valve: prenatal diagnosis using two-dimensional and pulsed Doppler echocardiography. JCU J Clin Ultrasound 1987; 15: 463–8.
Gaynor JW, Mahle WT, Cohen MI, et al. Risk factors for mortality after the Norwood procedure. Eur J Cardiothorac Surg 2002; 22: 82–9.
Krause M, Lunkenheimer A, Kohler W, Fischer T, Feige A. [Prenatal diagnosis of hypoplastic left heart syndrome: indications for abortion or transplantation; in German]. Z Geburtshilfe Perinatol 1995; 199: 42–5.
Mandorla S, Narducci PL, Migliozzi L, Pagliacci M, Cucchia G. Fetal echocardiography: prenatal diagnosis of hypoplastic left heart syndrome. G Ital Cardiol 1984; 14: 517–20.
Pizarro C, Davis DA, Galantowicz ME, Munro H, Gidding SS, Norwood WI. Stage I palliation for hypoplastic left heart syndrome in low birth weight neonates: can we justify it? Eur J Cardiothorac Surg 2002; 21: 716–20.
Sahn DJ, Shenker L, Reed KL, Valdes CL, Sobonya R, Anderson C. Prenatal ultrasound diagnosis of hypoplastic left heart syndrome in utero associated with hydrops fetalis. Am Heart J 1982; 104: 1368–72.
Vincent RN, Menticoglou S, Chanas D, Manning F, Collins GF, Smallhorn J. Prenatal diagnosis of an unusual form of hypoplastic left heart syndrome. J Ultrasound Med 1987; 6: 261–4.

Cardiac Rhabdomyomas

Definition: The cardiac rhabdomyoma is a benign tumor arising from the cardiac musculature.

Incidence: One in 20 000 births.

Sex ratio: M : F = 1 : 1.

Clinical history/genetics: Sporadic. Autosomal-dominant inheritance when associated with tuberous sclerosis of the brain.

Teratogens: Not known.

Embryology: Benign tumor of the heart musculature.

Associated malformations: In 50–86% of cases, cardiac tumors are associated with tuberous sclerosis of the brain. On the other hand, rhabdomyomas are detected in 50% of fetuses with tuberous sclerosis. Renal anomalies are also associated.

Ultrasound findings: Echocardiography demonstrates an intracardiac tumor with a connection to the ventricular septum. Tachyarrhythmias

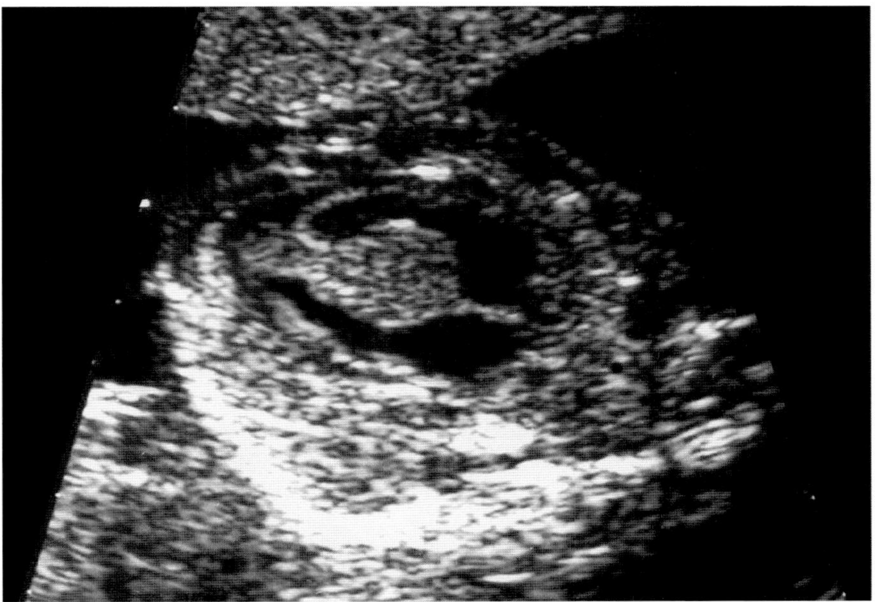

Fig. 5.26 **Cardiac rhabdomyoma.** Solitary cardiac rhabdomyoma of the ventricular septum, measuring approx. 10 mm in diameter, at 22 + 1 weeks.

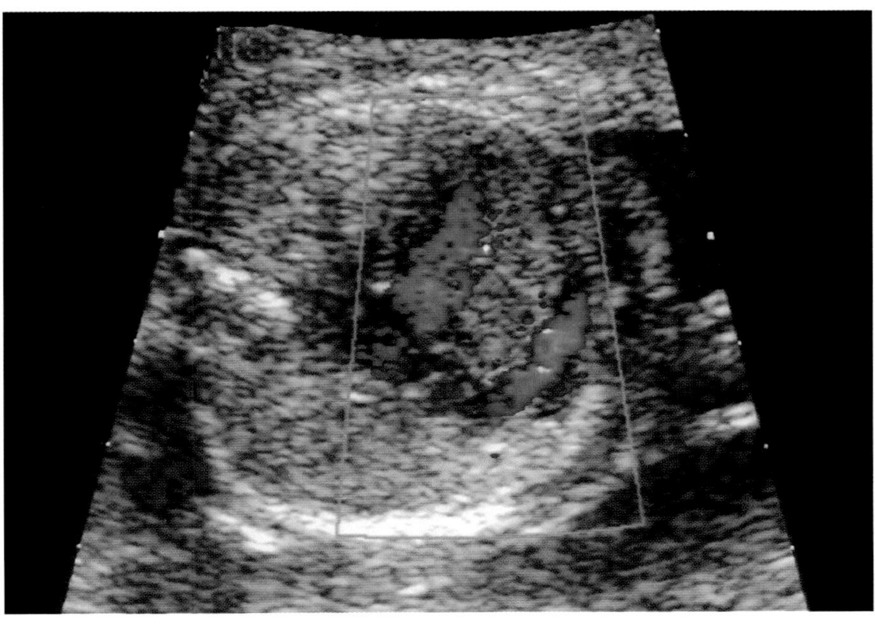

Fig. 5.27 **Cardiac rhabdomyoma.** Color flow mapping, showing blood flow into both ventricles.

2

occur concomitantly. In addition, cardiac failure or fetal hydrops may develop.

Differential diagnosis: Intracardiac fibromas, most frequently in the left ventricle, occasionally calcified. Teratomas, usually located outside of the cardiac cavity.

Clinical management: Further sonographic screening of other organs. Family history: is there a history of tuberous sclerosis? Ultrasound monitoring at regular intervals. Specific therapy if tachyarrhythmia develops. Diagnosis of cardiac insufficiency or fetal hydrops in the third trimester may make premature delivery necessary.

Procedure after birth: In small lesions not causing obstruction of the outflow tract, expectant management is advisable, as frequently these tumors regress spontaneously. Complete resection of larger lesions may not be always possible. Desperate cases have been reported in which heart transplantation had to be performed in the newborn.

Prognosis: The prognosis is usually good due to the possibility of spontaneous regression ("apoptosis"). As long as hemodynamic complications do not appear, specific therapy is not necessary. Large lesions may have deleterious effects. The overall mortality lies at 30%. In tuberous sclerosis of the brain, fits, mental retardation and various other types of tumor are associated.

References

Achiron R, Weissman A, Rotstein Z, Lipitz S, Mashiach S Hegesh J. Transvaginal echocardiographic examination of the fetal heart between 13 and 15 weeks' gestation in a low-risk population. J Ultrasound Med 1994; 13: 783–9

Calhoun BC, Watson PT, and Hegge F. Ultrasound diagnosis of an obstructive cardiac rhabdomyoma with severe hydrops and hypoplastic lungs: a case report. J Reprod Med 1991; 36: 317–9.

Deeg KH, Voigt HJ, Hofbeck M, Singer H, Kraus J. Prenatal ultrasound diagnosis of multiple cardiac rhabdomyomas. Pediatr Radiol 1990; 20: 291–2.

Green KW, Bors KR, Pollack P, Weinbaum PJ. Antepartum diagnosis and management of multiple fetal cardiac tumors. J Ultrasound Med 1991; 10: 697–9.

Guschmann M, Entezami M, Becker R, Vogel M. Intrauterine rhabdomyoma of the heart. Gen Diagn Pathol 1997; 143: 255–8.

Gushiken BJ, Callen PW Silverman NH. Prenatal diagnosis of tuberous sclerosis in monozygotic twins with cardiac masses. J Ultrasound Med 1999; 18: 165–8.

Hoadley SD, Wallace RL, Miller IF, Murgo JP. Prenatal diagnosis of multiple cardiac tumors presenting as an arrhythmia. JCU J Clin Ultrasound 1986; 14: 639–43.

Krapp M, Baschat AA, Gembruch U, Gloeckner K, Schwinger E, Reusche E. Tuberous sclerosis with intracardiac rhabdomyoma in a fetus with trisomy 21: case report and review of literature. Prenat Diagn 1999; 19: 610–3.

Sonigo P, Elmaleh A, Fermont L, Delezoide AL, Mirlesse V, Brunelle F. Prenatal MRI diagnosis of fetal cerebral tuberous sclerosis. Pediatr Radiol 1996; 26: 1–4.

Stanford W, Abu YM, Smith W. Intracardiac tumor (rhabdomyoma) diagnosed by in utero ultrasound: case report. JCU J Clin Ultrasound 1987; 15: 337–34.

Tachycardia

Definition: Fetal heart frequency of above 180 beats per minute (bpm).

Incidence: 0.5–1%, most frequently as supraventricular reentry tachycardia, over additional conduction points, rarely as a result of atrial flutter, atrial fibrillation or sinus tachycardia.

Clinical history/genetics: Supraventricular tachycardia or Wolff–Parkinson–White syndrome in the family, but usually sporadic. Sometimes there is a history of infections.

Associated malformations: Cardiac anomalies in 5% (Ebstein anomaly, corrected transposition) and rhabdomyoma, fetal hydrops.

Ultrasound findings: Diagnosis is made in B-mode and differentiation with M-mode.

Atrial fibrillation: atrial frequency of above 400 bpm, variable AV conduction (absolute arrhythmia).

Atrial flutter: atrial frequency of 280–320 bpm, frequently 1 : 2 AV conduction, frequency of chamber 160–300 bpm.

Supraventricular tachycardia: 1 : 1 conduction with a frequency of 200–300 bpm, occasionally only intermittent occurrence with a sudden change to normal frequency.

Sinus tachycardia: 1 : 1 conduction with a frequency of 180–190 bpm. Development of fetal hydrops unlikely. Seen typically in amnion infection, maternal fever, or medication with sympathomimetic agents.

Ventricular tachycardia: normal atrial rhythm with an increased frequency in the heart chamber. Mostly benign.

Clinical management: Further sonographic screening, including fetal echocardiography. Intermittent ultrasound monitoring. M-mode echocardiography. Depending on the form and cause of the tachyarrhythmia, initially therapy with transplacental medication (e.g., digoxin and flecainide, possibly sotalol). If this therapy is not successful, or in case of fetal hydrops, direct administration of agents into the umbilical vein (e.g., amiodarone is favorable due to its long half-life; side effects include hypothyroidism in the fetus). This treatment option should only be used in units with experience in prenatal cardiology. In a mature fetus, delivery and postnatal therapy is an option. Vaginal delivery is possible.

Procedure after birth: After birth, facilities for intensive medical treatment are required. In severe cases that do not respond to this, electrophysiological diagnosis and intervention with ablation of extra conduction points or other structures determining the cardiac rhythm using a catheter can be an option as the last resort.

Prognosis: Fetal hydrops develops within 48 h in case of fetal tachycardia of 220–240 bpm. The mortality is very high in these cases. The tachycardias are usually well treatable using medications.

References

Chang CL, Chao AS, Wu CD, Lien R, Cheng PJ. Ultrasound recognition and treatment of fetal supraventricular tachycardia with hydrops: a case report. Chang Keng I Hsueh Tsa Chih 1998; 21: 217–21.

Fyfe DA, Meyer KB, Case CL. Sonographic assessment of fetal cardiac arrhythmias. Semin Ultrasound CT MR 1993; 14: 286–97.

Gembruch U, Bald R, Hansmann M. Color-coded M-mode Doppler echocardiography in the diagnosis of fetal arrhythmia. Geburtshilfe Frauenheilkd 1990; 50: 286–90.

Gembruch U, Hansmann M, Bald R, Redel BA. Supraventricular tachycardia of the fetus in the 3rd trimester of pregnancy following persistent supraventricular extrasystole. Geburtshilfe Frauenheilkd 1987; 47: 656–9.

John JB, Bricker JT, Fenrich AL, et al. Fetal diagnosis of right ventricular aneurysm associated with supraventricular tachycardia with left bundle-branch block aberrancy. Circulation 2002; 106: 141–2.

Jouannic JM, Le Bidois J, Fermont L, et al. Prenatal ultrasound may predict fetal response to therapy in non-hydropic fetuses with supraventricular tachycardia. Fetal Diagn Ther 2002; 17: 120–3.

King CR, Mattioli L, Goertz KK, Snodgrass W. Successful treatment of fetal supraventricular tachycardia with maternal digoxin therapy. Chest 1984; 85: 573–5.

Krapp M, Baschat AA, Gembruch U, Geipel A, Germer U. Flecainide in the intrauterine treatment of fetal supraventricular tachycardia. Ultrasound Obstet Gynecol 2002; 19: 158–64.

Kühl PG, Ulmer HE, Schmidt W, Wille L. Non-immunologic hydrops fetalis: report of 14 cases and literature review. Klin Pädiatr 1985; 197: 282–7.

Shirley IM, Richards BA, Ward RH. Ultrasound diagnosis of hydrops fetalis due to fetal tachycardia. Br J Radiol 1981; 54: 815–7.

Simpson LL, Marx GR. Diagnosis and treatment of structural fetal cardiac abnormality and dysrhythmia. Semin Perinatol 1994; 18: 215–27.

Wester HA, Grimm G, Lehmann F. Echocardiographic diagnosis of fetal heart insufficiency caused by supraventricular tachycardia. Z Kardiol 1984; 73: 405–8.

Transposition of the Great Arteries (TGA)

Definition: In *D-TGA,* the aorta arises from the right ventricle and lies ventral and to the right (D, dextro-) of the pulmonary artery. The pulmonary artery arises posteriorly from the left ventricle. In *L-TGA* (corrected transposition; L, levo-), the atrioventricular and ventriculoarterial connections are discordant, so that the hemodynamic situation is corrected.

Incidence: One in 2000 births, 5% of all congenital heart disease.

Clinical history/genetics: Recurrence rate in case of one affected sibling is 1.5%, in case of two affected siblings 5%.

Teratogens: High doses of vitamin A, amphetamines, trimethadione, sexual steroids.

Associated malformations: Situs inversus.

Ultrasound findings: The two great vessels run parallel to each other instead of crossing. The *aorta* arises from the right ventricle and runs ventral to the pulmonary trunk, which arises from the left ventricle. The aorta is identified because of its arch and the branches arising from it. The pulmonary trunk is recognized due to its bifurcation into the right and left pulmonary arteries. The isthmus of the aorta may show stenosis. In 40% of cases, a concomitant VSD and

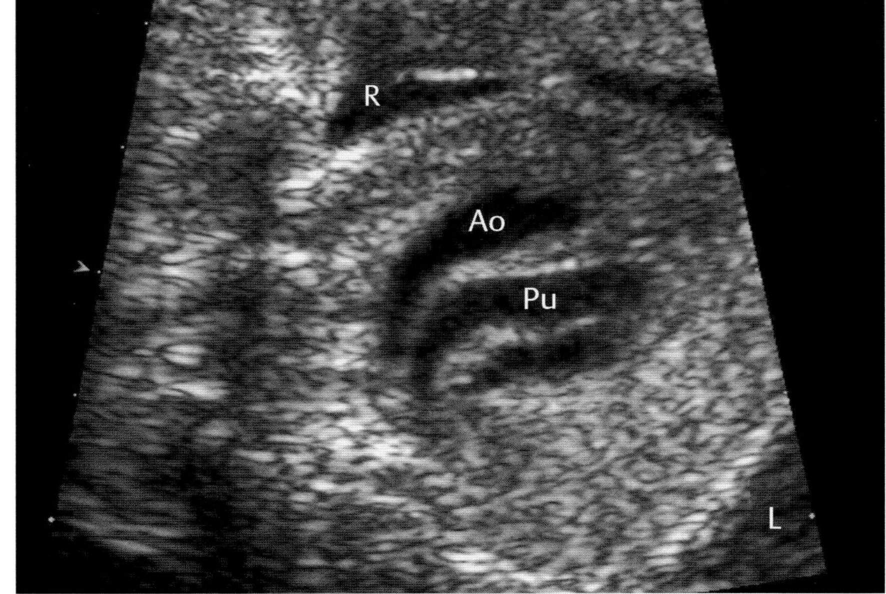

Fig. 5.**28** **Transposition of the great arteries.** Parallel course of the outgoing vessels in right-sided TGA (dextro-TGA). The aorta is coursing on the right. R: right, L: left.

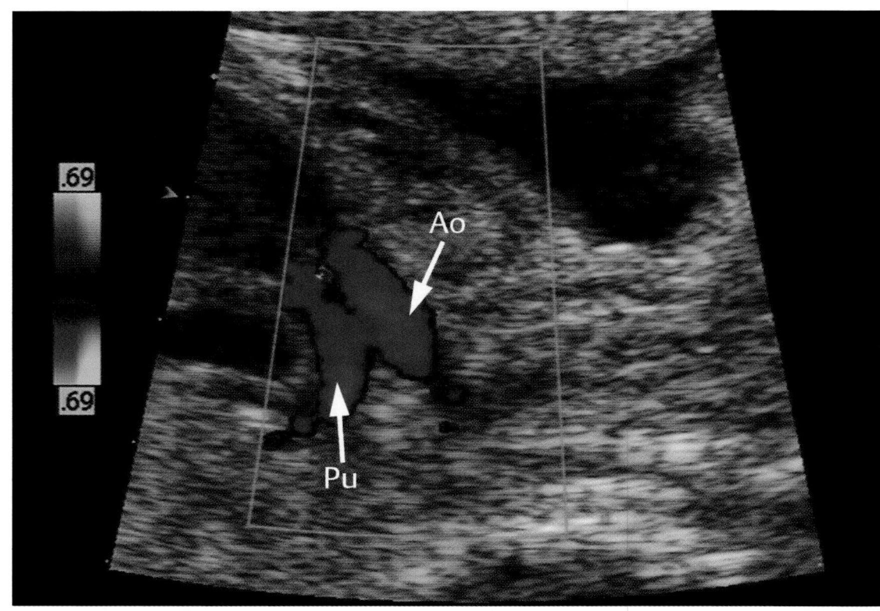

Fig. 5.**29** **Transposition of the great arteries.** The outflow tract of the heart at 21 + 5 weeks, shown using color flow mapping. The outflowing vessels do not cross, but run parallel to each other. (Ao: aorta, Pu: pulmonary artery.)

frequently also ASD are present. If a VSD is found, there is stenosis of the pulmonary artery in 35% of the cases.

Clinical management: Further sonographic screening. Karyotyping, regular ultrasound checks (if there is an obstruction of the outflow tracts, cardiac failure may develop). Vaginal delivery is possible.

Procedure after birth: This anomaly causes cyanosis. Prostaglandin is administered to keep the ductus arteriosus open; oxygen therapy should not exceed 40–60% in this case. If the oval foramen is constricted, widening of the atrial septum using a balloon catheter may be necessary prior to surgery. Surgical procedures such as the arterial switch operation are possible in the first 2 weeks of life.

Prognosis: The long-term prognosis after surgical correction is good. The mortality rate associated with the switch operation is 5% in the absence of other cardiac malformations.

References

Allan LD, Anderson RH, Cook AC. Atresia or absence of the left-sided atrioventricular connection in the fetus: echocardiographic diagnosis and outcome. Ultrasound Obstet Gynecol 1996; 8: 295–302.

Arias F, Retto H. The use of Doppler waveform analysis in the evaluation of the high-risk fetus. Obstet Gynecol Clin North Am 1988; 15: 265–81.

Bonnet D, Sidi D. What's new in pediatric cardiology? Arch Pediatr 1999; 6: 777–80.

Hafner E, Scholler J, Schuchter K, Sterniste W, Philipp K. Detection of fetal congenital heart disease in a low-risk population. Prenat Diagn 1998; 18: 808–15.

Hyett JA, Perdu M, Sharland GK, Snijders RS, Nicolaides KH. Increased nuchal translucency at 10–14 weeks of gestation as a marker for major cardiac defects. Ultrasound Obstet Gynecol 1997; 10: 242–6.

Kumar RK, Newburger JW, Gauvreau K, Kamenir SA, Hornberger LK. Comparison of outcome when hypoplastic left heart syndrome and transposition of the great arteries are diagnosed prenatally versus when diagnosis of these two conditions is made only postnatally. Am J Cardiol 1999; 83: 1649–53.

Shah MK, Morava E, Gill W, Marble MR. Transposition of the great arteries and hypocalcemia in a patient with fetal hydantoin syndrome. J Perinatol 2002; 22: 89–90.

Tennstedt C, Chaoui R, Korner H, Dietel M. Spectrum of congenital heart defects and extracardiac malformations associated with chromosomal abnormalities: results of a seven year necropsy study. Heart 1999; 82: 34–9.

Yagel S, Hochner CD, Hurwitz A, Paid Z, Gotsman MS. The significance and importance of prenatal diagnosis of fetal cardiac malformations by Doppler echocardiography. Am J Obstet Gynecol 1988; 158: 272–7.

Ventricular Septal Defect (VSD)

Definition: Partial absence of the interventricular septum, either in the muscular part (20%) or in the membranous part (80%) of the septum.

Incidence: One in 400 births, accounting for 20–30% of total congenital cardiac anomalies.

Sex ratio: M : F = 1 : 1.

Clinical history/genetics: Mostly sporadic. Multifactorial inheritance; there are recurrence rates of 3% and 10% in case of one or two affected siblings, respectively. If the mother has the condition, the likelihood of the child being affected is 9.5%, while if the father has it, it is 2.5%.

Teratogens: Alcohol, hydantoin, valproic acid.

Associated malformations: VSD is the most common associated malformation in complex heart disease (in about 50% of cases, it is associated with other cardiac anomalies).

Associated syndromes: Over 100 syndromes have been described in which VSD is a component. Chromosomal aberrations are present in 5–10%, more frequently in the membranous form, rarely in the muscular form of VSD.

Ultrasound findings: A *defect in the ventricular septum* is detected, but it is important to demonstrate it from different angles. In the apical axis of the four-chamber view, depletion of the septum may often be detected underneath the aorta, but this is an artefact. Using color flow Doppler mapping, it is possible to demonstrate a *shunt* over the VSD. This is usually in both directions, but may even be completely absent. Small defects are often missed in prenatal diagnosis.

Clinical management: Further sonographic screening. Karyotyping. Intrauterine complications are not expected. Vaginal delivery is possible.

Procedure after birth: There are no obvious clinical signs immediately after birth. Even larger lesions may cause first symptoms 4–6 weeks after birth. Surgical correction is carried out within the first year of life. Pulmonary hypertension is a feared complication. In certain cases, pulmonary banding is necessary to prevent this.

Prognosis: If there are no other malformations, the prognosis is excellent. In 25–30% of cases, closure of the defect occurs spontaneously in infancy.

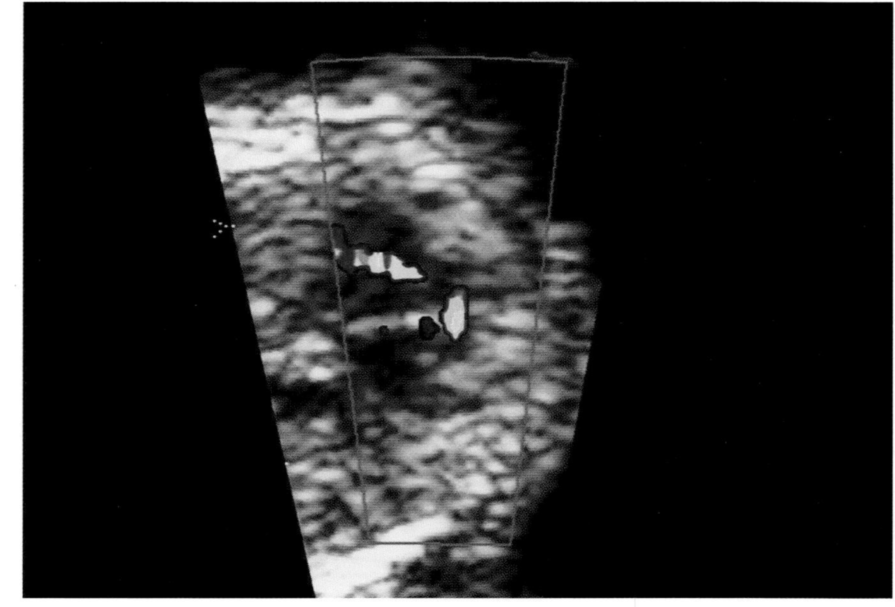

Fig. 5.**30** **Ventricular septal defect (VSD).** Demonstration of a ventricular septal defect (muscular part), combined with tricuspid incompetence at 14 + 2 weeks in trisomy 13. Color flow mapping.

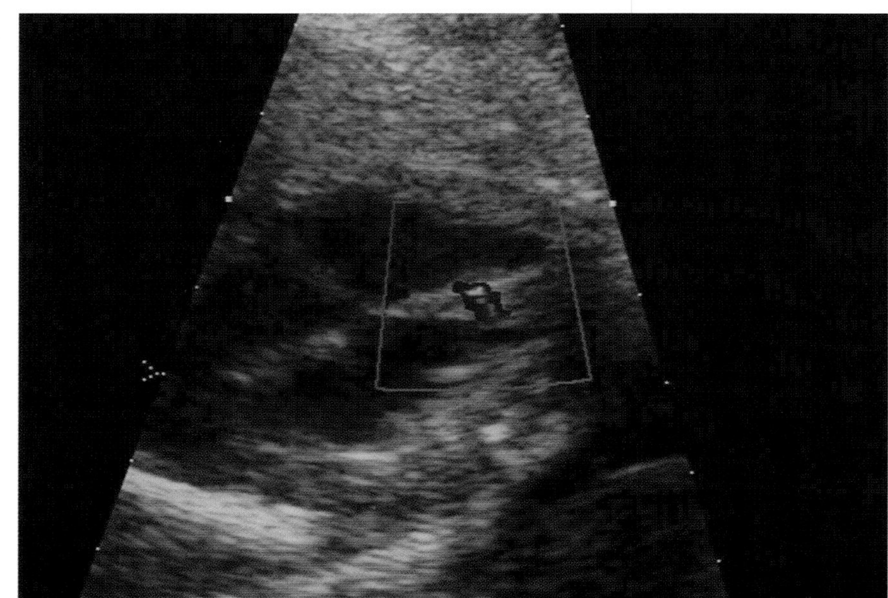

Fig. 5.**31** **Ventricular septal defect.** A small muscular VSD at 26 + 6 weeks. A flow jet is seen due to the presence of a right-to-left shunt, using color flow mapping.

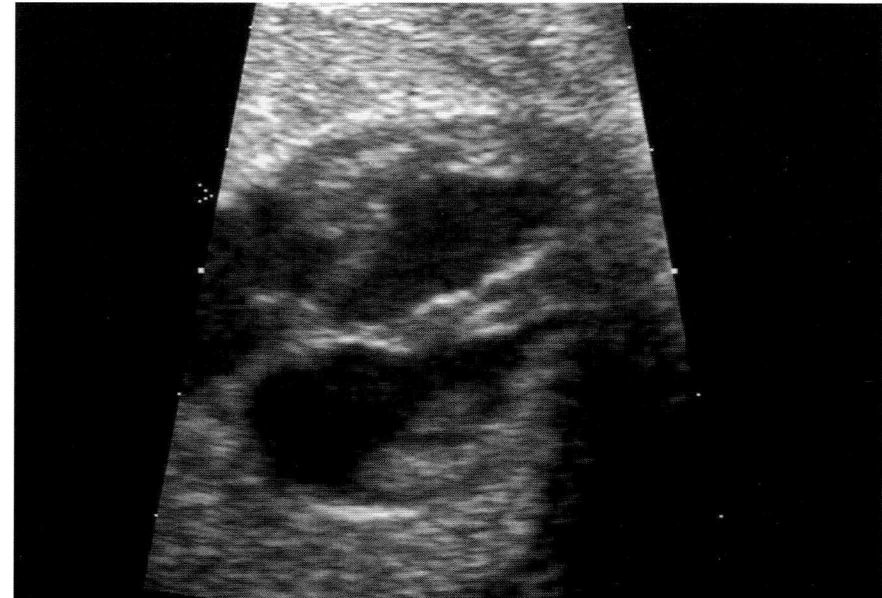

Fig. 5.**32** **Ventricular septal defect.** Same findings in B-mode. Without color flow mapping, the defect is not detectable.

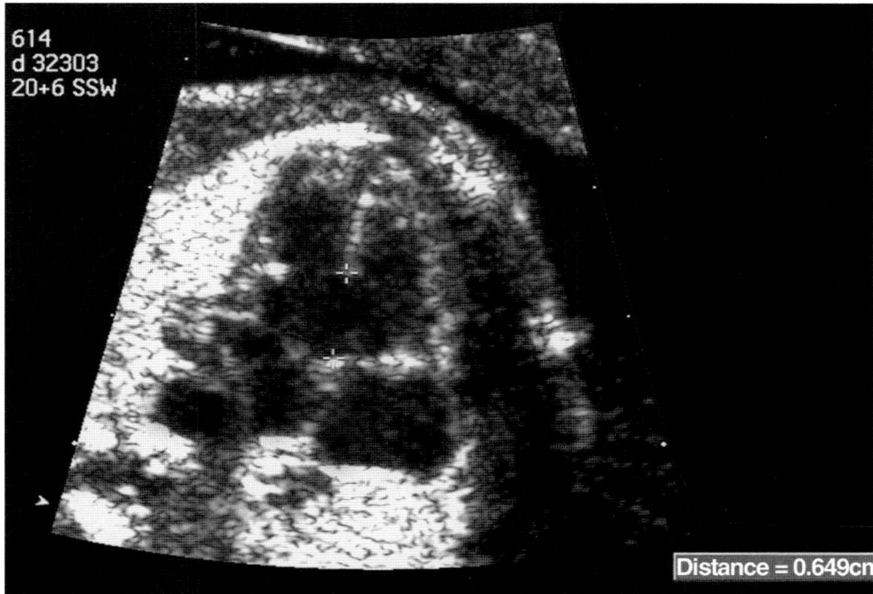

Fig. 5.**33** **Ventricular septal defect.** Extensive VSD, membranous part.

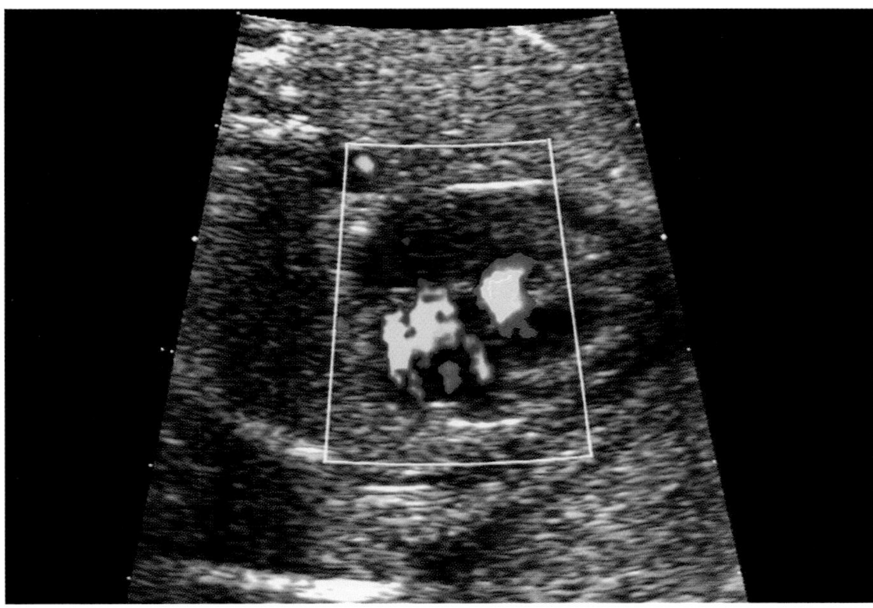

Fig. 5.**34** **Ventricular septal defect.** A large membranous VSD at 22 + 3 weeks. The right-to-left shunt is detected well using color flow mapping. The underlying disease in this case was Down syndrome.

2

References

Collinet P, Chatelet-Cheront C, Houze De L'Aulnoit D, Rey C. Prenatal diagnosis of an aorto-pulmonary window by fetal echocardiography. Fetal Diagn Ther 2002; 17: 302–7.

DeVore GR, Steiger RM, Larson EJ. Fetal echocardiography: the prenatal diagnosis of a ventricular septal defect in a 14-week fetus with pulmonary artery hypoplasia. Obstet Gynecol 1987; 69: 494–7.

Lethor JP, Marcon F, de Moor M, King ME. Physiology of ventricular septal defect shunt flow in the fetus examined by color Doppler M-mode. Circulation 2000; 101: E93.

Meyer WM, Simpson JM, Sharland GK. Incidence of congenital heart defects in fetuses of diabetic mothers: a retrospective study of 326 cases. Ultrasound Obstet Gynecol 1996; 8: 8–10.

Moene RJ, Sobotka PM, Oppenheimer DA, Lindhout D. Ventricular septal defect with overriding aorta in trisomy-18. Eur J Pediatr 1988; 147: 556–7.

Paladini D, Calabrò R, Palmieri S, D'Andrea T. Prenatal diagnosis of congenital heart disease and fetal karyotyping. Obstet Gynecol 1993; 81: 679–82.

Paladini D, Palmieri S, Lamberti A, Teodoro A, Martinelli P, Nappi C. Characterization and natural history of ventricular septal defects in the fetus. Ultrasound Obstet Gynecol 2000; 16: 118–22.

Wladimiroff JW, Stewart PA, Reuss A, Sachs ES. Cardiac and extra-cardiac anomalies as indicators for trisomies 13 and 18: a prenatal ultrasound study. Prenat Diagn 1989; 9: 515–20.

Yagel S, Sherer D, Hurwitz A. Significance of ultrasonic prenatal diagnosis of ventricular septal defect. JCU J Clin Ultrasound 1985; 13: 588–90.

6 Abdomen

Anal Atresia

Definition: Congenital absence of the opening of the anus.

Incidence: One in 5000 births.

Sex ratio: M : F = 3 : 2.

Clinical history/genetics: Sporadic, rarely familial forms with autosomal-recessive inheritance.

Embryology: Failure of division of the cloaca into the urogenital sinus and rectum, around 9 weeks after conception. Various lesions are recognized in which the rectum terminates above or below the puborectal sling. The higher the location of anal atresia, the more frequent the associated malformations. The level of atresia also determines whether primary surgical therapy is indicated after birth or whether a colostomy should be performed first, with definitive surgical correction at a later stage. This anomaly is commonly accompanied by esophageal atresia.

Teratogens: Alcohol, thalidomide, diabetes mellitus.

Associated malformations: These are found in 50%. Skeletal anomalies are associated in 30%, urogenital malformations in 38%, esophageal atresia in 10%, and cardiac anomalies in 5%.

Associated syndromes: Over 80 syndromes have been described in which anal atresia is found, including VACTERL association. Various chromosomal anomalies—e.g., partial trisomy 22 q and partial monosomy 10 q.

Ultrasound findings: The anus can be seen as an echogenic spot at the level of the genitals in transverse section. In the case of anal atresia, *the echogenic spot is missing*. Dilation of the large intestine and *calcification of meconium* within it may be an additional sign. These findings are first evident at a later gestational age (after 30 weeks).

Clinical management: Further sonographic screening, including fetal echocardiography. Karyotyping. Injection of contrast medium into the amniotic cavity followed by radiography of the fetus (amniofetography) have been performed in some cases historically.

Procedure after birth: Atretic anus is diagnosed at once at the first examination of the newborn after birth. Oral feeding is then contraindicated. A nasogastric tube should be inserted to relieve the secretions. In male infants, the anal fistula joins the urethra, and in the females the vagina. A blind ending of the rectum is an exception. An anus praeter is often established initially, so that definitive surgical treatment can follow at the age of 6–12 months.

Prognosis: This depends on the associated malformations. In the isolated form of anal atresia, 70% of cases show good functional capacity after surgical correction.

Self-Help Organizations

Title: The Pull-Thru Network

Description: A chapter of United Ostomy Association. Support and education of families with children born with anorectal malformations (including cloaca, VATER, cloacal exstrophy, or atretic anus and Hirschsprung's disease). Maintains a database for personal networking. Quarterly newsletter. Online discussion group. Phone support and literature.

Scope: National

Number of groups: Two affiliated groups

Founded: 1988

Address: 2312 Savoy Street, Hoover, AL 35226–1528, United States

Telephone: 205–978–2930

E-mail: pullthru@bellsouth.net

Web: http://www.pullthrough.org

Title: TEF/VATER Support Network (Connection)

Description: Offers support and encouragement for parents of children with tracheoesophageal fistula, esophageal atresia, and VATER. Aims to bring current information to parents and the medical community. Newsletter, information and referrals, phone support.

Scope: International

Number of groups: Six groups

Founded: 1992

Address: The VATER Connection, 1722 Yucca Lane, Emporia, KS 66801, United States

Telephone: 316-342-6954

Web: http://www.vaterconnection.org

References

Bean WJ, Calonje MA, Aprill CN, Geshner J. Anal atresia: a prenatal ultrasound diagnosis. JCU J Clin Ultrasound 1978; 6: 111–2.

Bronshtein M, Zimmer EZ. Early sonographic detection of fetal intestinal obstruction and possible diagnostic pitfalls. Prenat Diagn 1996. 16: 203–6.

Harris RD, Nyberg DA, Mack LA, Weinberger E. Anorectal atresia: prenatal sonographic diagnosis. AJR Am J Roentgenol 1987; 149: 395–400.

Lam YH, Shek T, Tang MH. Sonographic features of anal atresia at 12 weeks. Ultrasound Obstet Gynecol 2002; 19: 523–4.

Lomas FE, Dahlstrom JE, Ford JH. VACTERL with hydrocephalus: family with X-linked VACTERL-H. Am J Med Genet 1998; 76: 74–8.

Van Rijn M, Christaens GC, Hagenaars AM, Visser GH. Maternal serum alpha-fetoprotein in fetal anal atresia and other gastro-intestinal obstructions. Prenat Diagn 1998; 18: 914–21.

Stoll C, Alembik Y, Roth MP, Dott B. Risk factors in congenital anal atresias. Ann Genet 1997; 40: 197–204.

Tongsong T, Wanapirak C, Piyamongkol W Sudasana I. Prenatal sonographic diagnosis of VATER association. J Clin Ultrasound 1999, 27: 378–84.

Ascites

Definition: Ascites is defined as a collection of fluid within the peritoneal cavity.

Clinical history/causes: Fetal hydrops, fetal cardiac insufficiency, infections, mediastinal obstruction (pulmonary disease), gastrointestinal obstruction, meconium peritonitis; rarely, perforation in urinary tract obstruction, metabolic and hematological diseases of the fetus, hepatobiliary dysfunction, intra-abdominal tumors.

Ultrasound findings: The abdominal scan shows *fluid accumulation as an echo-free area* in the abdominal cavity. This is usually a clear diagnosis. The greater omentum may often falsely be confused with a cystic lesion in the abdomen. If only a narrow rim of ascites is found, then it is difficult to differentiate from certain artefacts.

Clinical management: Further sonographic screening, including fetal echocardiography. It is

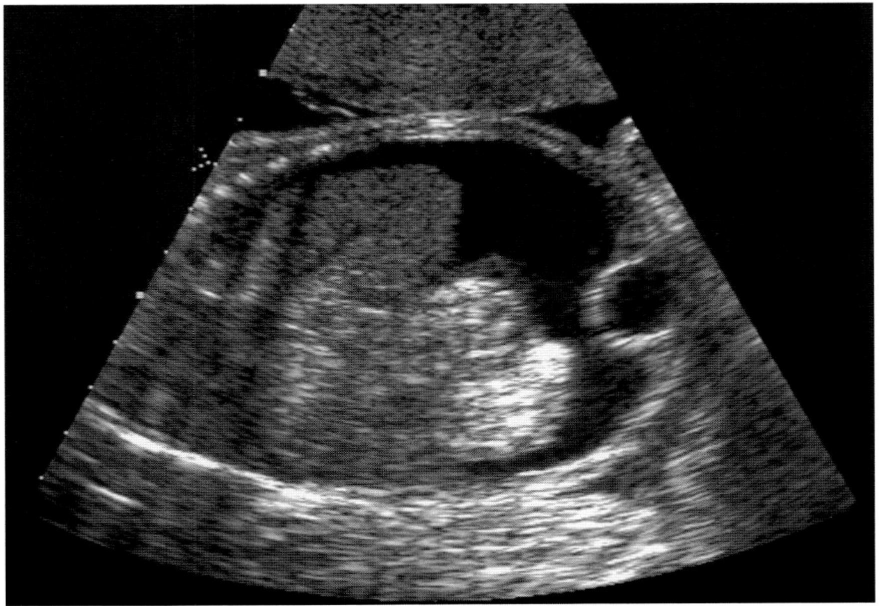

Fig. 6.**1** **Ascites.** Severe isolated fetal ascites at 25 + 6 weeks. The liver, urinary bladder and bowel loops with echoes due to meconium peritonitis are seen floating within it.

important to differentiate between isolated fetal ascites and ascites as a part of a generalized fetal hydrops. Are pleural and pericardial effusions present? Can edema of the fetal skin be demonstrated? TORCH serology (prenatal infection?), possibly amniocentesis for further clarification (infection? chromosomal anomaly? cystic fibrosis?).

Prognosis: Frequently no cause is found for isolated fetal ascites. Spontaneous remission may occur, with a very favorable prognosis.

References

Bettelheim D, Pumberger W, Deutinger J, Bernaschek G. Prenatal diagnosis of fetal urinary ascites. Ultrasound Obstet Gynecol 2000; 16: 473–5.

Domke N, Luckert G. Fetal ascites in the ultrasound B image. Zentralbl Gynäkol 1984; 106: 1582–6.

Gillan JE, Lowden JA, Gaskin K, Cutz E. Congenital ascites as a presenting sign of lysosomal storage disease. J Pediatr 1984; 104: 225–31.

Gross BH, Callen PW Filly RA. Ultrasound appearance of fetal greater omentum. J Ultrasound Med 1982; 1: 67–9.

Johnson TRJ, Graham D, Sanders RC, Smith N, Simmons MA, Winn K. Ultrasound-directed paracentesis of massive fetal ascites. JCU J Clin Ultrasound 1982; 10: 140–2.

Leppert PC, Pahlka BS, Stark RI, Yeh MN. Spontaneous regression of fetal ascites in utero in an adolescent. J Adolesc Health Care 1984; 5: 286–9.

Mazeron MC, Cordovi VL, Perol Y. Transient hydrops fetalis associated with intrauterine cytomegalovirus infection: prenatal diagnosis. Obstet Gynecol 1994; 84: 692–4.

Meizner I, Carmi R, Mares AJ, Katz M. Spontaneous resolution of isolated fetal ascites associated with extralobar lung sequestration. J Clin Ultrasound 1990; 18: 57–60.

Schmider A, Henrich W, Reles A, Vogel M, Dudenhausen JW. Isolated fetal ascites caused by primary lymphangiectasia: a case report. Am J Obstet Gynecol 2001; 184: 227–8.

Straub W, Zarabi M, Mazer J. Fetal ascites associated with Conradi's disease (chondrodysplasia punctata): report of a case. JCU J Clin Ultrasound 1983; 11: 234–6.

Vecchietti G, Borruto F. Ascites of the fetus: intrauterine diagnosis and puncture treatment using ultrasound. Ultraschall Med 1982; 3: 222–4.

Zelop C, Benacerraf BR. The causes and natural history of fetal ascites. Prenat Diagn 1994; 14: 941–6.

Duodenal Atresia

Definition: Complete obliteration of the lumen of the duodenum.

Incidence: One in 10 000 births.

Clinical history/genetics: Mostly sporadic, rarely familial disposition.

Teratogens: Diabetes mellitus, thalidomide.

Embryology: The lumen of the intestines is obliterated with epithelium in the 5 weeks after conception: this is a physiological finding. Up until 11 weeks of gestation, recanalization occurs. Duodenal atresia is caused by failure of recanalization.

Associated malformations: These are found in 50% of cases. Skeletal anomalies, other gastrointestinal anomalies, especially annular pancreas (20%), cardiac anomalies, and renal malformations.

Associated syndromes: Over 15 syndromes with duodenal atresia have been described. Up to a third of the cases have trisomy 21.

Ultrasound findings: *"Double bubble" sign*: the stomach is filled with fluid and next to it, the fluid-filled proximal duodenum can be seen as a second "bubble," with the pylorus separating the two cavities. The distal bowel is devoid of fluid. Hydramnios frequently coexists, and this is first apparent after 24 weeks.

Clinical management: Further sonographic screening, including fetal echocardiography. Karyotyping. Vaginal scan (cervical finding): premature labor? If there is hydramnios with premature contractions and maternal abdominal discomfort, drainage of the hydramnios may be necessary.

Procedure after birth: Placement of a nasogastric tube and removal of gastric secretions. The amniotic fluid appears green, due to bile reflux. Aspiration is similar to meconium aspiration. Intubation rather than mask respiration of the infant is preferred to avoid overdistension of the stomach, which facilitates aspiration. Withholding of fluid and nutrients. Early surgical correction with a duodenoduodenal or duodenojejunal anastomosis.

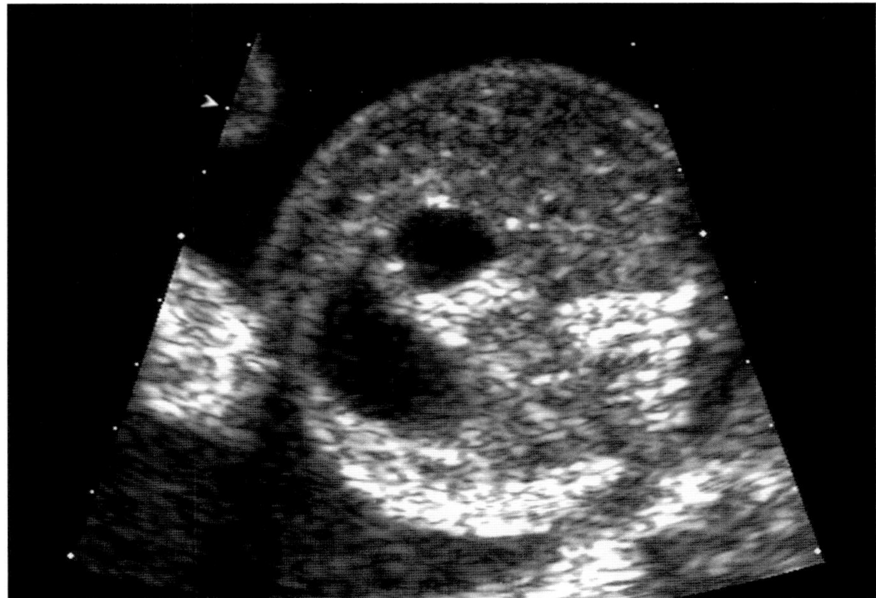

Fig. 6.2 **Duodenal atresia.** A cross-section of the fetus at the upper abdominal level at 27 weeks, showing two cystic lesions ("double bubble") following duodenal atresia in a fetus with trisomy 21.

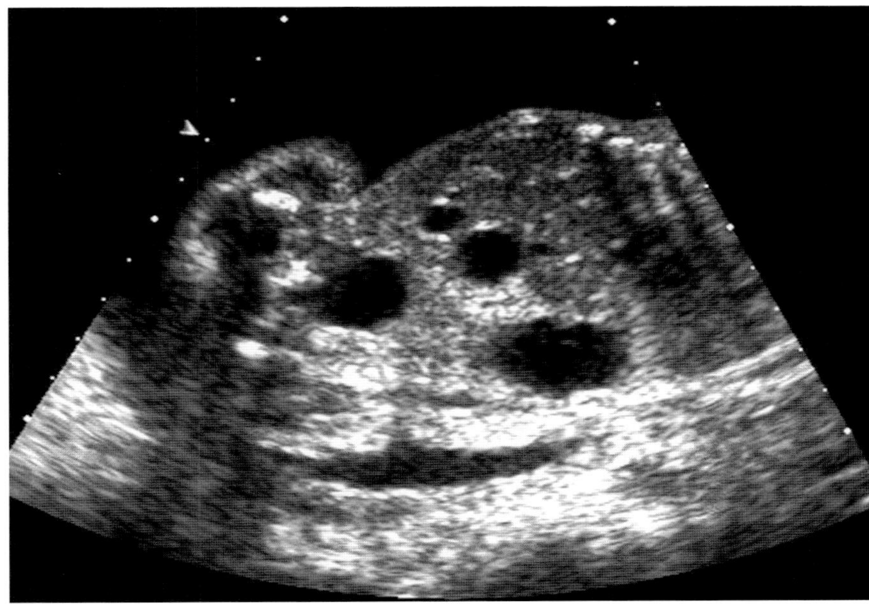

Fig. 6.3 **Duodenal atresia.** Same findings as above, in longitudinal section.

Prognosis: This depends on coexisting malformations and the maturity of the infant (premature labor due to hydramnios). Mortality can be as high as 36%. Surgical repair of isolated duodenal atresia is successful in almost all cases, with an overall survival rate of 95%.

References

Collier D. Antenatal diagnosis of duodenal atresia by ultrasound: a case report. Radiography 1982; 48: 102–3.

Dundas KC, Walker J, Laing IA. Oesophageal and duodenal atresia suspected at the 12 week booking scan. BJOG Br J Obstet Gynecol 2001; 108: 225–6.

Fletman D, McQuown D, Kanchanapoom V, Gyepes MT. "Apple peel" atresia of the small bowel: prenatal diagnosis of the obstruction by ultrasound. Pediatr Radiol 1980; 9: 118–9.

Grosfeld JL, Rescorla FJ. Duodenal atresia and stenosis: reassessment of treatment and outcome based on antenatal diagnosis, pathologic variance, and long-term follow-up. World J Surg 1993; 17: 301–9.

Hösli KI, Tercanli S, Nars PW, Holzgreve W. Combined esophageal atresia and duodenal stenosis in polyhydramnios: ante-, peri- and postpartum management. Z Geburtshilfe Neonatol 1996; 200: 161–5.

Lawrence MJ, Ford WD, Furness ME, Hayward T, Wilson T. Congenital duodenal obstruction: early antenatal ultrasound diagnosis. Pediatr Surg Int 2000; 16: 342–5.

Nelson LH, Clark CE, Fishburne JI, Urban RB, Penry MF. Value of serial sonography in the in utero detection of duodenal atresia. Obstet Gynecol 1982; 59: 657–60.

Nyberg DA, Resta RG, Luthy DA, Hickok DE, Mahony BS, Hirsch JH. Prenatal sonographic findings of Down syndrome: review of 94 cases. Obstet Gynecol 1990; 76: 370–7.

Ranzini AC, Guzman ER, Ananth CV, Day-Salvatore D, Fisher AJ, Vintzileos AM. Sonographic identification of fetuses with Down syndrome in the third trimester: a matched control study. Obstet Gynecol 1999; 93: 702–6.

Salihu HM, Boos R, Schmidt W. Antenatally detectable markers for the diagnosis of autosomally trisomic fetuses in at-risk pregnancies. Am J Perinatol 1997; 14: 257–61.

Stoll C, Alembik Y, Dott B, Roth MP. Evaluation of prenatal diagnosis of congenital gastro-intestinal atresias. Eur J Epidemiol 1996; 12: 611–6.

Tsukerman GL, Krapiva GA, Kirillova IA. First-trimester diagnosis of duodenal stenosis associated with oesophageal atresia. Prenat Diagn 1993; 13: 371–6.

Intestinal Atresia and Stenosis

Definition: Congenital atresia or stenosis of the small or large bowel.

Incidence: *Small-bowel atresia and stenosis* occur in one in 3000–5000 births (jejunum 50%, ileum 43%, multiple stenosis 7%). *Large-bowel atresia and stenosis* one in 20 000.

Clinical history/genetics: Mostly sporadic. Autosomal-recessive syndromes have been described in association with intestinal atresia and stenosis. Cystic fibrosis is found in 25% of cases of jejunal and ileum atresia.

Teratogen: Thalidomide, cocaine; application of methylene blue (e.g., amniocentesis in twin pregnancy).

Embryology: Most cases are attributed to a vascular accident (hypotension, vessel anomaly, volvulus) causing local ischemia. *Three types of stenosis* are described:

1. Bowel continuity is disturbed by a membrane consisting of mucous and submucous parts. The tunica muscularis is not involved.
2. Two blind-ending loops of bowel are connected through a fibrous band, while the mesentery remains intact.
3. Even this connection of the blind loops through a fibrous band is missing, and the continuity of the mesentery is also interrupted.

The most frequently found form is the second, followed by the third form of atresia. The proximal part of the bowel is distended, whereas the distal part is very thin. Atresias are three times more common than stenoses. In most cases, stenoses arise probably after perforation of a membranous bowel obstruction through the mucus membrane. Multiple atresias are especially feared, and are found in 10% of cases. Whereas duodenal atresia is considered to be a malformation in the embryonic stage, jejunal and ileal atresia occur in the fetal developmental phase (for example, due to arterial obstruction or other causes). This theory is supported by the fact that instillation of methylene blue in diagnostic amniocentesis in twin pregnancy often causes jejunal and ileal atresia, but not duodenal atresia.

Associated malformations: In 44% of cases, single anomalies or a combination of other anomalies are found: growth restriction (30%), meconium peritonitis (12%), meconium ileus (10%), cystic fibrosis (15%), omphalocele (7%), gastroschisis (12%), malrotation, anal atresia, cardiac anomaly (7%), chromosomal anomaly (7%). Over 15 syndromes have been described in association with intestinal atresia.

Ultrasound findings: Diagnosis is based on the presence of *dilated, fluid-filled loops of the intestines proximal to the atresia*. As the small and large bowel are difficult to distinguish in abdominal scanning, it may be difficult to locate the exact position of the lesion. Small-bowel atresia is more frequent. The more proximal the location of the atresia, the more frequently hydramnios develops. Large-bowel atresia is rarely associated with hydramnios. Ultrasound findings suggesting atresia are often first observed after 24 weeks of gestation. Meconium peritonitis is suspected if *ascites is combined with intestinal calcifications*. Other associated malformations such as malrotation, volvulus, and intestinal duplication can rarely be diagnosed at the prenatal stage.

Clinical management: Further sonographic screening, including fetal echocardiography. Karyotyping. If meconium ileus is suspected, cystic fibrosis should be excluded. A pediatric surgeon should be consulted for parental counseling regarding prognosis, management, and the optimal time of delivery. It is possible that early delivery of a fetus with considerable bowel distension may be advantageous, but there is no scientific evidence to support this.

Procedure after birth: The amniotic fluid may be stained green due to bile reflux. Aspiration of this fluid may be just as dangerous as aspiration of meconium. Superfluous gastric contents should be removed with nasogastric aspiration. In the presence of respiratory insufficiency, intubation of the infant is preferable to respiration using a nasopharyngeal mask; this helps prevent aspiration. In any case, surgical correction is necessary, the extent of lesion often being recognized at laparotomy. Frequently, part of the distended bowel has to be resected. If only a small length of bowel remains, short-bowel syndrome may develop, making it necessary to feed the infant intravenously over a long period.

Prognosis: This depends on the presence of other malformations. In isolated cases of intestinal atresia, a very good prognosis is expected in 95% of infants.

References

Benson IM, King PA. Multiple atresias in a low-birth-weight twin. J Pediatr Surg 1999; 34: 1040–2.

Boyd PA, Chamberlain P, Gould S, Ives NK, Manning N, Tsang T. Hereditary multiple intestinal atresia: ultrasound findings and outcome of pregnancy in an affected case. Prenat Diagn 1994; 14: 61–4.

Del'Agnola CA, Tomaselli V, Teruzzi E, Tadini B, Coran AG. Prenatal diagnosis of gastrointestinal obstruction: a correlation between prenatal ultrasonic findings and postnatal operative findings. Prenat Diagn 1993; 13: 629–32.

Font GE, Solari M. Prenatal diagnosis of bowel obstruction initially manifested as isolated hyperechoic bowel. J Ultrasound Med 1998; 17: 721–3.

Fourcade L, Shima H, Miyazaki E, Puri P. Multiple gastrointestinal atresias result from disturbed morphogenesis. Pediatr Surg Int 2001; 17: 361–4.

Garne E, Rasmussen L, Husby S. Gastrointestinal malformations in Funen county, Denmark: epidemiology, associated malformations, surgery and mortality. Eur J Pediatr Surg 2002; 12: 101–6.

Kubota A, Nakayama T, Yonekura T, et al. Congenital ileal atresia presenting as a single cyst-like lesion on prenatal sonography. J Clin Ultrasound 2000; 28: 206–8.

Lundkvist K, Ewald U, Lindgren PG. Congenital chloride diarrhoea: a prenatal differential diagnosis of small bowel atresia. Acta Paediatr 1996; 85: 295–8.

Miyakoshi K, Tanaka M, Miyazaki T, Yoshimura Y. Prenatal ultrasound diagnosis of small-bowel torsion. Obstet Gynecol 1998; 91: 802–3.

Muller F, Dommergues M, Ville Y, et al. Amniotic fluid digestive enzymes: diagnostic value in fetal gastrointestinal obstructions. Prenat Diagn 1994; 14: 973–9.

Müller R, Kohler R. Prenatal diagnosis of fetal small bowel stenosis: a case report. Zentralbl Gynäkol 1990; 112: 1047–50.

Voigt HJ, Hummer HP, Bowing B. Prenatal ultrasonic diagnosis of jejunal atresia. Z Geburtshilfe Perinatol 1985; 189: 144–6.

Gastroschisis

Definition: This is a prenatal evisceration of uncovered fetal bowel, through a paraumbilical defect in the anterior abdominal wall, into the amniotic cavity.

Incidence: One in 4000 births.

Sex ratio: M : F = 1 : 1.

Clinical history/genetics: Mostly sporadic. Rarely, single-gene autosomal-dominant inheritance. Alpha fetoprotein is increased in 75% of the cases; a level more than five times the median value is frequently found.

Teratogens: Not known.

Embryology: The cause of gastroschisis is not yet exactly known. The muscles of the abdominal wall are normal, but there is a defect of the aponeurosis of the rectus muscle, near the midline lying slightly to the right. A possible cause of this may be incomplete regression of the right umbilical vein, which is present only temporarily in the embryonic stage.

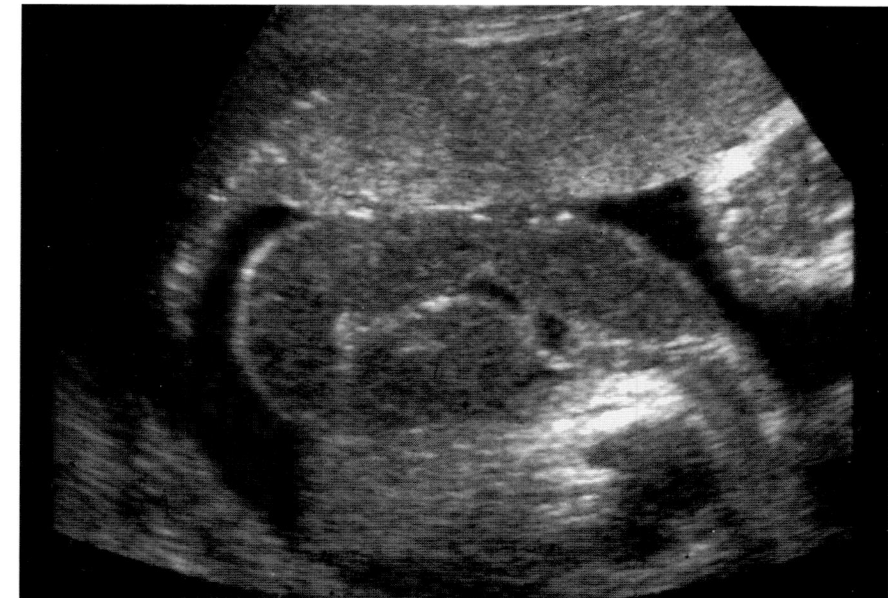

Fig. 6.4 **Gastroschisis.** Loops of bowel floating freely in the amniotic fluid in gastroschisis, at 35 + 5 weeks.

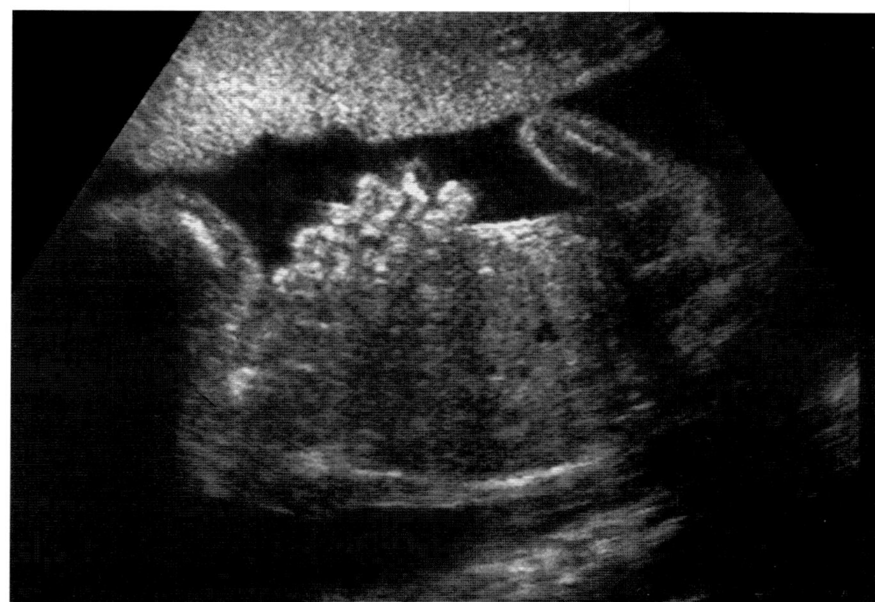

Fig. 6.5 **Gastroschisis in a twin,** 23 + 2 weeks. Eviscerated intestinal loops are seen, which—in contrast to an omphalocele—are not covered with peritoneum or skin.

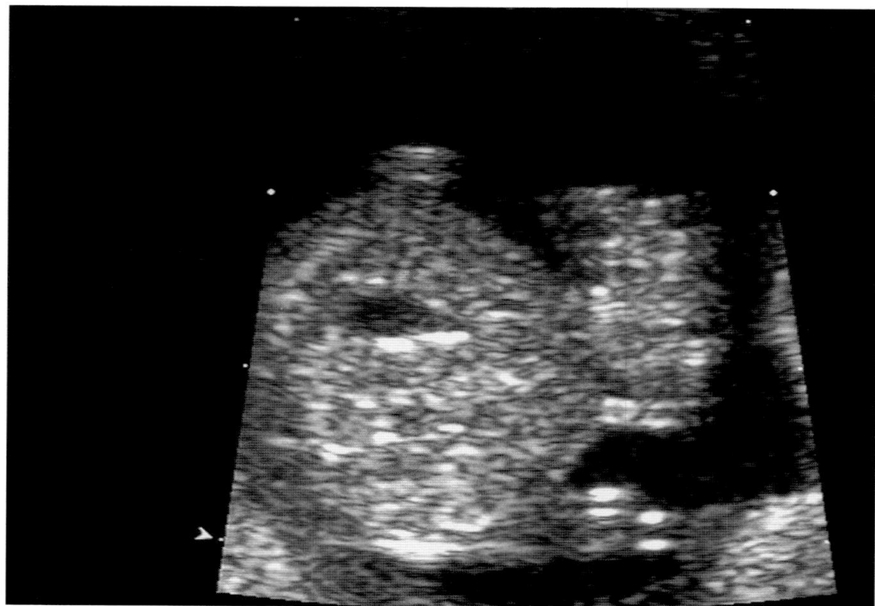

Fig. 6.6 **Gastroschisis.** Evisceration of the intestines, at 13 + 0 weeks.

Associated malformations: Malrotation of the intestines is almost always an accompanying feature. Intestinal atresia in 5–15% of cases and other extraintestinal anomalies (5%) are also detected.

Ultrasound findings: *Small-bowel and large-bowel loops* are found outside of the abdominal cavity *floating freely* in the amniotic fluid. The actual wall defect usually lies in the lower right quadrant of the abdomen, and is often difficult to pinpoint. The smaller the defect, the more severe is the restriction of blood flow to the intestines, and the greater damage that can be expected. If the small-bowel distension exceeds 1.8 cm, then a long-term damage of the intestines is probable. The assumption that in late pregnancy the intestinal wall is damaged due to contact with the amniotic fluid is disputed. Ischemia due to restricted blood flow or torsion of the mesentery may be a more likely cause of the bowel damage. In many cases, hydramnios develops as a result of bowel obstruction. *Intrauterine growth restriction* frequently coexists. Growth restriction may be diagnosed incorrectly, as the abdominal circumference appears too small due to evisceration of abdominal contents.

Differential diagnosis: It is often difficult to distinguish between gastroschisis and a ruptured omphalocele containing loops of bowel, as the location of the umbilical vessels relative to the abdominal wall defect cannot be determined exactly—a major criterion for differentiating be-

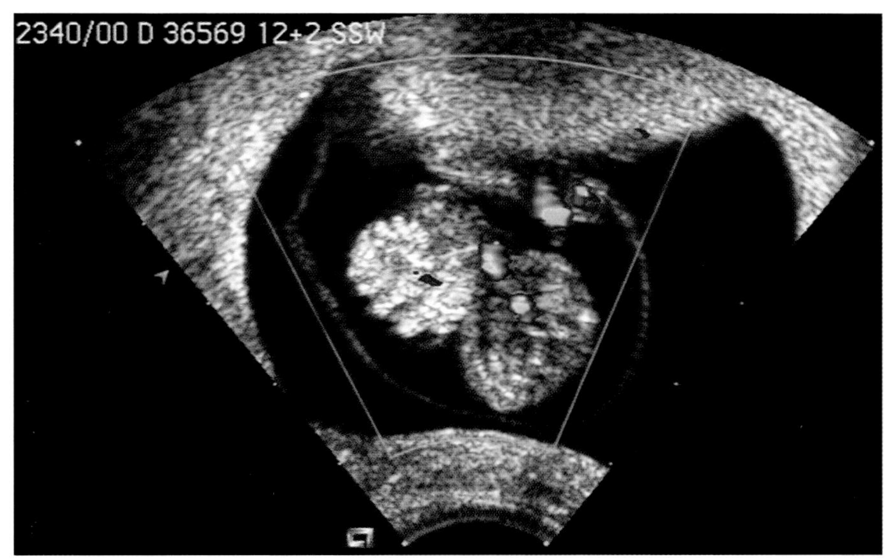

Fig. 6.**7** **Laparoschisis.** Cross-section of the fetal abdomen, showing a large defect in the anterior abdominal wall and evisceration of liver and bowel, at 12 + 2 weeks.

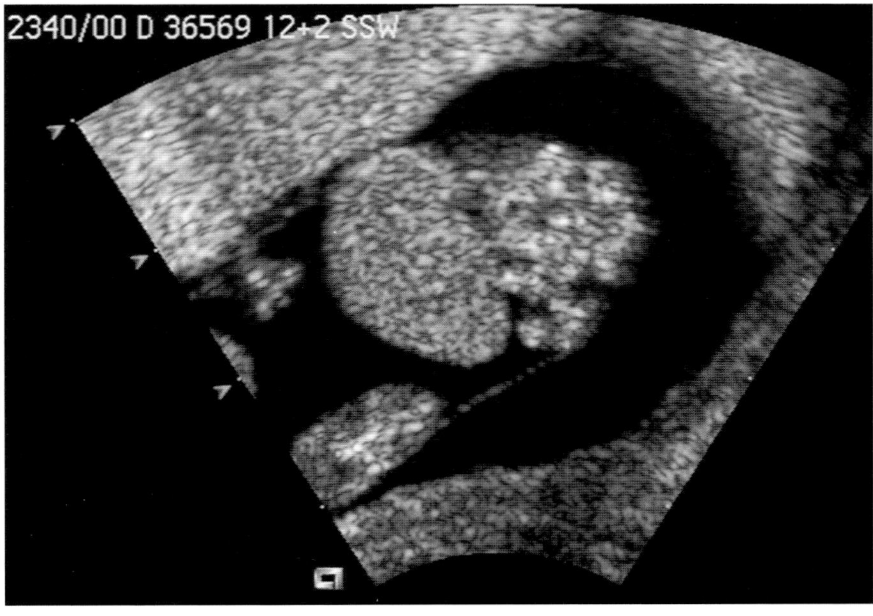

Fig. 6.**8** **Laparoschisis.** Same situation, showing a section at the frontal level through the herniated liver and small bowel.

tween the two conditions. If omphalocele is diagnosed, then the likelihood of other anomalies increases considerably.

Clinical management: Further sonographic screening, including fetal echocardiography. Karyotyping, as a ruptured omphalocele is more frequently associated with chromosomal anomaly, and as this cannot be excluded with certainty in a prenatal scan. A pediatric surgeon should counsel the parents regarding the severity of the condition. Regular scans are advisable, to monitor the thickness of the bowel wall, bowel distension, and fetal growth. If loops of bowel remain relatively normal in appearance, then the pregnancy can be continued up until the due date. Frequently, bowel distension begins 4–6 weeks before the due date, so that early delivery is the usual outcome. Some clinical studies have shown that cesarean section may be beneficial for the infant. Delivery should be attempted in a perinatal center with a pediatric surgical unit.

Procedure after birth: In case of respiratory distress, primary intubation is preferable to a nasopharyngeal mask, as the risk of distension of the bowel is greater in the latter form of ventilation. To avoid fluid loss, the loops should be covered immediately using a sterile plastic bag. It is usually also necessary to relieve the torsion of the bowel. A nasogastric tube is placed to remove excess secretion. Early surgical intervention is advised. If the intra-abdominal pressure increases above 20 mmHg after reposition of the bowel loops, then closure of the abdominal wall should be carried out in several stages.

Prognosis: The overall survival is above 90%. In some infants, short-bowel syndrome may result if intestinal atresia or severely damaged bowel wall are found.

References

Barisic I, Clementi M, Hausler M, Gjergja R, Kern J, Stoll C. Evaluation of prenatal ultrasound diagnosis of fetal abdominal wall defects by 19 European registries. Ultrasound Obstet Gynecol 2001; 18: 309–16.
Crombleholme TM, Dalton M, Cendron M, et al. Prenatal diagnosis and the pediatric surgeon: the impact of prenatal consultation on perinatal management. J Pediatr Surg 1996; 31: 156–62.
Durfee SM, Downard CD, Benson CB, Wilson JM. Postnatal outcome of fetuses with the prenatal diagnosis of gastroschisis. J Ultrasound Med 2002; 21: 269–74.
Grundy H, Anderson RI, Filly RA, et al. Gastroschisis: prenatal diagnosis and management. Fetal Ther 1987; 2: 144–7.
Haddock G, Davis CF, Raine PA. Gastroschisis in the decade of prenatal diagnosis: 1983–1993. Eur J Pediatr Surg 1996; 6: 18–22.
Hansen KH, Schachinger H, Kunze J. Pre- and postnatal diagnosis of abdominal wall defects (omphalocele and gastroschisis): case reports. Monatsschr Kinderheilkd 1983; 131: 228–31.
Lunzer H, Menardi G, Brezinka C. Long-term follow-up of children with prenatally diagnosed omphalocele and gastroschisis. J Matern Fetal Med 2001; 10: 385–92.
Nicholls EA, Ford WD, Barnes KH, Furness ME, Hayward C. A decade of gastroschisis in the era of antenatal ultrasound. Aust N Z J Surg 1996; 66: 366–8.
Nichols CR, Dickinson JE, Pemberton PJ. Rising incidence of gastroschisis in teenage pregnancies. J Matern Fetal Med 1997; 6: 225–9.
Raynor BD, Richards D. Growth retardation in fetuses with gastroschisis. J Ultrasound Med 1997; 16: 13–16.
Redford DH, McNay MB, Whittle MJ. Gastroschisis and exomphalos: precise diagnosis by midpregnancy ultrasound. Br J Obstet Gynaecol 1985; 92: 54–9.
Roberts JP, Burge DM. Antenatal diagnosis of abdominal wall defects: a missed opportunity? Arch Dis Child 1990; 65: 687–9.
Tannouri F, Avni EF, Lingier P, Donner C, Houben JJ, Struyven J. Prenatal diagnosis of atypical gastroschisis. J Ultrasound Med 1998; 17: 177–80.
Tawil A, Comstock CH, Chang CH. Prenatal closure of abdominal defect in gastroschisis: case report and review of the literature [review]. Pediatr Dev Pathol 2001; 4: 580–4.

Intra-Abdominal Calcification (Hepatic Calcification)

Definition: Focal calcifications of the liver are seen as echogenic structures with an absence of dorsal echoes. Ischemia, infections or neoplasia may be causative factors. Benacerraf reported that no pathological cause was found in 96% of the cases and that normal development of the infant can be expected.

Ultrasound findings: *Echogenic areas* within the liver are visible. The pattern of dorsal echoes in the scan is variable.

Clinical management: TORCH serology.

Prognosis: This is very good in the absence of infectious etiology.

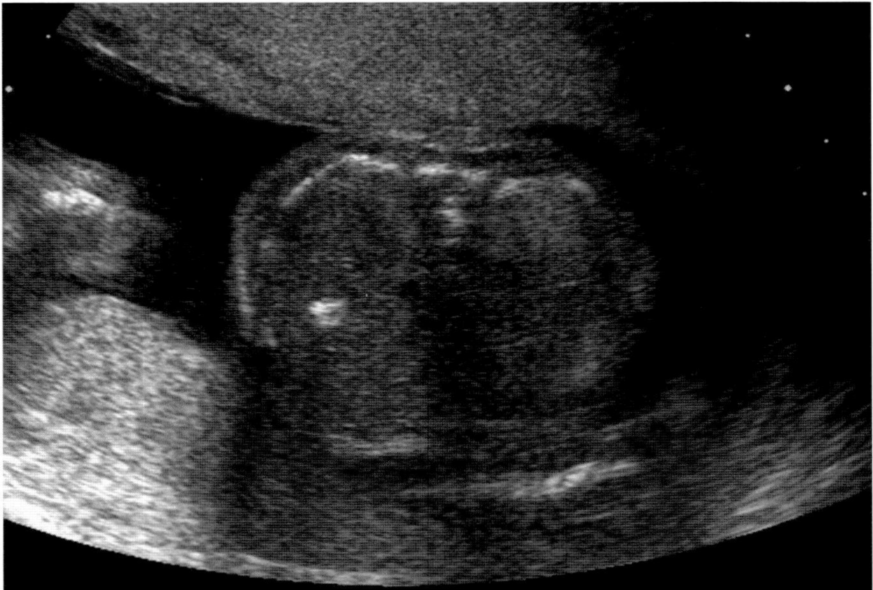

Fig. 6.**9** **Calcification of the liver.** Cross-section of the fetus (22 + 2 weeks) at the level of the upper abdomen. Liver with an echo-dense lesion ("liver calcification"). No abnormality was found after birth.

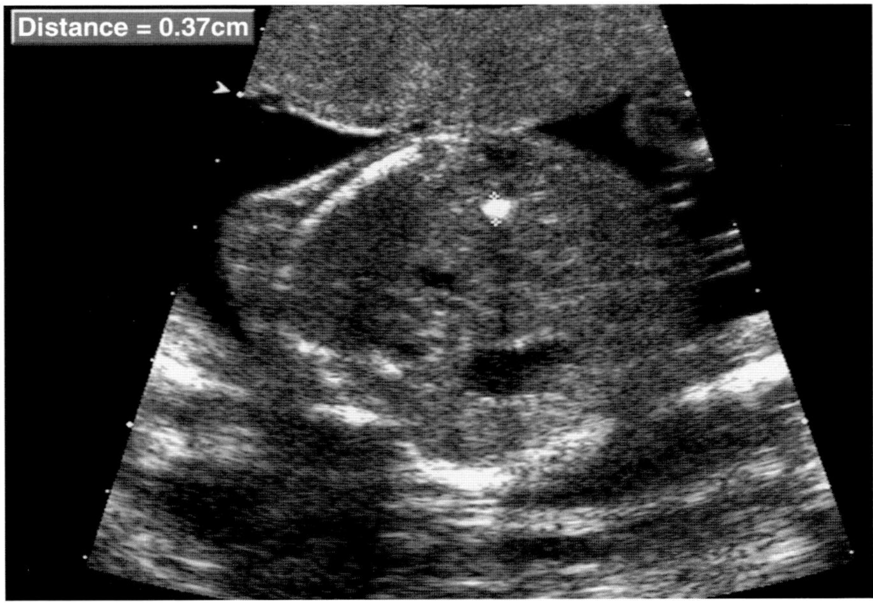

Fig. 6.**10** **Calcification of the liver,** 21 + 3 weeks. Cross-section of fetal abdomen at the level of the stomach, demonstrating an echo-dense lesion 3.7 mm in size in the liver.

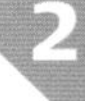

References

Arda K, Ozdemirel D, Tosun, Olcer T. Postpartum follow-up of hepatic calcification detected by prenatal ultrasound. JBR-BTR 2000; 83: 231–3.

Dirkes K, Crombleholme TM, Craigo SD, et al. The natural history of meconium peritonitis diagnosed in utero. J Pediatr Surg 1995; 30: 979–82.

Dreyfus M, Baldauf JJ, Dadoun K, Becmeur F, Berrut F, Ritter J. Prenatal diagnosis of hepatic hemangioma. Fetal Diagn Ther 1996; 11: 57–60.

Petrikovsky B, Klein V, Holsten N. Sludge in fetal gallbladder: natural history and neonatal outcome. Br J Radiol 1996; 69: 1017–8.

Sanders LD, Jequier S. Ultrasound demonstration of prenatal renal vein thrombosis. Pediatr Radiol 1989; 19: 733–5.

Spear R, Mack LA, Benedetti TJ, Cole RE. Idiopathic infantile arterial calcification: in utero diagnosis. J Ultrasound Med 1990; 9: 473–6.

Meconium Peritonitis

Definition: Intrauterine perforation of the intestines with leakage of meconium causing sterile peritonitis.

Incidence: One in 1500–2000 births.

Clinical history/genetics: Sporadic, except when associated with cystic fibrosis (autosomal-recessive inheritance).

Teratogens: Not known.

Embryology: There is a chemical peritonitis resulting from intrauterine bowel perforation due to varying causes. In case of fistula of the bowel, cystic lesions may also develop within the abdomen.

Associated malformations: Cystic fibrosis in 10%; cytomegalovirus infection; Down syndrome.

Ultrasound findings: *Echogenic areas resulting from calcifications* are found in the peritoneum, most frequently on the right side under the diaphragm. *Meconium pseudocysts* are found as echo-free lesions with irregular contours. Spontaneous remission is the usual course of these cysts. *Ascites* develops in 50% of the cases. This may be partly echo-dense due to mixing of bowel content with the amniotic fluid. In 25% of cases, *distended loops of bowel* are observed. The cause of meconium peritonitis here is the perforation of bowel secondary to obstruction. Calcifications are found only rarely in cystic fibrosis. Hydramnios coexists in 60%. The abdominal circumference may be increased. The diagnosis is usually made after 24 weeks of gestation.

Clinical management: Karyotyping, search for infections (cytomegalovirus). Cystic fibrosis should be excluded. Pediatric surgeon should be consulted. Early delivery may be indicated if severe distension of bowel is present. In case of a massive fetal ascites, delivery as well as immediate care of the newborn may be facilitated by prenatal puncture of the ascites.

Procedure after birth: A nasogastric tube is inserted and excess secretion is removed. Radiographic examination of the abdomen. Cystic fibrosis may not be excluded with certainty by the sweat test in the infant. If surgical correction is planned, a temporary anus praeter may be required.

Prognosis: Intrauterine spontaneous remission is seen frequently. Surgical treatment is required if torsion or perforation of the bowel are diagnosed. Depending on the cause and severity of the lesion, short bowel syndrome may develop. If the condition is diagnosed after birth, the mortality is as high as 62%.

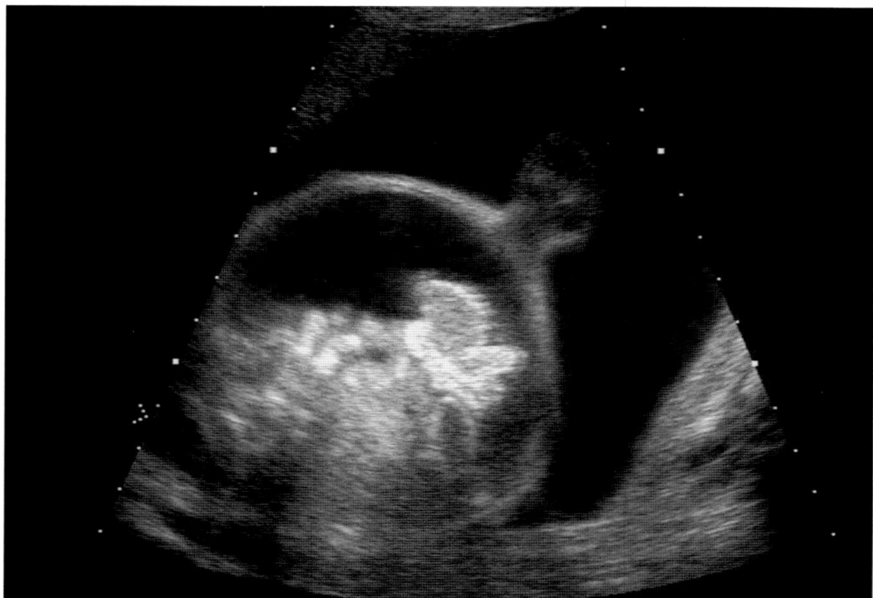

Fig. 6.**11** **Meconium peritonitis.** Cross-section of the fetal abdomen, 26 + 6 weeks; ascites, echogenic loops of bowel in a case of meconium peritonitis. Concomitant finding: hydramnios.

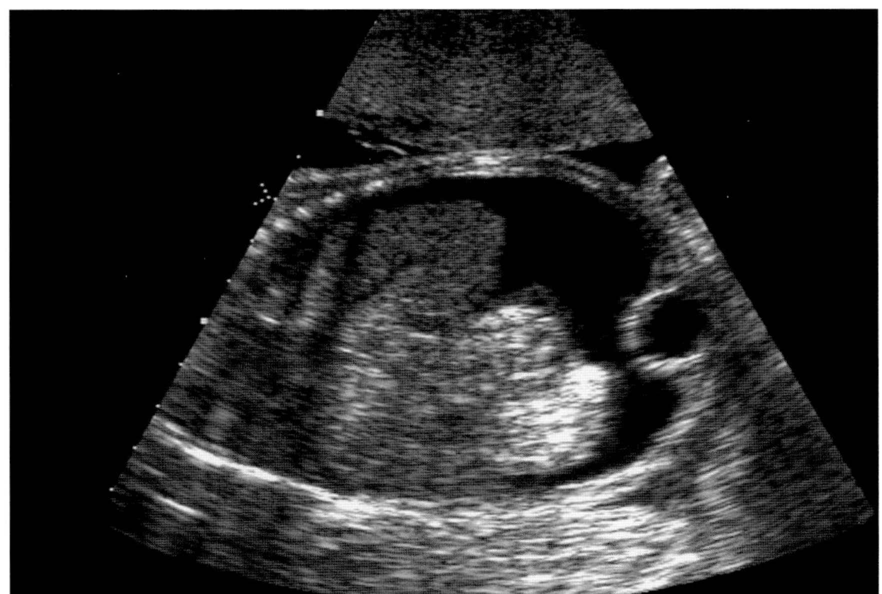

Fig. 6.**12** **Meconium peritonitis.** Same case as before, longitudinal section.

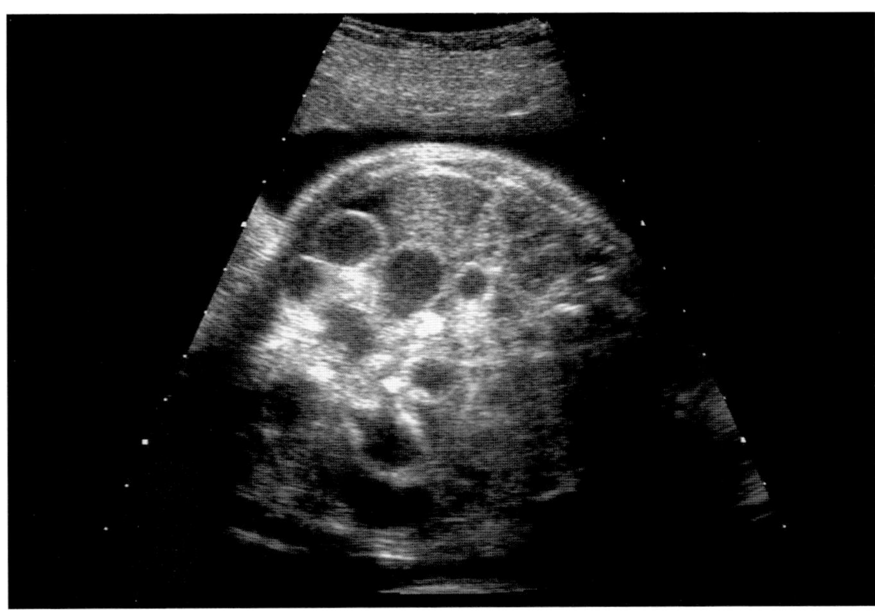

Fig. 6.**13** **Meconium peritonitis.** Same case at 27 + 6 weeks: distension of the bowel, a small amount of ascites, intra-abdominal calcifications.

References

Estroff JA, Bromley B, Benacerraf BR. Fetal meconium peritonitis without sequelae. Pediatr Radiol 1992; 22: 277–8.

Foster MA, Nyberg DA, Mahony BS, Mack LA, Marks WM, Raabe RD. Meconium peritonitis: prenatal sonographic findings and their clinical significance [review]. Radiology 1987; 165: 661–5.

She YY, Song LC. Meconium peritonitis: observations in 115 cases and antenatal diagnosis. Z Kinderchir 1982; 37: 2–5.

Stiemer B, Becker R, Waldschmidt J. Intrauterine Mekoniumperitonitis. Eine seltene Ursache des nicht immunologischen Hydrops fetalis: Fallbericht. Ultraschall Med 1993; 14: 44–7.

Omphalocele

Definition: Omphalocele is a median anterior wall defect characterized by the herniation of intra-abdominal contents into the base of the umbilical cord; in contrast to gastroschisis, the defect is covered by a transparent membrane (amnion and peritoneum). This membrane may be absent if the omphalocele is ruptured in the early stage. In umbilical hernia, on the other hand, the hernial sac is covered completely with skin.

Incidence: One in 4000 births.

Sex ratio: Contradictory reports, ranging from M : F = 1.6 : 1 to M : F = 1 : 5.

Clinical history/genetics: Mostly sporadic. Multifactorial inheritance; recurrence rate in isolated case of omphalocele in the sibling < 1%. Rarely inherited as autosomal-dominant or X-chromosome recessive forms. In connection with Beckwith–Wiedemann syndrome (omphalocele or umbilical hernia, macroglossia, acromegaly), autosomal-dominant inheritance is possible, with variable expression.

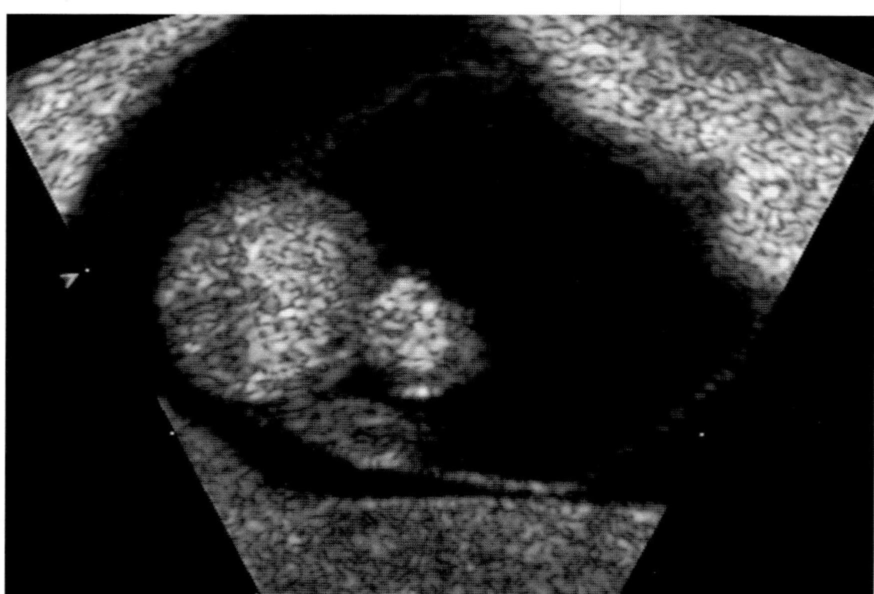

Fig. 6.**14** **Omphalocele.** Physiological omphalocele at 10 weeks of gestation. Spontaneous remission. Birth of a healthy neonate at term.

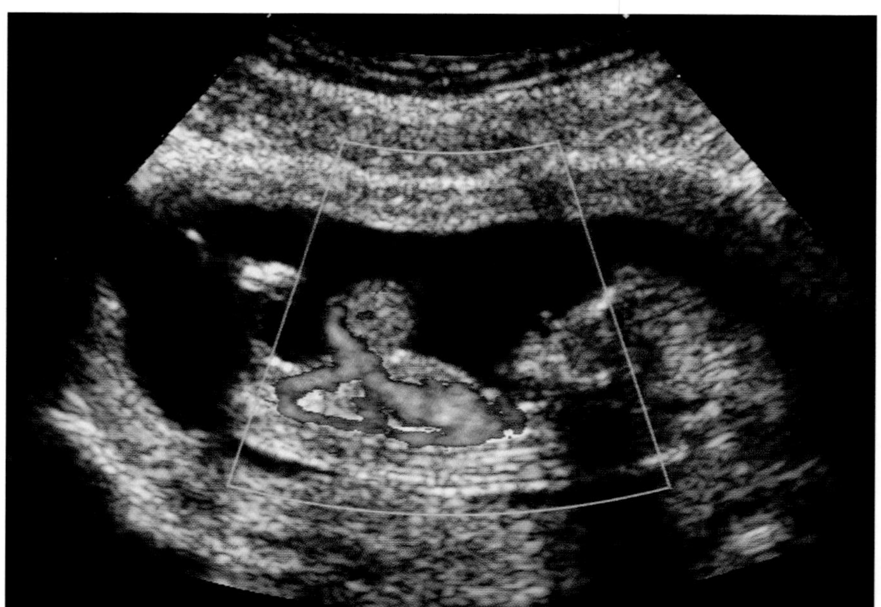

Fig. 6.**15** **Omphalocele.** Non-physiological omphalocele at 12 + 4 weeks. The fetal vessels are depicted using color Doppler energy, showing the umbilical vessels at the caudal pole of the omphalocele.

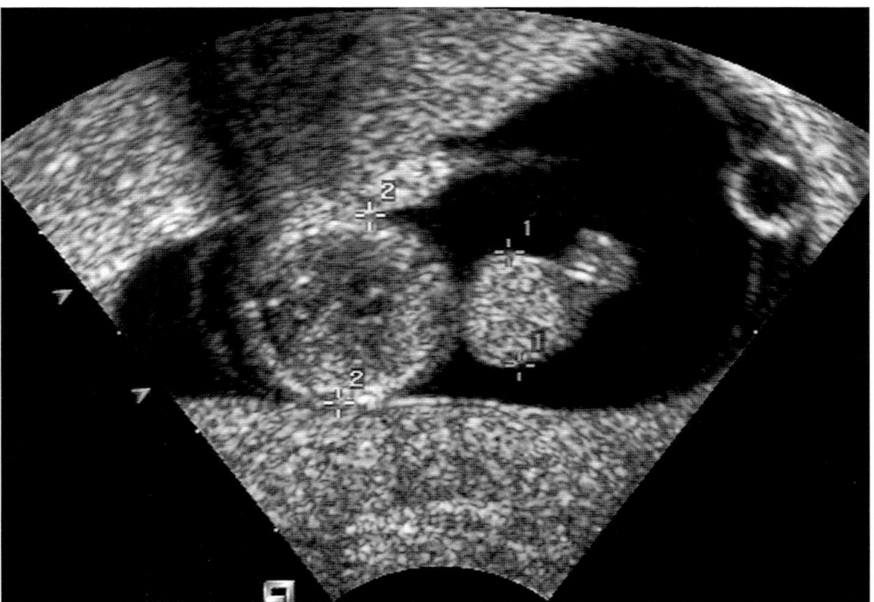

Fig. 6.**16** **Omphalocele.** Same fetus at 13 + 1 weeks. Oblique section through the fetal abdomen at the level of hernial canal and lower fetal thorax, with a section of fetal heart. The hernial canal appears much smaller than the hernial sac, with echogenic structures. Transabdominal chorionic villous sampling (TA-CVS) showed a normal karyotype. There were no other anomalies.

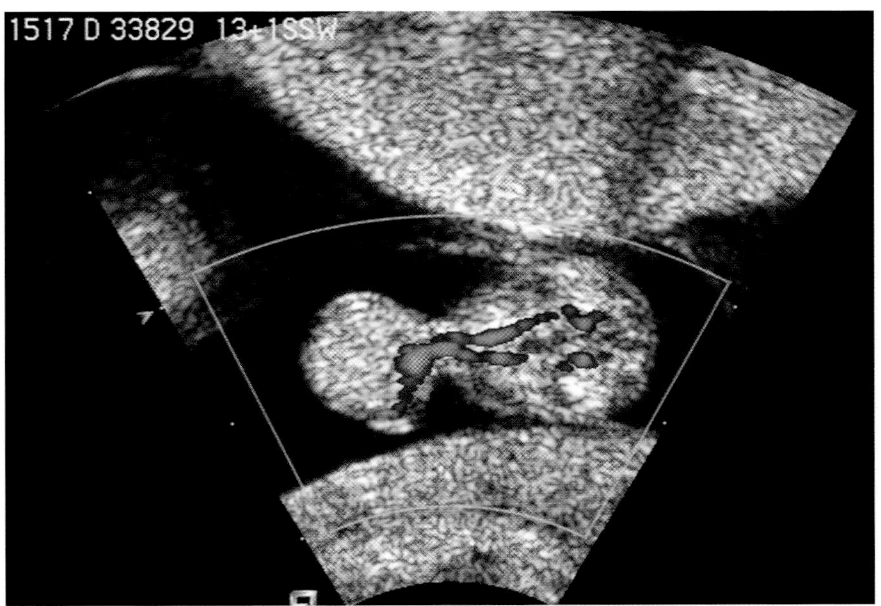

Fig. 6.**17** **Omphalocele.** Same fetus at 13 + 1 weeks. The transducer has been tilted caudally to obtain an oblique view of the umbilical vessels next to the fetal urinary bladder. Spontaneous abortion occurred at 16 weeks. "Isolated hepatic tissue" was found in the omphalocele.

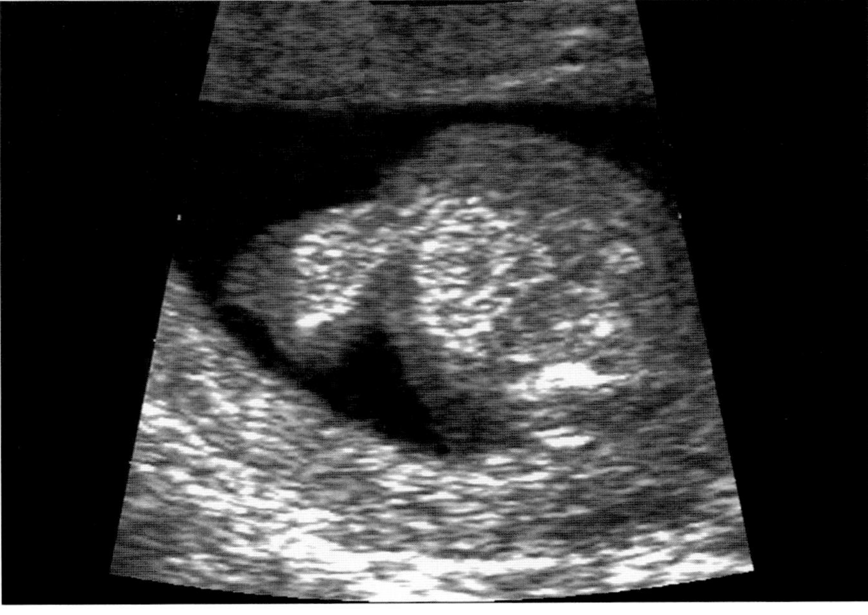

Fig. 6.**18** **Omphalocele**, 16 + 4 weeks. There is evidence of bowel in the hernial canal. Karyotype: trisomy 18.

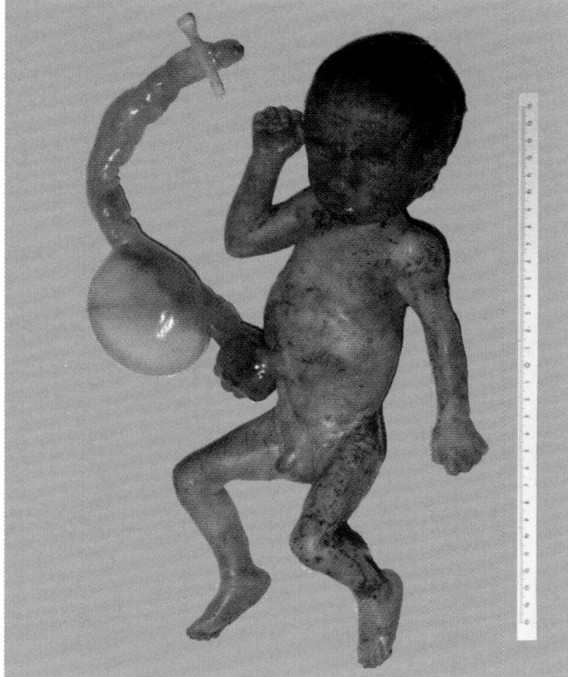

Fig. 6.**19** **Omphalocele.** Fetus with trisomy 18 after termination of the pregnancy; cystic lesion of the umbilical cord, small omphalocele.

Teratogens: Not known.

Embryology: Intestinal development takes place in three stages: 1, herniation of the bowel into the celom and rotation of the bowel; 2, repositioning of the intestines within the abdominal cavity; 3, fixation of the bowel to parietal peritoneum (from 12 weeks onwards). Each of these phases may be disturbed, causing specific dysfunctions. Omphalocele results when at the end of the first phase of rotation, the repositioning of the small-bowel loops into the abdominal cavity is incomplete. Some of the abdominal organs thus lie outside of the abdominal cavity. The hernia sac is covered with amnion and peritoneum. Loops of small bowel, liver, spleen, and pancreas may constitute the content of the hernia. Developmentally, omphalocele is detected up to 11 weeks of pregnancy. This "physiological omphalocele" is not considered to be a malformation, and should disappear at 13 weeks latest. The presence of liver outside of the abdomen excludes a physiological omphalocele.

Associated malformations: These are present in over 50%, especially if liver is found in the hernia sac. Cardiac anomalies (15–20%), bladder exstrophy, anal atresia, neural tube defects, facial clefts, diaphragmatic hernia and sirenomelia may also be found.

Associated syndromes: Twenty-five percent of cases are associated with chromosomal anomalies, especially if the content of the omphalocele is only intestines and umbilical cord cysts are present: triploidy, trisomy 13 and 18, Pallister–Killian syndrome. Other associated syndromes are Beckwith–Wiedemann syndrome, Shprintzen syndrome, Carpenter syndrome, and CHARGE association.

Ultrasound findings: Transverse and longitudinal scans of the abdomen show a *circular lesion at the navel,* which is connected to the abdomen with a wide base. It is covered with a *membranous layer* and appears *encapsulated.* The umbilical vessels can be followed up to the tip of

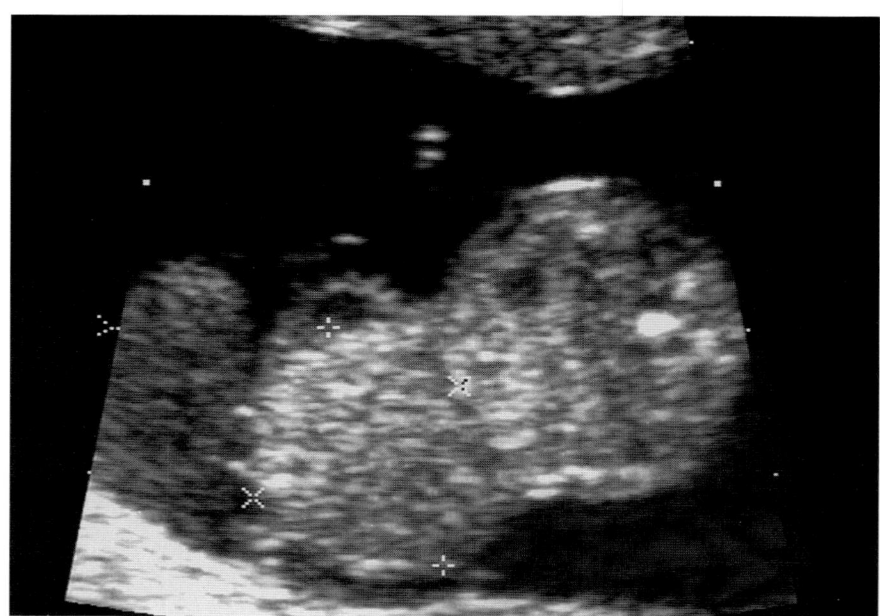

Fig. 6.**20** **Omphalocele.** Severe lesion found at 15 + 2 weeks in a fetus with trisomy 18.

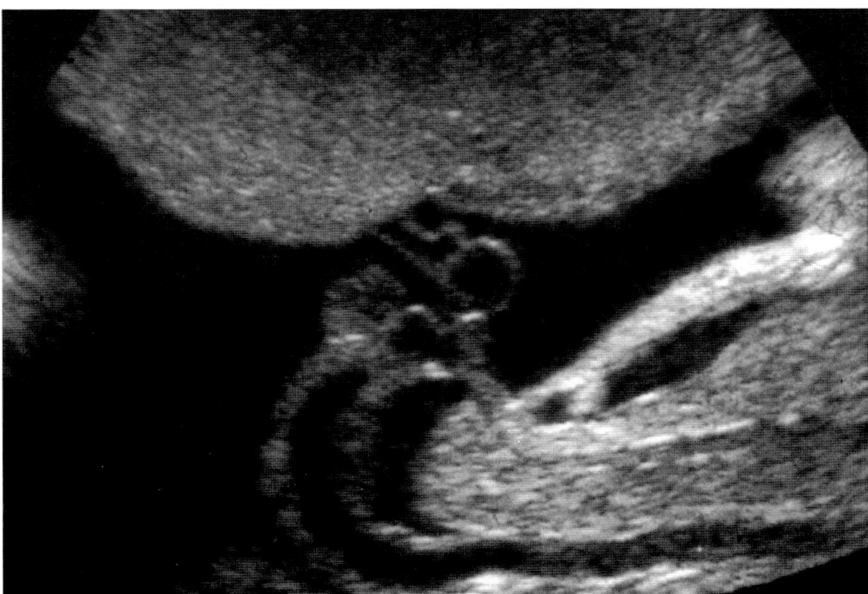

Fig. 6.**21** **Omphalocele.** Small lesion at 34 weeks of gestation.

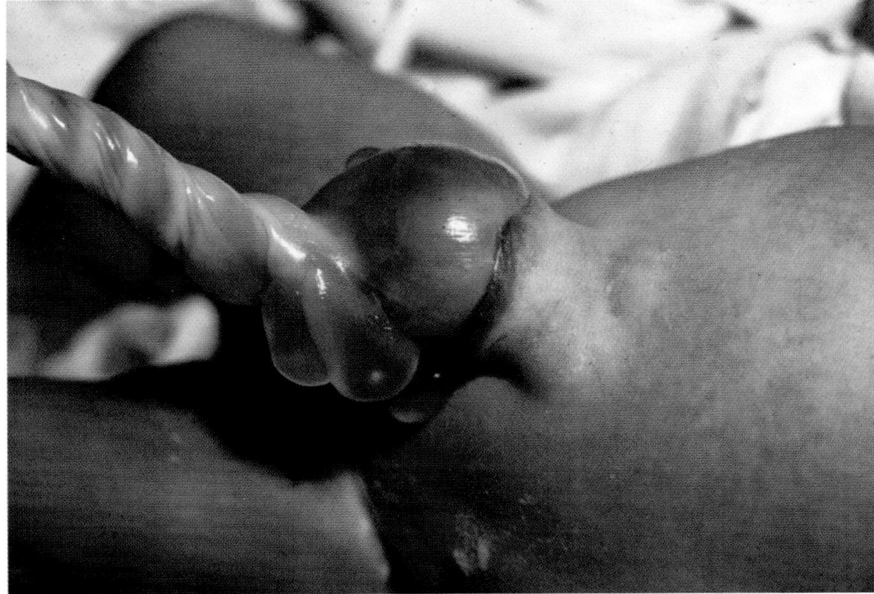

Fig. 6.**22** **Omphalocele.** Same finding after birth. Uncomplicated surgical correction.

the omphalocele. Freely floating loops of bowel are not seen as long as the omphalocele is intact. The hernia sac contains mainly *intestines* (seen in peristaltic motion). In a larger hernia, part of the stomach, liver (in 80%), bladder, and/or ascites may be found. These protrude through a defect at the insertion of the cord. Chromosomal anomalies are expected especially if only bowel and ascites are found within the hernia.

If *rupture of the omphalocele* occurs, insertion of the cord can be seen through the prolapsed abdominal content. If *liver is seen in front of the abdominal wall*, then this is most probably a ruptured omphalocele and not gastroschisis. Frequently hydramnios also develops.

The *physiological omphalocele* seen at 11 weeks contains only bowel. If liver is seen protruding out of the abdomen at this stage, then this is a pathological omphalocele.

Clinical management: Further sonographic screening including fetal echocardiography. Karyotyping. Consultation with a pediatric surgeon and parental counselling. Regular scan controls at 4-weekly intervals are recommended. The rate of stillbirths is 16–30%; intrauterine growth restriction occurs in 20%. If large parts of the liver are prolapsed out of the abdominal cavity, delivery per primary cesarean section is indicated to avoid rupture of the liver causing hemorrhage, which may occur during vaginal delivery, as the liver tissue is very vulnerable. In smaller omphaloceles, vaginal delivery is possible and here there is no indication for cesarean delivery.

Procedure after birth: The omphalocele should be covered immediately with a sterile plastic bag to avoid fluid loss. A nasogastric tube should be placed to remove stomach contents. Early surgical intervention within the first week. The earlier practice of smearing a sterile antiseptic solution on the lesion and delaying surgical intervention has ceased to be used except in rare cases of an extremely large omphalocele.

Prognosis: This is determined by the presence of associated anomalies and the extent of the lesion. The overall survival lies between 30–70%. In a small isolated case of omphalocele, the prognosis is very good (mortality below 5%). The mortality increases considerably (> 30%) if the defect is large (> 5 cm in the second trimester) and if the liver is prolapsed, even if no other anomalies are present.

Information for the mother: Surgical correction is very successful nowadays. If rare cases of large lesions with liver protrusion, associated malformations and chromosomal anomalies are excluded, then the long-term survival of the infant is very good, without significant long-term impairment.

References

Achiron R, Soriano D, Lipitz S, Mashiach S, Goldman B, Seidman DS. Fetal midgut herniation into the umbilical cord: improved definition of ventral abdominal anomaly with the use of transvaginal sonography. Ultrasound Obstet Gynecol 1995; 6: 256–60.

Bonilla-Musoles F, Machado LE, Bailao LA, Osborne NG, Raga F. Abdominal wall defects: two- versus three-dimensional ultrasonographic diagnosis. J Ultrasound Med 2001; 20: 379–89.

Curtis JA, Watson L. Sonographic diagnosis of omphalocele in the first trimester of fetal gestation. J Ultrasound Med 1988; 7: 97–100.

Hughes MD, Nyberg DA, Mack LA, Pretorius DH. Fetal omphalocele: prenatal US detection of concurrent anomalies and other predictors of outcome. Radiology 1989; 173: 371–6.

Kilby MD, Lander A, Usher SM. Exomphalos (omphalocele). Prenat Diagn 1998; 18: 1283–8.

Nyberg DA, Fitzsimmons J, Mack LA, et al. Chromosomal abnormalities in fetuses with omphalocele: significance of omphalocele contents. J Ultrasound Med 1989; 8: 299–308.

Pagliano M, Mossetti M, Ragno P. Echographic diagnosis of omphalocele in the first trimester of pregnancy. J Clin Ultrasound 1990; 18: 658–60.

Salvesen KA. Fetal abdominal wall defects: easy to diagnose—and then what? Ultrasound Obstet Gynecol 2001; 18: 301–4.

Skupski DW. Prenatal diagnosis of gastrointestinal anomalies with ultrasound: what have we learned? Ann NY Acad Sci 1998; 847: 53–8.

Towner D, Yang SP, Shaffer LG. Prenatal ultrasound findings in a fetus with paternal uniparental disomy 14q12-qter [review]. Ultrasound Obstet Gynecol 2001; 18: 268–71.

Tseng JJ, Chou MM, Ho ES. In utero sonographic diagnosis of a communicating enteric duplication cyst in a giant omphalocele. Prenat Diagn 2001; 21: 540–2.

van de Geijn EJ, van Vugt JM, Sollie JE, van Geijn HP. Ultrasonographic diagnosis and perinatal management of fetal abdominal wall defects. Fetal Diagn Ther 1991; 6: 2–10.

Wilson BR, Turner D, Langendoerfer S, Haverkamp AD. Prenatal diagnosis and subsequent team approach to the management of omphalocele. J Reprod Med 1980; 24: 134–6.

Wilson RD, McGillivray BC. Omphalocele: early prenatal diagnosis by ultrasound [letter]. JCU J Clin Ultrasound 1984; 12: A4.

7 Urogenital Tract

Bladder Exstrophy

Definition: Incomplete closure of the bladder, lower urinary tract, symphysis, and lower abdominal wall.

Incidence: One in 30 000 births.

Sex ratio: M : F = 3 : 1.

Clinical history/genetics: Mostly sporadic, rarely increased familial occurrence. Increase of alpha fetoprotein. If one parent is affected, there is a 1.5 % risk of occurrence.

Teratogens: Not known.

Embryology: The two halves of the bladder fail to close in the midline, so that this is not considered to be primarily a defect of the abdominal wall, but rather a disturbed development of the urogenital sinus at around 7–9 weeks after menstruation. The urethra and clitoris or penis are also affected.

Associated malformations: These are rarely found, except for the genital anomalies and clefting of the symphysis, which coexist with this malformation.

Ultrasound findings: The urinary bladder cannot be detected on repeated scans. A lesion is seen in the lower part of the abdomen (eversion of the posterior bladder wall). The insertion of the umbilical cord is lower than normal.

Clinical management: Further sonographic screening, including fetal echocardiography. Possibly karyotyping. Normal delivery.

Procedure after birth: The defect should be covered with sterile cloth. Early surgical correction. Additional operative procedures are necessary in the first years of life.

Prognosis: Surgical correction can restore urinary continence in 60–80 % of cases. The survival rate is > 90 %. Bladder cancers appear to occur more frequently in these patients.

Self-Help Organization

Title: Association for Bladder Exstrophy Community

Description: Mutual support for persons affected by bladder exstrophy, including parents of children with bladder exstrophy, adults, health-care professionals and others interested in exstrophy. Newsletter, literature, information and referrals, informal pen-pal program, conferences, advocacy, directory of members. Informal kids' e-mail exchange.

Scope: International network

Founded: 1991

Address: P.O. Box 1472, Wake Forest, NC 27 588–1472, United States

Telephone: 910-864-4308

E-mail: admin@bladderexstrophy.com

Web: http://www.bladderexstrophy.com/

References

Cacciari A, Pilu GL, Mordenti M, Ceccarelli PL, Ruggeri G. Prenatal diagnosis of bladder exstrophy: what counseling? J Urol 1999; 161: 259–61.

Gearhart JP, Ben Chaim J, Jeffs RD, Sanders RC. Criteria for the prenatal diagnosis of classic bladder exstrophy. Obstet Gynecol 1995; 85: 961–4.

Goldstein I, Shalev E, Nisman D. The dilemma of prenatal diagnosis of bladder exstrophy: a case report and a review of the literature. Ultrasound Obstet Gynecol 2001; 17: 357–9.

Langer JC, Brennan B, Lappalainen RE, et al. Cloacal exstrophy: prenatal diagnosis before rupture of the cloacal membrane. J Pediatr Surg 1992; 27: 1352–5.

Mirk P, Calisti A, Fileni A. Prenatal sonographic diagnosis of bladder exstrophy. J Ultrasound Med 1986; 5: 291–3.

Pinette MG, Pan YQ, Pinette SG, Stubblefield PG, Blastone J. Prenatal diagnosis of fetal bladder and cloacal exstrophy by ultrasound: a report of three cases. Reprod Med 1996; 41: 132–4.

Thomas DF. Prenatal diagnosis: does it alter outcome? Prenat Diagn 2001; 21: 1004–11.

Wilcox DT, Chitty LS. Non-visualisations of the fetal bladder: aetiology and management. Prenat Diagn 2001; 21: 977–83.

Genital Anomalies

Definition: In the prenatal scan, genital anomalies are diagnosed either as intersexual forms or as discrepancies between ultrasound findings and chromosomal findings.

Clinical history/genetics: Heterogeneous causes are known: 1, chromosomal anomalies; 2, gene mutation; 3, combined chromosomal and molecular defects; 4, multifactorial inheritance; 5, nongenetic causes (Table 7.**1**).

Incidence: With the exception of trisomy 13 and triploidy, chromosomal anomalies are rare. Single-gene anomalies such as the adrenogenital syndrome have an incidence of one in 15 000 births; hypospadias: one in 1000 male births.

Associated malformations: Xp duplication: facial clefts, ventricular septal defect. In addition to pseudohermaphroditism and actual intersexuality, intersexual genitals are found in trisomy 13, triploidy, 13q syndrome, camptomelic dysplasia, Smith–Lemli–Opitz syndrome, and in other very rare syndromes.

Ultrasound findings: Although the *genitals* are seen clearly, it is difficult to classify the gender correctly, the *penis* appearing too small or bent. The scrotal sac appears to be divided. A definite discrepancy is noted between the *ultrasound sex* determination and the *chromosomal sex.*

Clinical management: If the family history suggests adrenogenital syndrome, chorionic villous sampling should be performed, and HLA typing is also possible. An affected female fetus can thus be treated very early in the prenatal stage (even at the end of the first trimester) to minimize virilization.

Prognosis: This depends on the underlying disease; in adrenogenital syndrome, the prognosis is very favorable if therapy is started early.

Self-Help Organization

Title: Congenital Adrenal Hyperplasia

Description: Offers educational and emotional support to families of children with congenital adrenal hyperplasia. Provides information and referrals, pen-pal program, phone support, annual convention, networking. Quarterly newsletter. Assistance in starting new groups.

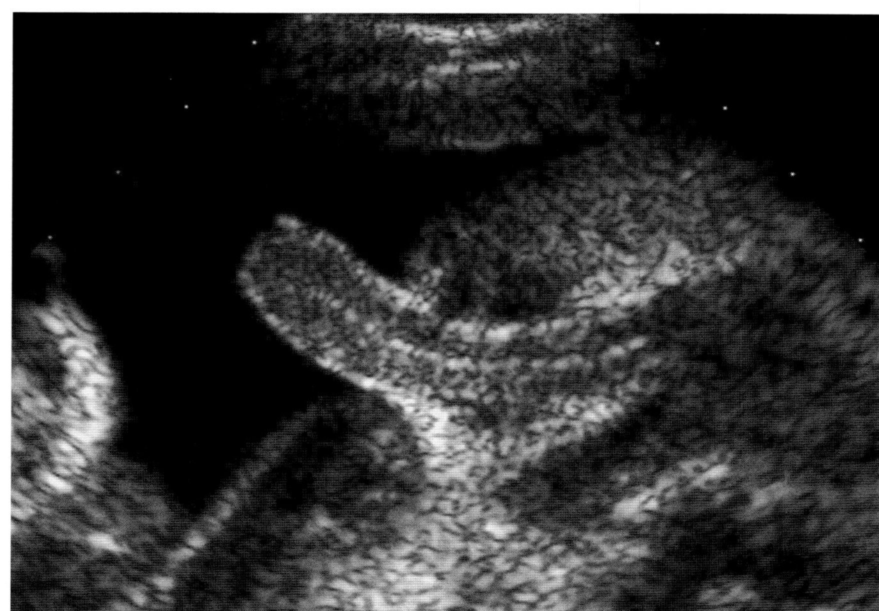

Fig. 7.**1** **Normal male genitals.** 33 weeks of gestation.

Table 7.**1** Heterogeneous genital anomalies arising from various causes

Chromosomal aberrations	
Xp, 1 p, 4 p, 9 p duplication; 10 q deletion; trisomy 13; 17 q aberration; triploidy; gonosomal mosaic (e.g., 45, X/6, XY)	Xp duplication: rare chromosomal aberration, genital anomalies of Y, double Xp chromosome: normal female genitalia or intersexual genitalia
Genetic mutations	
Adrenogenital syndrome (AGS)	Autosomal-recessive; the most common causes (in 70%) are mutations in the *CYP21* gene for 21-hydroxylase, gene locus 6 p21
Testicular feminization	Frequently X-recessive, gene mutation in the androgen receptor located at Xq11 – 12; any form between normal female genitals to intersexuality if 46,XY karyotype present
XY gonadal dysgenesis	Genetically heterogeneous; a frequent cause, in 10 – 15% of test persons, is a gene mutation in the testes-determining factor gene (*SRY* gene); a further 10 – 15% show deletion of the *SRY* gene, gene locus: Yp11.3. Depending on the expression of the gene mutation, there is either pure XY gonadal agenesis (Swyer syndrome) with normal female genitalia, or intersexual genitalia in incomplete gonadal dysgenesis. X-related recessive inheritance has been reported; autosomal-recessive inheritance with limited genital development is probable
Pure hermaphroditism	Possible combination of chromosomes: 46,XX, 46,XY or 46,XX/46,XY. Genetic cause largely unknown; *SRY* mutations have been seen in some cases, ovotestes or ovaries and testicles are present, external genitalia normal male or intersexual, presence of breasts
Smith–Lemli–Opitz syndrome, type II	Autosomal-recessive; hypospadias and cryptorchism if XY, no genital anomalies in female patients
Aarskog syndrome	X-related recessive, hypospadias
Genitopalatocardiac syndrome	Hypospadias or female genitalia in 46,XY karyotype, cardiac anomalies, cleft palate, club feet, kyphoscoliosis
Hypospadias	In rare cases, mutation in the *SRY* gene; mostly multifactorial inheritance (see below)
Denys–Drash syndrome	Gonadal dysgenesis; in 46,XY karyotype female or intersexual genitals, renal malformations, mutations in the Wilms tumor-1 gene (*WT1*)
Combined chromosomal aberration and molecular defect	
XX man	Normal female chromosomes. The gene for testes-determining factor (*SRY* gene) is incorrectly located on an X chromosome, a crossover that has failed in the germ-cell phase—this is the cause in 70% of XX men; the etiology for the rest is unclear. Normal male genitals are present
Camptomelic dysplasia	Two-thirds of patients have genital malformations with autosomal-dominant inheritance
Multifactorial inheritance	
Hypospadias	If hypospadias is not associated with a syndrome, the recurrence rate for male siblings is 10%
Nongenetic causes	
Vanishing twin	Early intrauterine death of a twin, with residual cellular components. This may be responsible for discrepancies in genital findings (especially in CVS diagnosis) that cannot be explained by contamination by maternal cells

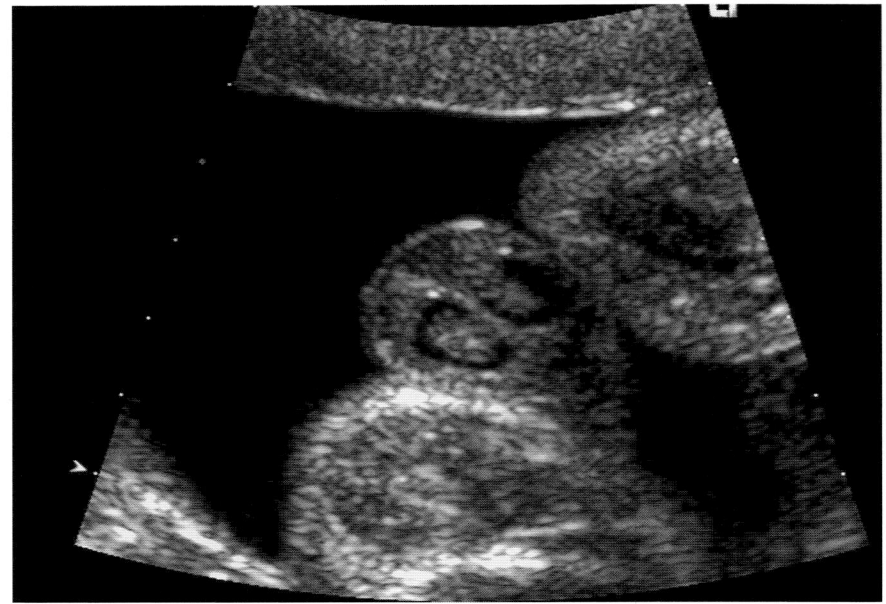

Fig. 7.2 **Hydrocele.** Fetal male gonads at 29 + 6 weeks. Bilateral hydroceles of the testes.

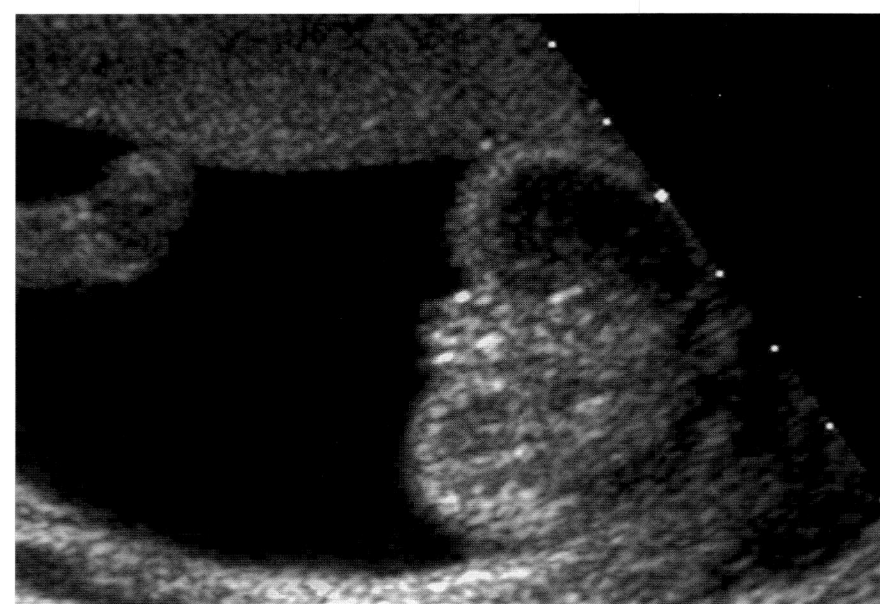

Fig. 7.3 **Normal female genitals,** 22 + 2 weeks. Cross-section showing labia majora and minora.

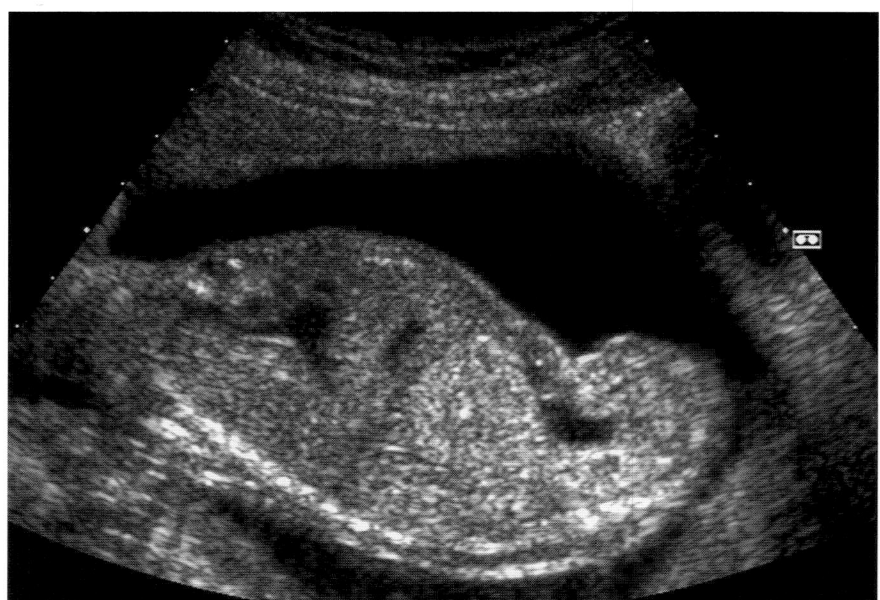

Fig. 7.4 **Normal female genitals,** 21 + 4 weeks. Longitudinal view showing the labia.

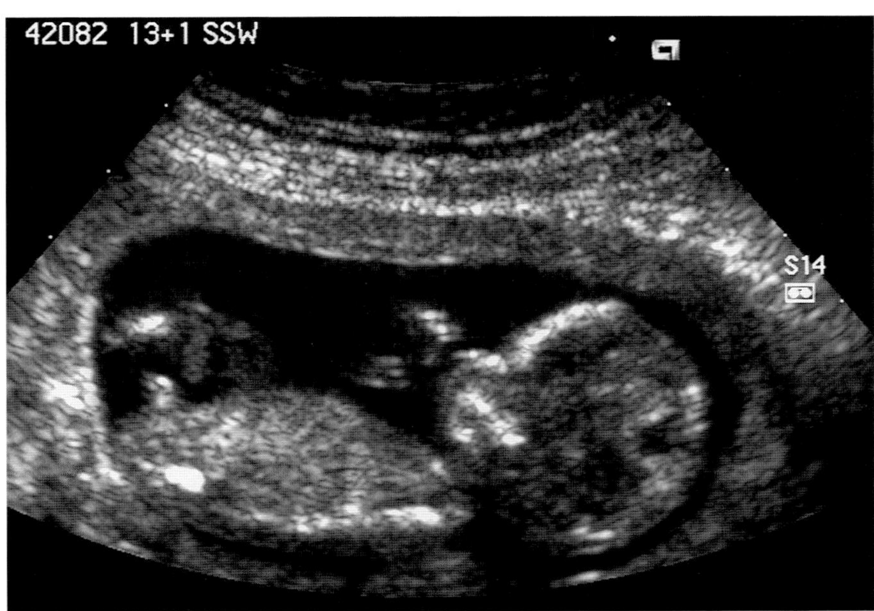

Fig. 7.5 **Normal male genitals,** 13 + 1 weeks. Longitudinal section. The penis is seen almost at right angles to the body surface.

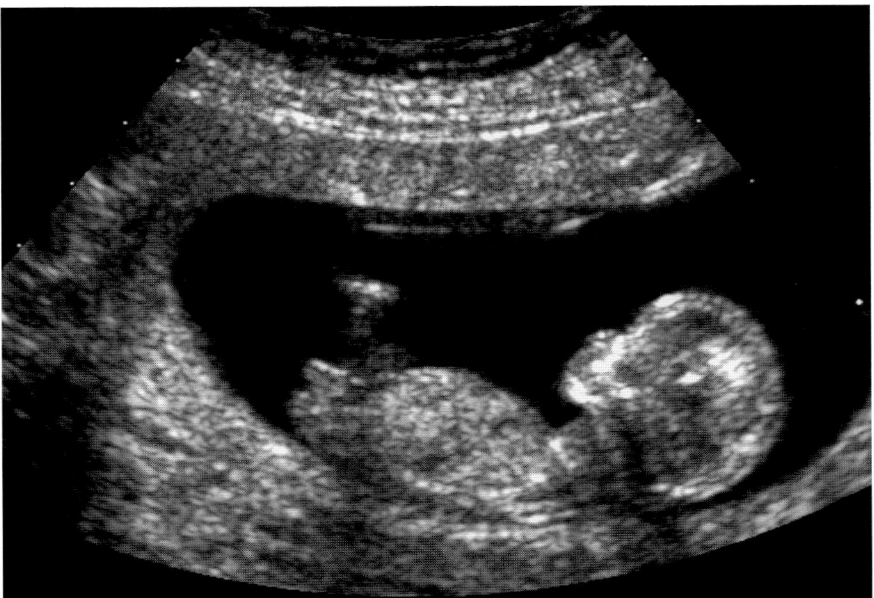

Fig. 7.6 **Normal female genitals,** 12 + 3 weeks. Longitudinal view. The clitoris is seen almost parallel to the body axis.

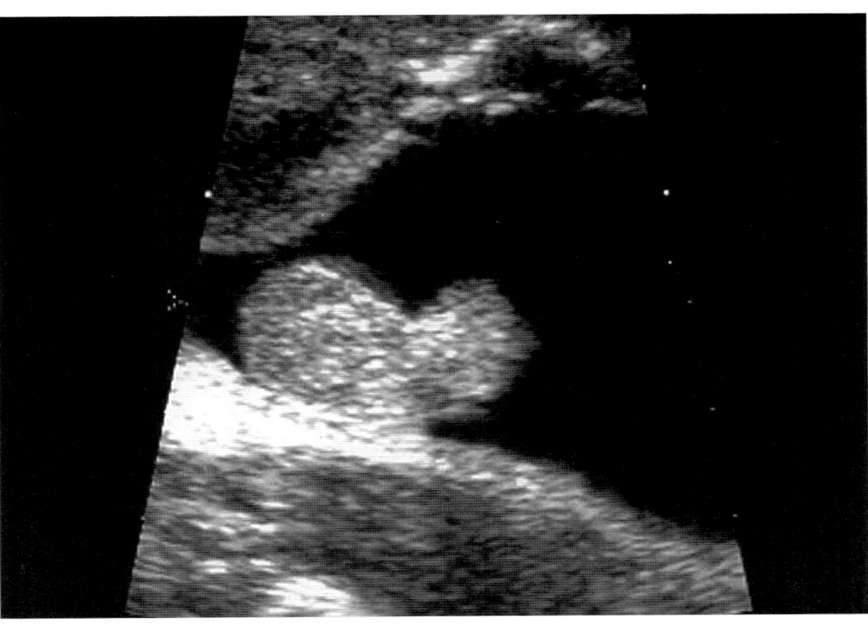

Fig. 7.7 **Scrotal hypospadias.** Genitals of a male fetus, longitudinal section. Atypical size and form of the penis: scrotal hypospadias, at 28 + 5 weeks.

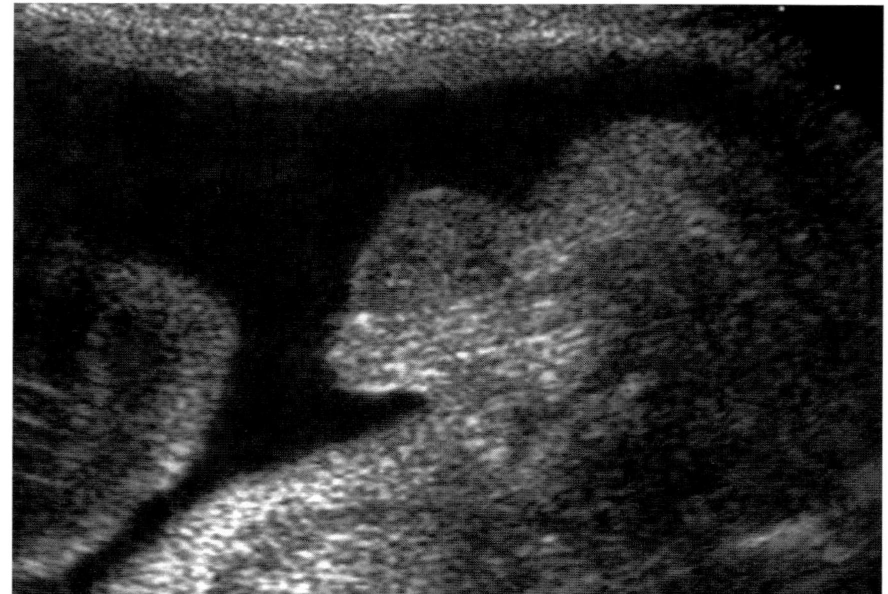

Fig. 7.**8** **Micropenis.** Male genitals, longitudinal section. Micropenis, 28 + 4 weeks.

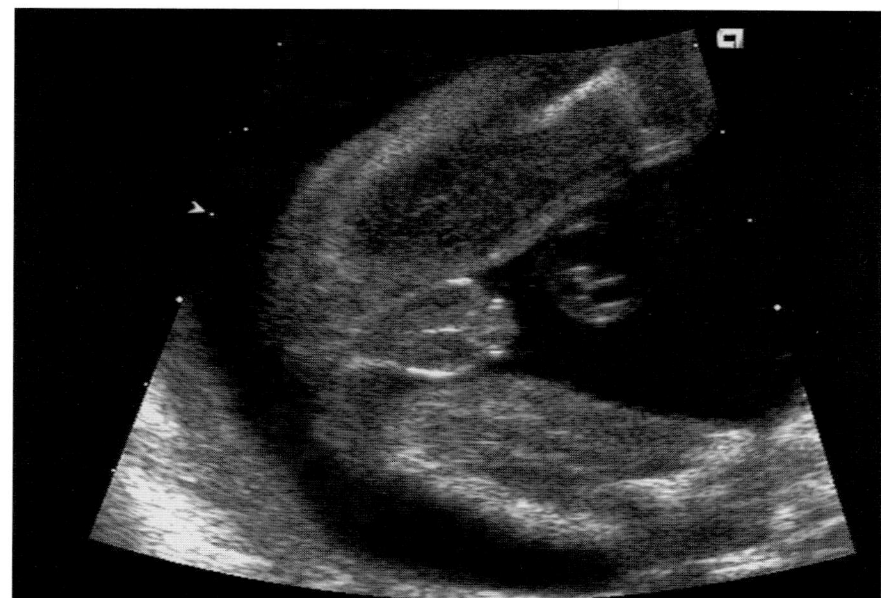

Fig. 7.**9** **Micropenis.** Male genitals 22 + 1 weeks, frontal view.

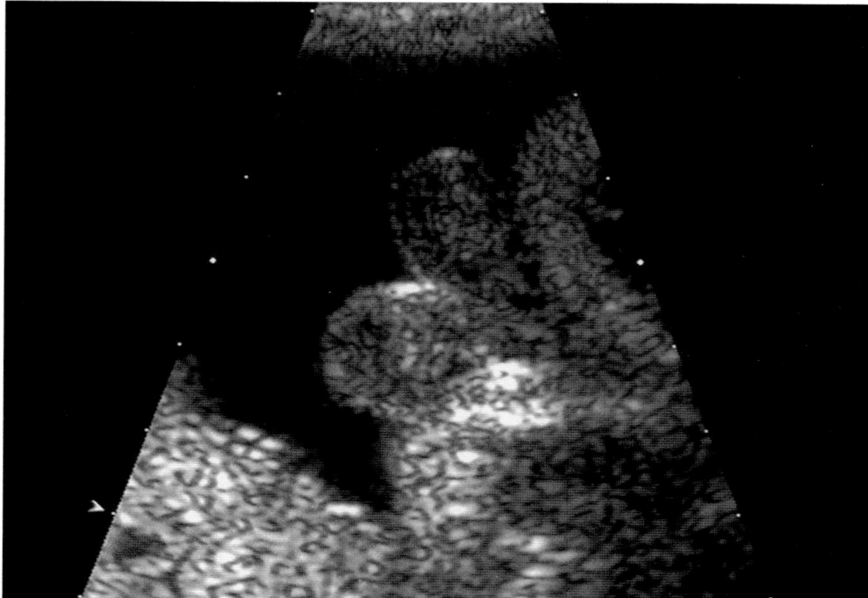

Fig. 7.**10** **Scrotum bipartitum,** at 30 + 2 weeks, in a fetus with anal atresia.

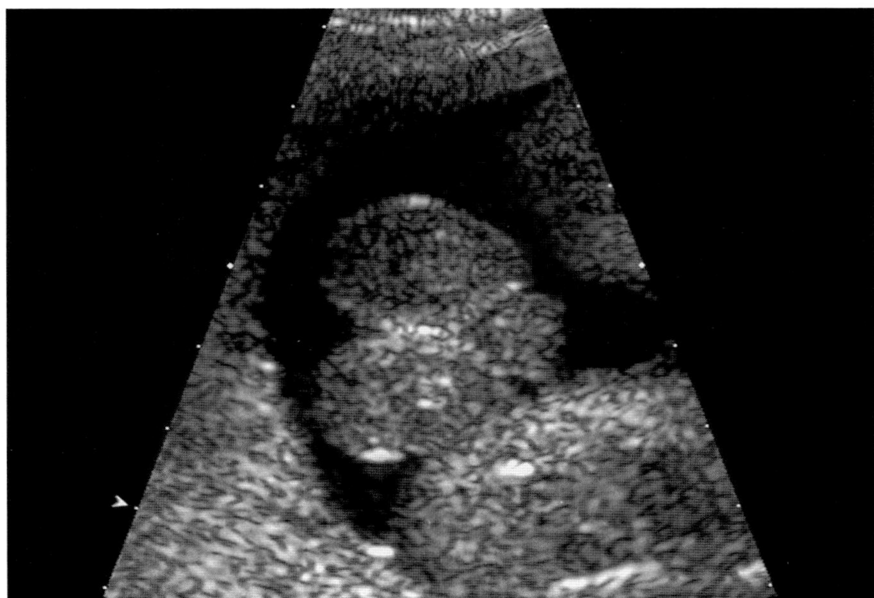

Fig. 7.**11** **Scrotum bipartitum, implying micropenis.** Frontal view at 30 + 2 weeks in a case of anal atresia. May be confused with female genitals.

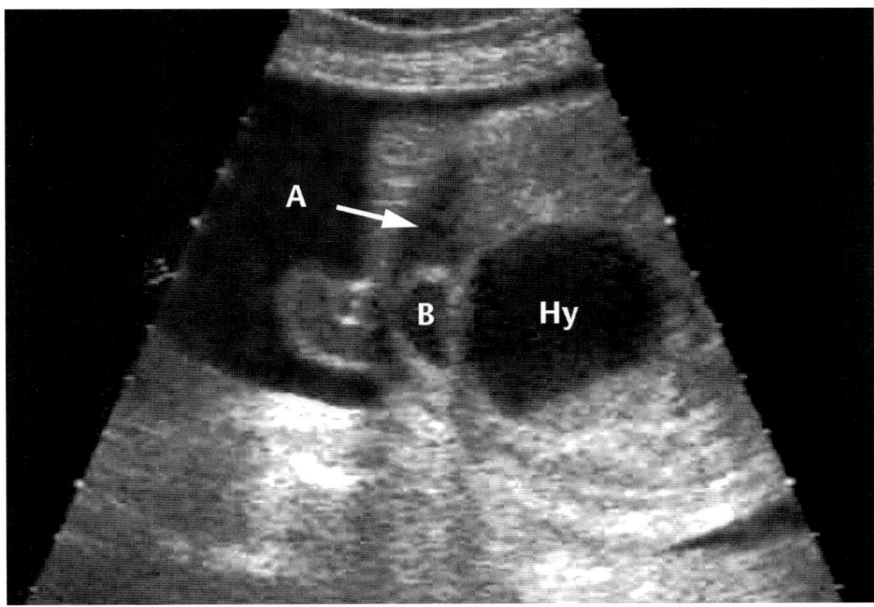

Fig. 7.**12** **Hydrometrocolpos in McKusick–Kaufmann syndrome,** 32 + 3 weeks. A: ascites, B: bladder, Hy: hydrometrocolpos.

Scope: National network of MAGIC

Founded: 1993

Address: CAH Division of MAGIC Foundation, 1327 N. Harlem Ave., Oak Park, IL 60302, United States

Telephone: 1-800-362-4423

Fax: 708-383-0899

E-mail: mary@magicfoundation.org

Web: http://www.magicfoundation.org

References

Angle B, Tint GS, Yacoub OA, Clark AL. Atypical case of Smith–Lemli–Opitz syndrome: implications for diagnosis. Am J Med Genet 1998; 80: 322–6.

Cerame BI, Newfield RS, Pascoe L, et al. Prenatal diagnosis and treatment of 11-beta-hydroxylase deficiency congenital adrenal hyperplasia resulting in normal female genitalia. J Clin Endocrinol Metab 1999; 84: 3129–34.

Cheikhelard A, Luton D, Philippe-Chomette P, et al. How accurate is the prenatal diagnosis of abnormal genitalia? J Urol 2000; 164: 984–7.

Kolon TF, Gray CL, Borboroglu PG. Prenatal karyotype and ultrasound discordance in intersex conditions. Urology 1999; 54: 1097.

Kratz LE, Kelley RI. Prenatal diagnosis of the RSH/Smith–Lemli–Opitz syndrome. Am J Med Genet 1998; 376–81.

Malini S, Valdes C, Malinak LR. Sonographic diagnosis and classification of anomalies of the female genital tract. J Ultrasound Med 1984; 3: 397–404.
Meizner I, Mashiach R, Shalev J, Efrat Z, Feldberg D. The "tulip sign": a sonographic clue for in-utero diagnosis of severe hypospadias. Ultrasound Obstet Gynecol 2002; 19: 250–3.
Neri G, Opitz J. Syndromal (and nonsyndromal) forms of male pseudohermaphroditism. Am J Med 1999: 89: 201–9.
Smith DP, Felker RE, Noe HN, Emerson DS, Mercer B. Prenatal diagnosis of genital anomalies. Urology 47: 114–7.
Speiser PW. Prenatal treatment of congenital adrenal hyperplasia. J Urol 1999; 162: 534–6.

Hydronephrosis

Definition: Dilation of the renal pelvis due to ureteropelvic, ureterovesical, vesicourethral stenosis or reflux. Hydronephrosis constitutes 75% of the renal anomalies detected prenatally. In 75% of cases, the finding is unilateral.

Incidence: One in 200 to 1 : 1000 births.

Sex ratio: M : F = 4 : 1 (ureteropelvic stenosis), M > F (ureterovesical stenosis).

Clinical history/genetics: Mostly sporadic, but may occur in association with 70 different syndromes.

Teratogens: Thalidomide, diabetes mellitus, cocaine, benzodiazepine.

Embryology: There are three different forms of obstruction—intrinsic, extrinsic, and secondary. The most common cause is the *intrinsic form*, due to an abnormal bundle of muscle leading to obstruction of the ureter. Over a certain period of time, this bundle degenerates, and the resulting fibrous tissue causes compression of the ureter. In the *extrinsic form*, the compression is caused primarily by a lesion outside of the ureter, usually a blood vessel anomaly (an accessory renal artery). The secondary form is due to ureterovesical reflux mimicking urinary tract obstruction.

Associated malformations: In 30% of cases, bilateral ureteropelvic stenoses are found. Other urogenital anomalies are found in a further 30%: cloaca formation, bladder exstrophy, ureterocele, megacystis, megaureter, urethral valve syndrome, ureter obstruction, vesicoureteral reflux. In addition, intra-abdominal tumors and cardiac anomalies may also be found.

Associated syndromes: In 20% of cases, multiple anomalies or syndromes coexist; chromosomal anomalies are found in 5%.

Ultrasound findings: *Widening of the renal pelvis* is well detected during abdominal scanning. The width of the renal pelvis should be measured in its anteroposterior diameter in a cross-sectional

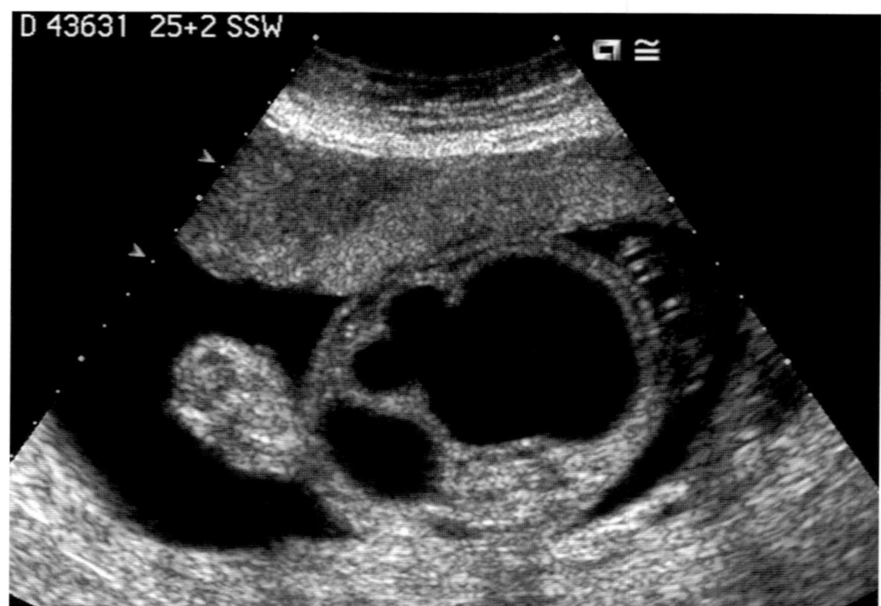

Fig. 7.**13** **Hydronephrosis.** Severe bilateral hydronephrosis at 25 + 2 weeks. The urinary bladder appears normal, and there is a normal amount of amniotic fluid.

scan. The transverse or oblique measurements give higher values, which are incorrect. It is difficult to detect *widening of the ureter*. In severe cases, the ureter can be followed up to its entry into the bladder. The upper limits for the widening of the renal pelvis are 5 mm around 20 weeks, and up to 10 mm after 30 weeks. The presence of *oligohydramnios* is an unfavorable sign.

Clinical management: Karyotyping; further sonographic screening, including fetal echocardiography. Regular scans to detect development of oligohydramnios so that early delivery may be considered if fetal maturity is achieved. In other cases, this is not necessary, as the renal parenchyma can recover very well even after weeks of renal congestion.

Procedure after birth: An ultrasound examination should be carried out on the second or the third day of life. Immediately after birth, diuresis is usually compromised due to the stress of labor, and renal congestion is not as pronounced as it is after a couple of days. Many cases do not require surgical correction. In these cases, an ultrasound check-up is recommended at 4 weeks. If reflux is diagnosed, antibiotics can be given prophylactically to prevent infection. Which surgical measures are taken (such as pyeloplasty or nephrostomy for decompression of obstruction over several months) depends on the severity of the findings and on the urologist's opinion.

Prognosis: After birth, spontaneous remission is seen in 40% of the cases diagnosed at the prenatal stage. In the first years of life, treatment-resistant reflux may cause irreversible renal damage due to recurrent urinary tract infection. Surgical corrections are very successful.

References

Bobrowski RA, Levin RB, Lauria MR, Treadwell MC, Gonik B, Bottoms SF. In utero progression of isolated renal pelvis dilation. Am J Perinatol 1997; 14: 423–6.

Chertin B, Rolle U, Farkas A, Puri P. Does delaying pyeloplasty affect renal function in children with a prenatal diagnosis of pelvi-ureteric junction obstruction? BJU Int 2002; 90: 72–5.

Cooper CS, Andrews JI, Hansen WF, Yankowitz J. Antenatal hydronephrosis: evaluation and outcome. Curr Urol Rep 2002; 3: 131–8.

Coplen DE. Prenatal intervention for hydronephrosis. J Urol 1997; 157: 2270–7.

Fugelseth D, Lindemann R, Sande HA, Refsum S, Nordshus T. Prenatal diagnosis of urinary tract anomalies; the value of two ultrasound examinations. Acta Obstet Gynecol Scand 1994; 73: 290–3.

Meizner I, Yitzhak M, Levi A, Barki Y, Barnhard Y, Glezerman M. Fetal pelvic kidney: a challenge in prenatal diagnosis? Ultrasound Obstet Gynecol 1995; 5: 391–3.

Nonomura K, Yamashita T, Kanagawa K, Itoh K, Koyanagi T. Management and outcome of antenatally diagnosed hydronephrosis. Int J Urol 1994; 1: 121–8.

Onen A, Jayanthi VR, Koff SA. Long-term follow-up of prenatally detected severe bilateral newborn hydronephrosis initially managed nonoperatively. J Urol 2002; 168: 1118–20.

Peters CA. The long-term follow-up of prenatally detected severe bilateral newborn hydronephrosis initially managed nonoperatively [editorial]. J Urol 2002; 168: 1121–2.

Philipson EH, Wolfson RN, Kedia KR. Fetal hydronephrosis and polyhydramnios associated with vesico-ureteral reflux. JCU J Clin Ultrasound 1984; 12: 585–7.

Podevin G, Mandelbrot L, Vuillard E, Oury JF, Aigrain Y. Outcome of urological abnormalities prenatally diagnosed by ultrasound. Fetal Diagn Ther 1996; 11: 181–90.

Quintero RA, Johnson MP, Arias F. In utero sonographic diagnosis of vesicoureteral reflux by percutaneous vesicoinfusion. Ultrasound Obstet Gynecol 1995; 6: 386–9.

Ransley PG, Dhillon HK, Gordon I, Duffy PG, Dillon MI, Barratt TM. The postnatal management of hydronephrosis diagnosed by prenatal ultrasound. J Urol 1990; 144: 584–7.

Thompson MO, Thilaganathan B. Effect of routine screening for Down's syndrome on the significance of isolated fetal hydronephrosis, Br J Obstet Gynaecol 1998; 105: 860–4.

Infantile Polycystic Kidney Disease (IPKD)

Definition: An autosomal-recessive disease in which normal renal tissue is replaced by widened renal tubules (1–2 mm). This causes symmetrical enlargement of the kidneys. Both kidneys are affected, resulting in renal failure.

Incidence: One in 20 000 to 1 : 50 000 births.

Sex ratio: M : F = 1 : 1.

Clinical history/genetics: Autosomal-recessive inheritance, rate of recurrence 25%.

Teratogens: Not known.

Associated malformation: Heart disease (VSD), cysts of the liver, Meckel–Gruber syndrome; also encephalocele and polydactyly. Trisomy 13.

Ultrasound findings: Both kidneys are considerably enlarged (above the 95th percentile for the gestational age). The renal parenchyma is very echogenic, and structural differentiation is absent. The bladder is almost empty. Severe oligohydramnios may develop, usually after 20 weeks of gestation. The circumference of the abdomen is increased due to enlarged kidneys.

Differential diagnosis: Bilateral polycystic renal dysplasia, Meckel–Gruber syndrome. Trisomy 13, adult or autosomal-dominant polycystic kidney disease.

Clinical management: Karyotyping, further sonographic screening, including fetal echocardiography. Ultrasound of the kidneys of both parents and siblings (adult form of polycystic kidney disease?). Exclude premature rupture of membranes causing amniotic fluid loss, regular scans to monitor amniotic fluid index. Vaginal delivery.

Procedure after birth: Hypoplasia of the lungs is expected. In the prenatal stage, a pediatrician should be consulted and the parents should be counseled regarding clinical management in the neonatal stage.

Prognosis: Intrauterine fetal death is the usual outcome. Only a small number survive the first year of life. All affected children develop renal insufficiency before adulthood.

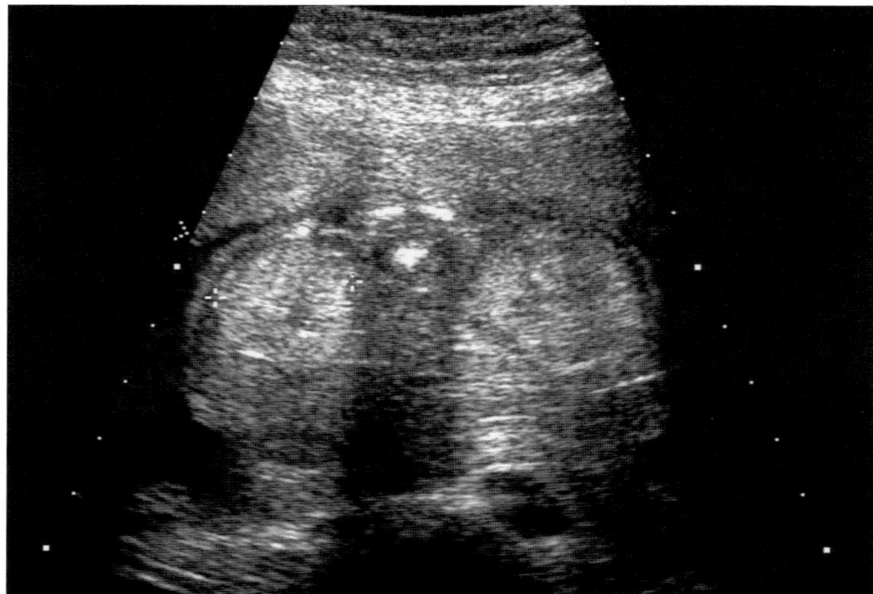

Fig. 7.**14** **Infantile polycystic kidney disease.** Cross-section of the fetal abdomen at the level of the kidneys, 23 + 0 weeks. Autosomal-recessive inheritance of the infantile form of polycystic kidney. Both kidneys are large and well visualized as echo-dense structures.

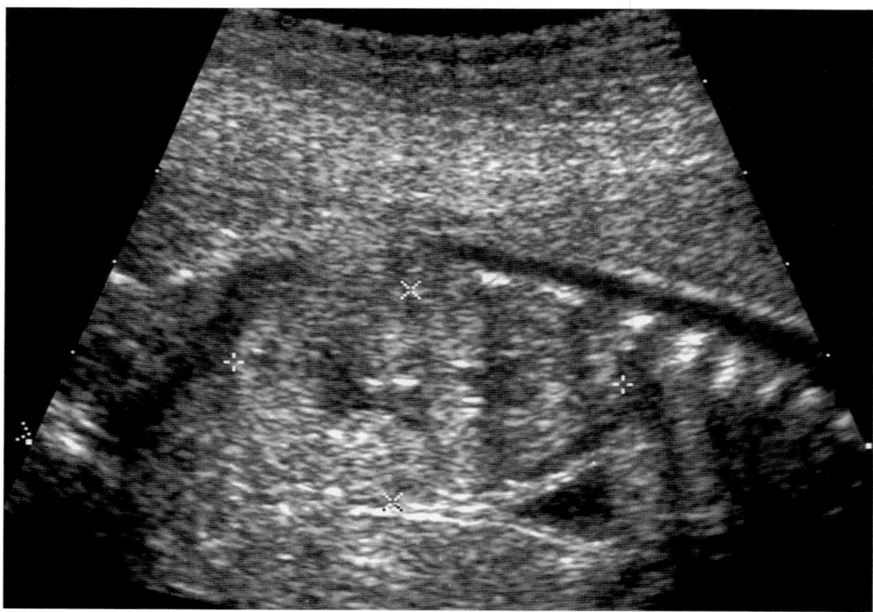

Fig. 7.**15** **Infantile polycystic kidney disease.** Same fetus, longitudinal section.

Self-Help Organization

Title: Polycystic Kidney Research Foundation

Description: Funds research and provides emotional support and education for persons with polycystic kidney disease and their families. Promotes public awareness. Holds medical seminars and fund-raisers. Conferences, phone support, newsletter, assistance in starting new groups.

Scope: International

Number of groups: 47 affiliated groups

Founded: 1982

Address: 4901 Main St., Suite 200, Kansas City, MO 64112, United States

Telephone: 1-800-753-2873 or 816-931-2600

Fax: 816-931-8655

E-mail: pkdcure@pkrfoundation.org

Web: http://www.pkdcure.org

References

Argubright KF, Wicks JD. Third trimester ultrasonic presentation of infantile polycystic kidney disease. Am J Perinatol 1987; 4: 1–4.

Bronshtein M, Bar HI, Blumenfeld Z. Clues and pitfalls in the early prenatal diagnosis of "late onset" infantile polycystic kidney. Prenat Diagn 1992; 12: 293–8.

Jung JH, Luthy DA, Hirsch JH, Cheng EY. Serial ultrasound of a pregnancy at risk for infantile polycystic kidney disease (IPKD). Birth Defects Orig Artic Ser 1982; 18: 173–9.

Ranke A, Schmitt M, Didier F, Droulle P. Antenatal diagnosis of multicystic renal dysplasia [review]. Eur J Pediatr Surg 2001; 11: 246–54.

Scott JE. Fetal, perinatal, and infant death with congenital renal anomaly. Arch Dis Child 2002; 87: 114–7.

Sessa A, Meroni M, Righetti M, Battini G, Maglio A, Puricelli SL. Autosomal-recessive polycystic kidney disease [review]. Contrib Nephrol 2001; 136: 50–6.

Tsuda H, Matsumoto M, Imanaka M, Ogita S. Measurement of fetal urine production in mild infantile polycystic kidney disease: a case report. Prenat Diagn 1994; 14: 1083–5.

Winyard P, Chitty L. Dysplastic and polycystic kidneys: diagnosis, associations and management [review]. Prenat Diagn 2001; 21: 924–35.

Multicystic Renal Dysplasia

Definition: Congenital renal dysplasia where the renal collecting tubules are extremely widened and thus appear as cysts. In 80% of cases, only one kidney is affected.

Incidence: One in 1000–1 : 5000 births.

Sex ratio: M > F.

Clinical history/genetics: Although most cases are sporadic, autosomal-dominant forms are described. In addition, the disease may occur in combination with at least 35 other syndromes.

Teratogens: Diabetes mellitus.

Associated malformations: Anencephalus, hydrocephalus, spina bifida, cleft lip and palate, microphthalmia, duodenal stenosis, tracheoesophageal fistula, anal atresia.

Ultrasound findings: This is characterized by evidence of *multiple cysts of various sizes in one, or rarely in both, kidneys*. The affected kidney is usually enlarged. The contralateral kidney may also be *enlarged, as it compensates* for the function of the affected kidney. The healthy kidney often shows a *slightly enlarged renal pelvis*. If both kidneys are affected, production of urine is decreased and oligohydramnios or even anhydramnios may result usually after 18 weeks. The volume of amniotic fluid remains normal if only one kidney is involved. The abdominal circumference may increase.

Clinical management: Karyotyping; further sonographic screening of other organs including fetal echocardiography. The kidneys of both parents should also be scanned to exclude or confirm autosomal-dominant forms. A pediatric urologist should be consulted and the parents should be counseled. In unilateral involvement, normal vaginal delivery is indicated, premature delivery does not offer any advantages. Bilateral disease is usually fatal after birth, due to hypoplasia of the lungs.

Procedure after birth: The diagnosis is confirmed through ultrasound scanning after birth. If only one side is affected, further treatment is

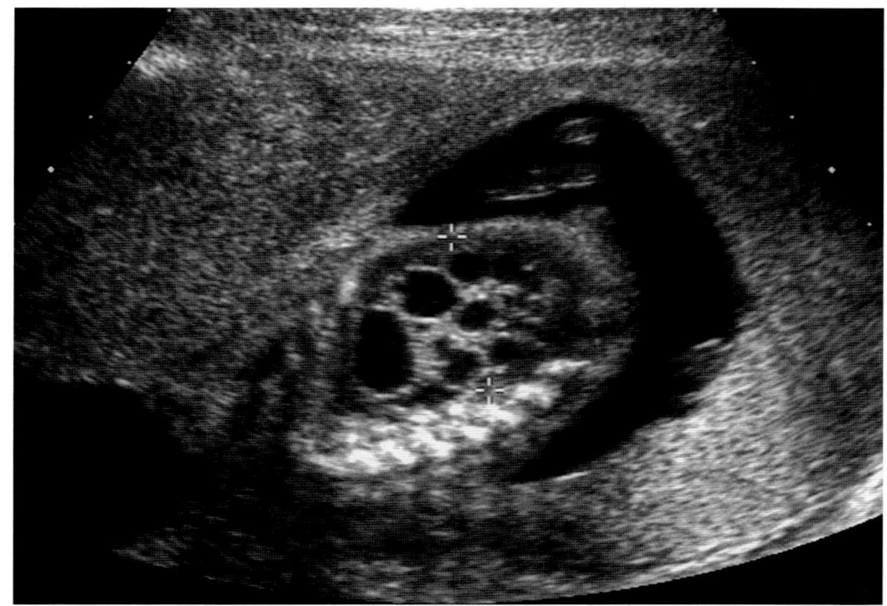

Fig. 7.**16** **Multicystic renal dysplasia.** Multicystic renal dysplasia, showing large cysts at 22 + 0 weeks. Longitudinal section.

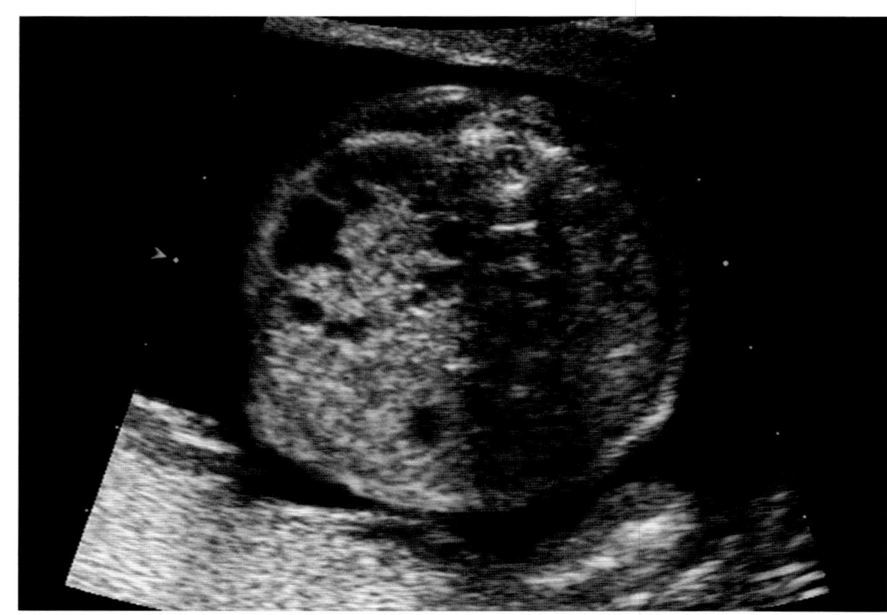

Fig. 7.**17** **Multicystic renal dysplasia.** Same case as before, with a cross-section of the fetal abdomen. The right kidney is affected, while the left is normal.

not necessary unless the enlarged kidney appears to be interfering with bowel motility. In these cases, the affected kidney is surgically removed.

Prognosis: One-sided renal disease does not restrict the quality of life in any way. The multicystic kidney usually decreases in size during the first year of life and after 2 years is often not detectable. Complete involvement of both kidneys has a fatal outcome. If only parts of both kidneys are affected, renal insufficiency may result.

Self-Help Organization

Title: National Potter Syndrome Support Group

Description: Support group and information network for families that have babies affected by Potter syndrome. Newsletter, information and referrals, phone support, parent match program.

Scope: National network

Founded: 1995

Address: 225 Louisiana Rd., Dyess AFB, TX 79607–1125, United States

Telephone: 915–692–0831

E-mail: potter_syndrome@hotmail.com

References

Aubertin G, Cripps S, Coleman G, et al. Prenatal diagnosis of apparently isolated unilateral multicystic kidney: implications for counselling and management. Prenat Diagn 2002; 22: 388–94.

Belk RA, Thomas DF, Mueller RF, Godbole P, Markham AF, Weston MJ. A family study and the natural history of prenatally detected unilateral multicystic dysplastic kidney. J Urol 2002; 167: 666–9.

Beretsky I, Lankin DH, Rusoff JH, Phelan L. Sonographic differentiation between the multicystic dysplastic kidney and the ureteropelvic junction obstruction in utero using high resolution real-time scanners employing digital detection. JCU J Clin Ultrasound 1984; 12: 429–33.

Diard F, Le Dosseur P, Cadier L, Calabet A, Bondonny JM. Multicystic dysplasia in the upper component of the complete duplex kidney. Pediatr Radiol 1984; 14: 310–3.

Dungan JS, Fernandez MT, Abbitt PL, Thiagarajah S, Howards SS, Hogge WA. Multicystic dysplastic kidney: natural history of prenatally detected cases. Prenat Diagn 1990; 10: 175–82.

Filion R, Grignon A, Boisvert J. Antenatal diagnosis of ipsilateral multicystic kidney in identical twins. J Ultrasound Med 1985; 4: 211–2.

Gordon AC, Thomas DF, Arthur RJ, Irving HC. Multicystic dysplastic kidney: is nephrectomy still appropriate? J Urol 1988; 140: 1231–4.

Nicolini U, Vaughan JI, Fisk NM, Dhillon HK, Rodeck CH. Cystic lesions of the fetal kidney: diagnosis and prediction of postnatal function by fetal urine biochemistry. J Pediatr Surg 1992; 27: 1451–4.

Ranke A, Schmitt M, Didier F, Droulle P. Antenatal diagnosis of multicystic renal dysplasia [review]. Eur J Pediatr Surg 2001; 11: 246–54.

Reuss A, Wladimiroff JW, Niermeyer ME Sonographic, clinical and genetic aspects of prenatal diagnosis of cystic kidney disease. Ultrasound Med Biol 1991; 17: 687–94.

Schifter T, Heller RM. Bilateral multicystic dysplastic kidneys. Pediatr Radiol 1988; 18: 242–4.

Sukthankar S, Watson AR. Unilateral multicystic dysplastic kidney disease: defining the natural history. Anglia Paediatric Nephrourology Group. Acta Paediatr 2000; 89: 811–3.

Renal Agenesis

Definition: Unilateral or bilateral absence of fetal kidneys.

Incidence: *Unilateral*: one in 600–1000, *bilateral*: one in 8000–40 000.

Sex ratio: *Unilateral:* M : F = 1 : 1, *bilateral:* M : F = 2.5 : 1.

Clinical history/genetics: Sporadic, rarely autosomal-dominant forms (unilateral).

Teratogens: Warfarin, cocaine, diabetes mellitus.

Embryology: Arises around 6–7 weeks after conception. It occurs due to failure of development of the ureteric buds of the mesonephros.

Associated malformations: Other renal malformations, gastrointestinal anomalies, cardiac anomalies. Over 50 malformation syndromes have been described.

Associated syndromes: Diabetic embryopathy, Smith–Lemli–Opitz syndrome, Fraser syndrome, EEC syndrome, short rib–polydactyly syndrome types I and III, caudal regression syndrome/sirenomelia, MURCS association, VACTERL association.

Ultrasound findings: A *reduction in amniotic fluid* results in poor visualization of internal structures, so that detection of the kidney is very difficult. One cannot visualize the kidney, but *the adrenal gland* may appear different in form and position, lying more caudally than normal. This may be *incorrectly interpreted* as renal tissue. The urinary bladder cannot be demonstrated in cases of bilateral agenesis. The diagnosis is confirmed *if a repeated ultrasound examination after an interval of 2 h fails to show the urinary bladder*. After about 18 weeks of gestation, oligohydramnios or anhydramnios may develop. *Color flow mapping* with an *angio-mode* is very useful in confirming the *absence of renal arteries*.

Clinical management: Karyotyping; further sonographic screening of other organs, including fetal echocardiography. Instillation of normal saline into the amniotic cavity improves the visualization of organs and thus helps confirm the diagnosis. In addition, this can, exclude premature rupture of the membranes causing amniotic fluid loss. Ultrasound examination of the kidneys of both parents and siblings. In unilateral renal agenesis, normal antenatal care and delivery.

Procedure after birth: Ultrasound examination of the kidneys after birth. In cases of unilateral agenesis, no further intervention is needed. In bilateral renal agenesis, the outcome is fatal and

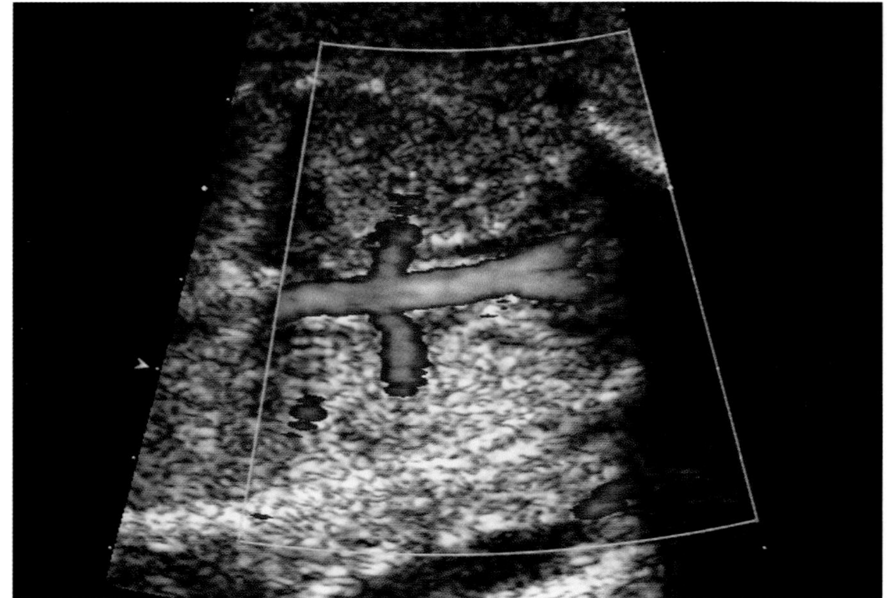

Fig. 7.**18** **Normal kidneys,** 21 + 4 weeks. Demonstration of one renal artery to each kidney.

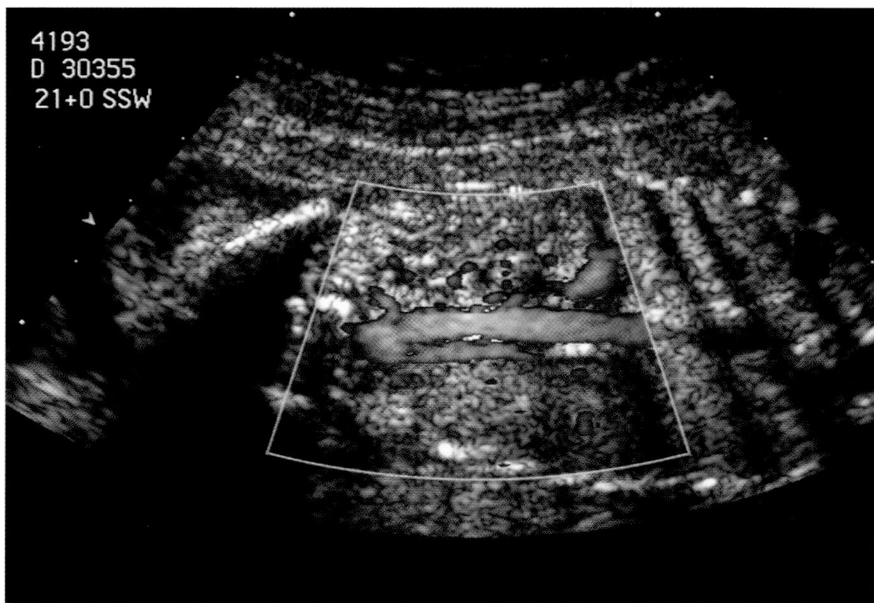

Fig. 7.**19** **Bilateral renal agenesis,** 21 + 0 weeks. Absence of renal tissue and renal arteries on both sides.

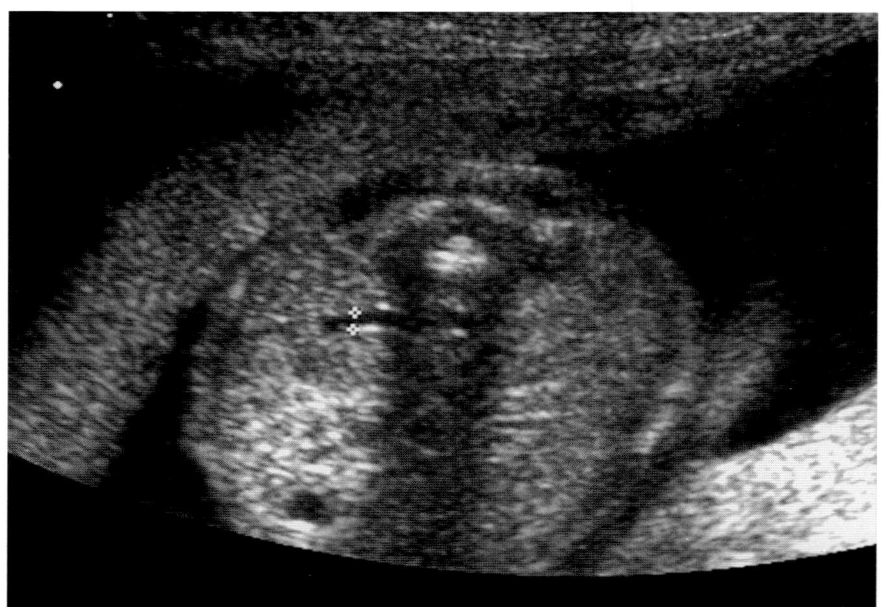

Fig. 7.**20** **Unilateral renal agenesis,** 21 + 6 weeks. There is a normal renal pelvis on the right, while the other side shows only bowel, with renal tissue being absent.

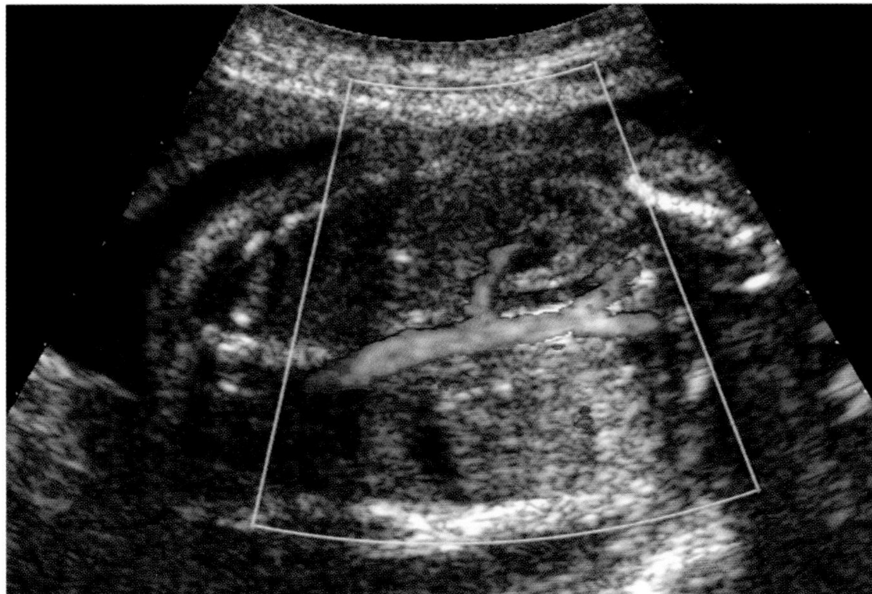

Fig. 7.21 **Unilateral renal agenesis,** 26 + 0 weeks. Color flow mapping shows only one renal artery. Renal tissue and the renal artery are absent on the contralateral side.

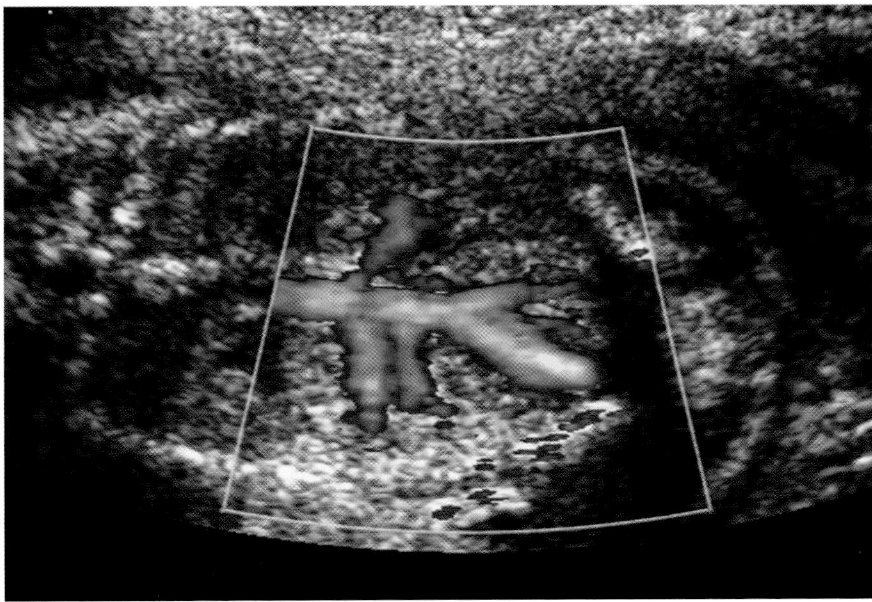

Fig. 7.22 **Unilateral double kidney.** One renal artery is demonstrated on the right, but two arteries branch off to the left.

death follows shortly after birth, due to hypoplasia of the lungs.

Prognosis: Bilateral renal agenesis results in intrauterine fetal death in 40 %. The rest die usually shortly after birth. Unilateral renal agenesis does not affect the further development of the infant and does not restrict the quality of life.

References

Curry CJ, Jensen K, Holland J, Miller L, Hall BD. The Potter sequence: a clinical analysis of 80 cases. Am J Med Genet 1984; 19: 679–702.

Dicker D, Samuel N, Feldberg D, Goldman JA. The antenatal diagnosis of Potter syndrome (Potter sequence): a lethal and not-so-rare malformation. Eur J Obstet Gynecol Reprod Biol 1984; 18: 17–24.

Dubbins PA, Kurtz AB, Wapner RJ, Goldberg BB. Renal agenesis: spectrum in utero findings. JCU J Clin Ultrasound 1981; 9: 189–93.

Hill LM, Rivello D. Role of transvaginal sonography in the diagnosis of bilateral renal agenesis. Am J Perinatol 1991; 8: 395–7.

Hitchcock R, Burge DM. Renal agenesis: an acquired condition? J Pediatr Surg 1994; 29: 454–5.

Hoffman CK, Filly RA, Callen PW The "lying down" adrenal sign: a sonographic indicator of renal agenesis or ectopia in fetuses and neonates. J Ultrasound Med 1992; 11: 533–6.

McCallum T, Milunsky J, Munarriz R, Carson R, Sadeghi-Nejad H, Oates R. Unilateral renal agenesis associated with congenital bilateral absence of the vas deferens: phenotypic findings and genetic considerations. Hum Reprod 2001; 16: 282–8.

Mackenzie FM, Kingston GO, Oppenheimer L. The early prenatal diagnosis of bilateral renal agenesis using transvaginal sonography and color Doppler ultrasonography. J Ultrasound Med 1994; 13: 49–51.

Morse RP, Rawnsley E, Crowe HC, Marin PM, Graham JMJ. Bilateral renal agenesis in three consecutive siblings. Prenat Diagn 1987; 7: 573–9.
Parikh CR, McCall D, Engelman C, Schrier RW. Congenital renal agenesis: case–control analysis of birth characteristics. Am J Kidney Dis 2002; 39: 689–94.
Romero R, Cullen M, Grannum P, et al. Antenatal diagnosis of renal anomalies with ultrasound, 3: bilateral renal agenesis. Am J Obstet Gynecol 1985; 1: 38–43.
Wilson RD, Hayden MR. Bilateral renal agenesis twins. Am J Med Genet 1985; 21: 147–9.

Hematoma of the Adrenal Gland

Definition: Bleeding into the tissues of adrenal gland resulting in calcification of the gland.

Incidence: Rare.

Clinical history/genetics: Congenital infection.

Associated malformations: Renal vein thromboses, leading to enlargement of the kidney and calcification.

Ultrasound findings: Cystic or echogenic lesions in the adrenal gland above the kidney. One or both adrenals may be involved. The ultrasound findings change in the course of the pregnancy. Occurrence usually in the third trimester.

Differential diagnosis: Neuroblastoma.

Clinical management: TORCH serology.

Procedure after birth: Function of the adrenal glands should be investigated (state of mineral balance).

Prognosis: Small lesions remain asymptomatic, whereas large lesions may lead to intrauterine fetal death.

References

Fang SB, Lee HC, Sheu JC, Lo ZJ, Wu BL. Prenatal sonographic detection of adrenal hemorrhage confirmed by postnatal surgery. J Clin Ultrasound 1999; 27: 206–9.
Gotoh T, Adachi Y, Nounaka O, Mori T, Koyanagi T. Adrenal hemorrhage in the newborn with evidence of bleeding in utero. J Urol 1989; 141: 1145–7.
Holgersen LO, Subramanian S, Kirpekar M, Mootabar H, Marcus JR. Spontaneous resolution of antenatally diagnosed adrenal masses. J Pediatr Surg 1996; 31: 153–5.
Janetschek G, Weitzel D, Stein W, Mijntefering H, Aiken P. Prenatal diagnosis of neuroblastoma by sonography. Urology 1984; 24: 397–402.
Lee W, Comstock CH, Jurcak ZS. Prenatal diagnosis of adrenal hemorrhage by ultrasonography. J Ultrasound Med 1992; 11: 369–71.
Nadler EP, Barksdale EM. Adrenal masses in the newborn. Semin Pediatr Surg 2000; 9: 156–64.
Rahman S, Ohlsson A, Fong KW, Glanc P. Fetal adrenal hemorrhage in a diamniotic, dichorionic twin: case report and review of controversies in diagnosis and management. J Ultrasound Med 1997; 16: 297–300.
Schwarzler P, Bernard JP, Senat MV, Ville Y. Prenatal diagnosis of fetal adrenal masses: differentiation between hemorrhage and solid tumor by color Doppler sonography. Ultrasound Obstet Gynecol 1999; 13: 351–5.
Speiser PW. Prenatal treatment of congenital adrenal hyperplasia. J Urol 1999; 162: 534–6.

Ovarian Cysts (Fetal)

Definition: Unilobular or multilobular cysts of the ovary, usually unilateral. Most frequently, these are benign functional cysts (theca lutein cysts).

Incidence: One in 6000 births.

Clinical history/genetics: Sporadic, except in McKusick–Kaufman syndrome (autosomal-recessive).

Teratogens: Not known.

Associated malformations: None.

Ultrasound findings: A *cystic lesion is visualized in the lower part of the abdomen* in a female fetus. Fetal ovarian cysts are mostly *without a septum, free of echoes, and with regular contours.* The cyst may be *displaced into the middle or upper abdomen.* This only rarely causes obstruction of the bowel resulting in hydramnios.

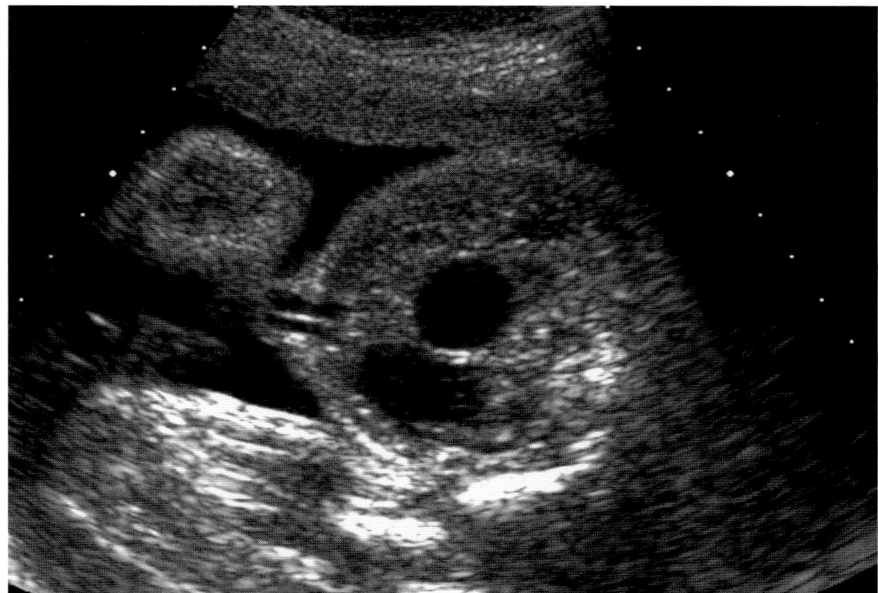

Fig. 7.**23** **Ovarian cysts.** Tilted cross-section of the lower abdomen of a female fetus at 27 + 5 weeks, showing two cystic lesions.

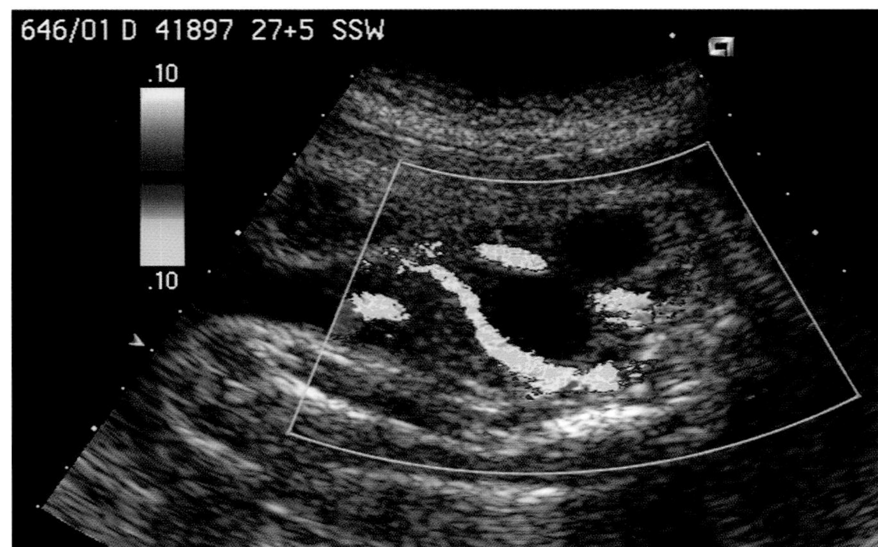

Fig. 7.**24** **Ovarian cysts.** Same fetus in the previous image, using color flow mapping: both umbilical arteries are seen on either side of the urinary bladder. A fetal ovarian cyst is seen next to it.

Differential diagnosis: Bowel duplication cysts, mesenteric cysts, cysts of the liver and the gallbladder.

Clinical management: Further sonographic screening, including fetal echocardiography. Karyotyping is advised to exclude cyst formation due to other causes. As spontaneous remission is known to occur frequently, aspiration of the cysts is controversial. Some authors advise intrauterine aspiration if the cyst is larger than 4 cm, as there is a danger of torsion of this mass.

Procedure after birth: Ultrasound scanning of the cyst after birth. Surgical treatment is only then indicated if the lesion is larger than 4–6 cm (to avoid possible torsion), if intra-abdominal bleeding is suspected, or if the lesion is causing bowel obstruction. Frequently, the cyst regresses spontaneously, but this may take a few months. Endoscopic removal of the cyst is also an option in the neonate, as long as an experienced team of surgeons is available to carry out this procedure. Histologically, these cysts are theca lutein and follicle cysts.

Prognosis: This is very good, as frequently the cyst regresses spontaneously. Endoscopic removal of the cyst with conservation of the rest of the ovary is usually possible.

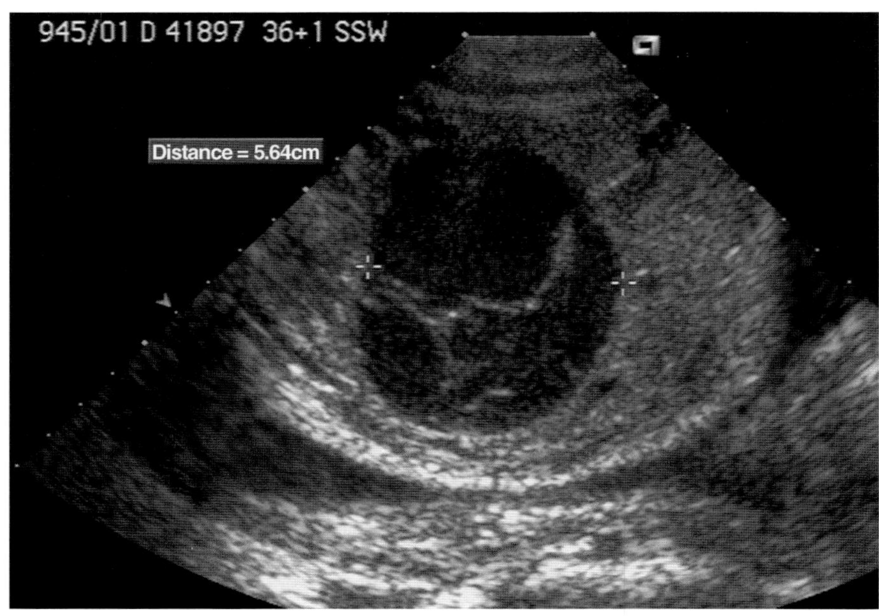

Fig. 7.**25** **Ovarian cysts.** Same fetus at 36 + 1 weeks. The cyst has increased in size to about 120 mL and contains low-level echoes representing internal bleeding. The hemoglobin level in the cystic fluid was 5.6 g%.

References

Abolmakarem H, Tharmaratnum S, Thilaganathan B. Fetal anemia as a consequence of hemorrhage into an ovarian cyst. Ultrasound Obstet Gynecol 2001; 17: 527–8.

Amodio J, Abramson S, Berdon W, et al. Postnatal resolution of large ovarian cysts detected in utero: report of two cases [published erratum in Pediatr Radiol 1988; 18: 178]. Pediatr Radiol 1987; 17: 467–9.

Bagolan P, Giorlandino C, Nahom A, et al. The management of fetal ovarian cysts. J Pediatr Surg 2002; 37: 25–30.

Bagolan P, Rivosecchi M, Giorlandino C, et al. Prenatal diagnosis and clinical outcome of ovarian cysts. Pediatr Surg 1992; 27: 879–81.

Born HJ, Kiihnert E, Halberstadt E. Diagnosis of fetal ovarian cysts: follow-up or differential diagnosis? Ultraschall Med 1997; 18: 209–13.

Crombleholme TM, Craigo SD, Garmel S, Dalton ME. Fetal ovarian cyst decompression to prevent torsion. J Pediatr Surg 1997; 32: 1447–9.

Giorlandino C, Rivosecchi M, Bilancioni E, et al. Successful intrauterine therapy of a large fetal ovarian cyst. Prenat Diagn 1990; 10: 473–5.

Heling KS, Chaoui R, Kirchmair F, Stadie S, Bollmann R. Fetal ovarian cysts: prenatal diagnosis, management and postnatal outcome. Ultrasound Obstet Gynecol 2002; 20: 47–50.

Mahomed A, Jibril A, Youngson G. Laparoscopic management of a large ovarian cyst in the neonate. Surg Endosc 1998; 12: 1272–4.

Perrotin F, Potin J, Haddad G, Sembely-Taveau C, Lansac J, Body G. Fetal ovarian cysts: a report of three cases managed by intrauterine aspiration [review]. Ultrasound Obstet Gynecol 2000; 16: 655–9.

van der Zee DC, van Seumeren IG, Bax KM, Rovekamp MH, ter Gunne AJ. Laparoscopic approach to surgical management of ovarian cysts in the newborn. J Pediatr Surg 1995; 30: 42–3.

von Schweinitz D, Habenicht R, Hoyer PF. Spontaneous regression of neonatal ovarian cysts: a prospective study. Monatsschr Kinderheilkd 1993; 141: 48–52.

Sacrococcygeal Teratoma

Definition: A teratoma localized in the sacrococcygeal region. Forty-seven percent are located externally, outside the pelvic cavity; 34% are external with some components reaching into the pelvis presacrally, and 19% are located only within the pelvic cavity in front of the sacrum. Eighty percent are benign, 20% are undifferentiated and malignant.

Incidence: One in 40 000 births.

Sex ratio: M : F = 1 : 3.

Clinical history/genetics: Mostly sporadic, rarely familial with an autosomal-dominant inheritance, sometimes aberration of chromosome 7 q-.

Teratogens: Not known.

Embryology: There are theories regarding the development of teratomas: 1, during the phase of migration from the yolk sac, there are some residual omnipotent cells that do not develop further into normal mesoderm, with the resulting teratomas lying axially or para-axially; 2, parthenogenetic cells that arise from a single germ cell are responsible—this would only explain ovarian teratomas, if any; 3, teratomas actually represent a degenerated twin—a theory that has been popularized in the lay media. If the latter theory is correct, it would also apply to brain teratomas, mediastinal and abdominal teratomas, and sacrococcygeal lesions.

Associated malformations: Obstruction of the urinary tract may arise secondary to compression from this type of teratoma. Arteriovenous anastomosis within the tumor may cause cardiac insufficiency and development of fetal hydrops. Malformations of the vertebral column and neural tube defects are found in 12–18% of cases. Anal atresia, esophageal atresia, and hydrocephalus have also been described.

Ultrasound findings: A *lesion is seen at the distal end of the vertebral column, which may appear as a cystic, partly solid, or purely solid lesion*. The lesions can be very large in size, sometimes even larger than the fetal torso. The lesion may be located either *externally, outside of the body surface behind the sacrum* or *inside the pelvic cavity in front of the sacrum*. Combined forms also exist involving both locations. Calcifications are often detected. Tumors lying inside the pelvis may displace the urinary bladder upwards. Hydramnios is a common feature. Arteriovenous anastomoses within the tumor can lead to an increase in volume load and cardiac failure, and fetal hydrops may follow.

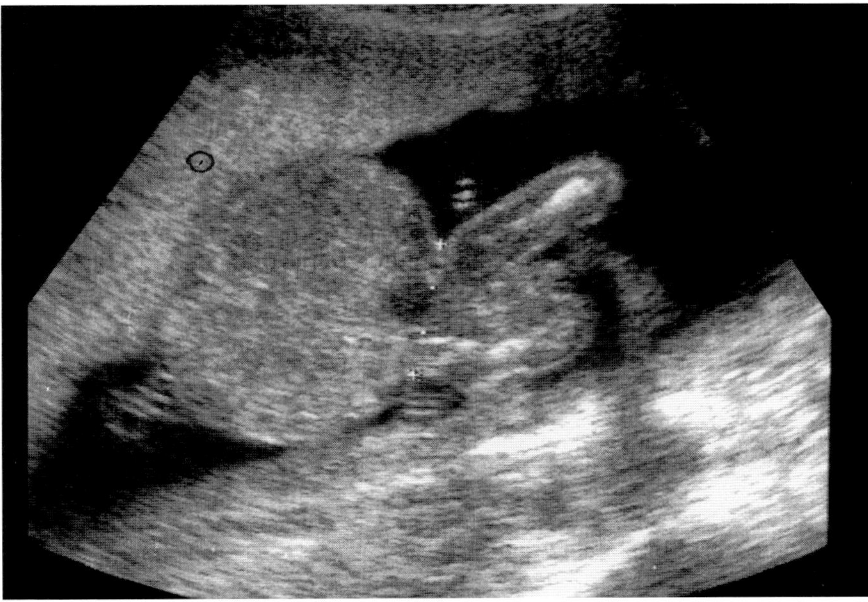

Fig. 7.**26** **Fetal sacrococcygeal teratoma,** 21 + 6 weeks.

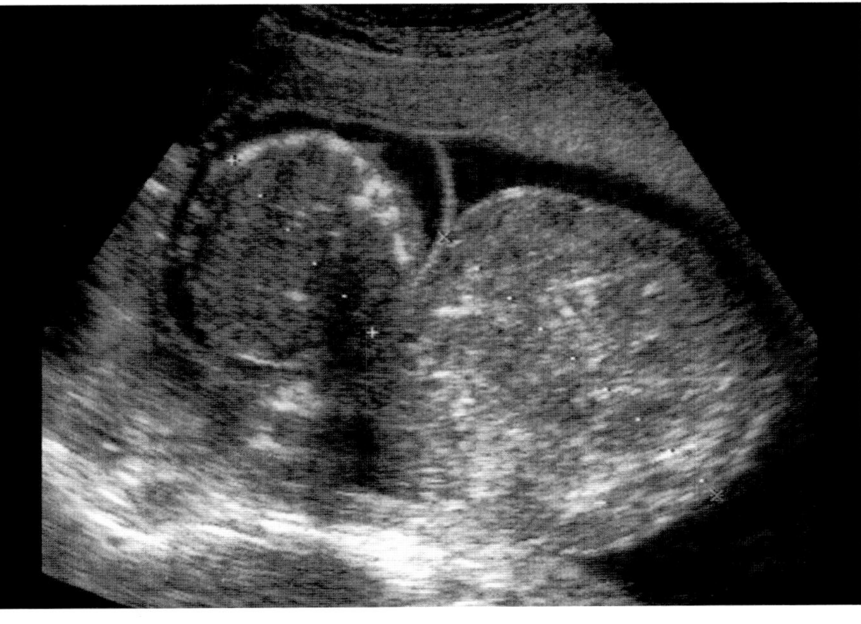

Fig. 7.**27** **Fetal sacrococcygeal teratoma.** Same fetus at 24 weeks, with nonimmune hydrops fetalis (NIHF) due to increased volume and overloading of the heart. Intrauterine fetal demise.

Differential diagnoses: Fibroma, myelomeningocele.

Clinical management: Karyotyping, further sonographic screening of other organs, including fetal echocardiography. Alpha fetoprotein may be increased, and acetylcholinesterase may be detected in the amniotic fluid. Regular ultrasound checks are needed to detect hydrops as soon as it begins to develop. If hydrops appears before 28–30 weeks of gestation, surgical intervention may be necessary, and premature delivery is therefore an option. Large tumors lying externally may bleed during vaginal delivery, and cesarean section is therefore advisable in order to reduce this risk.

Procedure after birth: The tumor should be covered using a sterile cloth and handled carefully, as minimal trauma may cause bleeding from tumor vessels, which may be life-threatening. Dangerous loss of fluid and heat may result if the tumor is covered by a very thin membrane. Measuring the level of alpha fetoprotein in the newborn may provide evidence of the malignancy of the lesion. Ultrasound, computed tomography, and magnetic resonance imaging can provide a good assessment of the extent of the tumor within the small pelvis. Surgical removal is required in all cases.

Prognosis: Two-thirds of the tumors lying within the pelvis that are not evident at birth are detected within the first 2 months of life. Ten percent of these are malignant. Tumors that are diagnosed at a later stage due to obstruction of the urinary tract or sub-ileus symptoms are malignant in 90% of cases. The perioperative mortality lies at 10% and depends on the size of the tumor. As these tumors compress the underlying nerves, urinary and fecal incontinence develops and may persist in 25% of newborns.

References

Alter DN, Reed KL, Marx GR, Anderson CF, Shenker L. Prenatal diagnosis of congestive heart failure in a fetus with a sacrococcygeal teratoma. Obstet Gynecol 1988; 71: 978–81.

Axt-Fliedner R, Hendrik HJ, Reinhard H, et al. Prenatal diagnosis of sacrococcygeal teratoma: a review of cases between 1993 and 2000. Clin Exp Obstet Gynecol 2002; 29: 15–8.

Bachmann G, Schtick R, Jovanovic V, Bauer T. The MRI in pre- and postnatal diagnosis of congenital sacrococcygeal teratoma. Radiologe 1995; 35: 504–7.

Bonilia-Musoles F, Machado LE, Raga F, Osborne NG, Bonilla F Jr. Prenatal diagnosis of sacrococcygeal teratomas by two- and three-dimensional ultrasound. Ultrasound Obstet Gynecol 2002; 19: 200–5.

Danzer E, Schier F, Paek B, Harrison MR, Albanese CT. [Fetal surgery for severe congenital abnormalities; in German; review.] Z Geburtshilfe Neonatol 2001; 205: 174–88.

De Backer A, Erpicum P, Philippe P, et al. Sacrococcygeal teratoma: results of a retrospective multicentric study in Belgium and Luxembourg. Eur J Pediatr Surg 2001; 11: 182–5.

Hecht F, Hecht BK, O'Keeffe D. Sacrococcygeal teratoma: prenatal diagnosis with elevated alphafetoprotein and acetylcholinesterase in amniotic fluid. Prenat Diagn 1982; 2: 229–31.

Lam YH, Tang MH, Shek TW. Thermocoagulation of fetal sacrococcygeal teratoma. Prenat Diagn 2002; 22: 99–101.

Montgomery ML, Lillehei C, Acker D, Benacerraf BR. Intra-abdominal sacrococcygeal mature teratoma or fetus in fetu in a third-trimester fetus. Ultrasound Obstet Gynecol 1998; 11: 219–21.

Morrow RJ, Whittle MJ, McNay MB, Cameron AD, Raine PA, Gibson AA. Prenatal diagnosis of an intra-abdominal sacrococcygeal teratoma. Prenat Diagn 1990; 10: 753–6.

Seeds JW, Mittelstaedt CA, Cefalo RC, Parker TFJ. Prenatal diagnosis of sacrococcygeal teratoma: an anechoic caudal mass. JCU J Clin Ultrasound 1982; 10: 193–5.

Shipp TD, Shamberger RC, Benacerraf BR. Prenatal diagnosis of a grade IV sacrococcygeal teratoma. J Ultrasound Med 1996; 15: 175–7.

Teal LN, Angtuaco TL, Jimenez JF, Quirk JGJ. Fetal teratomas: antenatal diagnosis and clinical management. JCU J Clin Ultrasound 1988; 16: 329–6.

Winderl LM, Silverman RK. Prenatal identification of a completely cystic internal sacrococcygeal teratoma (type IV). Ultrasound Obstet Gynecol 1997; 9: 425–8.

Ureterocele

Definition: Cystic dilation of the intravesical part of the ureter.

Incidence: One in 5000 births.

Sex ratio: M : F = 1 : 5.

Clinical history/genetics: Sporadic, sometimes multifactorial inheritance.

Teratogens: Not known.

Embryology: Duplication of the ureter is often the cause. In 10–20% of cases, the finding is bilateral.

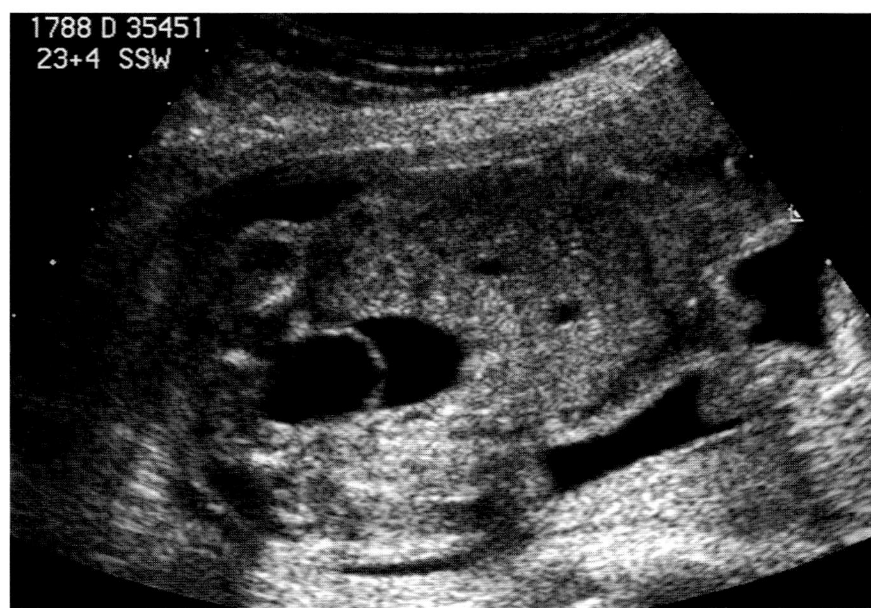

Fig. 7.**28** **Ureterocele.** Division of the fetal urinary bladder by a septum at 23 + 4 weeks, with a ureterocele and double ureter.

Ultrasound findings: Due to obstruction of the ureter, *hydronephroses and hydroureter* are diagnosed. If renal pelvis is duplicated (in 75% of cases), partial hydronephrosis is possible. A *cystic widening of the ureter* is seen within the urinary bladder (as a cystic lesion at the lateral bladder wall or a double contour within the bladder). If the findings are bilateral, oligohydramnios may develop.

Clinical management: Karyotyping; further sonographic screening, including fetal echocardiography. In cases of bilateral involvement and oligohydramnios, puncture of the urinary bladder may be useful in determining renal function. Sometimes this has a therapeutic effect. Regular ultrasound examinations. Premature delivery is only indicated if bilateral disease and oligohydramnios are diagnosed.

Procedure after birth: Urinary output has to be carefully monitored if both sides are involved. Ultrasound evaluation of the finding. Endoscopic surgical incision is possible and may relieve renal obstruction. In case of a double kidney, partial nephrectomy and resection of the second ureter is an alternative treatment.

Prognosis: Excellent. Usually, renal function recovers well. Reflux or urinary incontinence may result after surgical treatment.

References

Abuhamad AZ, Horton CEJ, Horton SH, Evans AT. Renal duplication anomalies in the fetus: clues for prenatal diagnosis. Ultrasound Obstet Gynecol 1996; 7: 174–7.

Athey PA, Carpenter RJ, Hadlock FP, Hedrick TD. Ultrasonic demonstration of ectopic ureterocele. Pediatrics 1983; 71: 568–71.

Caione P, Zaccara A, Capozza N, De Gennaro M. How prenatal ultrasound can affect the treatment of ureterocele in neonates and children. Eur Urol 1989; 16: 195–9.

Di Benedetto V, Morrison LG, Bagnara V, Monfort G. Transurethral puncture of ureterocele associated with single collecting system in neonates. J Pediatr Surg 1997; 32: 1325–7.

Hansen WF, Cooper CS, Yankowitz J. Ureterocele causing anhydramnios successfully treated with percutaneous decompression. Obstet Gynecol 2002; 99: 953–6.

Schoenecker SA, Cyr DR, Mack LA, Shuman WP, Lenke RR. Sonographic diagnosis of bilateral fetal renal duplication with ectopic ureteroceles. J Ultrasound Med 1985; 4: 617–8.

Sherer DM, Hulbert WC. Prenatal sonographic diagnosis and subsequent conservative surgical management of bilateral ureteroceles. Am J Perinatol 1995; 12: 174–7.

Upadhyay J, Bolduc S, Braga L, et al. Impact of prenatal diagnosis on the morbidity associated with ureterocele management. J Urol 2002; 167: 2560–5.

Vergani P, Ceruti P, Locatelli A, et al. Accuracy of prenatal ultrasonographic diagnosis of duplex renal system. J Ultrasound Med 1999; 18: 463–7.

Woodward M, Frank D. Postnatal management of antenatal hydronephrosis [review]. BJU Int 2002; 89: 149–56.

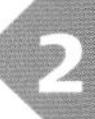

Urethral Valve Sequence

Definition: A membranous structure in the posterior urethra of male fetus causing urinary tract obstruction.

Incidence: Rare.

Sex ratio: Only males are affected.

Clinical history/genetics: Sporadic, rarely familial (multifactorial inheritance).

Teratogens: Not known.

Embryology: The development of the posterior urethral valves occurs usually at 5–7 weeks of gestation. In this embryonic stage, the lumen of the urethra is temporarily occluded. Absence of recanalization of the lumen or hypertrophy of these valves may cause obstruction.

Associated malformations: Trisomies are present in up to 20% of the cases. Megacystis–microcolon syndrome (also in females). It is still a matter of controversy whether *prune belly syndrome* (Eagle–Barrett syndrome, triad of hypotonic abdominal wall, urinary tract obstruction, and

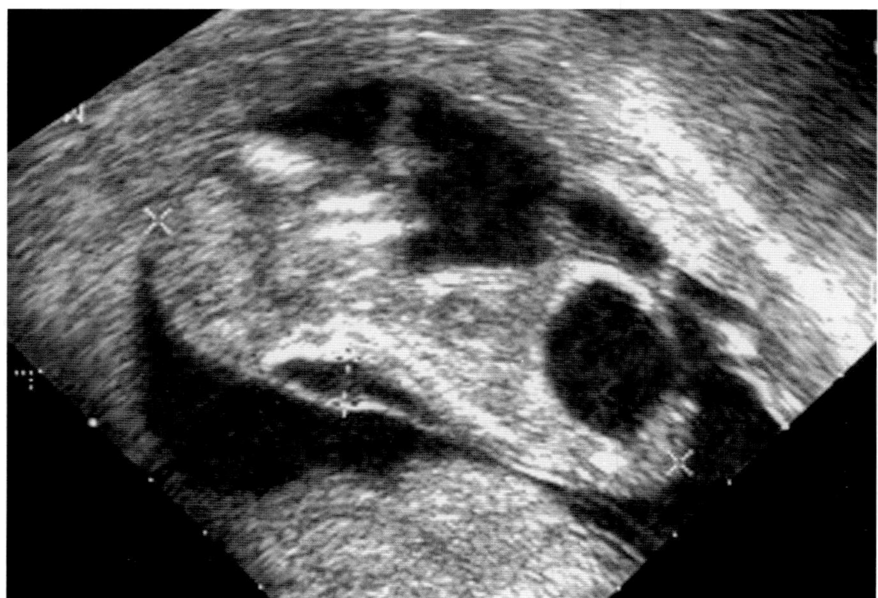

Fig. 7.**29** **Urethral valve sequence.** Megacystis in combination with hygroma colli at 14 weeks, in a case of trisomy 18.

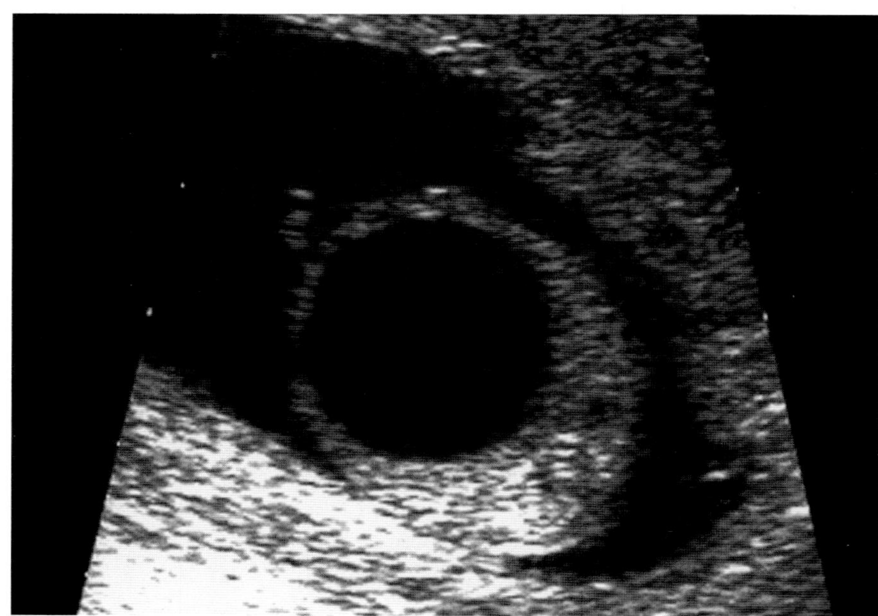

Fig. 7.**30** **Urethral valve sequence.** Same case. Cross-section of the lower fetal abdomen.

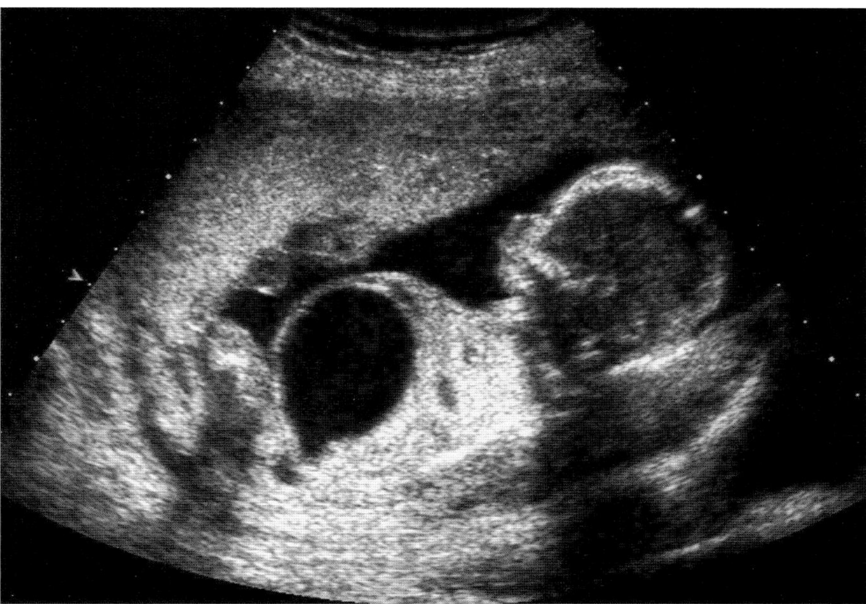

Fig. 7.**31** **Urethral valve sequence.** Megacystis at 15 weeks, longitudinal section. No other anomalies, normal male karyotype.

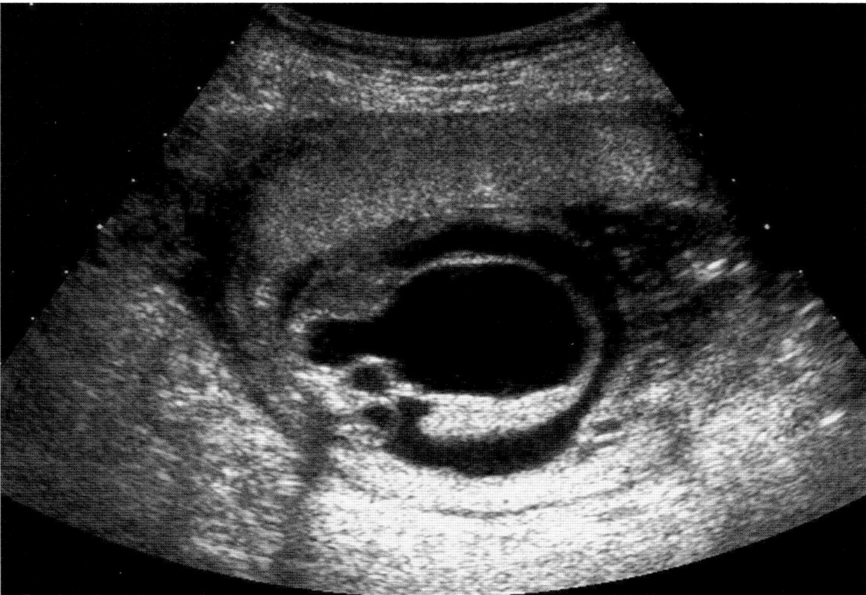

Fig. 7.**32** **Urethral valve sequence.** Same case, in a cross-section showing the “keyhole phenomenon.” There is a small amount of ascites due to a temporary vesicoabdominal fistula after bladder aspiration.

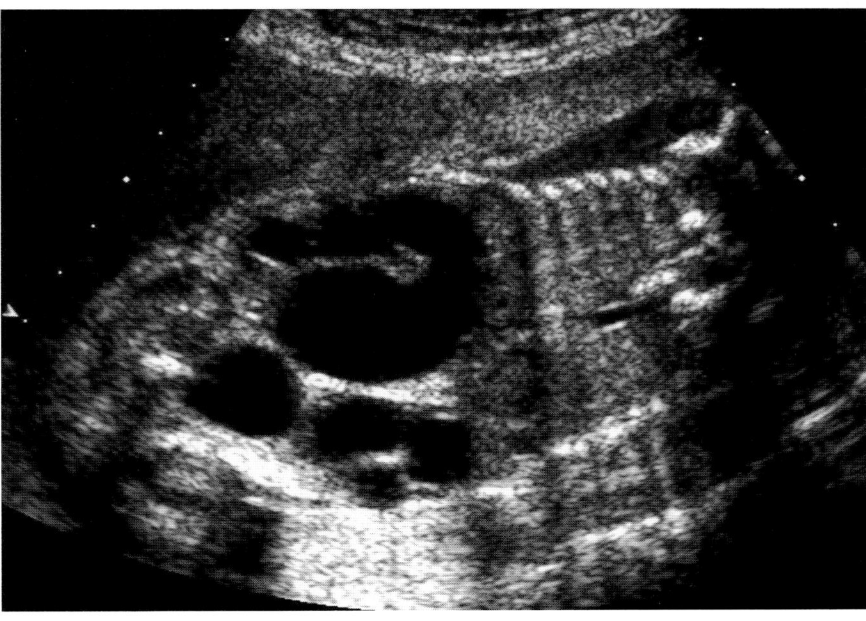

Fig. 7.**33** **Urethral valve sequence.** Same fetus, 23 + 1, with severe distension of the ureter and unilateral hydronephrosis.

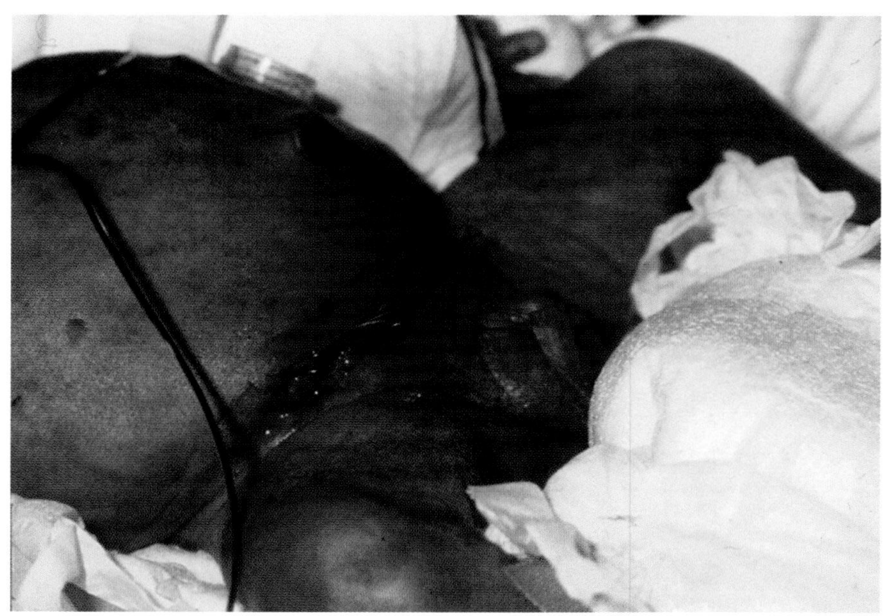

Fig. 7.**34** **Urethral valve sequence.** The same fetus after birth at 29 weeks of gestation.

cryptorchidism) is a distinct entity or forms part of the urethral valve sequence.

Ultrasound findings: These show signs of obstruction in the lower urinary tract: *distension of the urinary bladder* with thickening of the bladder wall and "keyhole" phenomenon, with *dilation of the renal pelvis and the ureter*, along with oligohydramnios or anhydramnios. Complications such as ascites secondary to rupture of the distended bladder, causing abdominal distension, may occur.

Caution: An extremely full bladder may be incorrectly interpreted as urethral obstruction. However, in this case the amniotic fluid index is normal and other signs of obstruction are not found.

Clinical management: Karyotyping; further sonographic screening, including fetal echocardiography. Consultation with a pediatric urologist to discuss the findings in the prenatal stage and to counsel the parents. Early delivery is an option after 32 weeks. Prior to this, puncture of the fetal urinary bladder and examination of the urine is helpful to obtain a rough estimate of renal function. Repeated puncture or insertion of a catheter to facilitate drainage may be required. Fetal therapy using laser is still at the experimental stage. Repeated instillation of fluid into the amniotic cavity may be considered, to prevent hypoplasia of the lungs resulting from anhydramnios.

Procedure after birth: If the anhydramnios has been present over a long period, hypoplasia of the lungs can be expected. Drainage of the urine is achieved by vesicotomy or ureterostomy. Renal function often recovers only gradually. Transurethral resection of the valve using endoscopic techniques is also a therapeutic option. Renal insufficiency and urinary incontinence may also develop.

Prognosis: This depends on the severity of renal function disturbance. The overall mortality is 50%; in the presence of oligo-anhydramnios it increases to 95%. Spontaneous recovery of the lesion in the prenatal stage has also been known to occur in 50% of cases if the diagnosis is made early.

References

Cohen HL, Zinn HL, Patel A, Zinn DL, Haller JO. Prenatal sonographic diagnosis of posterior urethral valves: identification of valves and thickening of the posterior urethral wall. J Clin Ultrasound 1998; 26: 366–70.

Gatti JM, Kirsch AJ. Posterior urethral valves: pre- and postnatal management [review]. Curr Urol Rep 2001; 2: 138–45.

Haecker FM, Wehrmann M, Hacker HW, Stuhldreier G, von Schweinitz D. Renal dysplasia in children with posterior urethral valves: a primary or secondary malformation? Pediatr Surg Int 2002; 18: 119–22.

McHugo J, Whittle M. Enlarged fetal bladders: aetiology, management and outcome [review]. Prenat Diagn 2001; 21: 958–63.

Meyer SM, Bedow W, Rascher W. Prenatal diagnosis and postnatal therapy of fetal obstructions related to the urinary tract. Acta Urol Belg 1990; 58: 39–54.

Shalev J, Itzchak Y, Blau H. The prenatal ultrasonic diagnosis of urethral obstruction and diverticulum of the urinary bladder. Pediatr Radiol 1982; 12: 48–50.

Sweeney I, Kang BH, Lin P, Giovanniello J. Posterior urethral obstruction caused by congenital posterior urethral valve; prenatal and postnatal ultrasound diagnosis. NY State J Med 1981; 81: 87–9.

8 Skeletal Anomalies

General information

Self-Help Organization

Title: Little People of America (English/Spanish)

Description: Provides mutual support to people of short stature (4 feet 10 inches/1.5 m and under) and their families. Information on physical and developmental concerns, employment, education, disability rights, medical issues, adaptive devices, etc. Newsletter. Provides educational scholarships and medical assistance grants, access to medical advisory board, assistance in adoption. Local, regional, and national conferences and athletic events. Online chat room.

Scope: National

Number of groups: 54 chapters

Founded: 1957

Address: P.O. Box 745, Lubbock, TX 79408, United States

Telephone: 1–888-LPA-2001

E-mail: LPADataBase@juno.com

Web: http://www.lpaonline.org

Achondrogenesis

Definition: Fatal skeletal dysplasia with a marked shortening of the torso and extremities and a comparatively large head.

Incidence: 0.2–0.5/10 000 births.

Sex ratio: M : F = 1 : 1.

Clinical history/genetics: Partly autosomal-recessive inheritance. Autosomal-dominant inheritance is also known (new mutations).

Teratogens: Not known.

Origin: In isolated cases, a defect in synthesis of collagen type II has been proved.

Ultrasound findings: There are various forms of achondrogenesis (type I and type II). *Severe shortening of the extremities*, a *narrow thorax* and *reduced ossification of the vertebral column and the skull* are characteristic features. In some cases, *hygroma colli or fetal hydrops* may also be present. *Thickening of the soft tissue of the arms* is typically seen. *Ascites* and *fetal hydrops* may also develop. The abdomen and head are very large compared to the chest and the limbs. In contrast to osteogenesis imperfecta, the skull is not compressible, and fractures of the long bones are not a feature; fractures of the ribs may sometimes be seen. The diagnosis is possible as early as 12 weeks of gestation, due to the appearance of a thickened nuchal fold (nuchal swelling) and skeletal malformations.

Clinical management: Molecular-genetic diagnosis, further ultrasound screening including fetal echocardiography. In cases of achondrogenesis, cardiac anomalies are seen rarely in comparison with other skeletal disorders. Radiographic examination of the skeletal system leads to further confirmation. Termination of pregnancy has to be considered, as the outcome is fatal. Management of the pregnancy and labor should not be influenced by fetal distress.

Procedure after birth: As the fetus is not viable, intensive medical interventions are not recommended.

Prognosis: Intrauterine fetal death usually occurs, resulting in stillbirth; if not, then death occurs within 24 h after birth due to hypoplasia of the lungs.

References

Benacerraf B, Osathanondh R, Bieber FR. Achondrogenesis type I: ultrasound diagnosis in utero. JCU J Clin Ultrasound 1984; 12: 357–9.

Gabrielli S, Falco P, Pilu G, Perolo A, Milano V, Bovicelli L. Can transvaginal fetal biometry be considered a useful tool for early detection of skeletal dysplasias in high-risk patients? Ultrasound Obstet Gynecol 1999;13 : 107–11.

Glenn LW, Teng SS. In utero sonographic diagnosis of achondrogenesis. JCU J Clin Ultrasound 1985; 13: 195–8.

Johnson VP, Yiu CV, Wierda DR, Holzwarth DR. Midtrimester prenatal diagnosis of achondrogenesis. J Ultrasound Med 1984; 3: 223–6.

Mahony BS, Filly RA, Cooperberg PL. Antenatal sonographic diagnosis of achondrogenesis. J Ultrasound Med 1984; 3: 333–5.

Ozeren S, Yüksel A, Tom T. Prenatal sonographic diagnosis of type I achondrogenesis with a large cystic hygroma [letter]. Ultrasound Obstet Gynecol 1999; 13: 75–6.

Sauer I, Klein B, Leeners B, Cotarelo C, Heyl W, Funk A. [Lethal osteochondrodysplasias: prenatal and postnatal differential diagnosis; in German.] Ultraschall Med 2000; 21: 112–21.

Soothill PW, Vuthiwong C, Rees H. Achondrogenesis type 2 diagnosed by transvaginal ultrasound at 12 weeks' gestation. Prenat Diagn 1993; 13: 523–8.

Tongsong T, Srisomboon J, Sudasna J. Prenatal diagnosis of Langer–Saldino achondrogenesis. J Clin Ultrasound 1995; 23: 56–8.

Wenstrom KD, Williamson RA, Hoover WW, Grant SS. Achondrogenesis type II (Langer–Saldino) in association with jugular lymphatic obstruction sequence. Prenat Diagn 1989; 9: 527–32.

Won HS, Yoo HK, Lee PR, et al. A case of achondrogenesis type II associated with huge cystic hygroma: prenatal diagnosis by ultrasonography. Ultrasound Obstet Gynecol 1999; 14: 288–90.

Achondroplasia

Definition: This is the most frequent heterozygous, nonfatal type of skeletal dysplasia (the homozygous form is fatal), with severe shortening of the limbs and a large head (dwarfism). Adult height: 116–140 cm.

Incidence: 0.5–1.5 per 10 000 births.

Sex ratio: M : F = 1 : 1.

Clinical history/genetics: Autosomal-dominant inheritance. New mutations are seen in 80%. Affected gene: *FGFR3*, gene locus: 4 p16.3.

Teratogens: Not known.

Pathogenesis: Reduced chondral ossification. Mutation of the fibroblast growth factor receptor. In the homozygous form, early manifestation and fatal outcome. In the heterozygous form, a normal ultrasound appearance is possible up to 20 weeks.

Ultrasound findings: Disproportionate hyposomia (dwarfism) with *short limbs, large head, and a typical facial profile—protruding forehead (also known as frontal bossing) and flattened nasal bridge.* The shortening of the bones of the extremities is apparent in the second half of pregnancy. The measurement of the long bones lies well below the fifth percentile, with accentuation of the proximal part. The hands and feet appear short and stubby. *Hydramnios* develops in the last trimester. The diagnosis is made with certainty after 24 weeks of gestation, the most reliable quotient being femur length to biparietal diameter, as the femur is often only minimally shortened, but the head is typically very large (macrocrania). In some cases, ventriculomegaly is also observed.

Differential diagnosis: Asymmetrical growth restriction, trisomy 21, hypochondroplasia, Kniest syndrome, Russell–Silver syndrome, Shprintzen syndrome, spondyloepiphyseal dysplasia, Turner syndrome.

Clinical management: Further ultrasound screening including fetal echocardiography, karyotyping, molecular-genetic diagnosis. There is a danger of cervical column compression due to narrowing of the foramen magnum. Thus, any clinical intervention that may cause manipulation in the neck region during labor and delivery, such as forceps or vacuum extraction, poses a high risk of complications. For this reason, a cesarean section may be an option for delivery.

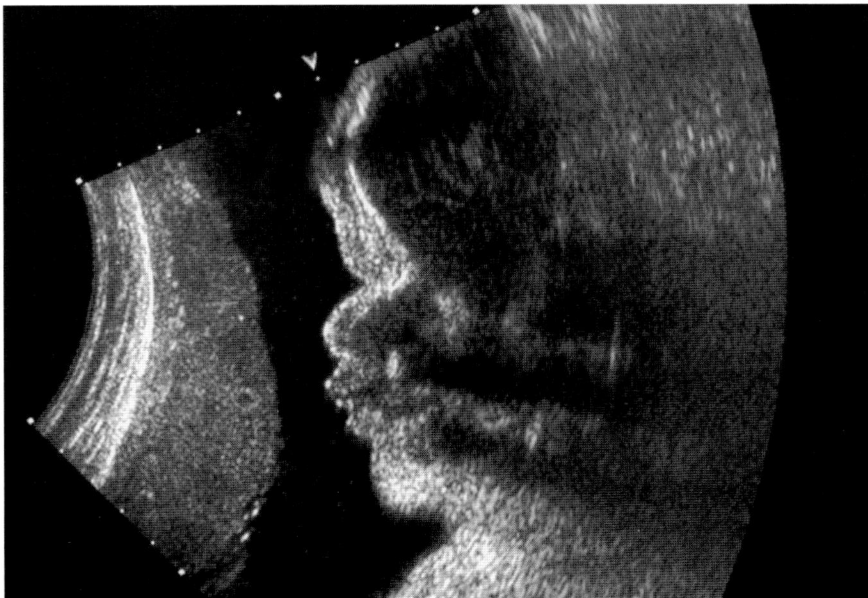

Fig. 8.1 **Achondroplasia.** Fetal profile in achondroplasia at 37 + 5 weeks, showing typical frontal bossing, flattened nasal bridge, and hypoplasia of the middle facial area.

Procedure after birth: Radiography of the skeletal system confirms the diagnosis. Hydrocephalus may develop secondary to occlusion of the foramen magnum. Surgical techniques involving lengthening of the bones of the extremities can lead to an increase in body height of about 20 to 25 cm.

Prognosis: Life expectancy in these children is normal. Intelligence is not restricted. Neurological complications, especially involving the cervical spine, are common. In homozygous cases (both parents affected), the outcome is fatal—stillbirth or neonatal death resulting from hypoplasia of the lungs.

References

Chitayat D, Fernandez B, Gardner A, et al. Compound heterozygosity for the achondroplasia–hypochondroplasia *FGFR3* mutations: prenatal diagnosis and postnatal outcome. Am J Med Genet 1999; 84: 401–5.

Gabrielli S, Falco P, Pilu G, Perolo A, Milano V, Bovicelli L. Can transvaginal fetal biometry be considered a useful tool for early detection of skeletal dysplasias in high- risk patients? Ultrasound Obstet Gynecol 1999; 13: 107–11.

Huggins MJ, Smith JR, Chun K, Ray PN, Shah JK, Whelan DT. Achondroplasia–hypochondroplasia complex in a newborn infant. Am J Med Genet 1999; 84: 396–400.

Kurtz AB, Filly RA, Wapner RJ, et al. In utero analysis of heterozygous achondroplasia: variable time of onset as detected by femur length measurements. J Ultrasound Med 1986; 5: 137–40.

Lemyre E, Azouz EM, Teebi AS, Glanc P, Chen MF. Achondroplasia, hypochondroplasia and thanatophoric dysplasia: review and update [review]. Can Assoc Radiol J 1999; 50: 185–97.

Mesoraca A, Pilu G, Perolo A, et al. Ultrasound and molecular mid-trimester prenatal diagnosis of de novo achondroplasia. Prenat Diagn 1996; 16: 764–8.

Modaff P, Horton VK, Pauli RM. Errors in the prenatal diagnosis of children with achondroplasia. Prenat Diagn 1996; 16: 525–30.

Moeglin D, Benoit B. Three-dimensional sonographic aspects in the antenatal diagnosis of achondroplasia. Ultrasound Obstet Gynecol 2001; 18: 81–3.

Schlotter CM, Pfeiffer RA. Prenatal ultrasonic diagnosis of achondroplasia. Ultraschall Med 1985; 6: 229–32.

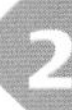

Amniotic Band Syndrome

Definition: Asymmetrical disruptive anomalies, with amputated limbs and splitting defects such as ventral wall defects. The cause is thought to be amniotic bands resulting from premature rupture of the amnion.

Incidence: One in 1300 births.

Sex ratio: M : F = 1 : 1.

Clinical history/genetics: Occurrence mostly sporadic. Rarely associated with congenital defects of fibrous tissue development, as in Ehlers–Danlos syndrome and epidermolysis bullosa.

Teratogens: None are known with any certainty. Smoking during pregnancy has been discussed as a possible teratogen.

Pathogenesis: The extent of malformations depends on the time at which the disturbances occur. Thus, anencephaly, encephalocele, facial clefts, abdominal wall defects and ectopia cordis may result. Later disturbance causes amputation of extremities and fusion of fingers, as in syndactyly.

Ultrasound findings: The findings are *extremely variable,* affecting many fetal structures. In mild forms, isolated fingers or toes may be missing. Club feet and malposition of the hands may be seen. Localized swellings of the distal parts of the limbs have also been observed ("constriction ring"). On scanning, amniotic bands can be detected in the amniotic cavity. Amniotic bands have to be differentiated from adhesions within the uterine cavity, which may also have connections to the amniotic cavity and are covered with amnion and chorion. These are often a result of curettage, but are not responsible for fetal malformations. In addition to *malformations of the limbs,* other severe defects are observed in amniotic band syndrome: abdominal wall defects, encephalocele, facial clefts, micrognathia, multiple anomalies of body surface (limb–body stalk anomaly, probably related in its pathogenesis to amniotic band syndrome).

Differential diagnosis: Gastroschisis, chromosomal aberrations, club feet, hypoplasia of femur, subcutaneous lymphangioma, Proteus syndrome, Klippel–Trenaunay–Weber syndrome, neural tube defect, omphalocele, Beckwith–Wiedemann syndrome, pentalogy of Cantrell.

Clinical management: Further ultrasound screening, including fetal echocardiography and karyotyping.

Prognosis: This depends on the severity of the malformations.

References

Abuhamad AZ, Romero R, Shaffer WK, Hobbins JC. The value of Doppler flow analysis in the prenatal diagnosis of amniotic sheets. J Ultrasound Med 1992; 11: 623–4.

Berlum KG. Amniotic band syndrome in second trimester associated with fetal malformations. Prenat Diagn 1984; 4: 311–4.

Chen CP. First-trimester sonographic demonstration of a mobile cranial cyst associated with anencephaly and amniotic band sequence. Ultrasound Obstet Gynecol 2001; 17: 360–1.

Daly CA, Freeman J, Weston W, Kovar I, Phelan M. Prenatal diagnosis of amniotic band syndrome in a methadone user: review of the literature and a case report. Ultrasound Obstet Gynecol 1996; 8: 123–5.

Fiske CE, Filly RA, Golbus MS. Prenatal ultrasound diagnosis of amniotic band syndrome. J Ultrasound Med 1982; 1: 45–7.

Herbert WN, Seeds JW, Cefalo RC, Bowes WA. Prenatal detection of intra-amniotic bands: implications and management. Obstet Gynecol 1985; 65: 36 S–38 S.

Hill LM, Kislak S, Jones N. Prenatal ultrasound diagnosis of a forearm constriction band. J Ultrasound Med 1988; 7: 293–5.

Jabor MA, Cronin ED. Bilateral cleft lip and palate and limb deformities: a presentation of amniotic band sequence? [review]. J Craniofac Surg 2000; 11: 388–93.

McGuirk CK, Westgate MN, Holmes LB. Limb deficiencies in newborn infants. Pediatrics 2001; 108: E64.

Merz E, Gerlach R, Hoffmann G, Goldhofer W. Amniotic band syndrome in ultrasound. Geburtshilfe Frauenheilkd 1984; 44: 576–8.

Pedersen TK, Thomsen SG. Spontaneous resolution of amniotic bands. Ultrasound Obstet Gynecol 2001; 18: 673–4.

Quintero RA, Morales WJ, Phillips J, Kalter CS, Angel JL. In utero lysis of amniotic bands. Ultrasound Obstet Gynecol 1997; 10: 316–20.

Wehbeh H, Fleisher J, Karimi A, Mathony A, Minkoff H. The relationship between the ultrasonographic diagnosis of innocent amniotic band development and pregnancy outcomes. Obstet Gynecol 1993; 81: 565–8.

Arthrogryposis Multiplex Congenita (Multiple Congenital Contractures)

Definition: This is a heterogeneous group of disorders all of which have multiple joint contractures present at birth. These may be caused by connective-tissue, muscular, or neurological abnormalities.

Incidence: One in 3000–10 000 births.

Sex ratio: M : F = 1 : 1.

Clinical history/genetics: Autosomal-dominant, autosomal-recessive or X-linked inheritance have all been observed. The distal forms are more likely to occur in families, but sporadic occurrence is also possible.

Teratogens: Hyperthermia, perinatal infections, mother suffering from myasthenia gravis.

Classification and ultrasound finding: The classification of arthrogryposis is still disputed. A primary condition is known, in addition to secondary, symptomatic disorders (of neuromuscular or central nervous system origin, mainly due to infections). Three basic forms of arthrogryposis are identified: 1, only the extremities are affected; 2, a generalized neuromuscular disorder is present; 3, the central nervous system is involved. The limbs are typically fixed in a certain position; the *legs may be stretched or bent*, the *arms are bent*. "Clenched fists" may be observed. The *feet are stretched or appear clubbed. Hypoplasia of muscular tissue* is evident. Fetal movement is restricted or totally absent. *Swelling of the limbs* is an accompanying feature. In some cases, the disorder first becomes evident as late as in the third trimester. *Hydramnios* is seen frequently. In 10% of the cases, anomalies of the central nervous system such as agenesis of the corpus callosum, lissencephaly, ventriculomegaly, or aplasia of the cerebellar vermis are associated.

Associated syndromes: Over 120 syndromes are known to occur concomitantly with arthrogryposis, such as Freeman–Sheldon syndrome, mul-

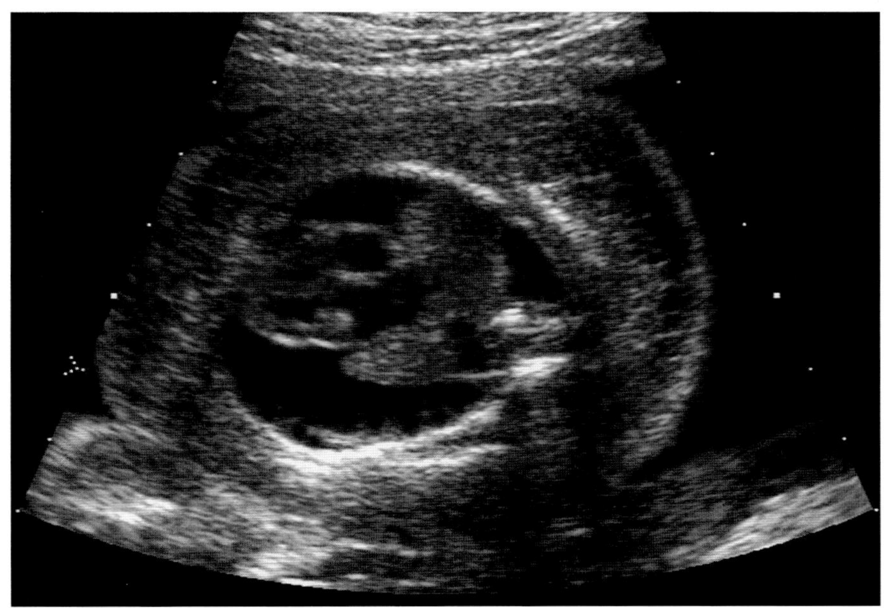

Fig. 8.**2** **Arthrogryposis multiplex congenita.** Cross-section of the fetal thorax at 21 + 6 weeks, with arthrogryposis sequence: hydrothorax, severe subcutaneous edema (anasarca).

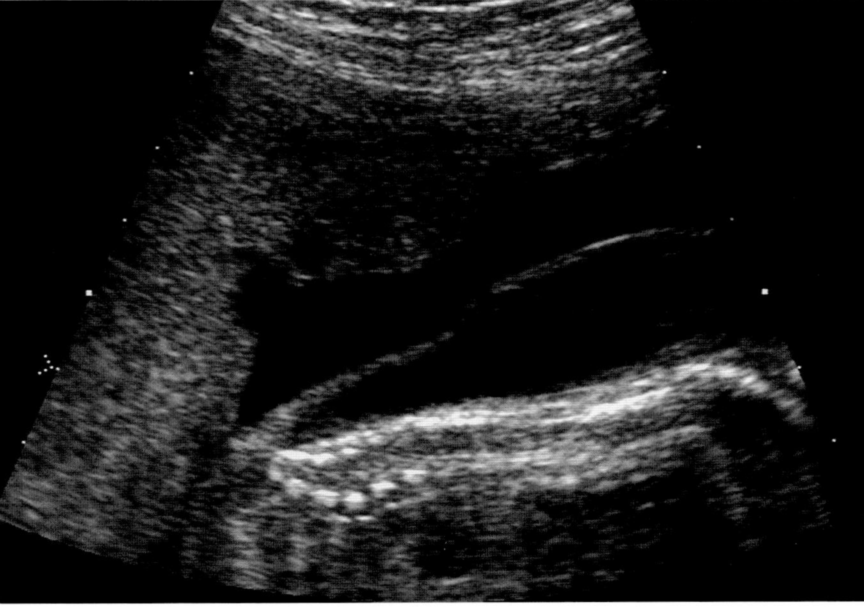

Fig. 8.**3** **Arthrogryposis multiplex congenita.** Dorsoanterior longitudinal section of a fetal thorax in fetal arthrogryposis sequence at 21 + 6 weeks, showing severe anasarca.

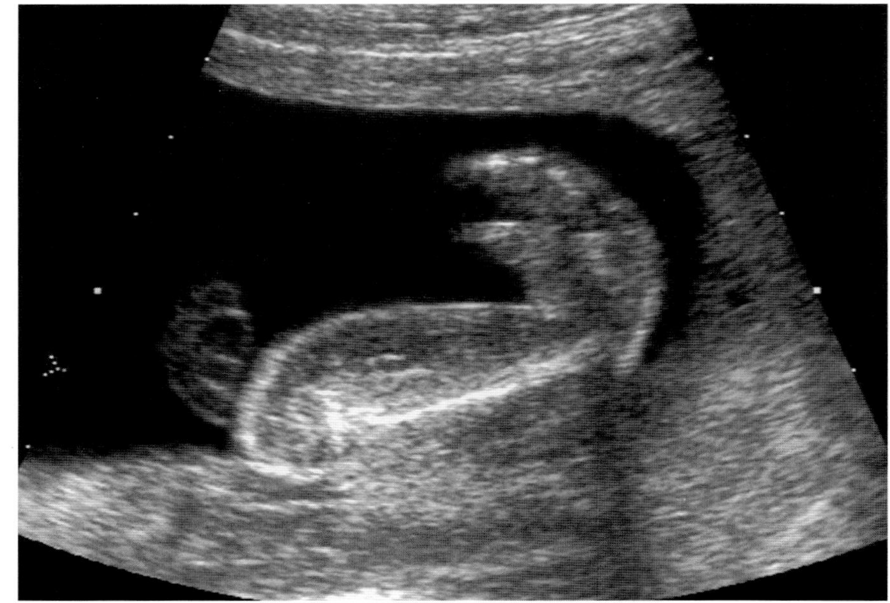

Fig. 8.4 **Arthrogryposis multiplex congenita.** Fixed positioning of the hand in fetal arthrogryposis sequence at 21 + 6 weeks.

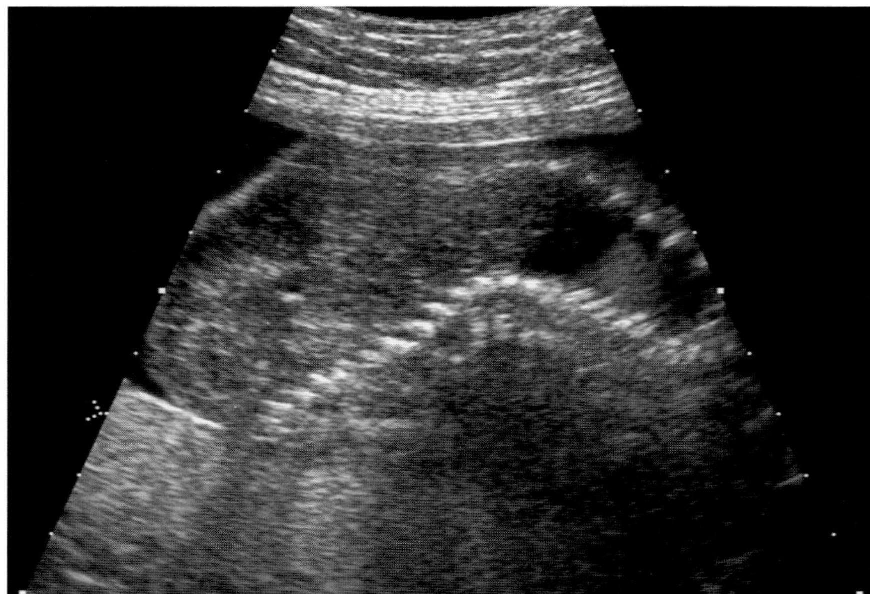

Fig. 8.5 **Arthrogryposis multiplex congenita.** Deformation of the vertebral column in fetal arthrogryposis sequence at 21 + 6 weeks.

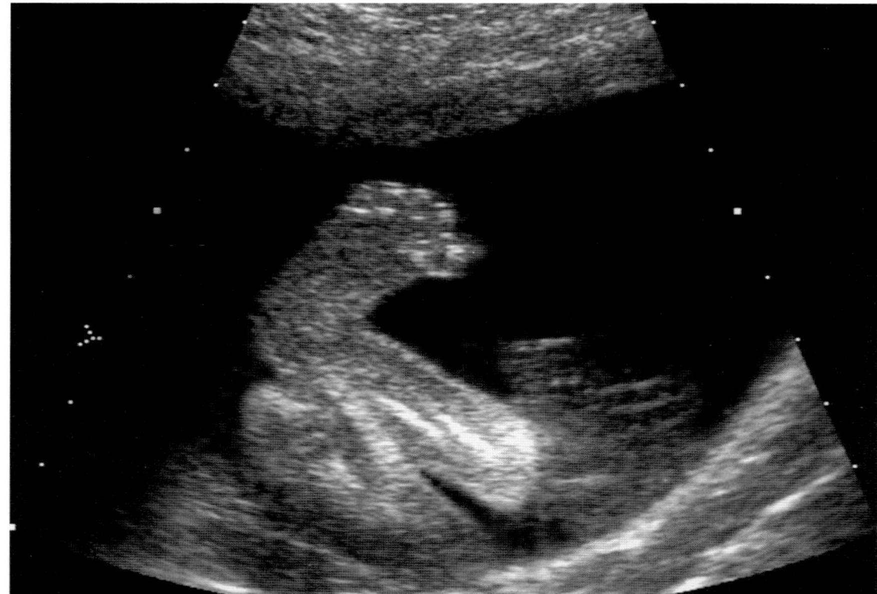

Fig. 8.6 **Arthrogryposis multiplex congenita.** Club foot in fetal arthrogryposis sequence at 21 + 6 weeks.

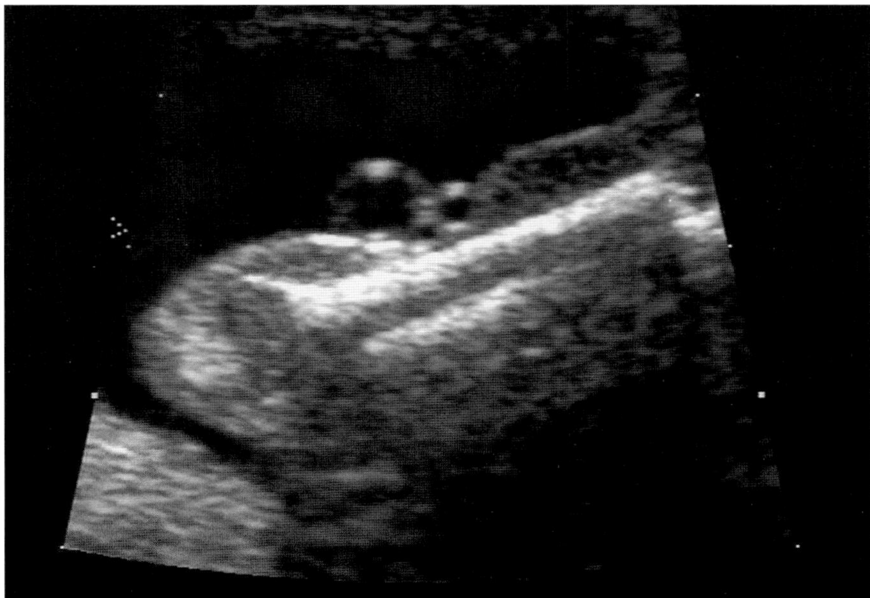

Fig. 8.7 **Arthrogryposis multiplex congenita.** The lower limb in fetal arthrogryposis multiplex congenita at 18 + 3 weeks. The umbilical cord is wrapped around the lower limb, giving the impression of a soft-tissue covering of the limb.

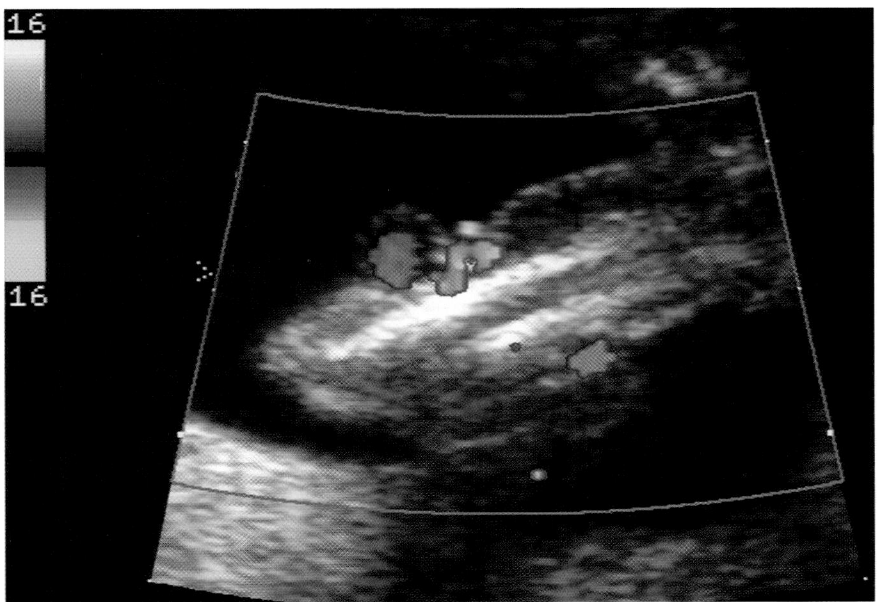

Fig. 8.8 **Arthrogryposis multiplex congenita.** Same case as before. Doppler color mapping shows coils of umbilical cord.

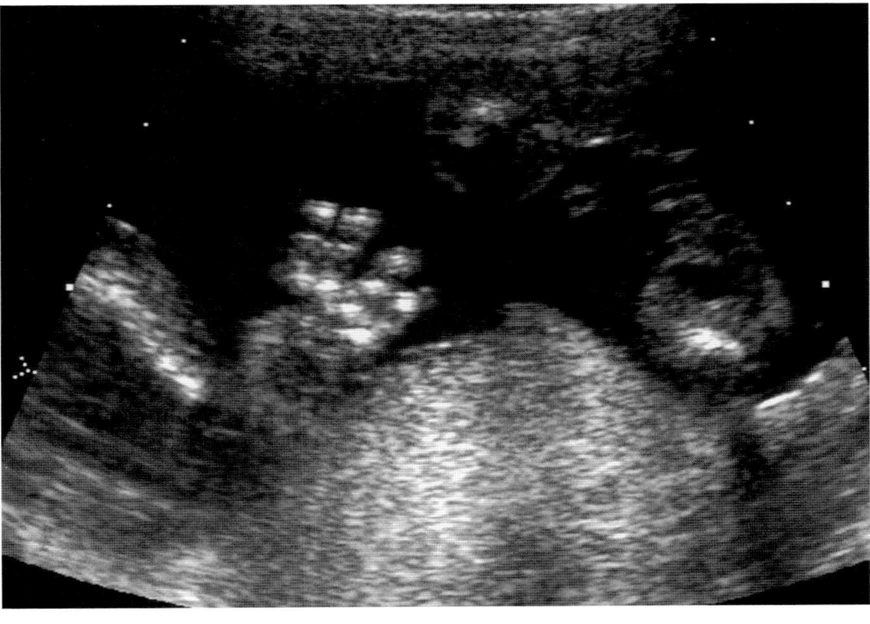

Fig. 8.9 **Arthrogryposis multiplex congenita.** Malpositioning of the fetal hand in arthrogryposis multiplex congenita at 18 + 3 weeks.

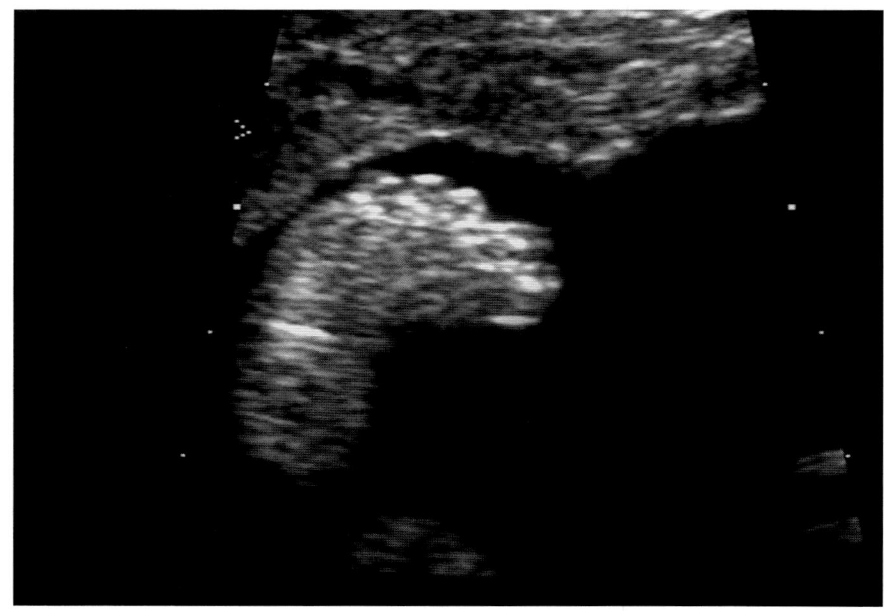

Fig. 8.**10** **Arthrogryposis multiplex congenita.** Club foot at 23 + 0 weeks in arthrogryposis multiplex congenita and fetal hypokinesia sequence.

tiple pterygium syndrome, Pena–Shokeir syndrome, Smith–Lemli–Opitz syndrome, trisomy 18, Larsen syndrome, trisomy 8 mosaic.

Clinical management: Further ultrasound screening, including fetal echocardiography and karyotyping. Search for infections (TORCH). A fixed breech position presents frequently, which may lead to complications during labor and delivery.

Procedure after birth: This is determined after an exact diagnosis is made.

Prognosis: This depends on the associated malformations and the severity of the disorder and can vary from a fatal outcome to minimal orthopedic handicap.

Self-Help Organization

Title: Avenues: A National Support Group for Arthrogryposis

Description: Connects families affected by arthrogryposis with each other for mutual support and sharing of information. Educates medical and social-service professionals. Semiannual newsletter $10/year.

Scope: National network

Founded: 1980

Address: P.O. Box 5192, Sonora, CA 95370, United States

Telephone: 209–928–3688 (PST)

E-mail: avenues@sonnet.com

Web: http://www.sonnet.com/avenues

References

Ajayi RA, Keen CE, Knott PD. Ultrasound diagnosis of the Pena–Shokeir phenotype at 14 weeks of pregnancy. Prenat Diagn 1995; 15: 762–4.

Baty BJ, Cubberley D, Morris C, Carey J. Prenatal diagnosis of distal arthrogryposis. Am J Med Genet 1988; 29: 501–10.

Bui TH, Lindholm H, Demir N, Thomassen P. Prenatal diagnosis of distal arthrogryposis type I by ultrasonography. Prenat Diagn 1992; 12: 1047–53.

Degani S, Shapiro I, Lewinsky R, Sharf M. Prenatal ultrasound diagnosis of isolated arthrogryposis of feet. Acta Obstet Gynecol Scand 1989; 68: 461–2.

Dudkiewicz I, Achiron R, Ganel A. Prenatal diagnosis of distal arthrogryposis type 1. Skeletal Radiol 1999; 28: 233–5.

Falsaperla R, Romeo G, Di Giorgio A, Pavone P, Parano E, Connolly AM. Long-term survival in a child with arthrogryposis multiplex congenita and spinal muscular atrophy. J Child Neurol 2001; 16: 934–6.

Goldberg JD, Chervenak FA, Lipman RA, Berkowitz RL. Antenatal sonographic diagnosis of arthrogryposis multiplex congenita. Prenat Diagn 1986; 6: 45–9.

Gorczyca DP, McGahan JP, Lindfors KK, Ellis WG, Grix A. Arthrogryposis multiplex congenita: prenatal ultrasonographic diagnosis. JCU J Clin Ultrasound 1989; 17: 40–4.

Madazli R, Tuysuz B, Aksoy F, Barbaros M, Uludag S, Ocak V. Prenatal diagnosis of arthrogryposis multiplex congenita with increased nuchal translucency but without any underlying fetal neurogenic or myogenic pathology. Fetal Diagn Ther 2002; 17: 29–33.

O'Flaherty P. Arthrogryposis multiplex congenita [review]. Neonatal Netw 2001; 20: 13–20.

Yau PW, Chow W, Li YH, Leong JC. Twenty-year follow-up of hip problems in arthrogryposis multiplex congenita. J Pediatr Orthop 2002; 22: 359–63.

Diastrophic Dysplasia

Definition: Skeletal dysplasia with short limbs, club foot, swelling of the ears, and progressive joint and spinal column deformities.

Incidence: Rare.

Sex ratio: M : F = 1 : 1.

Clinical history/genetics: Autosomal-recessive inheritance, single-gene heredity.

Teratogens: Not known.

Ultrasound findings: Micromelia involving all extremities, deviation of the hand medially, short fingers, "hitchhiker" thumb; club feet, microgenia; cleft palate in one-third of the cases; swelling of the pinna leads to "cauliflower ear" deformity; cervical kyphoscoliosis, flexion deformities of the elbow and knee. Hydramnios.

Differential diagnosis: Camptomelic dysplasia, distal arthrogryposis, Larsen syndrome, multiple pterygium syndrome, Roberts syndrome, spondyloepiphyseal dysplasia, thanatophoric dysplasia.

Clinical management: Further ultrasound screening including fetal echocardiography and karyotyping. Molecular-genetic diagnosis. The gene locus for diastrophic dysplasia is known, so that a definite prenatal diagnosis is possible. Hydramnios develops frequently, causing premature labor.

Procedure after birth: Respiratory distress develops frequently and may require intubation; however, this may be difficult due to microgenia. In this case, it is important to pull out the tongue and to visualize the pharynx for the intubation. Radiographic examination of the newborn will further confirm the diagnosis.

Prognosis: Neonatal death is rare. Life expectancy and mental function are usually normal. Adult height lies generally below 140 cm. Severe handicap due to orthopedic deformities. A variation of this disorder has been described with cardiac anomaly and intrauterine growth restriction; the affected child dies either shortly after birth or in the early infancy.

References

Gembruch U, Niesen M, Kehrberg H, Hansmann M. Diastrophic dysplasia: a specific prenatal diagnosis by ultrasound. Prenat Diagn 1988; 8: 539–45.

Gollop TR, Eigier A. Prenatal ultrasound diagnosis of diastrophic dysplasia at 16 weeks. Am J Med Genet 1987; 27: 321–4.

Jung C, Sohn C, Sergi C. Case report: prenatal diagnosis of diastrophic dysplasia by ultrasound at 21 weeks of gestation in a mother with massive obesity. Prenat Diagn 1998; 18: 378–83.

Kaitila I, Ammdld P, Karjalainen O, Liukkonen S, Rapola J. Early prenatal detection of diastrophic dysplasia. Prenat Diagn 1983; 3: 237–44.

Focal Femoral Hypoplasia

Definition: Shortening or distortion of the femur, usually unilateral.

Incidence: Rare.

Sex ratio: M : F = 2 : 3.

Clinical history/genetics: This anomaly may occur in association with a syndrome, or as an isolated finding.

Teratogens: Diabetes mellitus, high doses of vitamin A.

Ultrasound findings: The proximal part of the femur, including femoral head, is missing. Frequently, the femur is bowed or bent. On the affected side, the fibula may also be missing and the tibia may be bowed. In addition, other long bones or fingers may be partly or completely absent.

Differential diagnosis: This anomaly has been described in over 25 syndromes.

Clinical management: Further ultrasound screening, including fetal echocardiography and karyotyping. Regular scans. Femoral growth var-

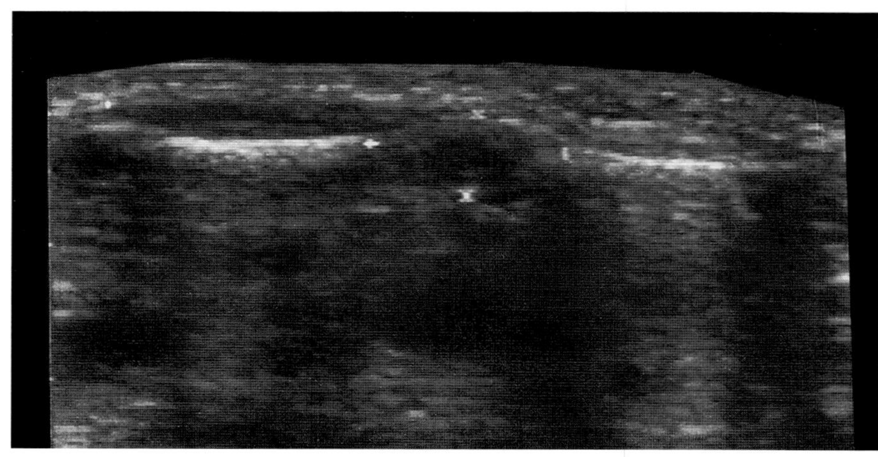

Fig. 8.**11** **Focal femur hypoplasia.** The continuity of the femur is interrupted in focal femur hypoplasia at 18 weeks.

ies during the course of pregnancy, and determines the final femoral length after birth.

Procedure after birth: No specific intervention is needed immediately after birth. Radiography of the newborn confirms the diagnosis. Orthopedic surgery is required at a later stage.

Prognosis: This depends on the associated anomalies. In an isolated finding, orthopedic surgery shows a good success.

References

Bohring A, Oppermann HC. A further case of vertical transmission of proximal femoral focal deficiency? Am J Med Genet 1997; 71: 194–6.

Court C, Carlioz H. Radiological study of severe proximal femoral focal deficiency. J Pediatr Orthop 1997; 17: 520–4.

Gonçalves LF, De Luca GR, Vitorello DA, et al. Prenatal diagnosis of bilateral proximal femoral hypoplasia. Ultrasound Obstet Gynecol 1996; 8: 127–30.

Gul D, Ozturk H. Unilateral proximal femoral focal deficiency and Hirschsprung disease. Clin Dysmorphol 2000; 9: 149–50.

Shetty AK, Khubchandani RP. Proximal femoral focal deficiency (PFFD). Indian J Pediatr 1998; 65: 766–9.

Stormer SV. Proximal femoral focal deficiency [review]. Orthop Nurs 1997; 16: 25–31.

Hypochondroplasia

Definition: Moderate hyposomia (dwarfism), with disproportionate shortening of the limbs (first manifestation may occur even after birth). There is an increase in head circumference. Other symptoms include lumbar lordosis and bowing of the bones of the lower limbs.

First described in 1961 by Lamy and Maroteaux.

Clinical history/genetics: Autosomal-dominant inheritance; genetically heterogeneous; gene locus: 4 p16.3. Gene defect: a mutation in the fibroblast growth factor receptor-3 gene (*FGFR3*) is detected in 60% of the patients. At least one other gene is known to exist, mutation of which may also cause hypochondroplasia.

Ultrasound findings: Disproportionate hyposomia (dwarfism) with shortened extremities.

Clinical management: Further ultrasound screening, including fetal echocardiography and karyotyping. Molecular-genetic diagnosis.

Prognosis: The children have a normal life expectancy. Mental function is not affected.

References

Huggins MJ, Mernagh JR, Steele L, Smith JR, Nowaczyk MJ. Prenatal sonographic diagnosis of hypochondroplasia in a high-risk fetus. Am J Med Genet 1999; 87: 226–9.

Huggins MJ, Smith JR, Chun K, Ray PN, Shah JK, Whelan DT. Achondroplasia–hypochondroplasia complex in a newborn infant. Am J Med Genet 1999; 84: 396–400.

Ramaswami U, Rumsby G, Hindmarsh PC, Brook CGD. Genotype and phenotype in hypochondroplasia. J Pediatr 1998; 133: 99–102.

Stoilov I, Kilpatrick, MW, Tsipouras P. Possible genetic heterogeneity in hypochondroplasia [letter]. J Med Genet 1995; 32: 492–3.

Camptomelic Dysplasia

Definition: Skeletal dysplasia with typical bowing of the femur and tibia. This may be associated with other extraskeletal anomalies in cases of genetic mutation.

Incidence: Rare.

Sex ratio: *Phenotype:* M : F = 1.0 : 2.3; *chromosomal*: M : F = 1 : 1 (frequently seen in 46 XY boys with intersexual or female genitals).

Etiology: New mutation with autosomal-dominant inheritance; gene localization on chromosome 17, gene locus 17 q24.3 –q25.1. Altered collagen synthesis.

Teratogen: Not known.

Ultrasound findings: Characteristic features are *bowing and shortening of the lower extremities* (femur, tibia) and hypoplasia of fibula. In many cases, hydramnios develops. Anomalies such as hydrocephalus, a flat facial profile, microgenia, hypertelorism, cleft palate, and esophageal malformations have also been observed. In addition, a "bell-shaped" thorax (thoracic circumference much smaller than the abdominal measurement), cardiac anomalies, omphalocele, dilation of renal calyces, and club feet are present. Intersexual genitalia are frequently seen.

Differential diagnosis: Diastrophic dysplasia, femur–fibula–ulna (FFU) syndrome, hypophosphatasia, osteogenesis imperfecta, Roberts syndrome, thanatophoric dysplasia.

Clinical management: Molecular-genetic diagnosis. Further ultrasound screening, including fetal echocardiography. Premature birth is likely, due to hydramnios. Intervention based on a fetal indication is controversial.

Procedure after birth: Intensive medical interventions should be avoided. Radiography of the newborn.

Prognosis: Extremely unfavorable. In most cases, the outcome is already fatal in the neonatal stage (respiratory insufficiency); rarely, some survive the infancy stage, but die usually in early childhood. Restriction in physical and mental development is to be expected.

References

Garjian KV, Pretorius DH, Budorick NE, Cantrell CJ, Johnson DD, Nelson TR. Fetal skeletal dysplasia: three-dimensional US—initial experience. Radiology 2000; 214: 717–23.

Redon JY, Le Grevellec JY, Marie F, Le Coq E, Le Guern H. Prenatal diagnosis of camptomelic dysplasia. J Gynecol Obstet Biol Reprod 1984; 13: 437–41.

Soell J. Camptomelic dysplasia: a case study [review]. Neonatal Netw 1999; 18: 41–8.

Wasant P, Waeteekul S, Rimoin DL, Lachman RS. Genetic skeletal dysplasia in Thailand: the Siriraj experience. Southeast Asian J Trop Med Public Health 1995; 26 (Suppl 1): 59–67.

2

Club Foot (Talipes), Rocker-Bottom Foot

Definition of club foot: In this condition, the foot is plantar flexed, internally rotated and adducted (the sole of the foot points medially). Anomalies in the lower limb musculature are usually associated.

Definition of rocker-bottom foot: This is characterized by a prominent heel and convex sole.

Incidence: Club foot one in 1000 births; rocker-bottom foot is rarer.

Teratogens: Not known.

Associated malformations: In case of neural tube defects, this anomaly may be secondary to paralysis of the muscles of the lower extremities.

Associated syndrome: Club foot has been described in over 200 syndromes. Rocker-bottom foot has been associated with over 30 syndromes, most frequently with trisomy 18. Other syndromes are: hydrolethalus, Nager syndrome, atelosteogenesis type 1, camptomelic dysplasia, diastrophic dysplasia, Ellis–van Creveld syndrome, Freeman syndrome, Larsen syndrome, triploidy, trisomy 13, arthrogryposis, caudal regression syndrome, Pena–Shokeir syndrome.

Ultrasound findings in club foot: In sagittal section, the long bones of the lower limb and the foot can be visualized in one plane. The position of the foot is fixed.

Ultrasound findings in rocker-bottom foot: The heel is prominent, extending well beyond the posterior limit of the lower limb. The plantar arch shows convex bending.

Clinical management: Further ultrasound screening, including fetal echocardiography and karyotyping. Counseling with a pediatrician and/or an orthopedic surgeon.

Procedure after birth: Careful search for other anomalies, which may have been missed in prenatal screening, is advised. Orthopedic intervention is needed. At least 50% of the children require surgical correction, as conservative measures such as casts are not sufficient. The optimal time for operative intervention is 6–12 months after birth.

Prognosis: This depends on the cause of the malformation. An isolated condition can generally be successfully treated, and normal anatomy and function can be expected.

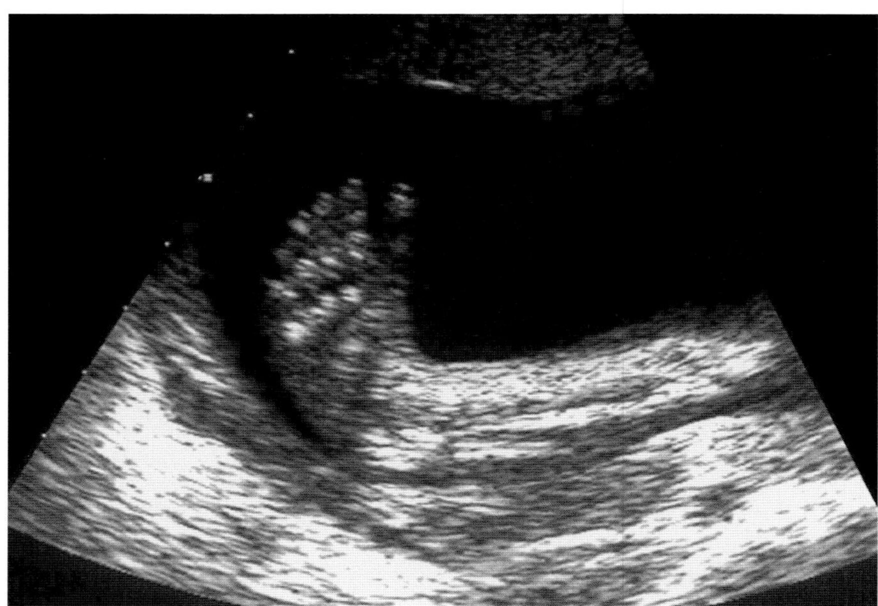

Fig. 8.**12** **Pes equinovarus.** Club foot at 23 + 6 weeks.

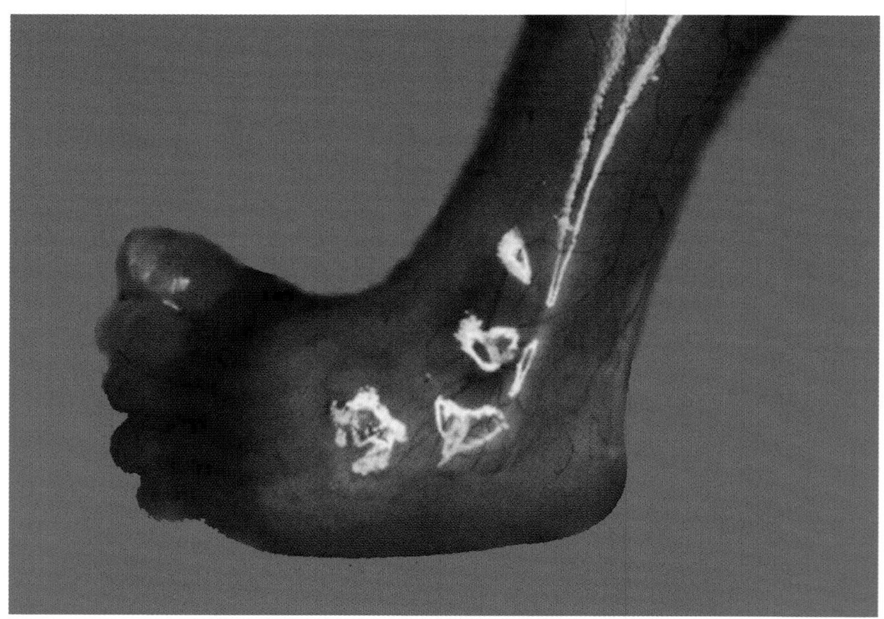

Fig. 8.**13** **Pes equinovarus.** Seen after termination of pregnancy due to other anomalies at 22 weeks.

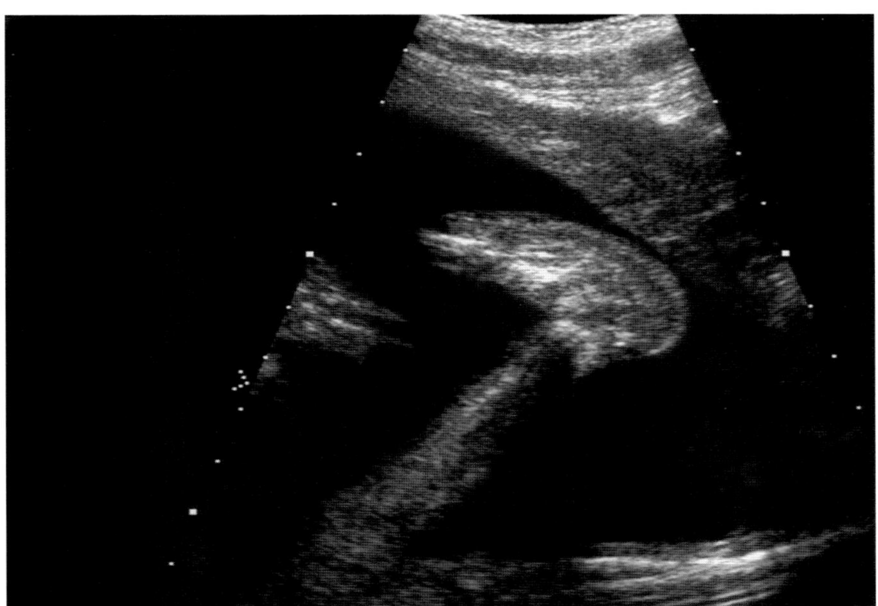

Fig. 8.**14** **Rocker-bottom foot.** Seen in trisomy 18 at 24 + 4 weeks.

Self-Help Organization

Title: Club foot Mailing List

Description: Support group for parents of children with club foot/feet, persons with club foot/feet, or anyone needing support on this topic. Operates through an e-mail mailing list.

Scope: Online

Web: http://www.onelist.com/community/clubfoot

References

Anonymous. Randomised trial to assess safety and fetal outcome of early and midtrimester amniocentesis. The Canadian Early and Mid-trimester Amniocentesis Trial (CEMAT) Group. Lancet 1998; 351: 242–7.

Benacerraf BR, Frigoletto FD. Prenatal ultrasound diagnosis of clubfoot. Radiology 1985; 155: 211–3.

Bronshtein M, Zimmer EZ. Transvaginal ultrasound diagnosis of fetal clubfeet at 13 weeks, menstrual age. JCU J Clin Ultrasound 1989; 17: 518–20.

Burgan HE, Furness ME, Foster BK. Prenatal ultrasound diagnosis of clubfoot. J Pediatr Orthop 1999; 19: 11–3.

Chesney D. Clinical outcome of congenital talipes equinovarus diagnosed antenatally by ultrasound. J Bone Joint Surg Br 2001; 83: 462–3.

Foster BK, Furness ME, Mulpuri K. Prenatal ultrasonography in antenatal orthopaedics: a new subspecialty. J Pediatr Orthop 2002; 22: 404–9.

Hashimoto BE, Filly RA, Callen PW Sonographic diagnosis of clubfoot in utero. J Ultrasound Med 1986; 5: 81–3.

Katz K, Meizner I, Mashiach R, Soudry M. The contribution of prenatal sonographic diagnosis of clubfoot to preventive medicine. J Pediatr Orthop 1999; 19: 5–7.

Malone FD, Marino T, Bianchi DW, Johnston K, D'Alton ME. Isolated clubfoot diagnosed prenatally: is karyotyping indicated? Obstet Gynecol 2000; 95: 437–40.

Pagnotta G, Maffulli N, Aureli S, Maggi E, Mariani M, Yip KM. Antenatal sonographic diagnosis of clubfoot: a six-year experience. J Foot Ankle Surg 1996; 35: 67–71.

Rijhsinghani A, Yankowitz J, Kanis AB, Mueller GM, Yankowitz DK, Williamson RA. Antenatal sonographic diagnosis of club foot with particular attention to the implications and outcomes of isolated club foot. Ultrasound Obstet Gynecol 1998; 12: 103–6.

Treadwell MC, Stanitski CL, King M. Prenatal sonographic diagnosis of clubfoot: implications for patient counseling. J Pediatr Orthop 1999; 19: 8–10.

Osteogenesis Imperfecta

Definition: This is a heterogeneous group of disorders affecting the bones, characterized by multiple fractures. Certain subtypes may be diagnosed even in the prenatal stage due to fractures and shortening of the bones, and increased bone transparency. The disorder can be divided into four subtypes following Sillence's classification:

Type I: is diagnosed frequently after birth; fractures, blue sclera, and impaired hearing are present.

Type II: is characterized even at the prenatal stage by severe findings and has a fatal prognosis, with death resulting at the early neonatal stage.

Type III: shows a slow progression and leads to severe handicap; it is diagnosed in the early adult stage.

Type IV: is a mild form with a very high tendency to fractures. Sclera are normal.

Incidence: One in 30 000–70 000 births.

Sex ratio: M : F = 1 : 1.

Etiology: Inheritance is most frequently autosomal-dominant; recessive forms are also known. Type II is due to a new mutation, rarely inherited. The disorder is caused by a defect in the synthesis of type I collagen. Prenatal detection using molecular-genetic diagnosis is possible.

Teratogens: Not known.

Associated malformation: Cataracts.

Ultrasound findings: *Types I and IV:* isolated fractures of the slightly shortened long bones. Callus formation in the fracture region. Bowing and bending of the long bones. *Type II* is diagnosed if detection is possible in the prenatal stage. Earliest prenatal diagnosis at 14 weeks. Generalized significant undermineralization, with multiple deformities of the ribs. The skull is compressible and devoid of echo. The bones of the extremities are shortened with multiple fractures.

Clinical management: Further ultrasound screening, including fetal echocardiography. If a cardiac anomaly is detected, then the diagnosis has to be questioned. Possible radiographic examination. Hydramnios may develop. In the nonfatal forms, delivery by cesarean section should be considered, in order to avoid fractures and intracranial bleeding due to soft skull bones.

Procedure after birth: The fatal type II disorder is suspected in the presence of multiple fractures and blue coloring of the sclera. In this case, "minimal handling" is indicated; due to the fragility of the bones and risk of fractures, the newborn should be handled extremely carefully.

Prognosis: This depends on the type of disorder. Death is the usual outcome in type II, due to respiratory failure. In the nonfatal forms, the infants survive with considerable disability, 30% of cases requiring a wheelchair if the fractures occur before the child has learned to walk. Healing of the fractures is complicated with pseudoarthrosis in 20% of cases.

Self-Help Organization

Title: Osteogenesis Imperfecta Foundation

Description: Support and resources for families dealing with osteogenesis imperfecta. Provides information for medical professionals. Supports research. Literature, bimonthly newsletter. Telephone support network.

Scope: National

Number of groups: 21 affiliated groups

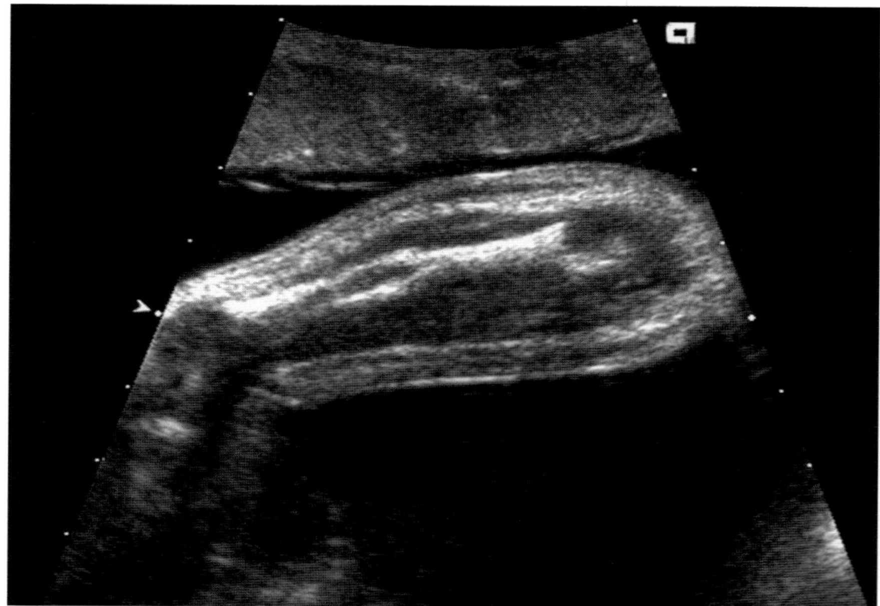

Fig. 8.**15** **Osteogenesis imperfecta.** Loss of continuity of the humerus due to fractures at 32 + 4 weeks.

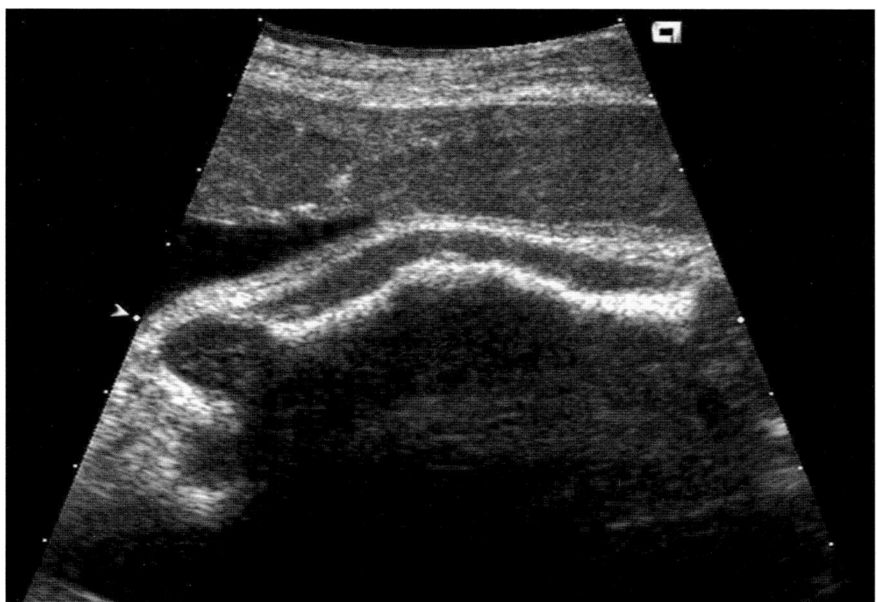

Fig. 8.**16** **Osteogenesis imperfecta.** Fetal femur showing severe bowing at 32 + 4 weeks.

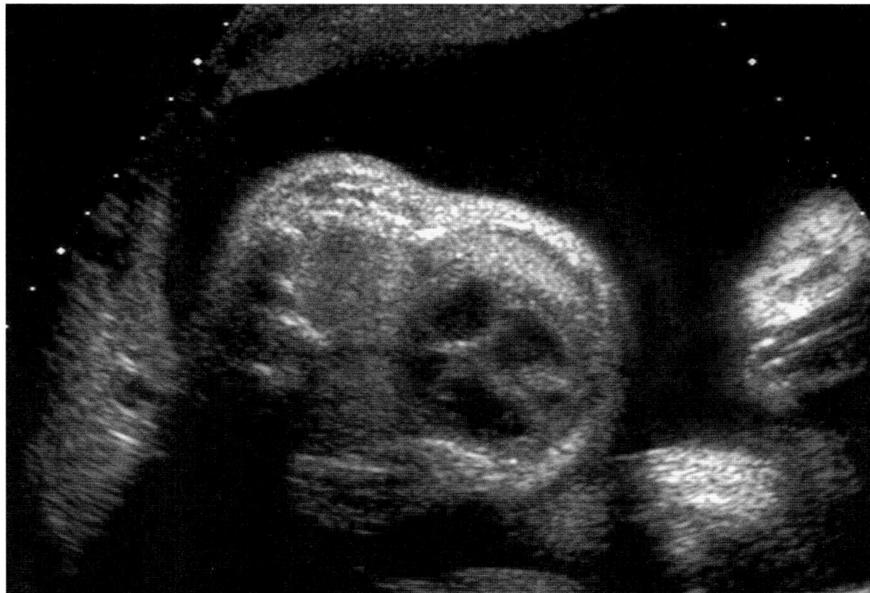

Fig. 8.**17** **Osteogenesis imperfecta.** Cross-section of the fetal thorax in osteogenesis imperfecta at 32 + 4 weeks, showing deformation due to fractured ribs.

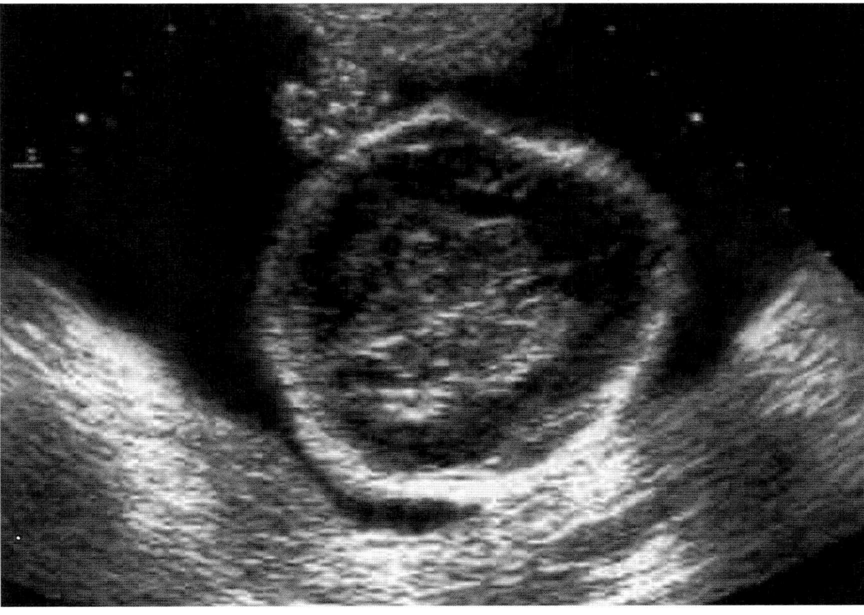

Fig. 8.**18** **Osteogenesis imperfecta.** Fetal head with a deformed skull bone at 23 + 1 weeks.

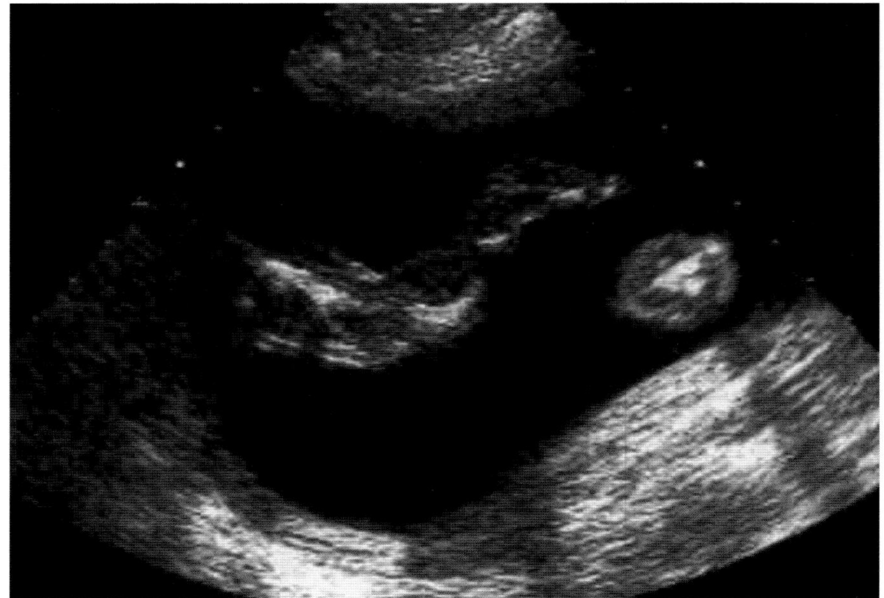

Fig. 8.**19** **Osteogenesis imperfecta.** Fetal leg with shortening and bowing of the long bones at 23 + 1 weeks.

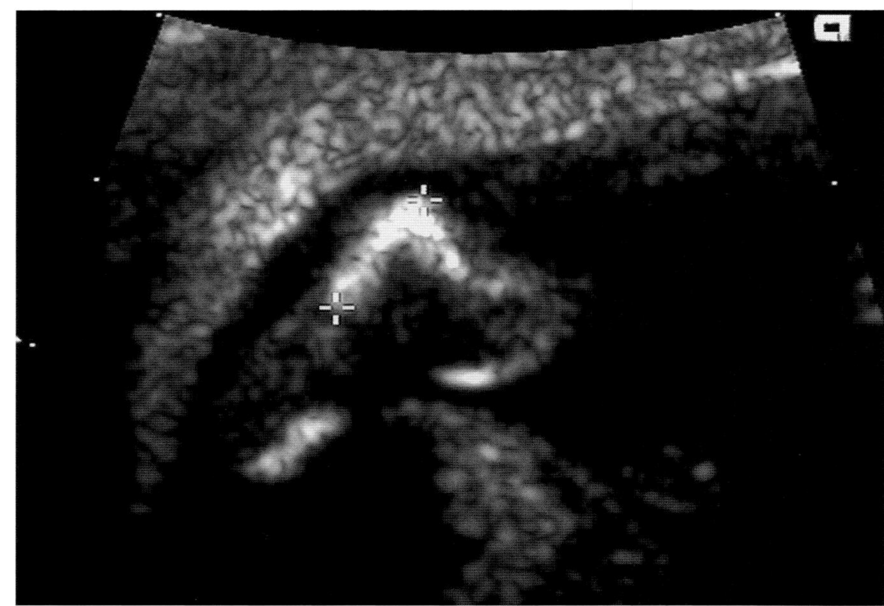

Fig. 8.**20** **Osteogenesis imperfecta.** Fetal femur at 13 + 4 weeks. Complete change of axis due to a fracture.

Founded: 1970

Address: 804 W. Diamond Ave., Suite 210, Gaithersburg, MD 20878, United States

Telephone: 1-800-981-2663 or 301-947-0083

TTY: TDD: 202-466-4315

Fax: 301-947-0456

E-mail: bonelink@oif.org brittle

Web: http://www.oif.org

References

Aylsworth AS, Seeds JW Guilford WB, Burns CB, Washburn DB. Prenatal diagnosis of a severe deforming type of osteogenesis imperfecta. Am J Med Genet 1984; 19: 707–14.

Chalubinski K, Plenk HI, Schaller A. Prenatal diagnosis of osteogenesis imperfecta: report of a case classified as the classical Vrolik lethal type. Ultraschall Med 1995; 16: 25–8.

Chang LW, Chang CH, Yu CH, Chang FM. Three-dimensional ultrasonography of osteogenesis imperfecta at early pregnancy. Prenat Diagn 2002; 22: 77–8.

DiMaio MS, Barth R, Koprivnikar KE. First-trimester prenatal diagnosis of osteogenesis imperfecta type II by DNA analysis and sonography. Prenat Diagn 1993; 13: 589–96.

Gabrielli S, Falco P, Pilu G, Perolo A, Milano V, Bovicelli L. Can transvaginal fetal biometry be considered a useful tool for early detection of skeletal dysplasias in high-risk patients? Ultrasound Obstet Gynecol 1999; 13: 107–11.

Heller RH, Winn KJ, Heller RM. The prenatal diagnosis of osteogenesis imperfecta congenita. Am J Obstet Gynecol 1975; 121: 572–3.
Munoz C, Filly RA, Golbus MS. Osteogenesis imperfecta type II: prenatal sonographic diagnosis. Radiology 1990; 174: 181–5.
Ogita S, Kamei T, Matsumoto M, Shimamoto T, Shimura K. Prenatal diagnosis of osteogenesis imperfecta congenita by means of fetography. Eur J Pediatr 1976; 123: 179–86.
Pepin M, Atkinson M, Starman BJ, Byers PH. Strategies and outcomes of prenatal diagnosis for osteogenesis imperfecta: a review of biochemical and molecular studies completed in 129 pregnancies. Prenat Diagn 1997; 17: 559–70.
Sanders RC, Greyson FR, Hogge WA, Blakemore KJ, McGowan KD, Isbister S. Osteogenesis imperfecta and camptomelic dysplasia: difficulties in prenatal diagnosis. J Ultrasound Med 1994; 13: 691–700.
Sharma A, George L, Erskin K. Osteogenesis imperfecta in pregnancy: two case reports and review of literature [review]. Obstet Gynecol Surv 2001; 56: 563–6.
Tongsong T, Wanapirak C, Siriangkul S. Prenatal diagnosis of osteogenesis imperfecta type II. Int J Gynaecol Obstet 1998; 61: 33–8.
Viora E, Sciarrone A, Bastonero S, et al. Increased nuchal translucency in the first trimester as a sign of osteogenesis imperfecta. Am J Med Genet 2002; 109: 336–7.
Virdi AS, Loughlin JA, Irven CM, Goodship J, Sykes BC. Mutation screening by a combination of biotin-SSCP and direct sequencing. Hum Genet 1994; 93: 287–90.

Polydactyly

Definition: This is defined as extra fingers or toes. It may be postaxial (findings on the ulna or fibula side), or preaxial (findings on the side of radius or tibia).

Incidence: Postaxial: one in 3000; in those with African ancestry, one in 300. Preaxial: one in 7000.

Sex ratio: M : F = 1.5 : 1.

Clinical history/genetics: *Postaxial* forms are mostly autosomal-dominant; *preaxial* forms are usually unilateral and sporadic.

Teratogens: Alcohol, valproic acid, diabetes mellitus.

Associated malformations: Over 100 syndromes have been described featuring polydactyly.

Associated syndromes: Trisomy 13, Smith–Lemli–Opitz syndrome, hydrolethalus, Joubert syndrome, Meckel–Gruber syndrome, orofaciodigital syndrome type II, Mohr syndrome, Ellis–van Creveld syndrome, hypochondroplasia, short rib–polydactyly syndrome, Carpenter syndrome, VACTERL association.

Ultrasound findings: The hands and/or feet show an extra finger or toe, which may consist of bony parts and appear normal, or may be bent. If the bony part is absent, it is difficult to diagnose this anomaly in a prenatal scan.

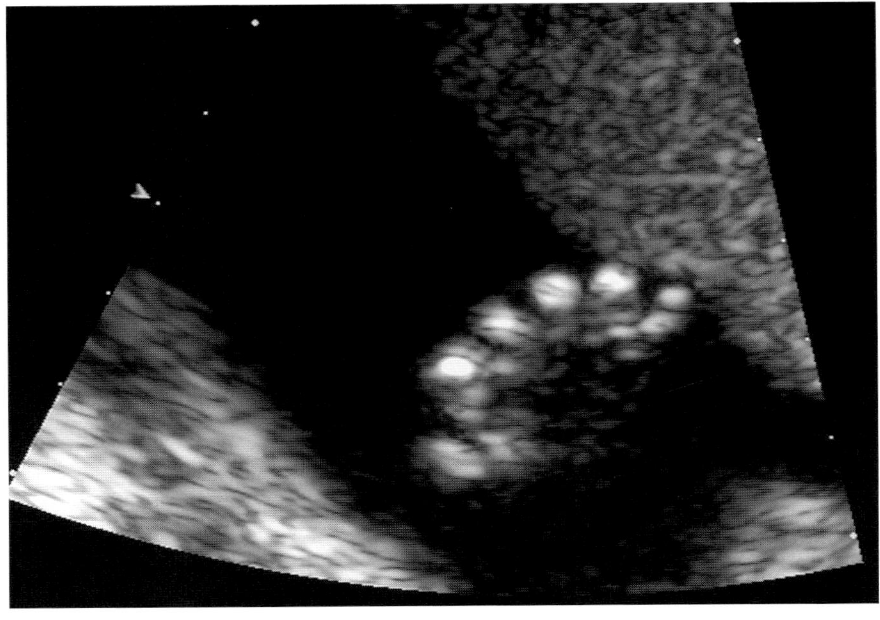

Fig. 8.**21** **Polydactyly.** Isolated familial postaxial hexadactyly involving all limbs at 25 + 2 weeks. This figure shows a hand. No other anomalies were found.

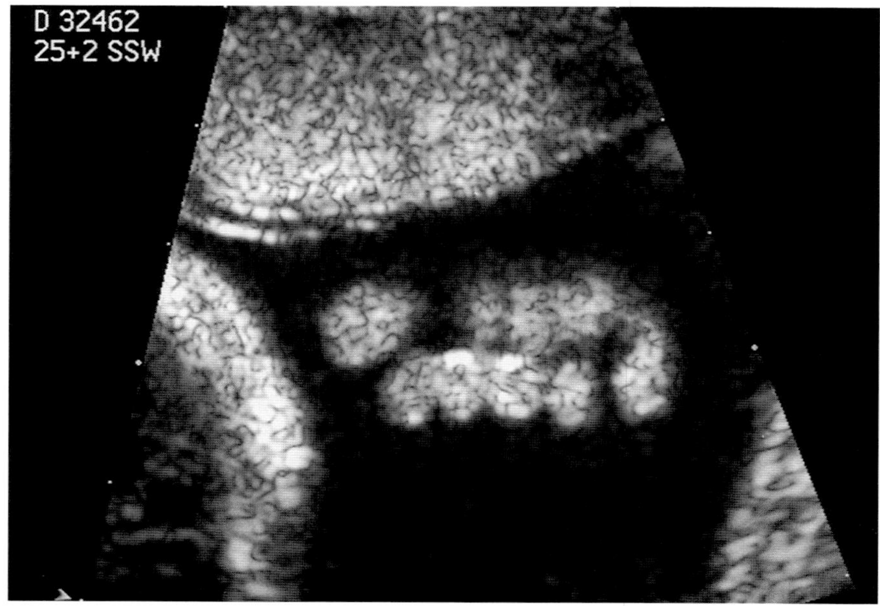

Fig. 8.**22** **Polydactyly.** Same fetus as before. Hexadactyly of the foot is seen here.

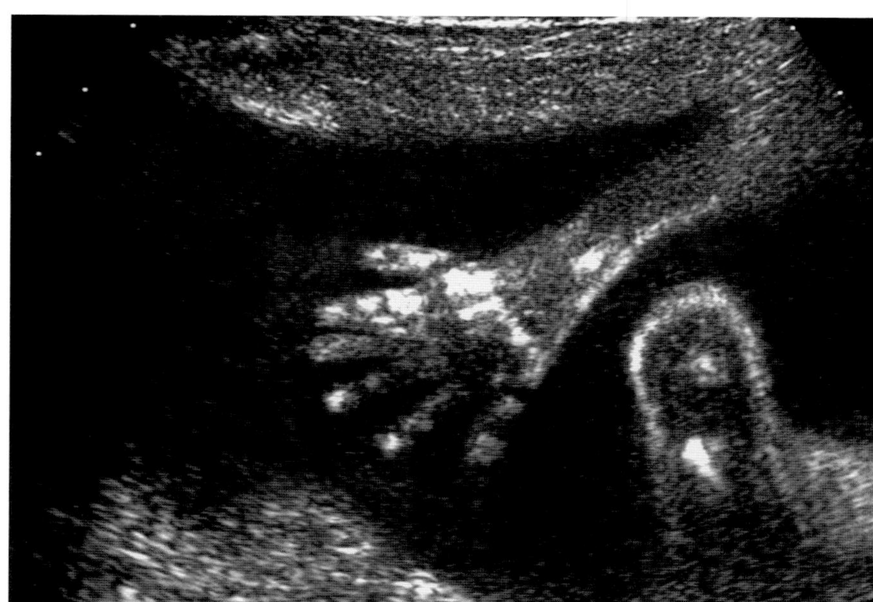

Fig. 8.**23** **Polydactyly.** Hexadactyly in a case of otocephaly at 21 + 3 weeks.

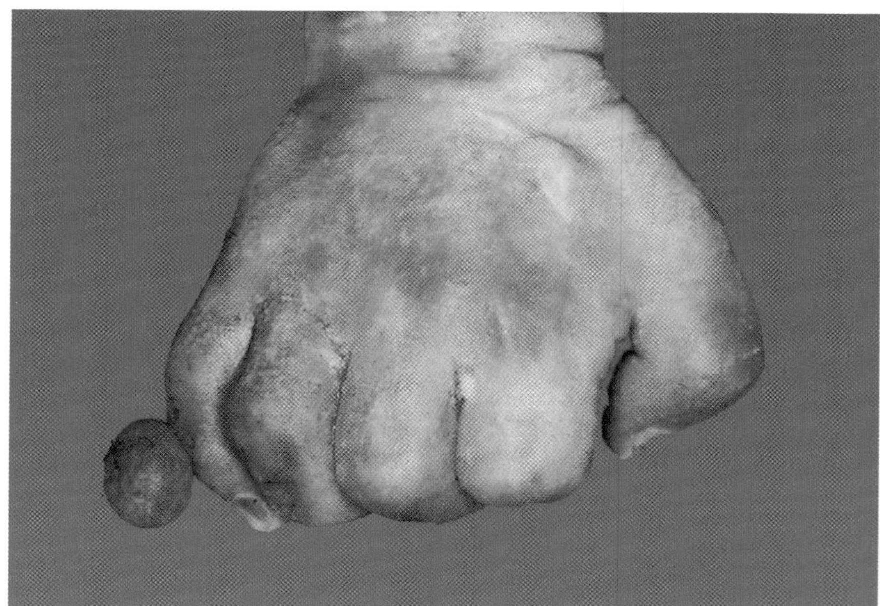

Fig. 8.**24** **Polydactyly.** Postaxial hexadactyly seen in trisomy 13 after termination of pregnancy.

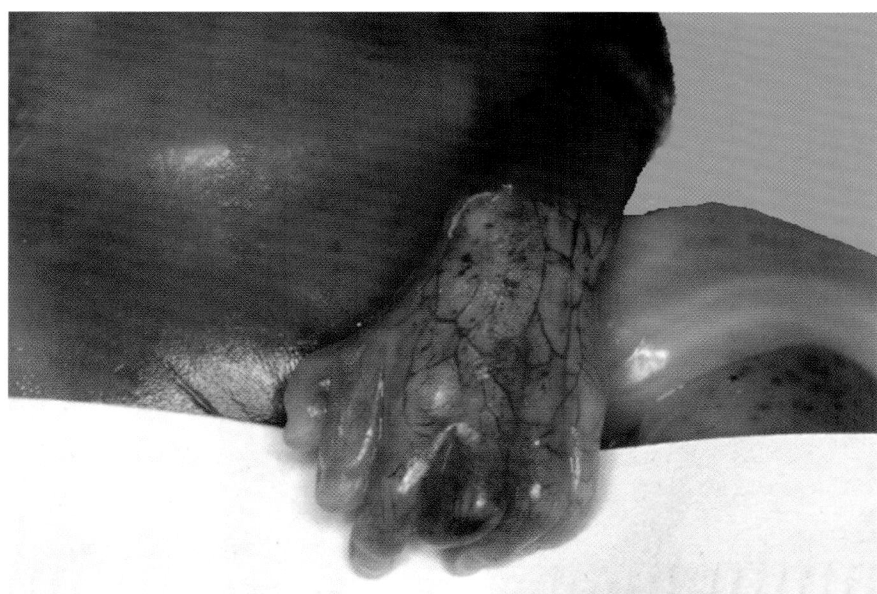

Fig. 8.**25** **Polydactyly.** Preaxial hexadactyly seen in a fetus after termination of pregnancy.

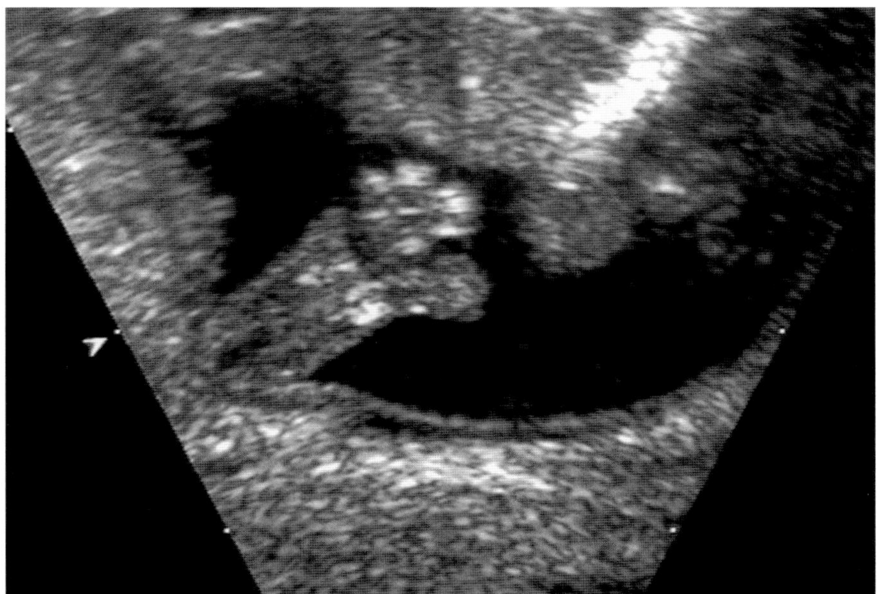

Fig. 8.**26** **Oligodactyly.** Tetradactyly in a fetus with triploidy at 14 + 5 weeks.

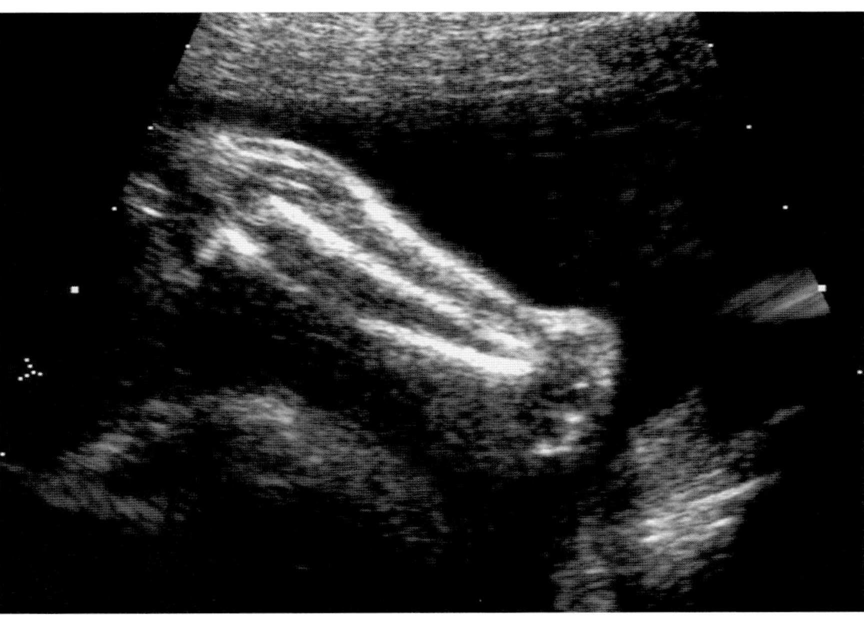

Fig. 8.**27** **Adactyly.** Seen at 22 weeks, in a fetus with Adams–Oliver syndrome.

Clinical management: Further ultrasound screening, including fetal echocardiography and karyotyping.

Procedure after birth: Special treatment is not required if the anomaly is isolated.

Prognosis: The isolated anomaly does not interfere with a normal healthy life.

References

Braithwaite JM, Economides DL. First-trimester diagnosis of Meckel–Gruber syndrome by transabdominal sonography in a low-risk case. Prenat Diagn 1995; 15: 1168–70.

Bromley B, Shipp TD, Benacerraf B. Isolated polydactyly: prenatal diagnosis and perinatal outcome. Prenat Diagn 2000; 20: 905–8.

Bronshtein M, Stahl S, Zimmer EZ. Transvaginal sonographic diagnosis of fetal finger abnormalities in early gestation. J Ultrasound Med 1995; 14: 591–5.

Hill LM, Leary J. Transvaginal sonographic diagnosis of short-rib polydactyly dysplasia at 13 weeks' gestation. Prenat Diagn 1998; 18: 1198–201.

Lavanya R, Pratap K. Short rib polydactyly syndrome: a rare skeletal dysplasia. Int J Gynaecol Obstet 1995; 50: 291–2.

Meizner I, Bar ZJ. Prenatal ultrasonic diagnosis of short rib polydactyly syndrome (SRPS) type HI: a case report and a proposed approach to the diagnosis of SRPS and related conditions. JCU J Clin Ultrasound 1985; 13: 284–7.

Salamanca A, Padilla MC, Sabatel RM, Motos MA, Stemper K, Gonzalez GF. Prenatal diagnosis of holoprosencephaly with postaxial polydactyly, cardiopathy with normal karyotype. Geburtshilfe Frauenheilkd 1992; 52: 783–5.

Wladimiroff JW, Stewart PA, Reuss A, Sachs ES. Cardiac and extra-cardiac anomalies as indicators for trisomies 13 and 18: a prenatal ultrasound study. Prenat Diagn 1989; 9: 515–20.

Zimmer EZ, Bronshtein M. Fetal polydactyly diagnosis during early pregnancy: clinical applications. Am J Obstet Gynecol 2000; 183: 755–8.

Radius Aplasia, Radius Hypoplasia

Definition: Complete or partial absence of the radius or distal end of it (base of the hand, thumb). Usually unilateral.

Incidence: One in 12 000–30 000 births.

Clinical history: Mostly sporadic, but autosomal-dominant, autosomal-recessive, and X-linked inheritance are also observed. It may also be associated with some syndromes.

Teratogens: Thalidomide, cocaine, valproic acid, high doses of vitamin A.

Associated malformations: Cardiac anomaly, thrombocytopenia.

Associated syndromes: Bilateral malformation is associated more frequently with a syndrome—e.g., Fanconi anemia, Aase syndrome, thrombocytopenia–absent radius (TAR) syndrome, VACTERL association, Goldenhar syndrome, some forms of trisomy, acrofacial dysostosis, Baller–Gerold syndrome, Cornelia de Lange syndrome, Townes–Brock syndrome, Holt–Oram syndrome.

Ultrasound findings: The *radius* is bowed or missing completely. The *ulna* may also be either bent, shortened, or absent. The *hand* is turned, and the thumb may be missing. In TAR syndrome, the disorder is bilateral. The lower extremities may also be involved. The findings are unilateral in Holt–Oram syndrome, without involvement of the lower limb. The humerus may also be absent.

Clinical management: Family history is important—is the marriage consanguineous? Was the mother exposed to any teratogens? Further ultrasound screening, including fetal echocardiography and karyotyping. Fetal blood sample (hemoglobin, platelets): if the platelet count is below 50 000 (Fanconi anemia, TAR syndrome), platelet infusion and/or delivery by cesarean section is indicated.

Procedure after birth: Hematological investigation: is anemia or thrombocytopenia present?

Prognosis: This depends on the underlying disorder. Good functional results are usually obtained after orthopedic surgery.

Self-Help Organization

Title: Thrombocytopenia Absent Radius Syndrome Association

Description: Information, networking and support for families with children with

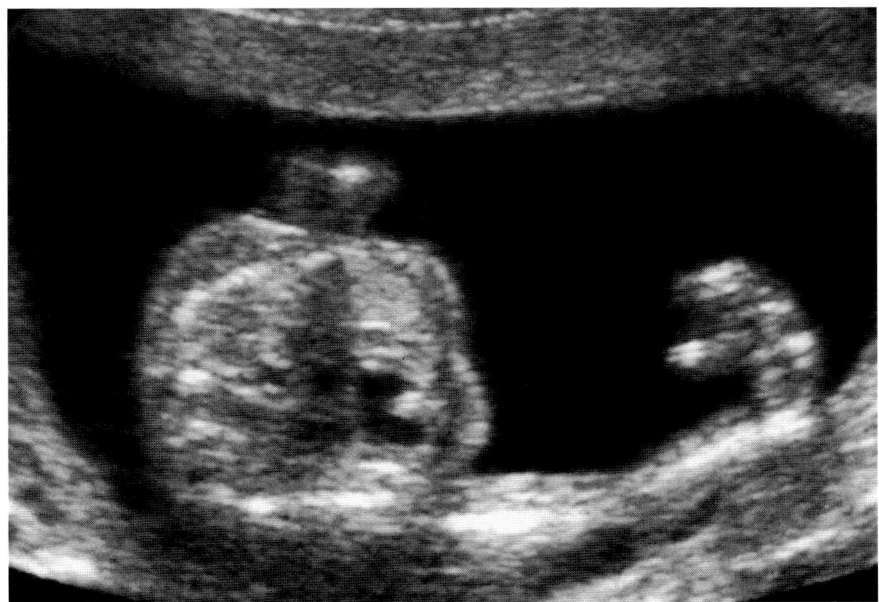

Fig. 8.**28** **Radius aplasia.** Fetal arm at 19 + 1 weeks in trisomy 18. Malposition of the hand due to aplasia of the radius.

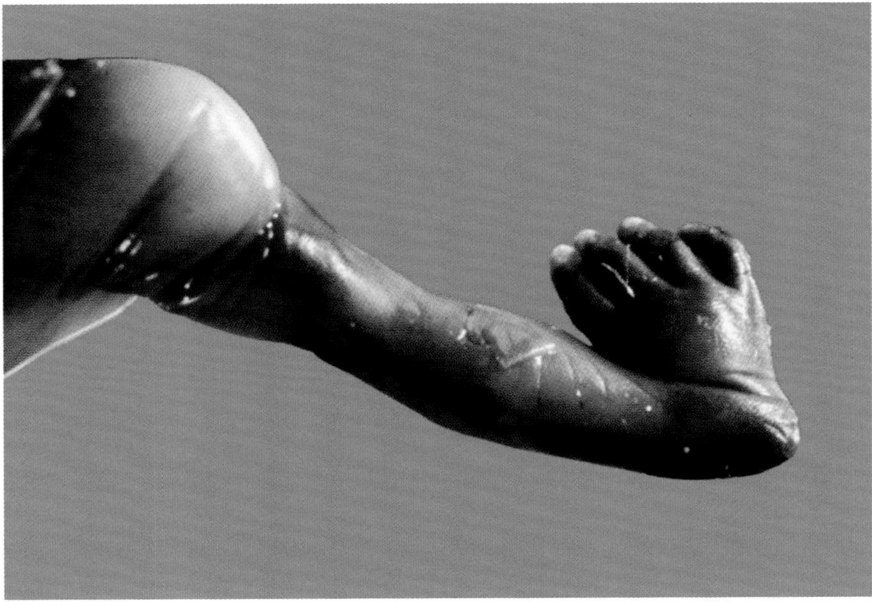

Fig. 8.**29** **Radius aplasia.** Same fetus shown after termination of pregnancy.

thrombocytopenia–absent radius syndrome (a shortening of the arms), and for affected adults. (Does not include ITP). Newsletter, pen-pal program, phone network.

Scope: International

Founded: 1981

Address: 212 Sherwood Dr., Egg Harbor Township, NJ 08234-7658, United States

Telephone: 609-927-0418

Fax: 609-653-8639

E-mail: purinton@earthlink.net

References

Hume RFJ, Gingras JL, Martin LS, Hertzberg BS, O'Donnell K, Killam AP. Ultrasound diagnosis of fetal anomalies associated with in utero cocaine exposure: further support for cocaine-induced vascular disruption teratogenesis. Fetal Diagn Ther 1994; 9: 239–45.

Schinzel A, Savoldelli G, Briner J, Sigg P, Massini C. Antley–Bixler syndrome in sisters: a term newborn and a prenatally diagnosed fetus. Am J Med Genet 1983; 14: 139–47.

Sepulveda W, Treadwell MC, Fisk NM. Prenatal detection of preaxial upper limb reduction in trisomy 18. Obstet Gynecol 1995; 85: 847–50.

Shelton SD, Paulyson K, Kay HH. Prenatal diagnosis of thrombocytopenia absent radius (TAR) syndrome and vaginal delivery. Prenat Diagn 1999; 19: 54–7.

Tongsong T, Wanapirak C, Piyamongkol W, Sudasana J. Prenatal sonographic diagnosis of VATER association. J Clin Ultrasound 1999; 27: 378–84.

Short Rib–Polydactyly Syndrome (SRPS) Type I (Saldino–Noonan) and Type III (Naumoff)

Definition: This is a disorder with anomalies consisting of short ribs, polydactyly, and short limbs. Facial clefts are not seen here (as in SRPS type II). SRPS types I and III are dealt with together here, as it is believed to be the same syndrome with varying expression.

Etiology/genetics: Autosomal-recessive inheritance.

Ultrasound findings: Head measurements seem large. *Short ribs* and a *narrow thorax* are typically seen. Anomalies of the vertebral bodies, such as distortion, may also be observed. Characteristic findings are *shortening of the extremities* and *polydactyly*. Other associated symptoms include: intestinal occlusion, anal atresia, renal hypoplasia, polycystic kidneys, intersexual genitalia, cardiac anomaly (DORV, AV canal, transposition). It is possible to diagnose SRPS type I at 17 weeks, with narrowed thorax, shortening of the long bones and polydactyly. The diagnosis of type III is made at 20 weeks due to micromelia, anomaly of the vertebral bodies, and polydac-

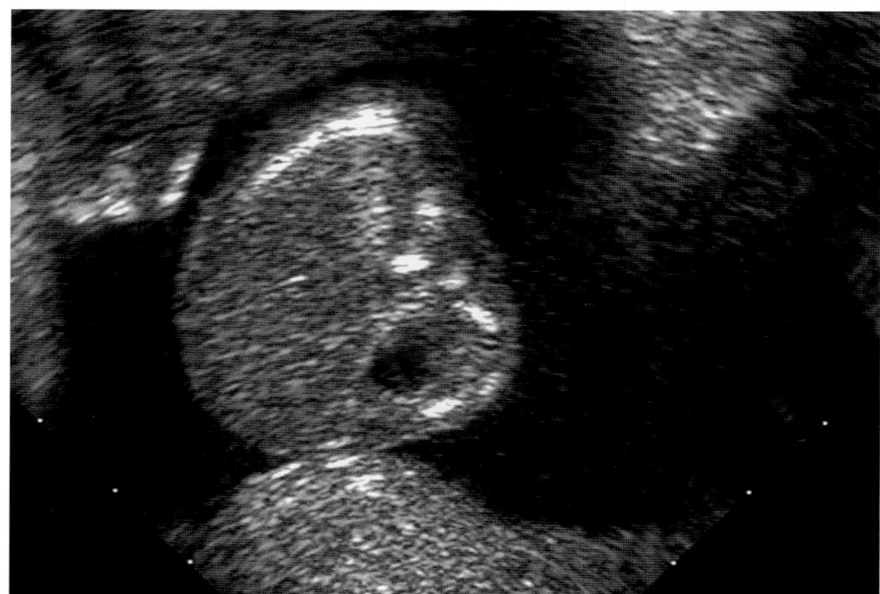

Fig. 8.**30** **Short rib–polydactyly syndrome type I.** Cross-section of the lower thoracic aperture at 16 + 3 weeks in a fetus with SRPS type I: shortening of the ribs and deformation of the rib cage are seen.

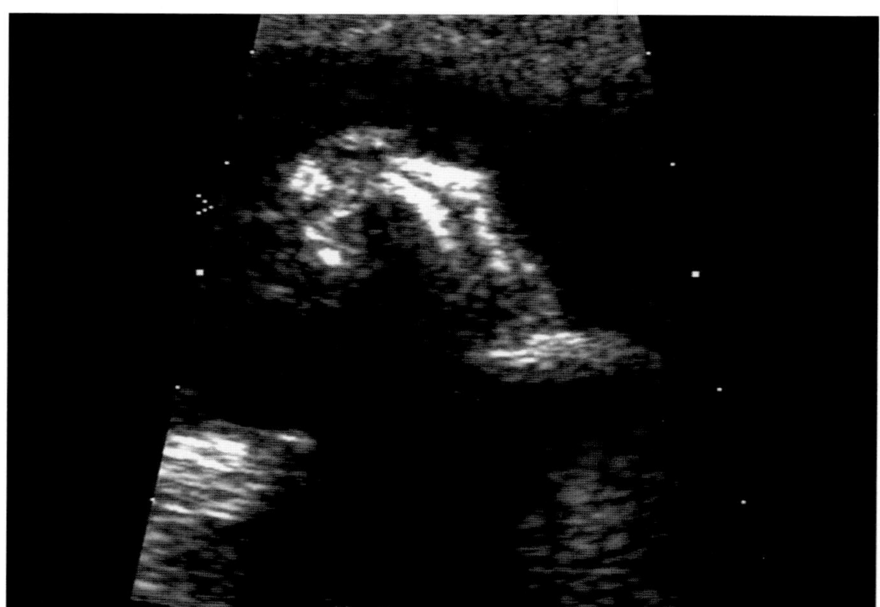

Fig. 8.**31** **Short rib–polydactyly syndrome type I.** Same fetus as before. The lower limb is seen, with shortening and atypical shapes of the tibia and fibula.

tyly. Hydramnios usually develops in the third trimester.

Differential diagnosis: Dysplasia of the thorax causing asphyxia, Ellis–van Creveld syndrome, SRPS II, thanatophoric dysplasia.

Prognosis: This condition is fatal, due to hypoplasia of the lungs causing respiratory failure.

References

Bronstein M, Reichler A, Borochowitz Z, Bejar J, Drugan A. Early prenatal diagnosis of polycystic pancreas with narrow thorax and short limb dwarfism. Am J Med Genet 1994; 49: 6–9.
de Sierra TM, Ashmead G, Bilenker R. Prenatal diagnosis of short rib (polydactyly) syndrome with situs inversus. Am J Med Genet 1992; 44: 555–7.
Golombeck K, Jacobs VR, von Kaisenberg C, Oppermann HC, Reinecke-Luthge A, et al. Short rib–polydactyly syndrome type III: comparison of ultrasound, radiology, and pathology findings. Fetal Diagn Ther 2001; 16: 133–8.
Hill LM, Leary J. Transvaginal sonographic diagnosis of short rib polydactyly dysplasia at 13 weeks' gestation. Prenat Diagn 1998; 18: 1198–201.
Lavanya R, Pratap K. Short rib polydactyly syndrome: a rare skeletal dysplasia. Int J Gynaecol Obstet 1995; 50: 291–2.
Meizner I, Bar ZJ. Prenatal ultrasonic diagnosis of short-rib polydactyly syndrome (SRPS) type III: a case report and a proposed approach to the diagnosis of SRPS and related conditions. JCU J Clin Ultrasound 1985; 13: 284–7.
Sarafoglou K, Funai EF, Fefferman N, et al. Short rib–polydactyly syndrome: more evidence of a continuous spectrum. Clin Genet 1999; 56: 145–8.
Shindel B, Wise S. Recurrent short rib–polydactyly syndrome with unusual associations. J Clin Ultrasound 1999; 27: 143–6.
Wu MH, Kuo PL, Lin SJ. Prenatal diagnosis of recurrence of short rib–polydactyly syndrome. Am J Med Genet 1995; 55: 279–84.

Short Rib–Polydactyly Syndrome Type II (Majewski Syndrome)

Definition: This is a fatal syndrome characterized by restricted growth, short ribs and polydactyly.

First described in 1971 by Majewski.

Genetics: Autosomal-recessive inheritance.

Ultrasound findings: *Severe shortening of the long bones* (detectable from 17 weeks), *narrowed thorax with very short ribs*, (in cross-section, the ribs encase less than half of the thoracic cavity), *hydramnios* (seen from the second trimester onwards), *postaxial polysyndactyly* of hands and feet. The following malformations may also be associated: hypoplasia of the cerebellar vermis,

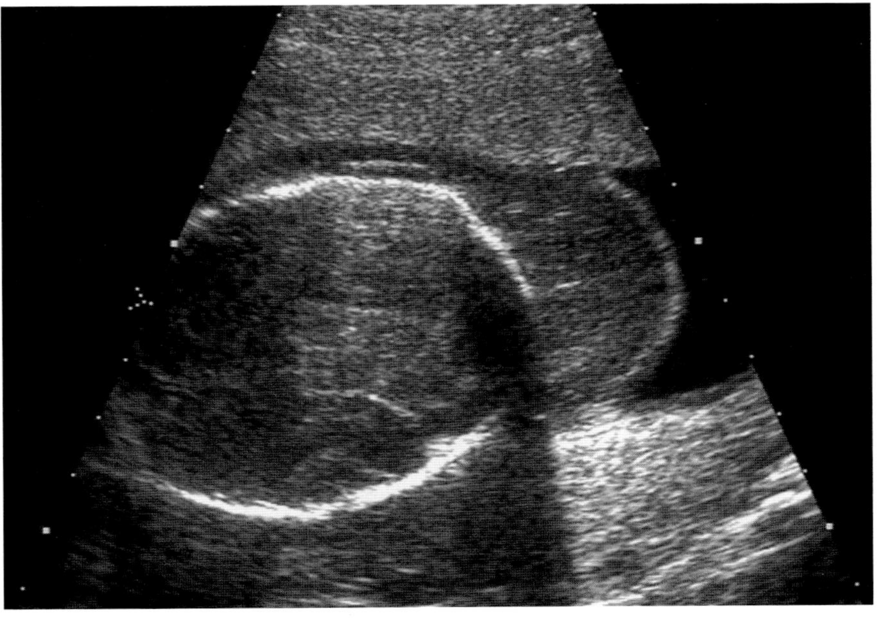

Fig. 8.32 **Short rib–polydactyly syndrome type II** (Majewski syndrome). Severe edema of the neck associated with nonimmune hydrops fetalis (NIHF) in a fetus with SRPS type II at 21 + 1 weeks.

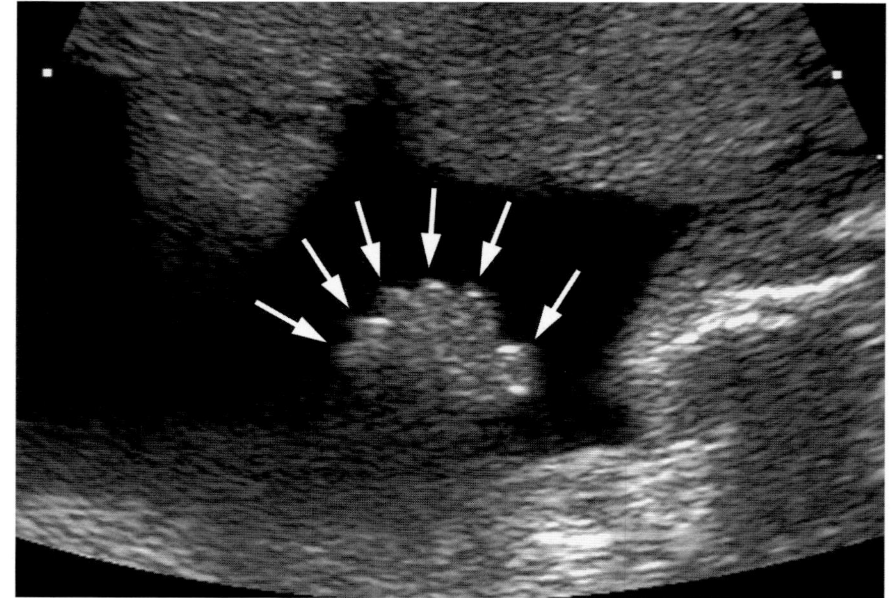

Fig. 8.33 . **Short rib–polydactyly syndrome type II** (Majewski syndrome). Same fetus, showing hexadactyly.

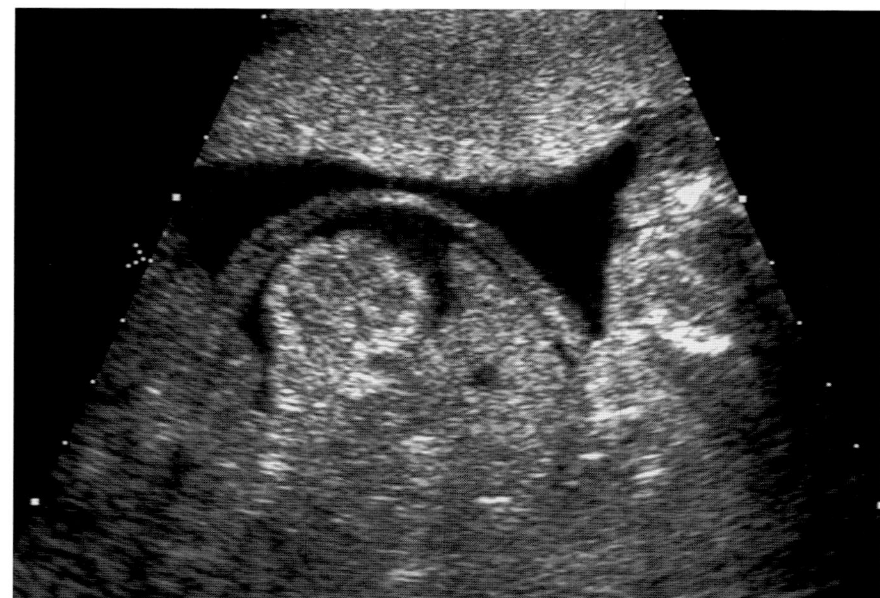

Fig. 8.34 **Short rib–polydactyly syndrome type II** (Majewski syndrome). Same fetus as before. Ascites and moderate pleural effusion are seen.

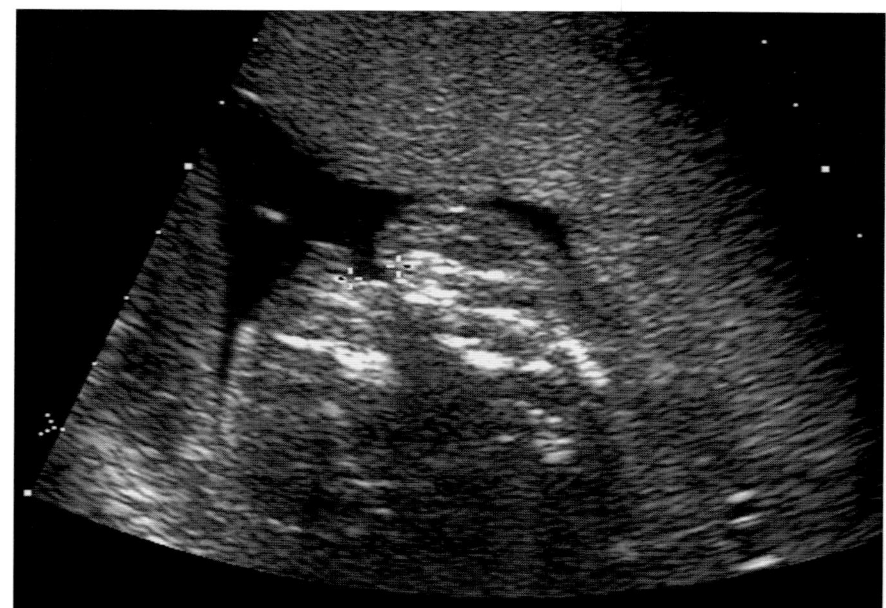

Fig. 8.35 **Short rib–polydactyly syndrome type II** (Majewski syndrome). Same fetus: cleft lip and palate; the defect measures 6 mm.

median facial cleft, cardiac malformations, renal anomalies, disorders of the genitalia, fetal hydrops.

Differential diagnosis: Asphyxiating thoracic dystrophy (absence of cleft palate and cleft lip), Ellis–van Creveld syndrome (in 60% cardiac anomalies), short rib–polydactyly syndrome type I (absence of facial clefts), thanatophoric dysplasia (absence of polydactyly).

Prognosis: Fatal outcome, due to hypoplasia of the lungs.

References

Benacerraf BR. Prenatal sonographic diagnosis of short rib–polydactyly syndrome type II, Majewski type. J Ultrasound Med 1993; 12: 552–5.

Bronstein M, Reichler A, Borochowitz Z, Bejar J, Drugan EA. Early prenatal diagnosis of polycystic pancreas with narrow thorax and short limb dwarfism. Am J Med Genet 1994; 49: 6–9.

de Sierra TM, Ashmead G, Bilenker R. Prenatal diagnosis of short rib (polydactyly) syndrome with situs inversus. Am J Med Genet 1992; 44: 555–7.

Gembruch U, Hansmann M, Fodisch HJ. Early prenatal diagnosis of short rib–polydactyly (SRP) syndrome type I (Majewski) by ultrasound in a case at risk. Prenat Diagn 1985; 5: 357–62.

Hill LM, Leary J. Transvaginal sonographic diagnosis of short-rib polydactyly dysplasia at 13 weeks' gestation. Prenat Diagn 1998; 18: 1198–201.

Lavanya R, Pratap K. Short rib polydactyly syndrome: a rare skeletal dysplasia. Int J Gynaecol Obstet 1995; 50: 291–2.

Meizner I, Bar ZJ. Prenatal ultrasonic diagnosis of short rib polydactyly syndrome (SRPS) type III: a case report and a proposed approach to the diagnosis of SRPS and related conditions. JCU J Clin Ultrasound 1985; 13: 284–7.

Sirichotiyakul S, Tongsong T, Wanapirak C, Chanprapaph P. Prenatal sonographic diagnosis of Majewski syndrome. J Clin Ultrasound 2002; 30: 303–7.

Thomson GS, Reynolds CP, Cruickshank J. Antenatal detection of recurrence of Majewski dwarf (short rib polydactyly syndrome type II Majewski). Clin Radiol 1982; 33 : 509–17.

Wu MH, Kuo PL, Lin SJ. Prenatal diagnosis of recurrence of short rib–polydactyly syndrome. Am J Med Genet 1995; 55: 279–84.

Thanatophoric Dysplasia

Definition: This fatal skeletal disorder is characterized by short extremities (micromelia), a narrowed thorax and comparatively large head and can be divided into type I and II.

Incidence: About one in 40 000 births; the most frequent type of fatal skeletal dysplasia.

Clinical history/genetics: sporadic occurrence; new mutation; autosomal-dominant inheritance; affected gene: *FGFR3*; gene locus: 4 p16.3. *Type I*: various gene mutations, *type II*: until now, only identical mutations have been found.

Teratogens: Not known.

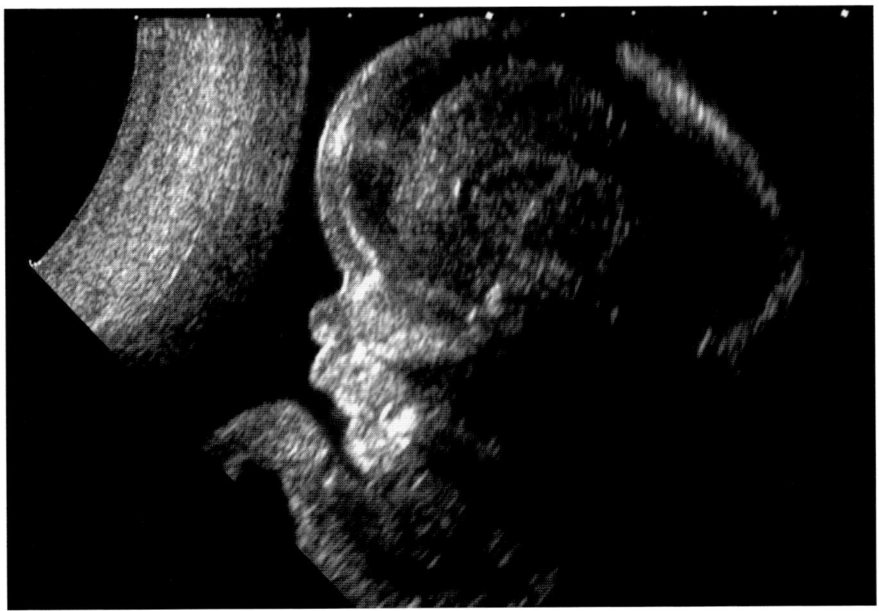

Fig. 8.**36** **Thanatophoric dysplasia.** Fetal profile: flattened nasal bridge, frontal bossing.

2

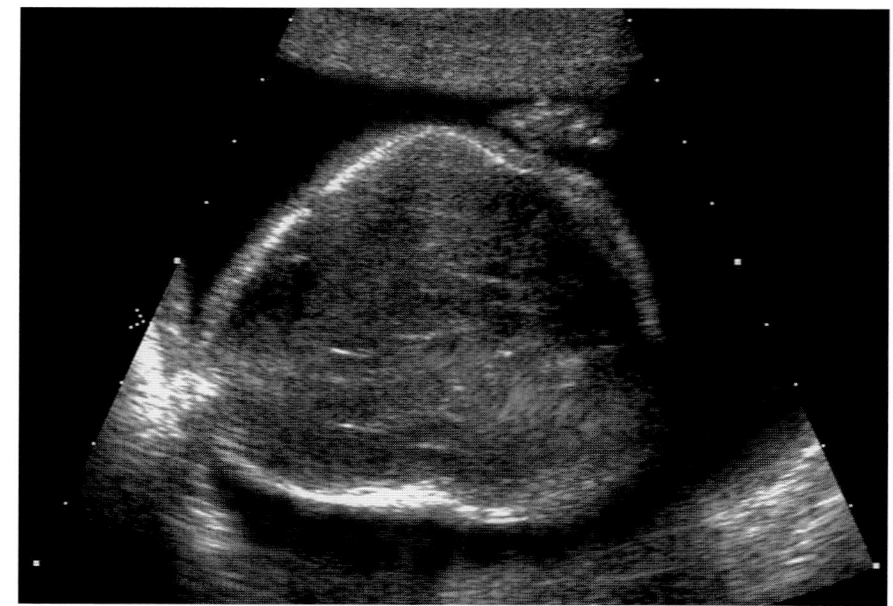

Fig. 8.**37** **Thanatophoric dysplasia.** Atypical shape of the fetal head at 21 + 3 weeks.

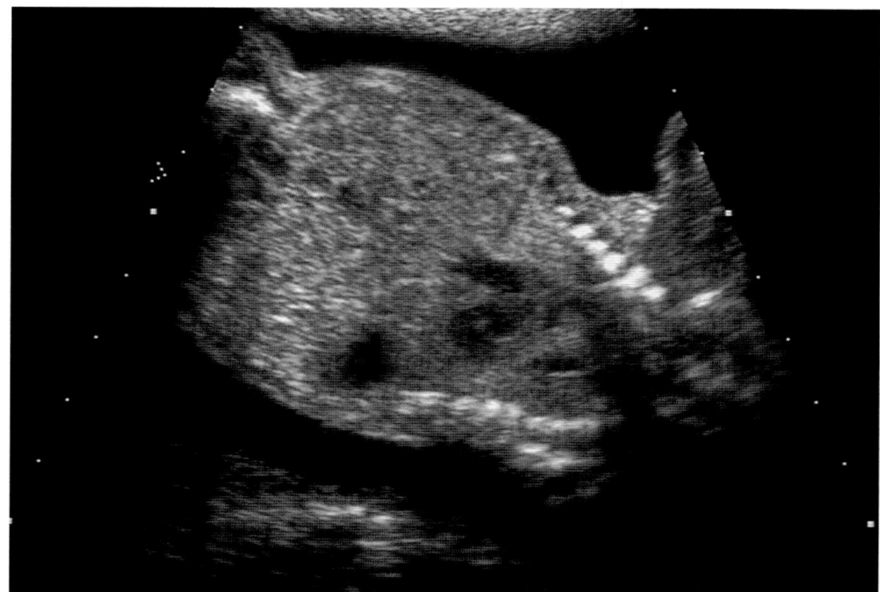

Fig. 8.**38** **Thanatophoric dysplasia.** Frontal plane, showing thoracic and abdominal cavities in fetus with thanatophoric dysplasia at 21 + 3 weeks: "champagne cork" appearance.

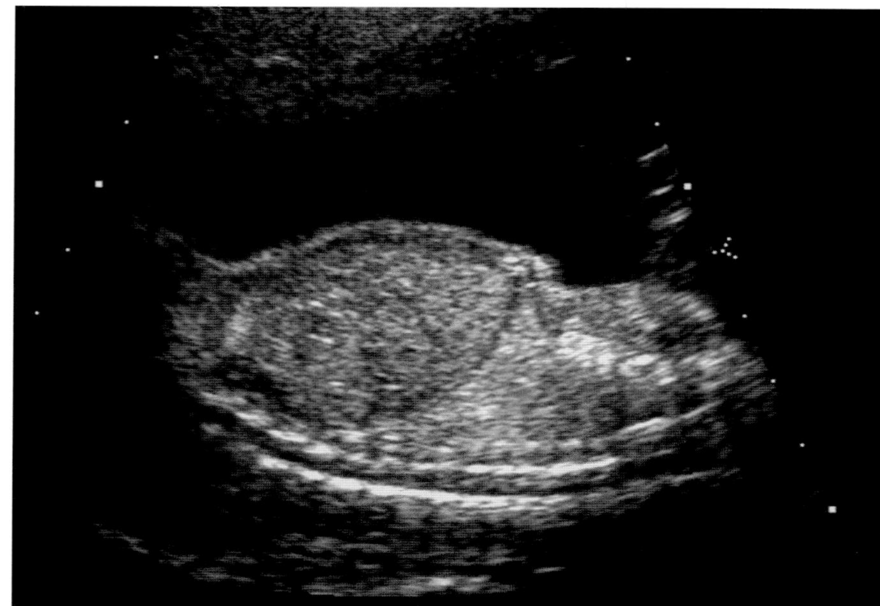

Fig. 8.**39** **Thanatophoric dysplasia.** Dorsoposterior longitudinal section in a fetus with thanatophoric dysplasia at 21 + 3 weeks. The circumferences of the thoracic (dysplastic) and abdominal cavities differ considerably.

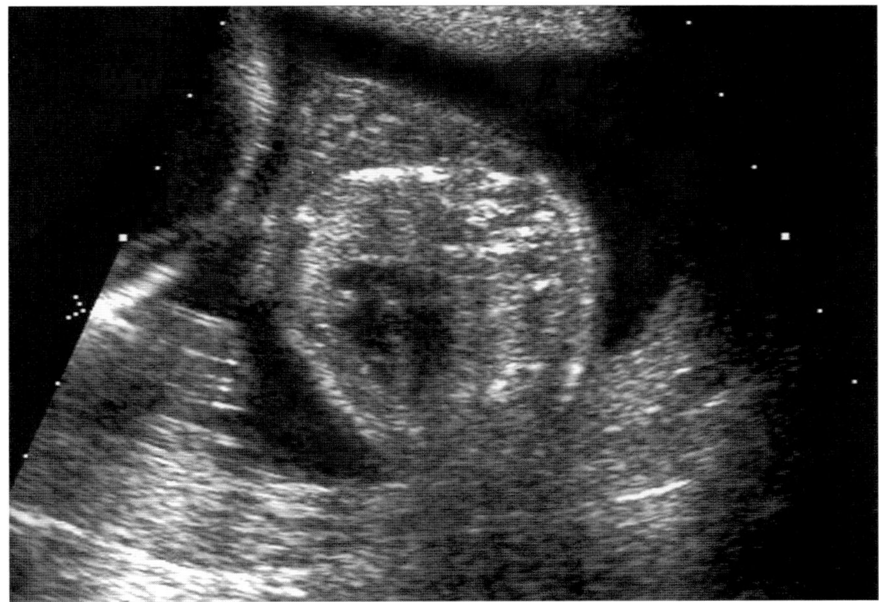

Fig. 8.**40** **Thanatophoric dysplasia.** Cross-section of the thorax at 21 + 3 weeks in a fetus with thanatophoric dysplasia. The plane of the heart is displaced. The normal-sized heart appears large within the thorax, due to dysplasia of the thorax.

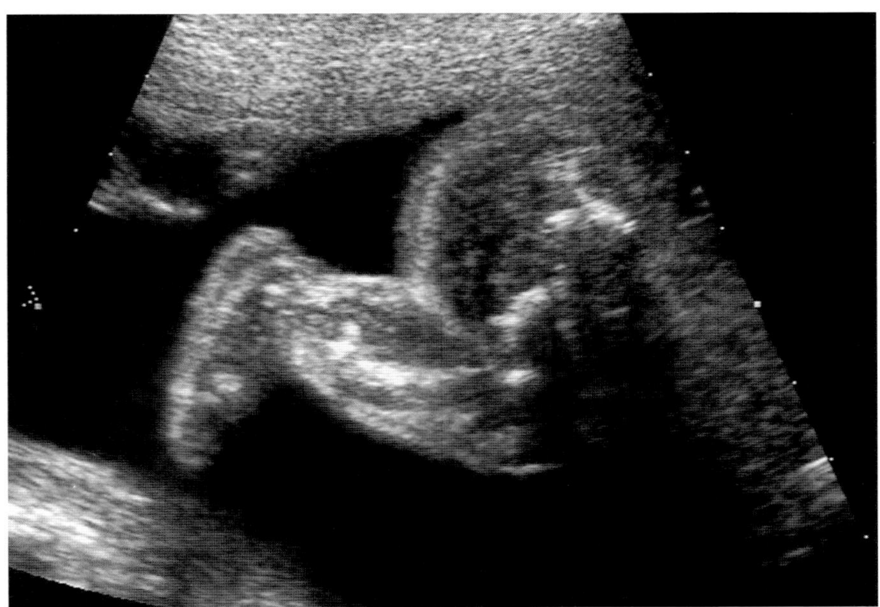

Fig. 8.**41** **Thanatophoric dysplasia.** Fetal lower limbs at 21 + 3 weeks, showing severe shortening of the long bones.

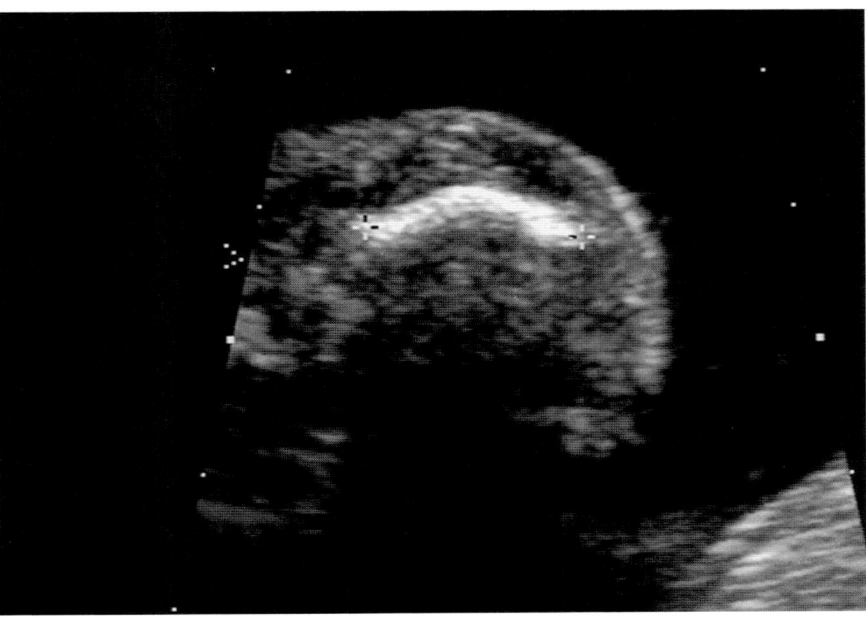

Fig. 8.**42** **Thanatophoric dysplasia.** Shortening and bowing of the femur at 21 + 3 weeks.

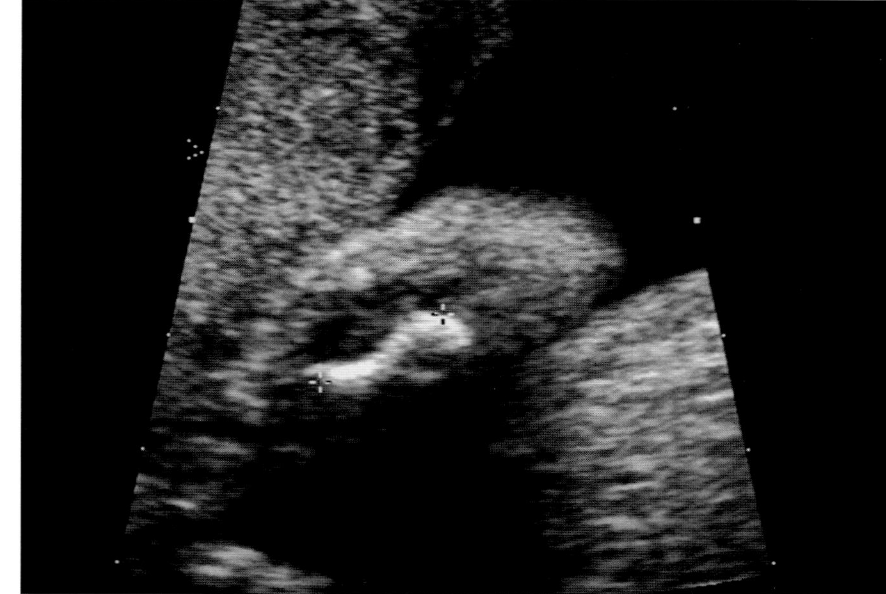

Fig. 8.**43** **Thanatophoric dysplasia.** Shortening and bowing of the tibia at 21 + 3 weeks.

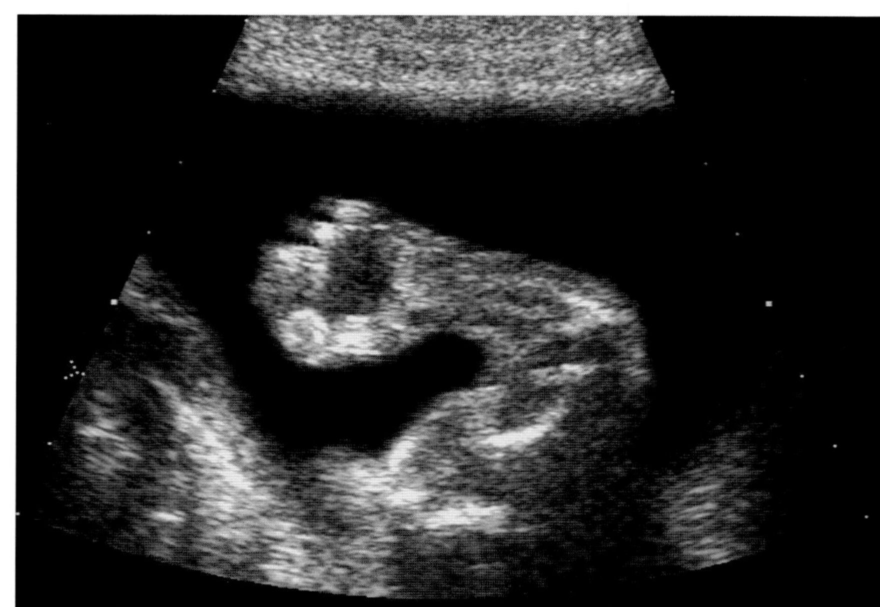

Fig. 8.**44** **Thanatophoric dysplasia.** Upper limb of a fetus at 21 + 3 weeks.

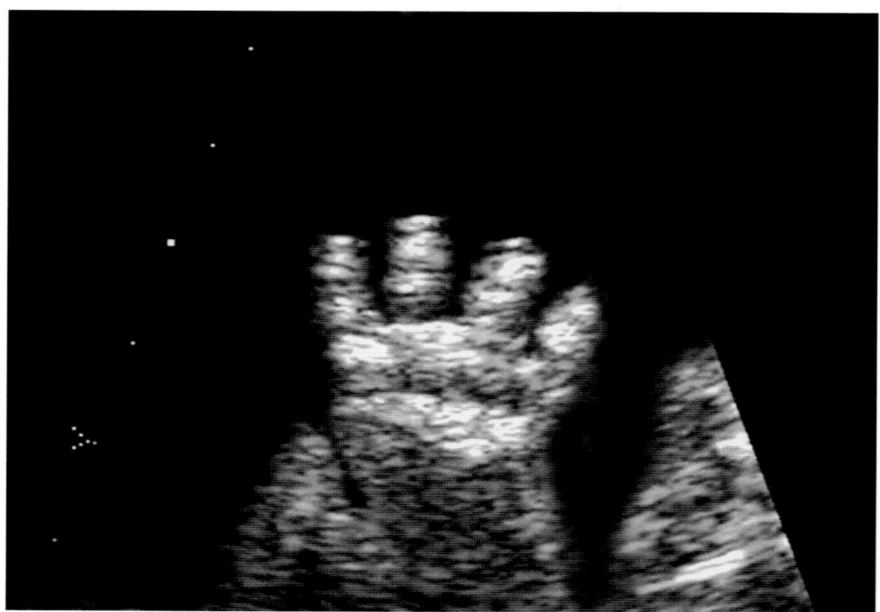

Fig. 8.**45** **Thanatophoric dysplasia.** Fetal hand at 21 + 3 weeks, showing short, stubby fingers.

Ultrasound findings: *Extremely short extremities with a typical bowing of the femur, resembling a "telephone receiver"* are characteristic features. A *narrow, "bell-shaped" thorax* and *short stubby fingers with wide inter digital spaces ("sausage-shaped" fingers)* are also typical. In 14% of cases, a *"cloverleaf" skull* is detected. *Hydrocephalus* may also be present. The vertebral column is shortened. Severe hydramnios develops in the late second or third trimester. The abdomen and head appear relatively large. Cardiac anomalies and hydronephrosis may be associated. It is possible to detect this disorder as early as at 14 weeks during prenatal screening.

Clinical management: Molecular-genetic diagnosis is possible. If diagnosis made with certainty, intervention due to fetal indication is not recommended. Cephalocentesis may be required to facilitate vaginal delivery.

Procedure after birth: Respiratory insufficiency is to be expected immediately after birth. Radiography of the skeletal system is advised to confirm the diagnosis.

Prognosis: The outcome is inevitably fatal, due to hypoplasia of the lungs.

References

Camera G, Dodero D, Camandona F, Camera A. Prenatal diagnosis of thanatophoric dysplasia at 21st week of pregnancy. Pathologica 1993; 85: 215–9.

Chen CP, Chern SR, Chang TY, Lin CJ, Wang W, Tzen CY. Second trimester molecular diagnosis of a stop codon *FGFR3* mutation in a type I thanatophoric dysplasia fetus following abnormal ultrasound findings. Prenat Diagn 2002; 22: 736–7.

Elejalde BR, de Elejalde MM. Thanatophoric dysplasia: fetal manifestations and prenatal diagnosis. Am J Med Genet 1985; 22: 669–83.

Gerihauser H, Schuster C, Immervoll H, Sochor G. Pränatal diagnosis of thanatophoric dwarfism. Ultraschall Med 1992; 13: 41–5.

Hall C. Pre-natal diagnosis of lethal dwarfism using ultrasound. Radiogr Today 1991; 57: 22–3.

Kassanos D, Botsis D, Katassos T, Panayotopoylos N, Zourlas P. Prenatal sonographic diagnosis of thanatophoric dwarfism. Int J Gynaecol Obstet 1991; 34: 373–6.

Kolble N, Sobetzko D, Ersch J, et al. Diagnosis of skeletal dysplasia by multidisciplinary assessment: a report of two cases of thanatophoric dysplasia. Ultrasound Obstet Gynecol 2002; 19: 92–8.

Machado LE, Bonilla-Musoles F, Osborne NG. Thanatophoric dysplasia. Ultrasound Obstet Gynecol 2001; 18: 85–6.

Mahony BS, Filly RA, Callen PW, Golbus MS. Thanatophoric dwarfism with the cloverleaf skull: a specific antenatal sonographic diagnosis. J Ultrasound Med 1985; 4: 151–4.

Schild RL, Hunt GH, Moore J, Davies H, Horwell DH. Antenatal sonographic diagnosis of thanatophoric dysplasia: a report of three cases and a review of the literature with special emphasis on the differential diagnosis. Ultrasound Obstet Gynecol 1996; 8: 62–7.

Stamm ER, Pretorius DH, Rumack CM, Manco JM. *Kleeblattschädel* anomaly: in utero sonographic appearance. J Ultrasound Med 1987; 6: 319–24.

Weiner CP, Williamson RA, Bonsib SM. Sonographic diagnosis of cloverleaf skull and thanatophoric dysplasia in the second trimester. JCU J Clin Ultrasound 1986; 14: 463–5.

Chromosomal Disorders and their Soft Markers

9 Chromosomal Disorders

General Considerations

Chromosomal aberrations are the most frequent and significant disorders and are detected in five per 1000 live births. The forms vary widely, ranging from those causing no clinical symptoms (for example, balanced translocation), to those of little significance for the affected individual (e.g., Klinefelter syndrome), up to those with a fatal outcome (trisomy 13, 18). As the consequences for the affected families are serious, diagnosis of chromosomal anomalies has always been the main aim of prenatal screening, taking into account all the ethical considerations involved.

Amniocentesis was developed over 30 years ago and has been increasingly included in antenatal care for older pregnant women. In Germany, this has had legal consequences. In effect, the gynecologist is obliged to guarantee a chromosomally healthy child and to document the fact that adequate patient information regarding invasive prenatal diagnosis has been provided if the mother is going to be over the age of 34 at the expected date of delivery.

In fact, however, only a small percentage of affected fetuses are detected prenatally on the basis of the age indication. In order to offer younger mothers the option of detecting the most frequent chromosomal anomaly—Down syndrome—without the risks of amniocentesis, the *triple test* was first developed some 10 years ago. The disadvantage of this test is that, at a cutoff level of 1 : 350, it has a false-positive rate of 5–10%, with a detection rate of 60–65%.

In recent years, the measurement of *nuchal translucency* (NT) at 11–13 weeks has been increasingly carried out for early detection of genetic and organ anomalies in younger mothers. The sensitivity of this method for detecting Down syndrome, is 70–80%, with a 5% rate of false-positive findings. In addition to ultrasound scanning, determination of *PAPP-A* and *free* β*-HCG* raises the sensitivity to 90%. This allows many pregnant women above the age of 35 years to avoid invasive prenatal diagnosis, which have their own risks. However, it should be borne in mind here that a sensitivity of 90% means that one in 10 affected fetuses will not be detected.

Self-Help Organizations

Title: The Genetic Alliance

Description: Consortium of support groups dedicated to helping individuals and families affected by genetic disorders. Information and referrals to support groups and genetic services.

Scope: National network

Telephone: 1-800-336-4363 or 202-966-5557

Fax: 202-966-8553

E-mail: info@geneticalliance.org

Web: http://geneticalliance.org

Title: Chromosome 22 Central

Description: Networking and support for parents of children with any chromosome disorder. Supports research. Offers newsletter, literature, phone support and pen pals.

Scope: International network

Founded: 1996

Address: 2327 Kent Ave., Timmons, Ontario P4 N 3 C3, Canada

Telephone: 705-268-3099

Fax: 705-268-3099

Web: http://www.c22 c.org

Jacobsen Syndrome (11 q Deletion)

Definition: This is a structural chromosomal anomaly with a deletion, of varying size, of the distal long arm of chromosome 11. It is associated with multiple congenital malformations and mental retardation.

First described in 1973.

Etiology: Deletion of the long arm of chromosome 11, as a new mutation or due to balanced translocation in one of the parents.

Ultrasound findings: Intrauterine growth restriction, trigonocephaly, microcephaly, dilation of ventricles, holoprosencephaly, hypertelorism, micrognathia, ear anomaly, cardiac and renal anomalies, anomalies of the genitals, clinodactyly, joint contractures.

Differential diagnosis: Trisomy 13, trisomy 18, craniostenosis, spina bifida.

Prognosis: This depends on the severity of the cardiac anomaly. Survivors suffer moderate to severe mental impairment.

Self-Help Organization

Title: 11 q Research and Resource Group

Description: Mutual support for families of children with structural abnormalities of chromosome 11, including deletions, duplications and translocations. Networking of families, researchers and organizations. Newsletter, conferences, books, videos.

Scope: Online

Address: Melanie 11 q Research and Resource Group, 6123 A Duncan Rd., Petersberg, VA 23 803, United States

Web: http://www.11 q.net

References

Fernandez Gonzalez N, Prieto Espunes S, Ibanez Fernandez A, Fernandez Colomer B, Lopez Sastre J, Fernandez Toral J. [Deletion 11q23→qter (Jacobsen Syndrome) associated with duodenal atresia and annular pancreas; in Spanish.] An Esp Pediatr 2002; 57: 249–52.

Chen CP, Chern SR, Tzen CY, et al. Prenatal diagnosis of de novo distal 11 q deletion associated with sonographic findings of unilateral duplex renal system, pyelectasis and orofacial clefts. Prenat Diagn 2001; 21: 317–20.

Chen CP, Liu FF, Jan SW, Chen CP, Lan CC. Partial duplication of 3 q and distal deletion of 11 q in a stillbirth with an omphalocele containing the liver, short limbs, and intrauterine growth retardation. J Med Genet 1996; 33: 615–7.

Pallister–Killian Syndrome (Tetrasomy 12 p)

Definition: This is a severe chromosomal disorder, clinically characterized by a severe decrease in muscle tension, severe mental retardation and other anomalies. Mosaic with tetrasomy 12 p.

Incidence: Rare condition; only 50 cases have been described.

Etiology: Sporadic occurrence. Chromosomal mosaic is difficult to detect in the lymphocytes, but not in fibroblasts and amniotic cells. It correlates with advanced maternal age.

Ultrasound findings: Growth restriction, hydramnios, singular umbilical artery and microcephaly are possible findings. Cerebellar hypoplasia, hydrocephalus, craniofacial anomalies such as large forehead, coarse facial features, hypertelorism, ear dysplasia, macrostomia, and elevated palate may also be present. Cardiac anomalies such as VSD, aortic isthmus stenosis, PDA, ASD, and others occur in 25% of cases. Diaphragmatic hernia is seen in 50% of cases, and anal atresia may also be seen. Other anomalies include renal and genital malformations. Extremities may also be involved: shortening of the bones, small, stubby hands and feet, doubling of the big toes. Skin disorders, alopecia and skin pigmentation may also be seen.

Differential diagnosis: Wolf–Hirschhorn syndrome, Fryns syndrome, trisomy 9 mosaic, trisomy 18.

Clinical management: Karyotyping of various cellular types may be necessary, as in mosaic disorders only 1–3% of lymphocytes from fetal blood may be abnormal. Analyses of amniocytes or placental tissue shows a higher proportion of abnormal cells.

Prognosis: 50% die in the prenatal or perinatal stage. The survivors may reach the age of 10–15 years; the oldest patient known is 45 years old, with severe mental retardation.

References

Chiesa J, Hoffet M. Rousseau O, et al. Pallister–Killian syndrome [i(12p)]: first prenatal diagnosis using cordocentesis in the second trimester confirmed by in situ hybridization. Clin Genet 1998; 54: 294–302.

Choo S, Teo SH, Tan M, Yong MH, Ho LY. Tissue-limited mosaicism in Pallister–Killian syndrome: a case in point. J Perinatol 2002; 22: 420–3.

Doray B, Girard-Lemaire F, Gasser B, et al. Pallister–Killian syndrome: difficulties of prenatal diagnosis. Prenat Diagn 2002; 22: 470–7.

Langford K, Hodgson S, Seller M, Maxwell D. Pallister–Killian syndrome presenting through nuchal translucency screening for trisomy 21. Prenat Diagn 2000; 20: 670–2.

Mathieu M, Piussan C, Thepot F, et al. Collaborative study of mosaic tetrasomy 12 p or Pallister–Killian syndrome (nineteen fetuses or children). Ann Genet 1997; 40: 45–54.

Mowery RP, Stadler MP, Kochmar SJ, McPherson E, Surti U, Hogge WA. The use of interphase FISH for prenatal diagnosis of Pallister–Killian syndrome. Prenat Diagn 1997; 17: 255–65.

Paladini D, Borghese A, Arienzo M, Teodoro A, Martinelli P, Nappi C. Prospective ultrasound diagnosis of Pallister–Killian syndrome in the second trimester of pregnancy: the importance of the fetal facial profile. Prenat Diagn 2000; 20): 996–8.

Sharland M, Hill L, Patel R, Patton M. Pallister–Killian syndrome diagnosed by chorionic villus sampling. Prenat Diagn 1991; 11: 477–9.

Wilson RD, Harrison K, Clarke LA, Yong SL. Tetrasomy 12 p (Pallister–Killian syndrome): ultrasound indicators and confirmation by interphase fish. Prenat Diagn 1994; 14: 787–92.

Triploidy

Definition: This is the third most frequent fatal chromosomal disorder seen in the prenatal stage. The chromosomes are tripled (instead of the normal doubling), such that the cell nuclei have 69 instead of 46 chromosomes.

Incidence: Some 1–2% of all conceptions have triploidy; these cases end mostly as early spontaneous miscarriages. Six percent of fetuses lost as spontaneous abortions up to 28 weeks show triploidy. Birth of a live infant is extremely rare.

Sex ratio: M : F = 1.5 : 1.

Clinical history: Sporadic occurrence. Elevation of β-HCG and α-fetoprotein (up to four times the median value) is detected.

Etiology: An additional complete set of chromosomes leads to a karyotype of 69,XXX or 69,XXY or 69,XYY. Sixty percent of cases are due to fertilization of one ovum with two sperms (paternal origin); 40% arise due to fertilization of a diploid ovum (maternal origin).

Teratogens: Not known.

Ultrasound findings: Severe intrauterine growth restriction is detected early (beginning at 12–14 weeks). Oligohydramnios, enlarged placenta with cystic regions (partial molar degeneration in triploidy of paternal origin, that of maternal origin usually of normal appearance). *CNS*: hydrocephalus, holoprosencephaly, neural tube defects, agenesis of the corpus callosum, Arnold–Chiari malformation. *Facial features*: hypertelorism, cleft palate, cleft lip. *Extremities* : syndactyly of the third and fourth fingers, club feet. *Others*: cardiac anomalies, omphalocele, hydronephrosis, genital anomalies.

Caution: The placenta may appear normal; the pattern of anomalies is very variable.

Differential diagnosis: Trisomy 9, 13, and 18, infections, Neu–Laxova syndrome, Russell–Silver syndrome, Seckel syndrome.

Clinical management: Karyotyping and further ultrasound screening, including fetal echocardiography. If the mother decides to continue with

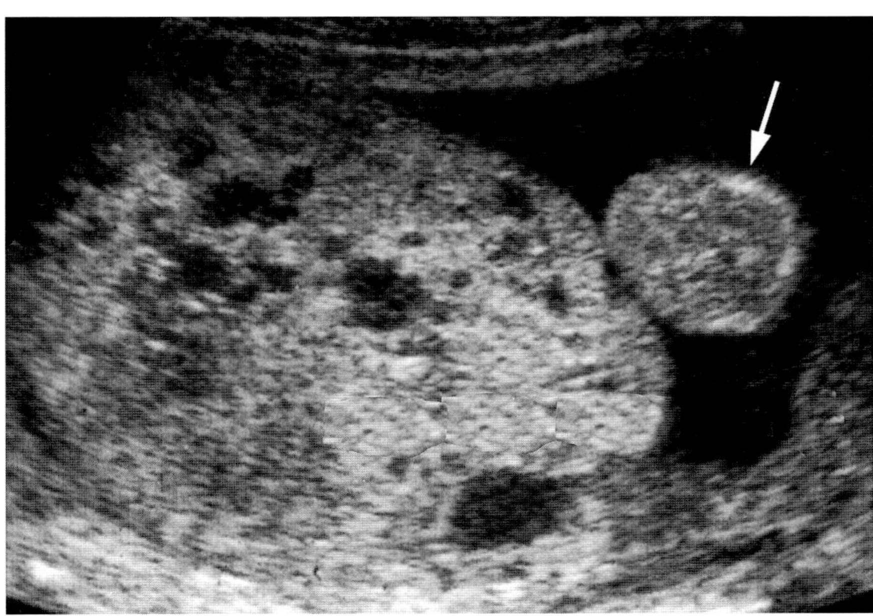

Fig. 9.1 **Triploidy** at 16 + 3 weeks, showing an enlarged placenta with molar degeneration and vacuoles of various sizes. A fetus with severe growth restriction (arrow) is also seen.

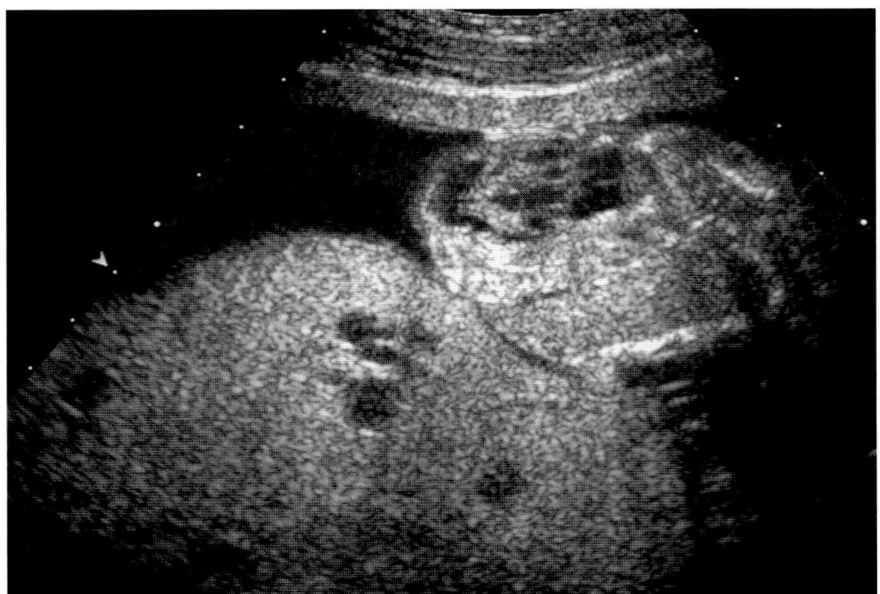

Fig. 9.2 **Triploidy.** Cardiac effusion at 17 + 1 weeks in a fetus with triploidy.

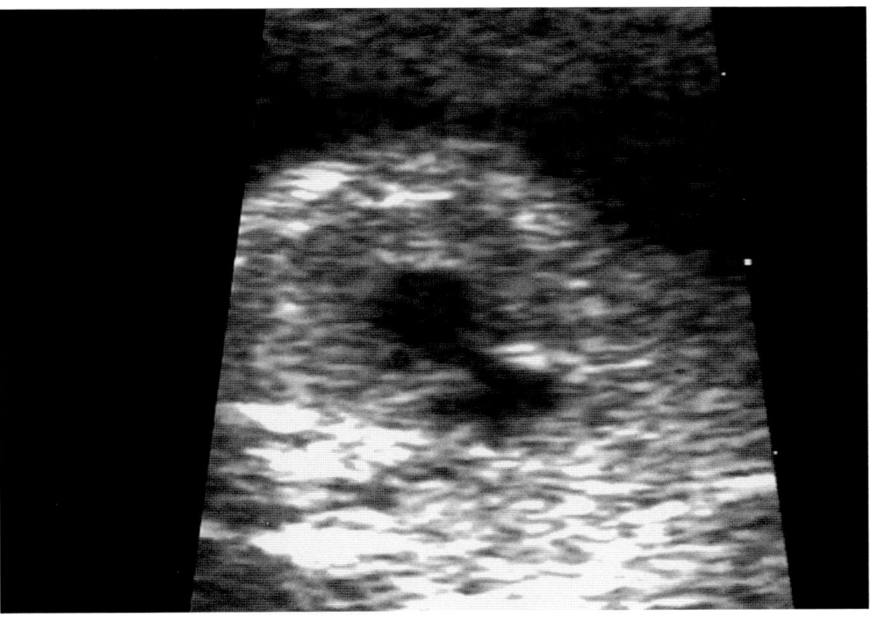

Fig. 9.3 **Triploidy.** Fetal heart showing "single ventricle" in triploidy, at 21 + 3 weeks.

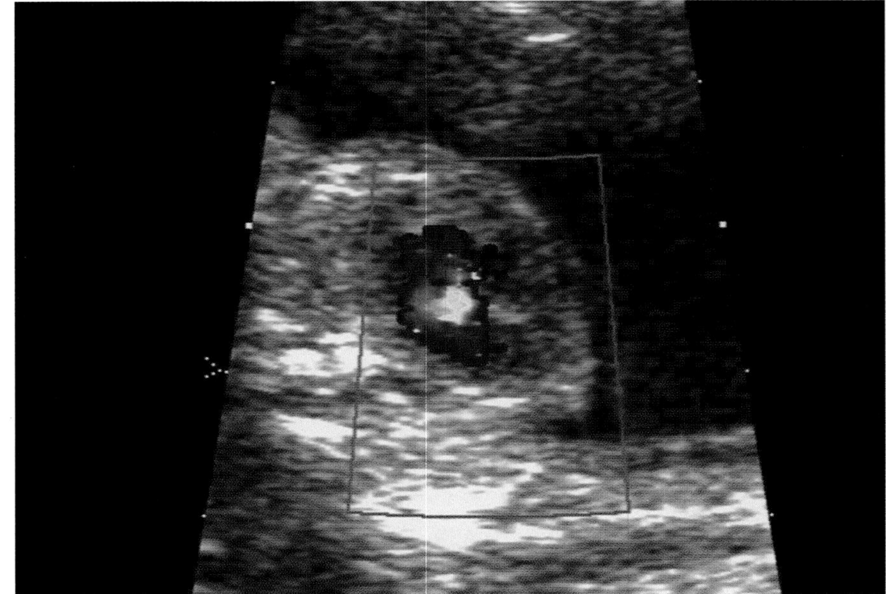

Fig. 9.**4** **Triploidy.** Doppler color mapping of the fetal heart at 21 + 3 weeks, showing a "single ventricle" in a fetus with triploidy.

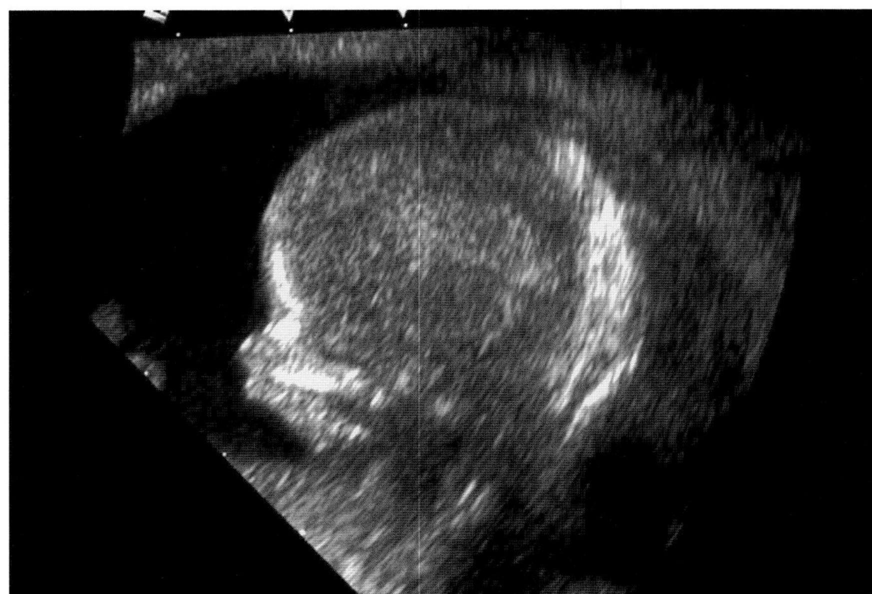

Fig. 9.**5** **Triploidy.** Fetal profile at 14 + 5 weeks, showing severe micrognathia in a fetus with triploidy (69,XXX).

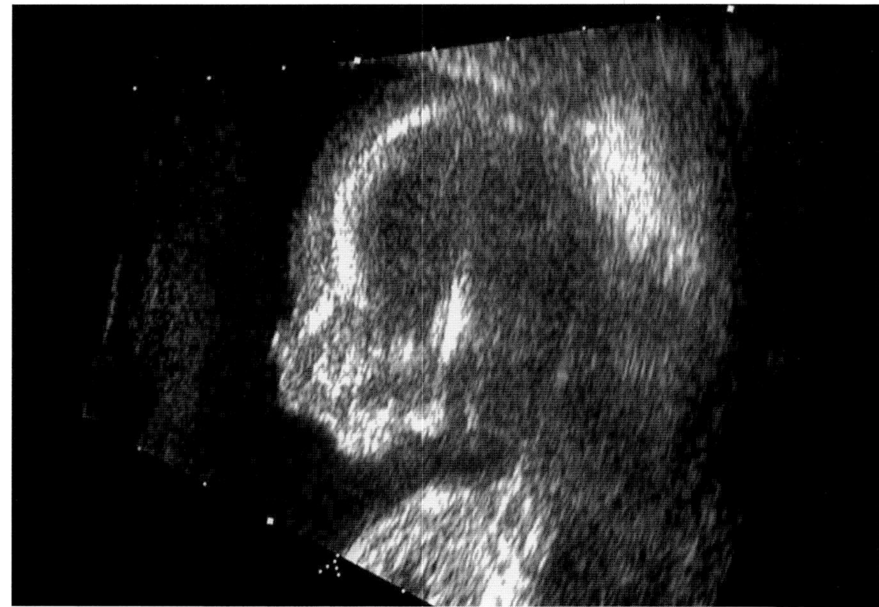

Fig. 9.**6** **Triploidy.** Fetal profile with severe micrognathia in triploidy at 21 + 3 weeks.

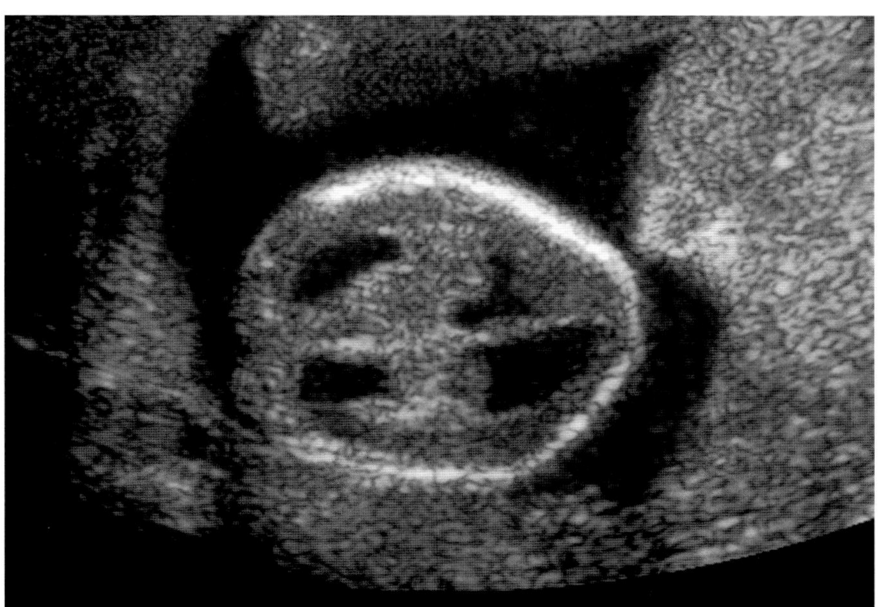

Fig. 9.**7** **Triploidy.** Marginal dilation of cerebrospinal fluid space and strawberry sign in a fetus with triploidy at 17 + 1 weeks.

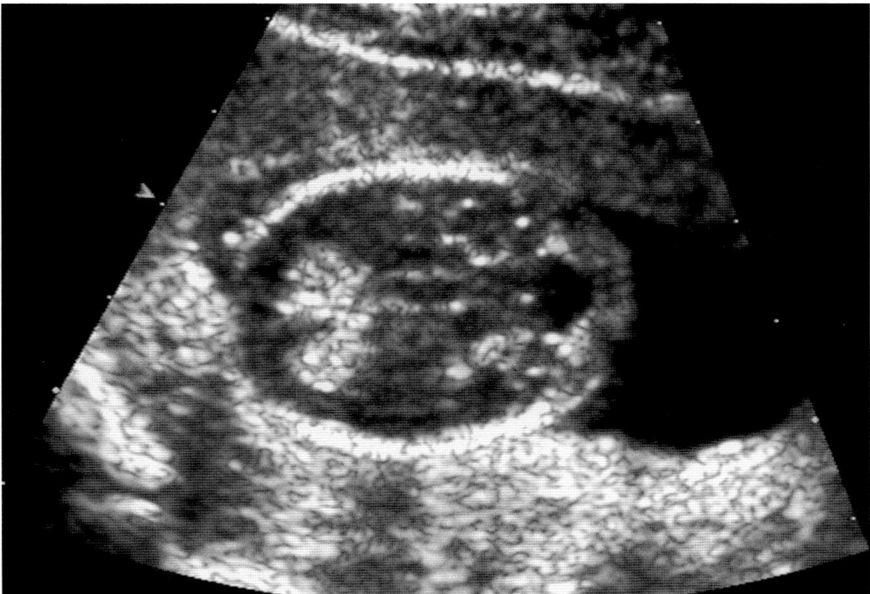

Fig. 9.**8** **Triploidy.** Dilation of the cerebellomedullary cistern at 14 + 5 weeks.

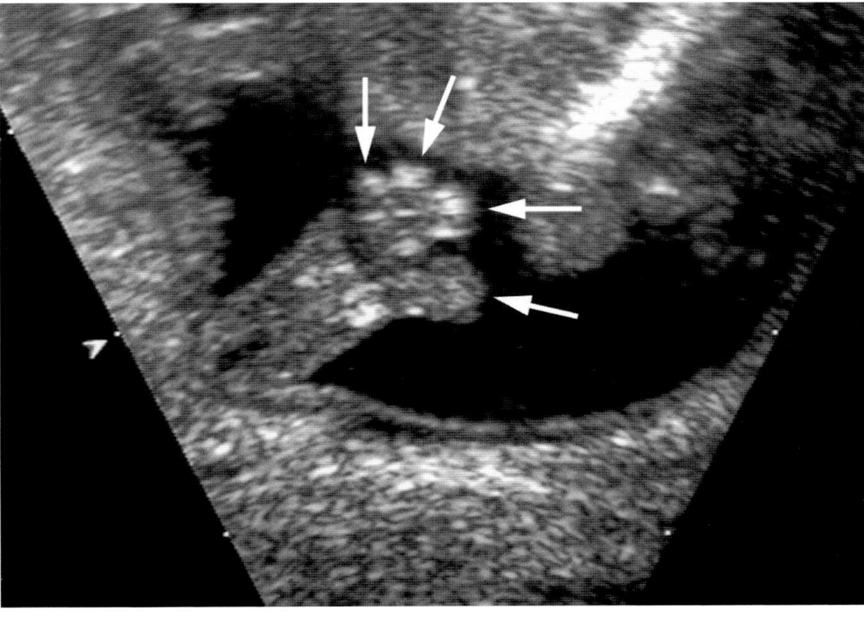

Fig. 9.**9** **Triploidy.** Tetradactyly in a fetus with triploidy at 14 + 5 weeks.

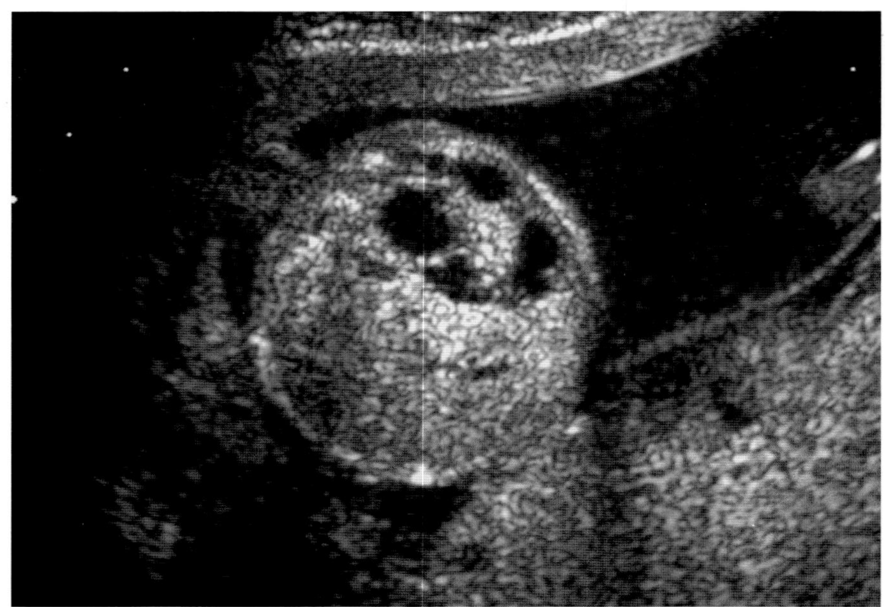

Fig. 9.**10** **Triploidy.** Unilateral multicystic renal dysplasia in a case of triploidy at 17 + 1 weeks.

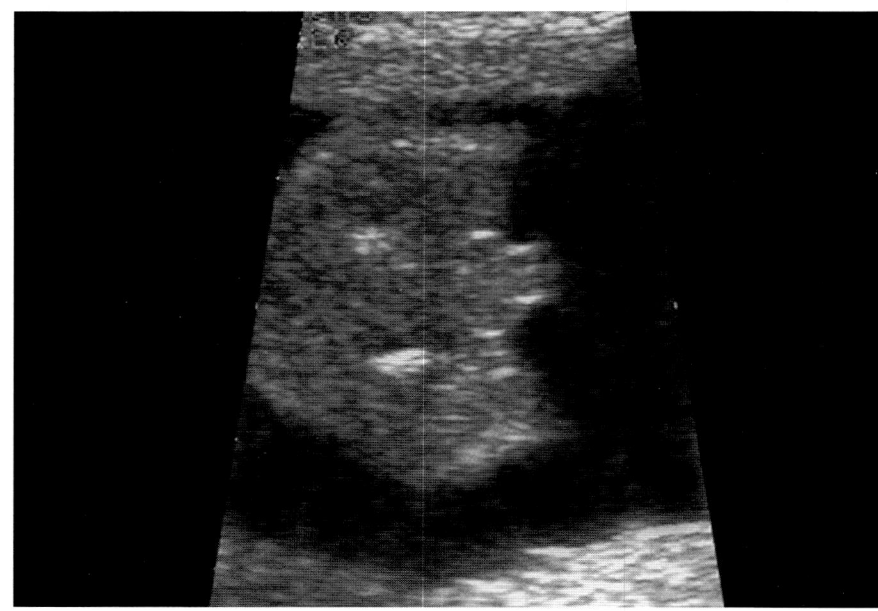

Fig. 9.**11** **Triploidy.** Genitals in a fetus with 69,XXX with hypertrophy of the clitoris at 21 + 3 weeks.

the pregnancy, she should be warned of the high risk of developing preeclampsia and hyperthyroidism. Hyperemesis gravidarum and theca lutein cysts of the ovaries are frequent. The β-HCG level is increased, but only in 80% of cases in case of a partial mole. Cesarean section on the basis of a fetal indication should be avoided.

Procedure after birth: Intensive medical measures are not indicated.

Prognosis: The pregnancy usually ends with an early miscarriage. Otherwise intrauterine demise or death in the early neonatal stage is the general outcome. In case of mosaic, survival into early childhood is rare, with severe mental retardation.

Information for the parents: The risk of recurrence is not increased.

References

Beinder E, Voigt HJ, Jager W, Wildt L. Partial hydatidiform mole in a cytogenetically normal fetus. Geburtshilfe Frauenheilkd 1995; 55: 351–3.

Benacerraf BR. Intrauterine growth retardation in the first trimester associated with triploidy. J Ultrasound Med 1988; 7: 153–4.

Blaicher W, Ulm B, Ulm MR, Hengstschlager M, Deutinger J, Bernaschek G. Dandy–Walker malformation as sonographic marker for fetal triploidy. Ultraschall Med 2002; 23: 129–33.

Harper MA, Ruiz C, Pettenati MJ, Rao PN. Triploid partial molar pregnancy detected through maternal serum alpha-fetoprotein and HCG screening. Obstet Gynecol 1994; 83: 844–6.

1
2
3
4
5

Holzgreve W, Miny P, Holzgreve A, Rehder H. Ultrasound findings as a sign of fetal triploidy. Ultraschall 1986; 7: 169–71.
Jauniaux E. Partial moles: from postnatal to prenatal agnosis. Placenta 1999; 20: 379–88.
Jauniaux E, Haider A, Partington C. A case of partial m associated with trisomy 13. Ultrasound Obstet Gynecol 1998; 11: 62–4.
Mittal TIC, Vujanic GM, Morrissey BM, Jones A. Triploidy: antenatal sonographic features with postmortem correlation. Prenat Diagn 1998; 18: 1253–62.
Pecile V, Demori E, Gambel Benussi D, Dolce S, Amoroso A. Diagnosis of triploidy in metaphases from uncultured amniocytes. Prenat Diagn 2002; 22: 78–9.
Philipp T, Kalousek DK. Neural tube defects in missed abortions: embryoscopic and cytogenetic findings. Am J Med Genet 2002; 107: 52–7.
Pircon RA, Porto M, Towers CV, Crade M, Gocke SE. Ultrasound findings in pregnancies complicated by fetal triploidy. J Ultrasound Med 1989; 8: 507–11.
Ranzini AC, Sharma S, Soriano C, Vintzileos AM. Early diagnosis of triploidy [letter]. Ultrasound Obstet col 1997; 10: 443–4.
Rubenstein JB, Swayne LC, Dise CA, Gersen SL, Schwartz JR, Risk A. Placental changes in fetal triploidy syndrome. J Ultrasound Med 1986; 5: 545–50.
Wasserman SA, Bofinger MK, Saldana LR. Ultrasound and genetic features of a term triploid pregnancy J Perinatol 1991; 8: 398–401.
Yaron Y, Heifetz S, Ochshorn Y, Lehavi O, Orr-Urtreger A. Decreased first trimester PAPP-A is a predictor of adverse pregnancy outcome. Prenat Diagn 2002; 22: 778–82.

Trisomy 8

Definition: Chromosomal disorder with a tripled chromosome 8; postnatal diagnosis is usually a mosaic; patients with pure trisomy 8 are rare.

Incidence: As far as chromosomal aberrations are concerned, this is quite a frequent anomaly (> 100 cases have been described); overall, it is a rare disorder.

Clinical history/genetics: The occurrence of trisomy 8 and trisomy 8 mosaic is relatively common after chorionic villus sampling. Prognosis of the disorder, only relating to the placenta and that of a real fetal mosaicism is uncertain.

Anomalies/ultrasound findings: The clinical manifestations differ considerably; completely normal patients have also been described. Symptoms: overweight, cardiac anomalies, renal and skeletal malformations, often mild to moderate mental retardation. Patients with a low proportion of mosaicism and with normal intelligence have also been described. In addition: arthrogryposis, tetra-amelia, high risk of cancer, in the prenatal stage: thickened nuchal translucency, dilation of the renal calices.

Differential diagnosis: Syndromes with arthrogryposis.

Prognosis: This is difficult to predict, and depends on the malformations and the proportion of pathological cells (affecting mental development).

References

Campbell S, Mavrides E, Prefumo F, Presti F, Carvalho JS. Prenatal diagnosis of mosaic trisomy 8 in a fetus with normal nuchal translucency thickness and reversed end-diastolic ductus venosus flow. Ultrasound Obstet Gynecol 2001; 17: 341–3.
Danesino C, Pasquali F, Dellavecchia C, Maserati E, Minelli A, Seghezzi L. Constitutional trisomy 8 mosaicism: mechanism of origin, phenotype variability, and risk of malignancies. Am J Med Genet 1998; 80: 540.
Gotze A, Krebs P, Stumm M, Wieacker P, Allhoff EP. Trisomy 8 mosaicism in a patient with tetraamelia. Am J Med Genet 1999; 86: 497–8.
Jay A, Kilby MD, Roberts E, et al. Prenatal diagnosis of mosaicism for partial trisomy 8: a case report including fetal pathology. Prenat Diagn 1999; 19: 976–9.
van Haelst MM, Van Opstal D, Lindhout D, Los FJ. Management of prenatally detected trisomy 8 mosaicism. Prenat Diagn 2001; 21: 1075–8.

Trisomy 9, Partial Trisomy 9 p

Definition: An extra triple chromosome 9, frequently as trisomy 9 p. It is associated with multiple anomalies. Usually occurs as mosaic forms, as pure trisomy usually leads to early fetal demise.

First described in 1973 by Feingold and Atkins.

Ultrasound findings: Growth restriction. *Head and face:* microcephaly, cerebellar anomaly, ventriculomegaly, Dandy–Walker cysts, neural tube defect, facial clefts, micrognathia, microphthalmia. *Extremities:* flexion anomaly of the fingers, abnormal fixation of the feet. *Thorax and abdomen:* cardiac anomaly, liver calcification, singular umbilical artery, renal anomalies, maldescent of the testis.

Differential diagnosis: Trisomy 13, trisomy 18, Wolf–Hirschhorn syndrome, triploidy

Prognosis: Intrauterine demise or neonatal death is the frequent outcome. Survivors are severely mentally impaired. In mosaic forms, the severity depends on the percentage of affected cells and the organ systems involved.

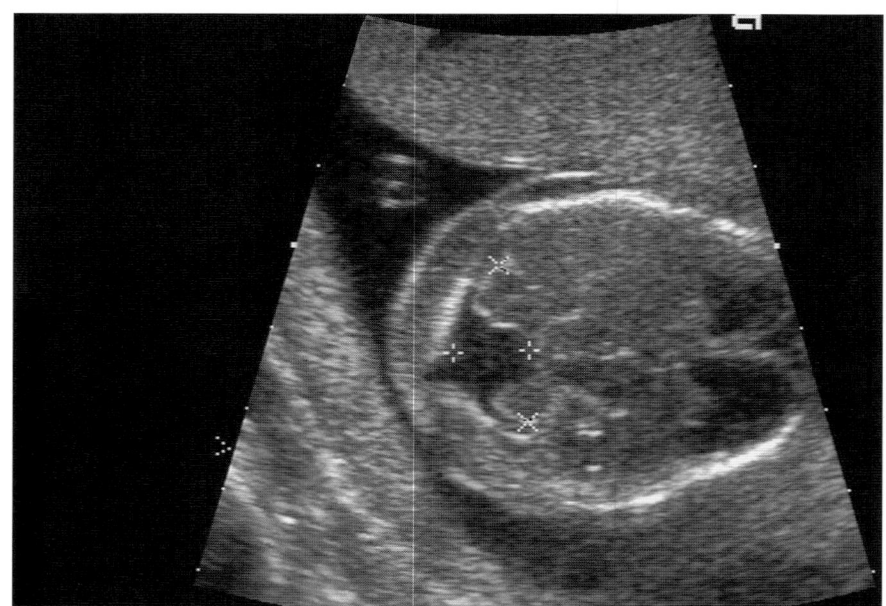

Fig. 9.**12** **Trisomy 9.** Widening of the cerebellomedullary cistern at 16 + 1 weeks (Dandy–Walker variant).

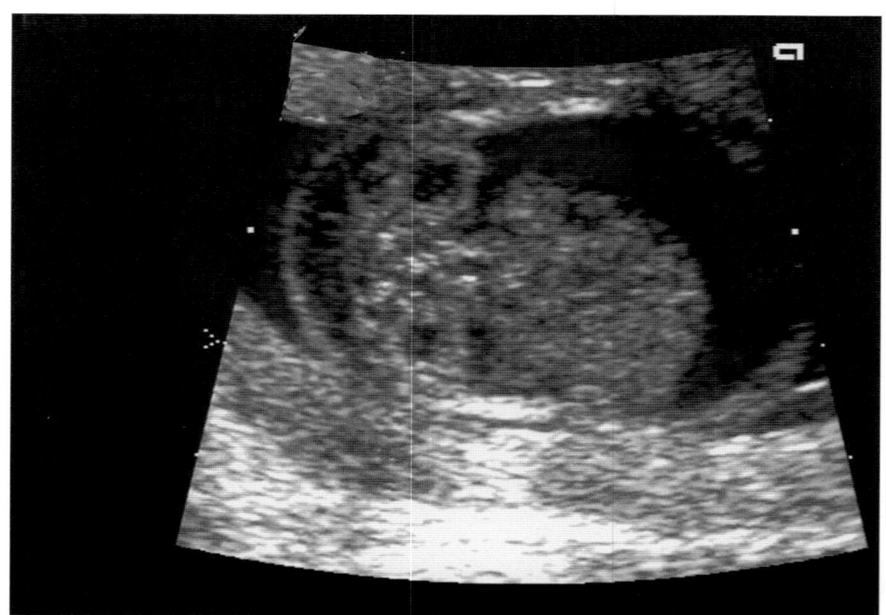

Fig. 9.**13** **Trisomy 9.** Echogenic kidneys, with dilation of renal pelvis as well as fetal ascites at 16 + 1 weeks.

References

Hengstschlager M, Bettelheim D, Repa C, Lang S, Deutinger J, Bernaschek G. A fetus with trisomy 9 p and trisomy 10 p originating from unbalanced segregation of a maternal complex chromosome rearrangement t(4;10;9). Fetal Diagn Ther 2002; 17: 243–6.

McDuffie RSJ. Complete trisomy 9: case report with ultrasound findings. Am J Perinatol 1994; 11: 80–4.

Merino A, De Perdigo A, Nombalais F, Yvinec M, Le Roux MG, Bellec V. Prenatal diagnosis of trisomy 9 mosaicism: two new cases. Prenat Diagn 1993; 13: 1001–7.

Murta C, Moron A, Avila M, Franca L, Vargas P. Reverse flow in the umbilical vein in a case of trisomy 9. Ultrasound Obstet Gynecol 2000; 16: 575–7.

Pinette MG, Pan Y, Chard R, Pinette SG, Blackstone J. Prenatal diagnosis of nonmosaic trisomy 9 and related ultrasound findings at 11.7 weeks. J Matern Fetal Med 1998; 7: 48–50.

Saura R, Traore W, Taine L, et al. Prenatal diagnosis of trisomy 9: six cases and a review of the literature. Prenat Diagn 1995; 15: 609–14.

Tseng JJ, Chou MM, Shih-Chu Ho E. Varix of the portal vein: prenatal diagnosis in a fetus with mosaic trisomy 9 syndrome. Prenat Diagn 2002; 22: 495–7.

von Kaisenberg CS, Caliebe A, Krams M, Hackeloer BJ, Jonat W. Absence of 9 q22–9 qter in trisomy 9 does not prevent a Dandy–Walker phenotype. Am J Med Genet 2000; 95: 425–8.

Trisomy 10

Definition: Additional chromosome 10; usually fatal except when mosaicism is present.

Incidence: Seen in about 2% of spontaneous miscarriages. Postnatally, extremely rare.

Ultrasound findings: Intrauterine growth restriction, nuchal edema, hypertelorism, cardiac anomaly, cryptorchism. In *complete trisomy 10* additionally facial clefts, micrognathia, polydactyly, syndactyly of the toes.

Differential diagnosis (of nuchal edema): Trisomy 18, trisomy 21, Turner syndrome, multiple pterygium syndrome, Pena–Shokeir syndrome, Roberts syndrome, Smith–Lemli–Opitz syndrome, and others.

Prognosis: Complete trisomy 10 is fatal; infants with mosaic forms may survive with mental impairment and short growth, but life expectancy is severely reduced.

References

Brizot ML, Schultz R, Patroni LT, Lopes LM, Armbruster-Moraes E, Zugaib M. Trisomy 10: ultrasound features and natural history after first trimester diagnosis. Prenat Diagn 2001; 21: 672–5.

Hengstschlager M, Bettelheim D, Repa C, Lang S, Deutinger J, Bernaschek G. A fetus with trisomy 9 p and trisomy 10 p originating from unbalanced segregation of a maternal complex chromosome rearrangement t(4;10;9). Fetal Diagn Ther 2002; 17: 243–6.

Knoblauch H, Sommer D, Zimmer C, et al. Fetal trisomy 10 mosaicism: ultrasound, cytogenetic and morphologic findings in early pregnancy. Prenat Diagn 1999; 19: 379–82.

Martin-Denavit T, Attia-Sobol J, Theuil J, et al. First prenatal diagnosis of partial trisomy 10 and partial monosomy 15 derived from a maternal translocation (10;15)(q11;q13). Prenat Diagn 2002; 22: 487–8.

Schwarzler P, Moscoso G, Bernard JP, Hill L, Senat MV, Ville Y. Trisomy 10: first-trimester features on ultrasound, fetoscopy and postmortem of a case associated with increased nuchal translucency. Ultrasound Obstet Gynecol 1999; 13 : 67–70.

Trisomy 13 (Patau syndrome)

Definition: Additional chromosome 13. The phenotype is characterized by severe anomalies and development disorder.

Clinical history/genetics: Free trisomy 13 correlates with maternal age. The risk of recurrence is about 1% above the expected risk due to maternal age. In the rare cases of translocation trisomy, which is a result of familial balanced translocation, a much higher risk of recurrence is to be expected (depending on the chromosome involved in the Robertson translocation and the sex of the carrier). The triple test does not give any indication of trisomy 13. Trisomy 13 is the third most frequent trisomy in live-born cases. Three forms are known:

Free trisomy 13: chromosome 13 is present as independent copies.

Translocation trisomy 13: Chromosome 13 is a part of translocation chromosome. Usually, this type of translocation results from fusion of the long arm of chromosome 13 with the long arm of another acrocentric chromosome, such as chromosomes 14, 15, 21, or 22. Exception: a translocation chromosome arising from two long arms of chromosome 13. All of the above-mentioned rearrangements belong to the group of Robertson translocations.

Mosaic trisomy 13: In addition to pathological cells, another cell line is present (generally with a normal set of chromosomes).

Teratogens: Not known.

Ultrasound findings: Mostly fetal growth restriction, especially very early. Hydramnios in 15%; oligohydramnios may rarely be present. Head and face: hygroma colli (21%), microcephaly (12%), holoprosencephaly (40%), microphthalmia or anophthalmia, neural tube defect, widening of cisterna magna (15%), cleft palate and cleft lip (45%), nasal malformation, low set and dysplasia of ears. Extremities: postaxial polydactyly. Thorax: cardiac anomalies in 80%; the commonest are ASD or VSD, in many cases complex cardiac anomalies. Echogenic intracardiac foci (white spots, echogenic chordae tendineae are seen in 35%). In 30% of cases, polycystic kidneys and other urogenital anomalies are seen. Omphalocele is seen in less than 20%. In very rare cases, specific ultrasound anomalies are not detected.

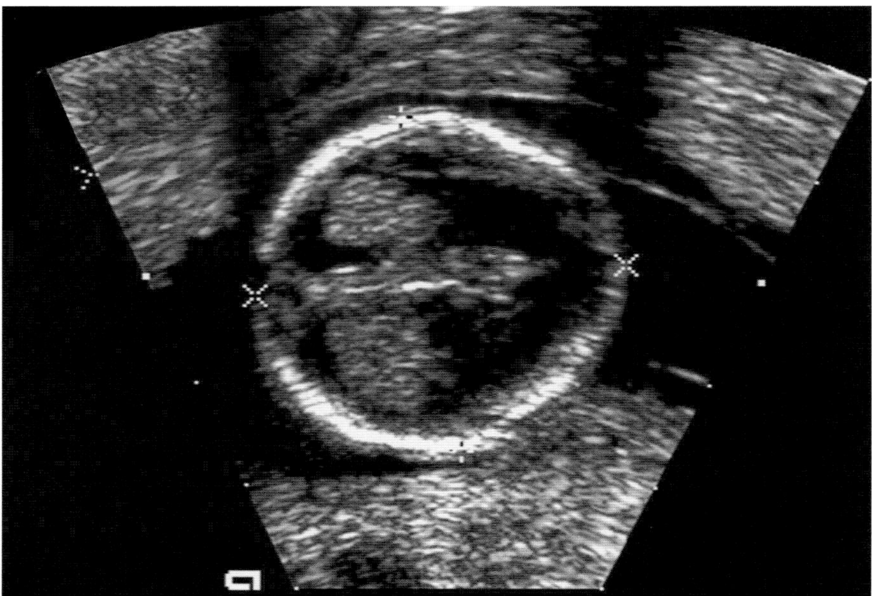

Fig. 9.**14** **Trisomy 13.** Brachycephaly at 14 + 2 weeks.

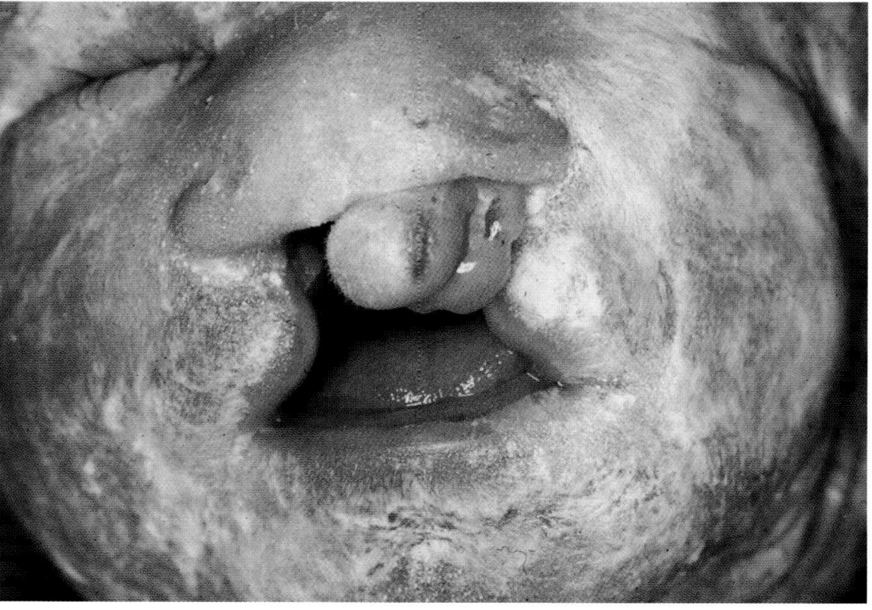

Fig. 9.**15** **Trisomy 13.** Bilateral cleft lip and cleft palate seen after termination of pregnancy at 27 + 6 weeks.

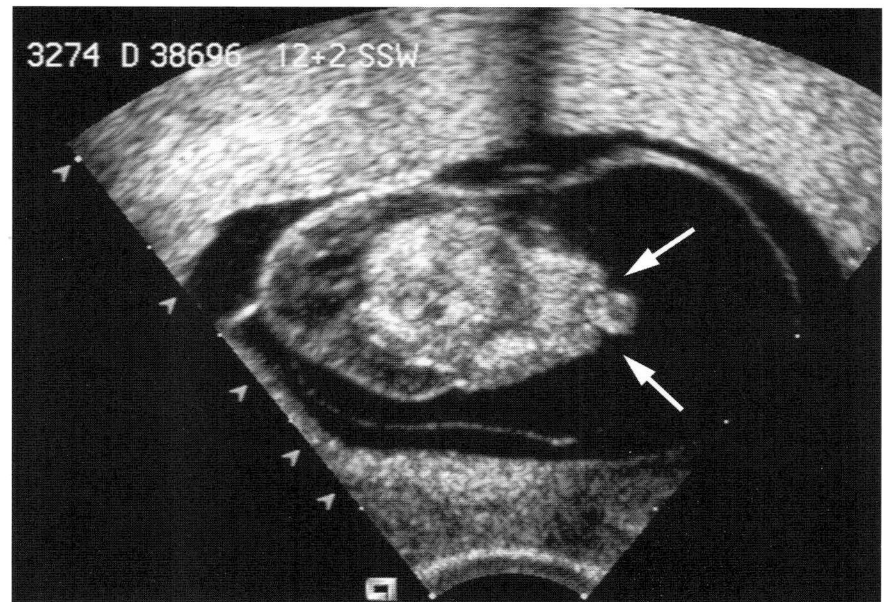

Fig. 9.**16** **Trisomy 13.** Bilateral clefts of the lip and the palate seen at 12 + 1 weeks in a fetus with translocation trisomy 13.

Differential diagnosis: Meckel–Gruber syndrome, and many other syndromes, depending on the pattern of malformations.

Clinical management: Karyotyping, as well as further ultrasound screening, including fetal echocardiography. If the mother decides to carry on with the pregnancy, obstetric intervention on the basis of fetal indications (especially cesarean section) is not justified.

Procedure after birth: Generally, intensive medical measures should not be taken. The pediatrician present at birth should be informed in advance of the anomalies that are to be expected.

Prognosis: In most cases of trisomy 13, the outcome is fatal in the early neonatal stage; survivors show severe mental impairment. Fifty percent are stillborn or die within the first 6 months of life; 85% have died by the end of the first year of life.

Information for the mother: If both parents have a normal set of chromosomes, then the risk of recurrence lies 1% above that for the maternal age. Karyotyping in early pregnancy (chorionic villus sampling at 11–12 weeks of gestation) allows exclusion of this chromosomal disorder in the following pregnancy.

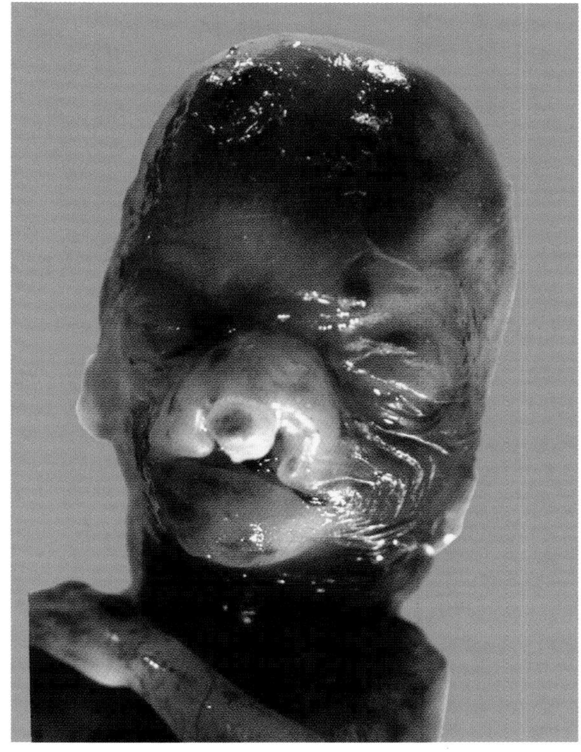

Fig. 9.**17** **Trisomy 13.** Finding after termination of pregnancy (courtesy of Prof. Vogel).

Self-Help Organization

Title: SOFT: Support Organization for Trisomy

Description: Support and education for families of children with trisomy 18 and 13 and related genetic disorders. Education for professionals. Bimonthly newsletter. Pen-pal program, phone network. Regional gatherings. Annual international conference, booklets.

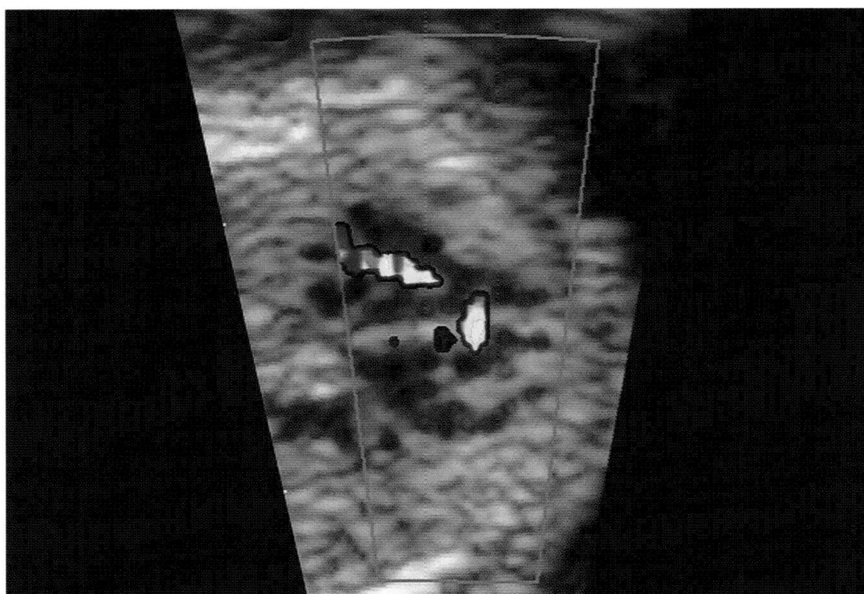

Fig. 9.**18** **Trisomy 13.** Muscular VSD as well as tricuspid incompetence at 14 + 1 weeks.

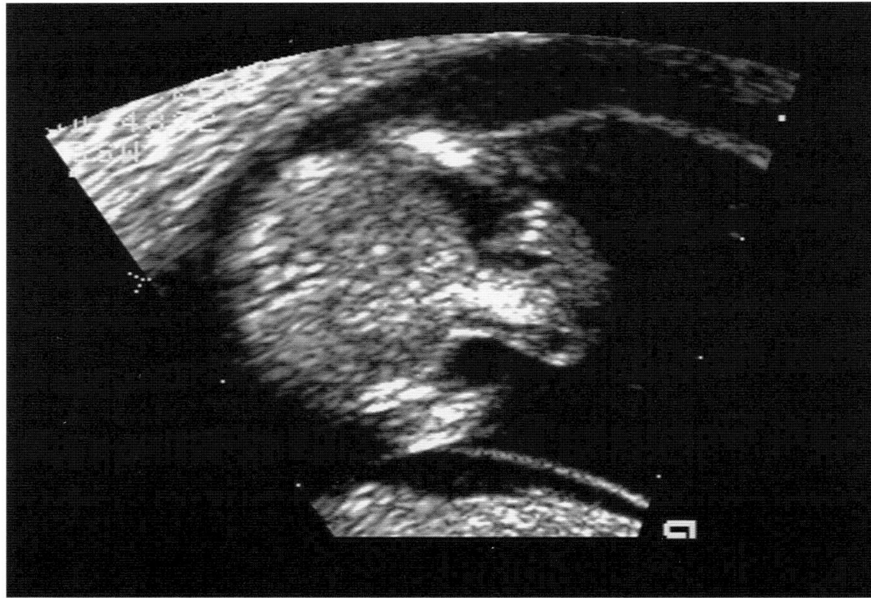

Fig. 9.**19** **Trisomy 13.** Omphalocele seen at 14 + 1 weeks.

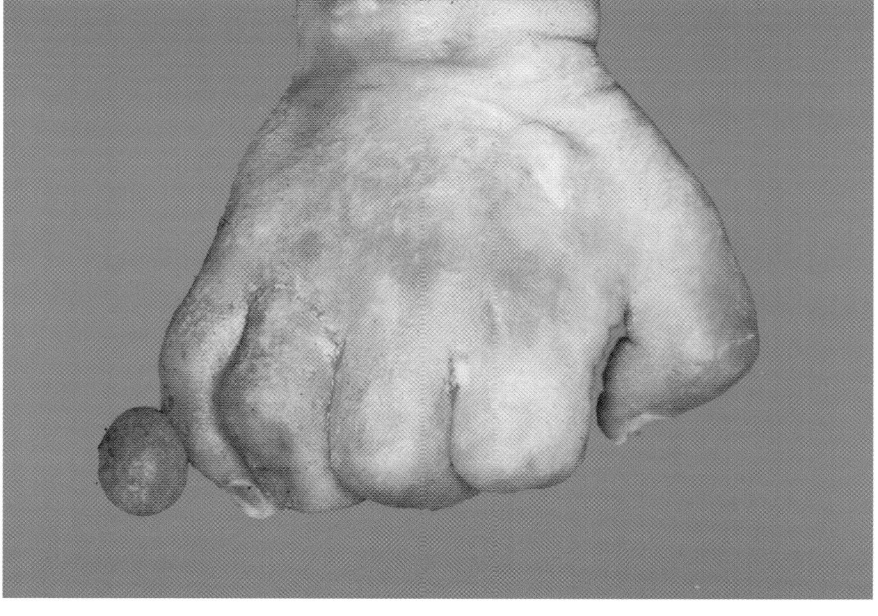

Fig. 9.**20** **Trisomy 13.** Hexadactyly. Finding after termination of pregnancy.

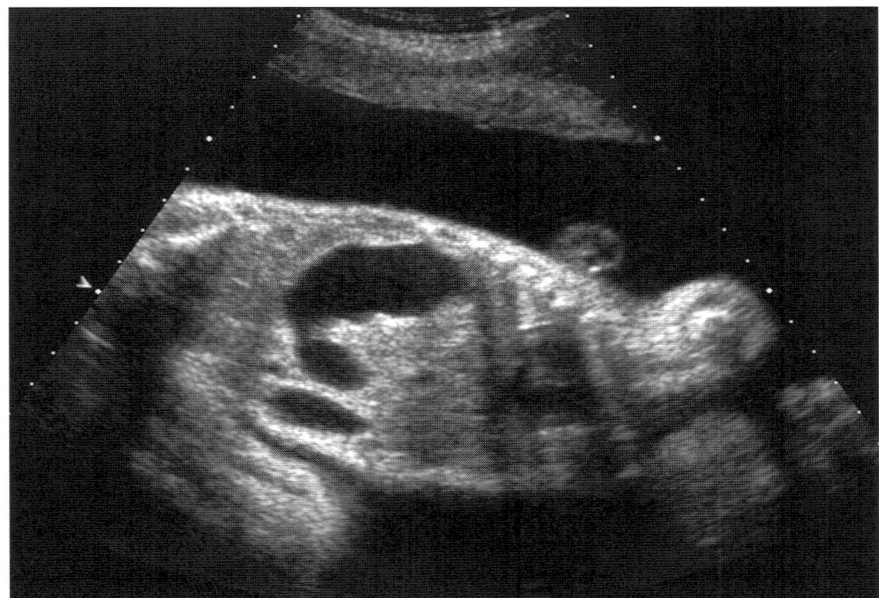

Fig. 9.**21** **Trisomy 13.** Double-bubble sign secondary to duodenal atresia, causing hydramnios.

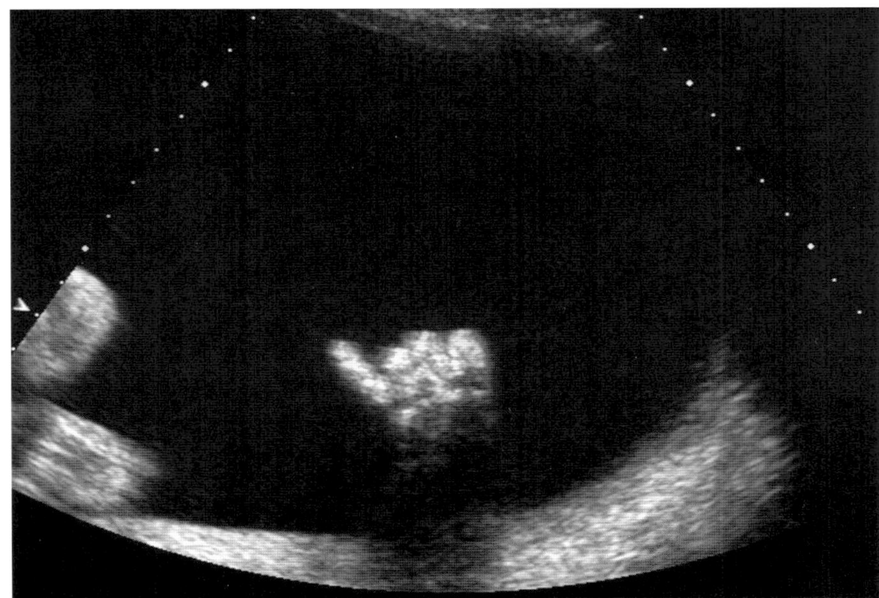

Fig. 9.**22** **Trisomy 13.** Same fetus as before. Severe hydramnios. A hand is seen with overlapping fingers, showing the typical clenched fist.

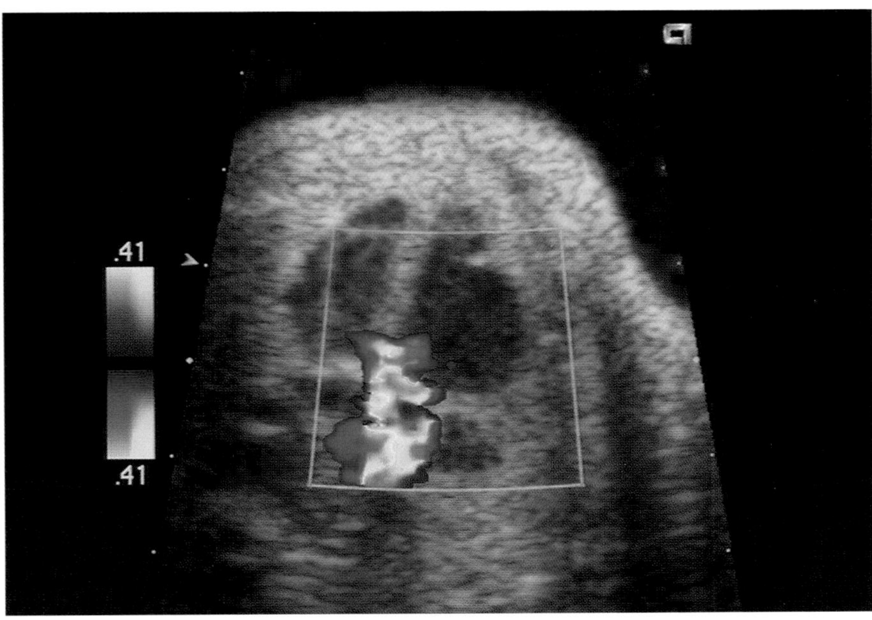

Fig. 9.**23** **Trisomy 13.** Same fetus. AV valve incompetence in the presence of an AV canal.

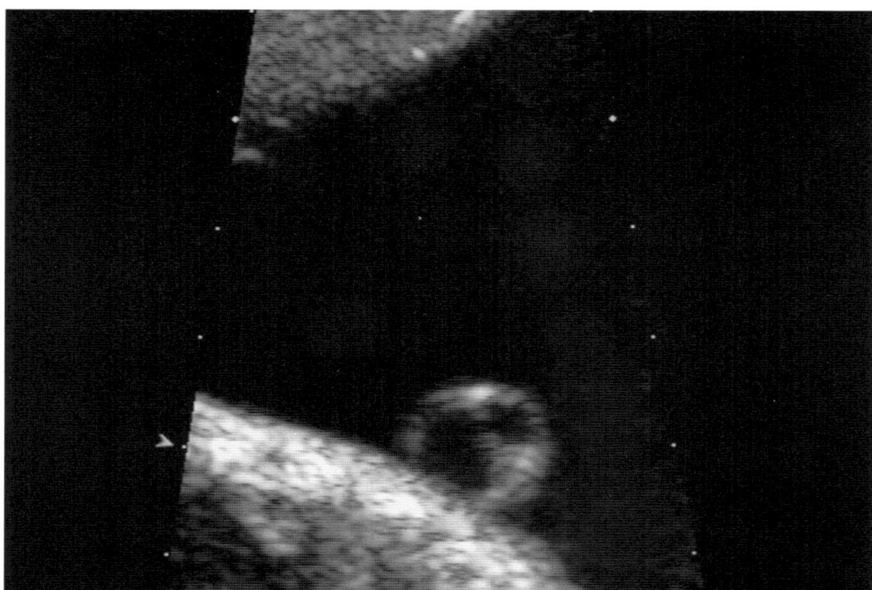

Fig. 9.**24** **Trisomy 13.** Same fetus. A single umbilical artery is detected.

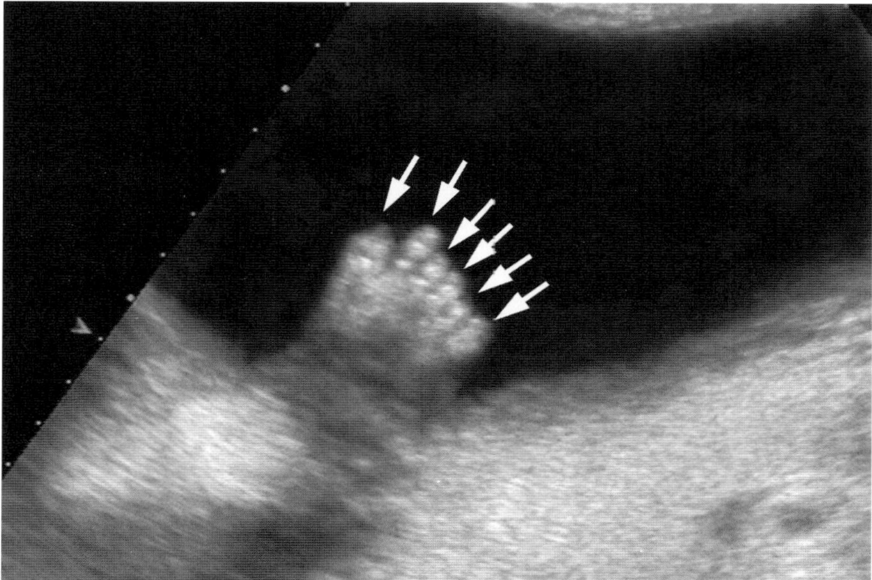

Fig. 9.**25** **Trisomy 13.** Same fetus. Hexadactyly of the foot.

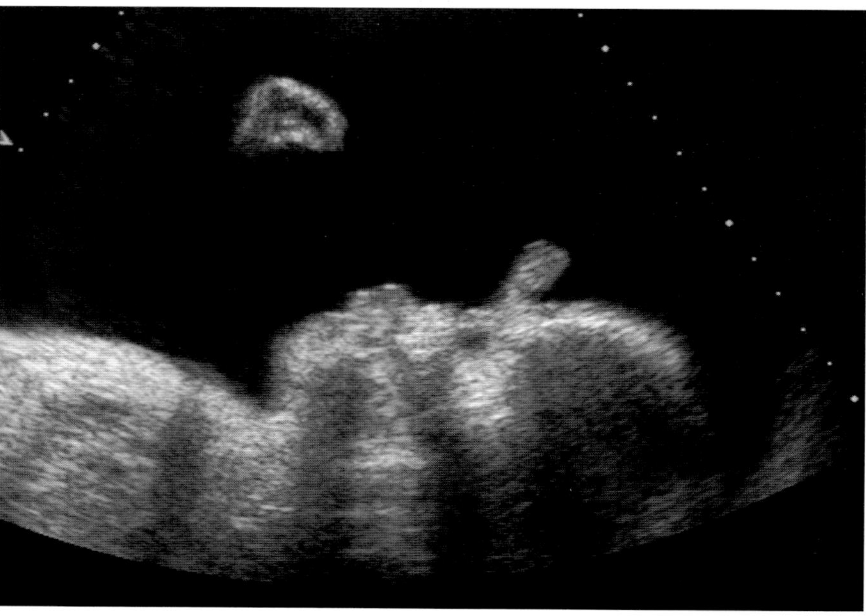

Fig. 9.**26** **Trisomy 13.** Same fetus. Highly pathological facial profile, showing only one eye in the midline (cyclopia) and spouting of tissue above it (proboscis).

Scope: National

Number of groups: 50 chapters

Founded: 1979

Address: 2982 S. Union St., Rochester, New York, 14624, United States

Telephone: 716-594-4621 or 1-800-716-SOFT

Fax: 716-594-1957

E-mail: barbsoft@aol.com

Web: http://www.trisomy.org

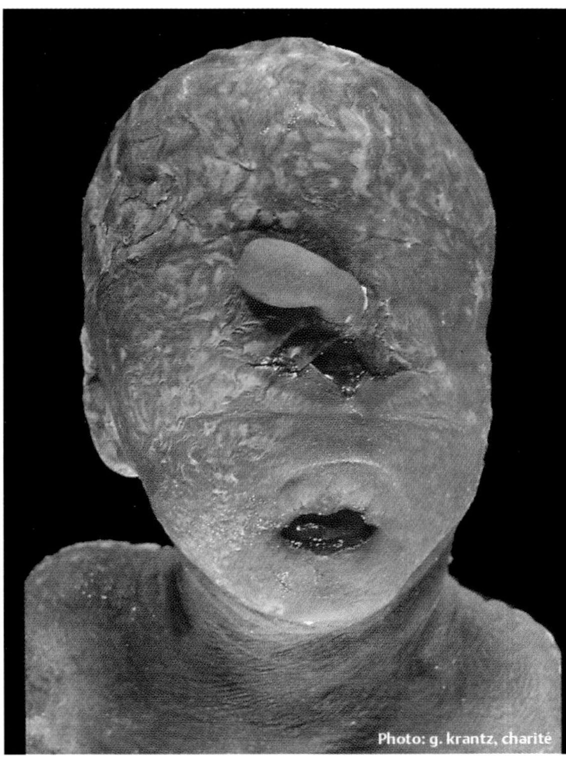

Fig. 9.**27** **Trisomy 13.** Same fetus after termination of pregnancy. Cyclopia, proboscis (courtesy of Prof. Vogel).

References

Aubry JP, Aubry MC, Henrion R, Boué J, Labbe I. Echographic detection of chromosomal anomalies apropos of trisomy 13 and 18. J Genet Hum 1982; 30: 233–53.

Benacerraf BR, Miller WA, Frigoletto FDJ. Sonographic detection of fetuses with trisomies 13 and 18: accuracy and limitations. Am J Obstet Gynecol 1988; 158: 404–9.

Berge SJ, Plath H, Van de Vondel PT, et al. Fetal cleft lip and palate: sonographic diagnosis, chromosomal abnormalities, associated anomalies and postnatal outcome in 70 fetuses. Ultrasound Obstet Gynecol 2001; 18: 422–31.

Brewer CM, Holloway SH, Stone DH, Carothers AD, FitzPatrick DR. Survival in trisomy 13 and trisomy 18 cases ascertained from population based registers. J Med Genet 2002; 39: e54.

Eubanks SR, Kuller JA, Amjadi D, Powell CM. Prenatal diagnosis of mosaic trisomy 13: a case report. Prenat Diagn 1998; 18: 971–4.

Greenberg F, Carpenter RJ, Ledbetter DH. Cystic hygroma and hydrops fetalis in a fetus with trisomy 13. Clin Genet 1983; 24: 389–91.

Has R, Ibrahimoglu L, Ergene H, Ermis H, Basaran S. Partial molar appearance of the placenta in trisomy 13. Fetal Diagn Ther 2002; 17: 205–8.

Jauniaux E, Haider A, Partington C. A case of partial mole associated with trisomy 13. Ultrasound Obstet Gynecol 1998; 11: 62–4.

Wax JR, Pinette MG, Blackstone J, Cartin A. Isolated multiple bilateral echogenic papillary muscles: a unique sonographic feature of trisomy 13. Obstet Gynecol 2002; 99: 902–3.

Wladimiroff JW, Stewart PA, Reuss A, Sachs ES. Cardiac and extra-cardiac anomalies as indicators for trisomies 13 and 18: a prenatal ultrasound study. Prenat Diagn 1989; 9: 515–20.

Trisomy 18 (Edwards Syndrome)

Definition: Numerical chromosomal aberration with an extra chromosome 18. This is the second most common trisomy in live born neonates. The phenotype is characterized by severe malformations and growth disorder.

Incidence: One in 3000 births.

Sex ratio: M : F = 1 : 3.

Clinical history/genetics: Trisomy 18 correlates with maternal age. The risk of recurrence after an affected child lies 1 % above that for the given age.

Etiology: In majority of cases, complete trisomy is present, but mosaic may also be found.

Ultrasound findings: Abnormal ultrasound findings are observed in at least 80 % of fetuses. *Early growth restriction* is seen in 50 % (frequently before 18 weeks). In 25%, *hydramnios* is detected. A *singular umbilical artery* is a common finding. Fifteen percent show *hygroma colli. Microcephaly,* with a typical *"strawberry-shaped head,"* is characteristic. Other anomalies are: *neural tube defects* (20%), *cysts of the choroid plexus* (25%), widening of the *cisterna magna* (more than 10 mm) and *agenesis of the corpus callosum*. Other frequently associated malformations are: *microgenia, overlapping fingers—"clenched fist"* (the fourth finger lies over the third and the fist cannot be opened), diaphragmatic hernia (10%), omphalocele (25%; typically the hernia contents are solely intestines) and renal anomalies. Eight percent of cases have *cardiac anomalies*, especially VSD, tetralogy of Fallot, and aortic isthmus stenosis. Shortening of the extremities is common, and other limb anomalies may be seen in 50%. *Rocker-bottom foot* is a typical feature (convexity of foot soles and prominent heel). Club feet, malformation or absence of the thumb and radius aplasia can also be detected. Ninety percent of trisomy 18 cases can be diagnosed at the prenatal stage by an abnormal measurement of nuchal translucency and screening for organ anomalies.

Differential diagnosis: Freeman–Sheldon syndrome, Pena–Shokeir syndrome, Smith–Lemli–Opitz syndrome, triploidy, trisomy 9 mosaic, and other syndromes showing growth restriction.

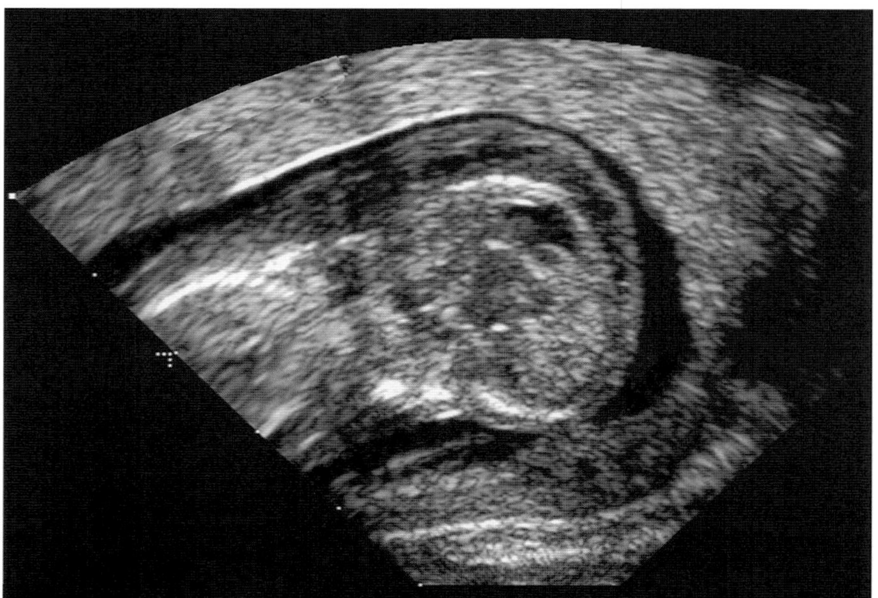

Fig. 9.**28** **Trisomy 18.** Early fetal hydrops, 12 + 3 weeks.

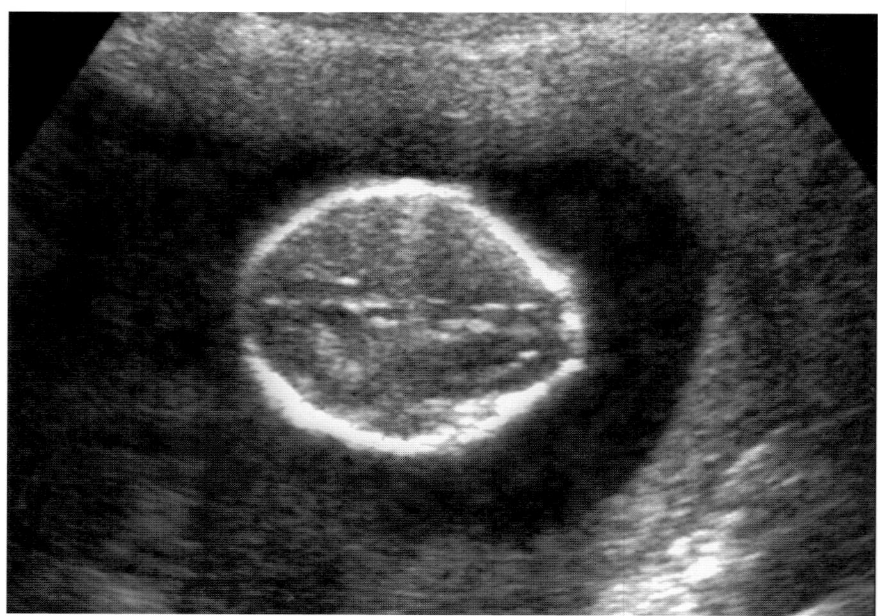

Fig. 9.**29** **Trisomy 18.** Fetal head at 19 + 1 weeks, showing the strawberry sign.

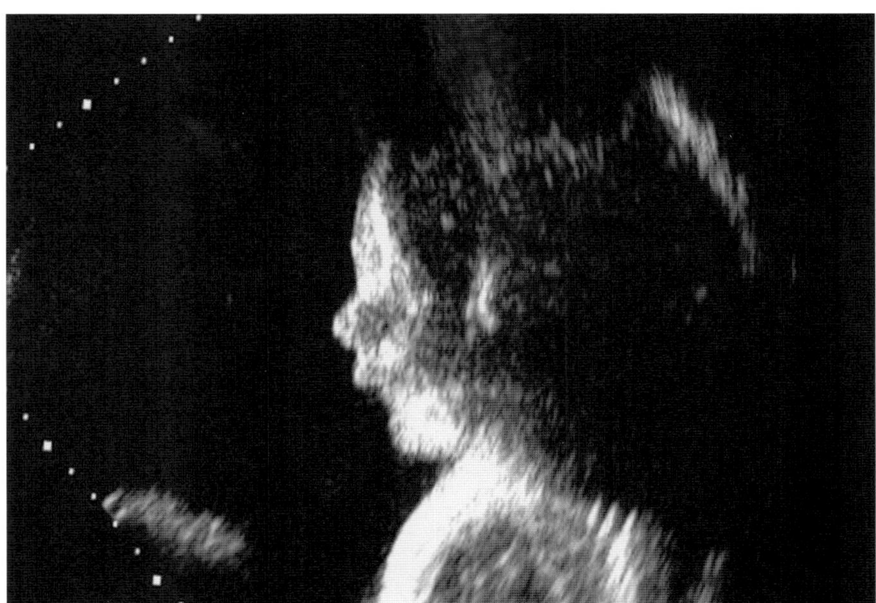

Fig. 9.**30** **Trisomy 18.** Fetal profile with retraction of the lower jaw at 40 + 1 weeks.

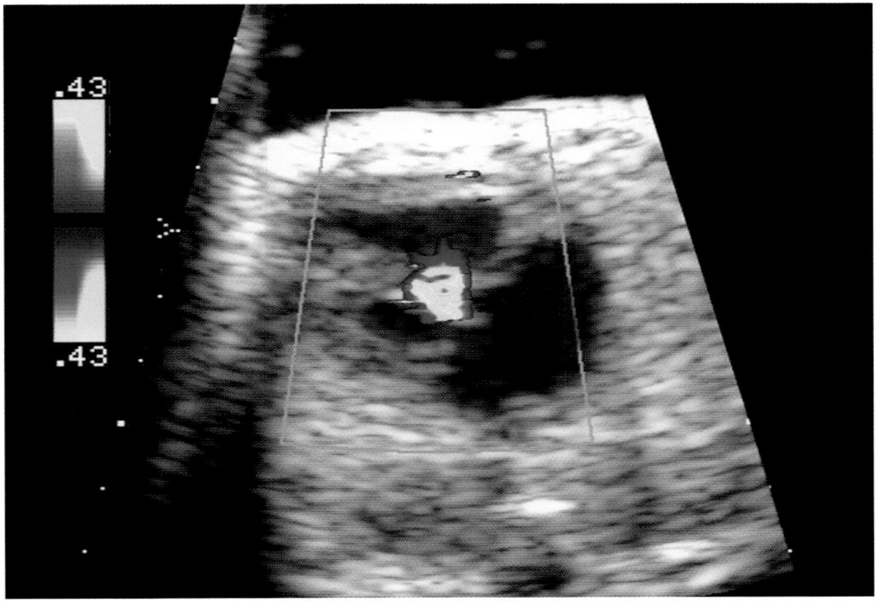

Fig. 9.**31** **Trisomy 18.** Membranous VSD at 40 + 1 weeks in a fetus with trisomy 18.

Clinical management: Karyotyping, as well as further ultrasound screening, including fetal echocardiography. If the mother opts to continue the pregnancy, intrauterine growth restriction and fetal distress during labor can be expected. Cesarean section due to fetal distress is not recommended.

Procedure after birth: After parental consent, intensive medical treatment should be withheld. The pediatrician present at birth should be informed in advance of the anomalies that are to be expected.

Prognosis: Trisomy 18 has a fatal outcome in most cases. Surviving infants are severely mentally impaired. Fifty percent die within the first 2 months of life, and 90% within the first year.

Information for the mother: The sporadic form of trisomy 18 has a recurrence risk of 1% above that for the maternal age. In a subsequent pregnancy, prenatal diagnosis can be made early by chorionic villus sampling at 11–12 weeks of gestation.

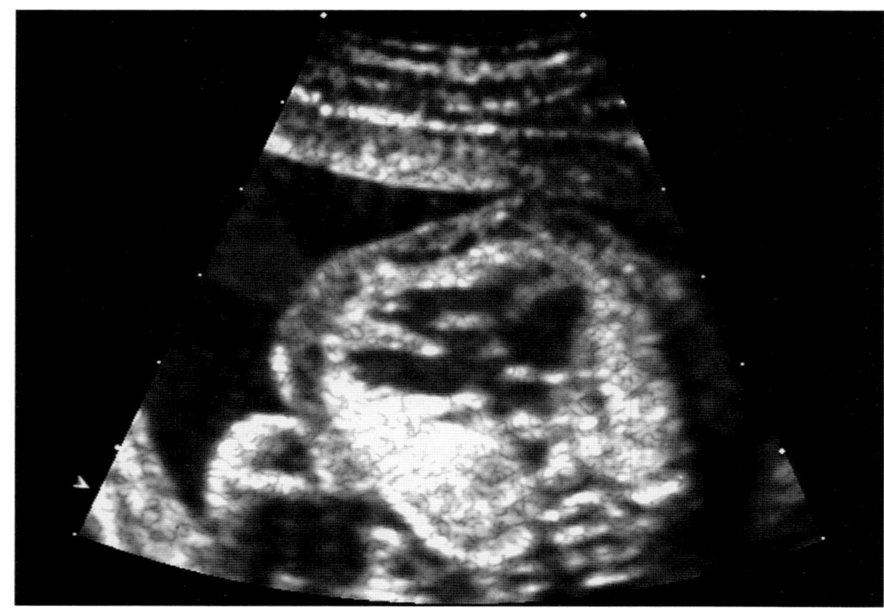

Fig. 9.**32** **Trisomy 18.** AV canal at 20 + 6 weeks.

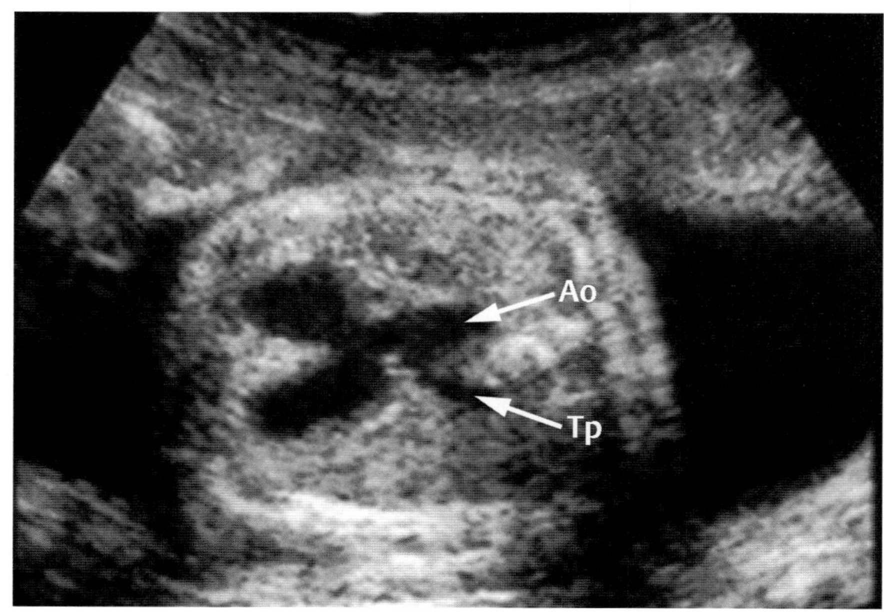

Fig. 9.**33** **Trisomy 18.** Fetal heart showing a large VSD and overriding of the aorta (Ao): this has a larger circumference than the pulmonary trunk (Tp). Tetralogy of Fallot in trisomy 18.

Self-Help Organization

Title: SOFT: Support Organization for Trisomy

Description: Support and education for families of children with trisomy 18 and 13 and related genetic disorders. Education for professionals. Bimonthly newsletter. Pen-pal program, phone network. Regional gatherings. Annual international conference, booklets.

Scope: National

Number of groups: 50 chapters

Founded: 1979

Address: 2982 S. Union St., Rochester, NY 14624, United States

Telephone: 716–594–4621 or 1–800–716-SOFT

Fax: 716–594–1957

E-mail: barbsoft@aol.com

Web: http://www.trisomy.org

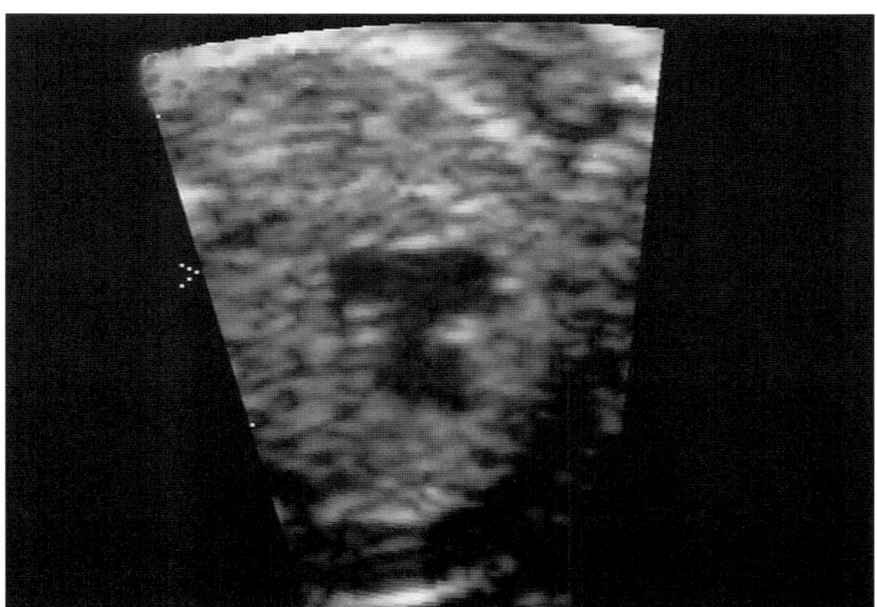

Fig. 9.**34** **Trisomy 18.** Fetal heart at 12 + 3 weeks, showing an AV canal in trisomy 18.

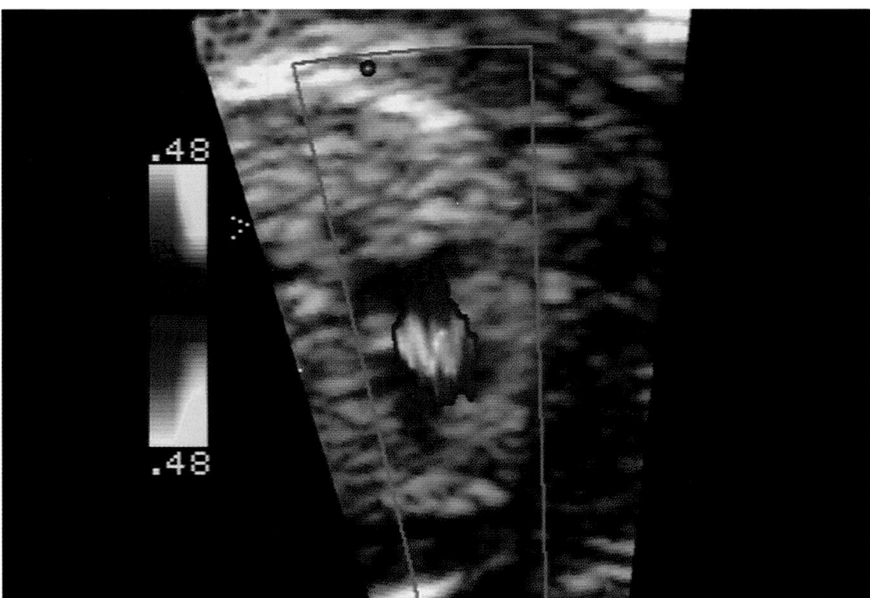

Fig. 9.**35** **Trisomy 18.** Same case, shown using Doppler color mapping.

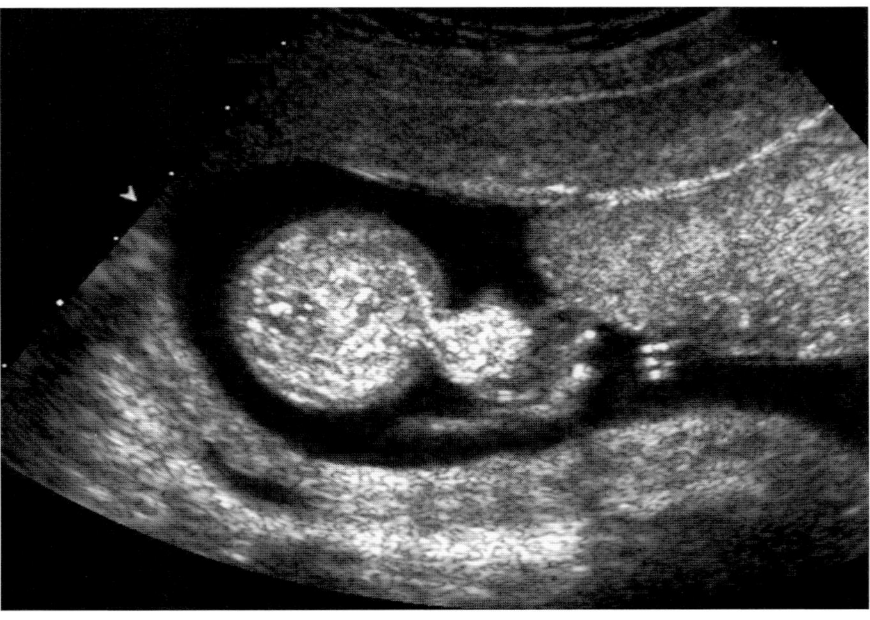

Fig. 9.**36** **Trisomy 18.** Omphalocele at 16 + 4 weeks.

3

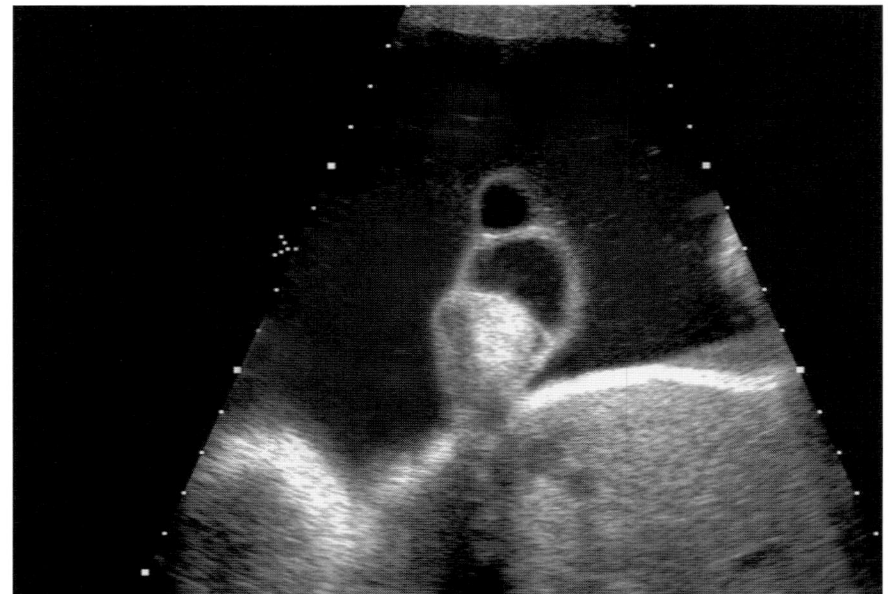

Fig. 9.**37** **Trisomy 18.** A large omphalocele at 16 weeks.

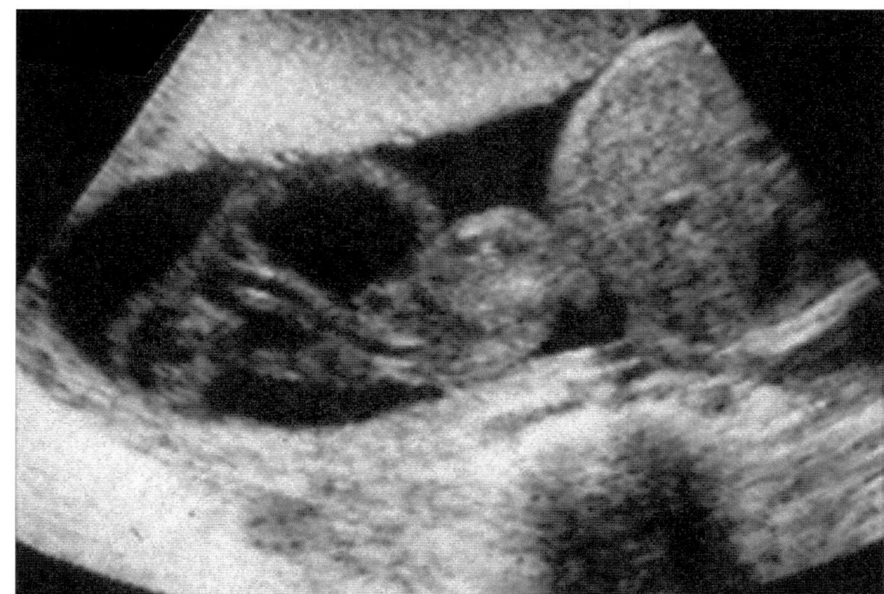

Fig. 9.**38** **Trisomy 18.** Cross-section of fetal abdomen at 30 + 5 weeks, demonstrating an omphalocele as well as a large cyst of the umbilical cord in a fetus with trisomy 18.

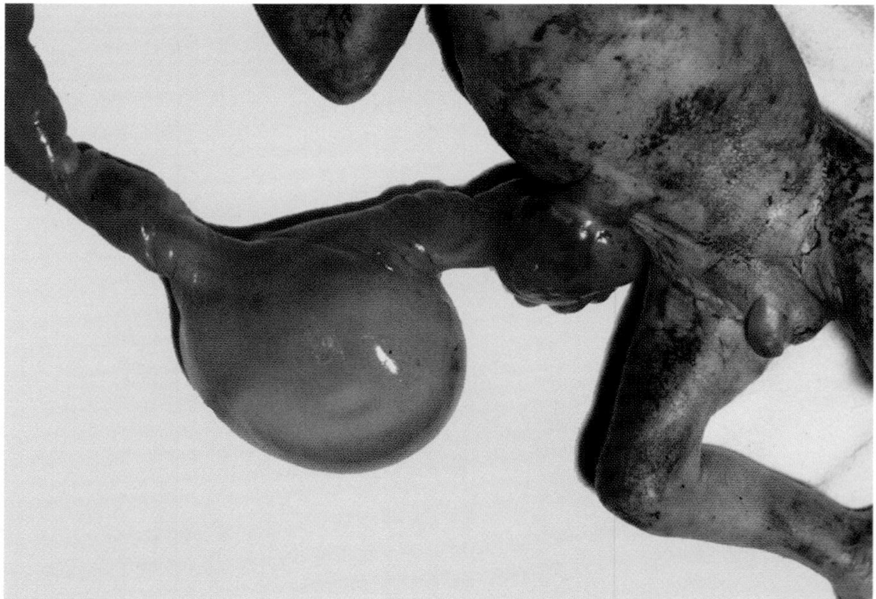

Fig. 9.**39** **Trisomy 18.** Same fetus after termination of pregnancy.

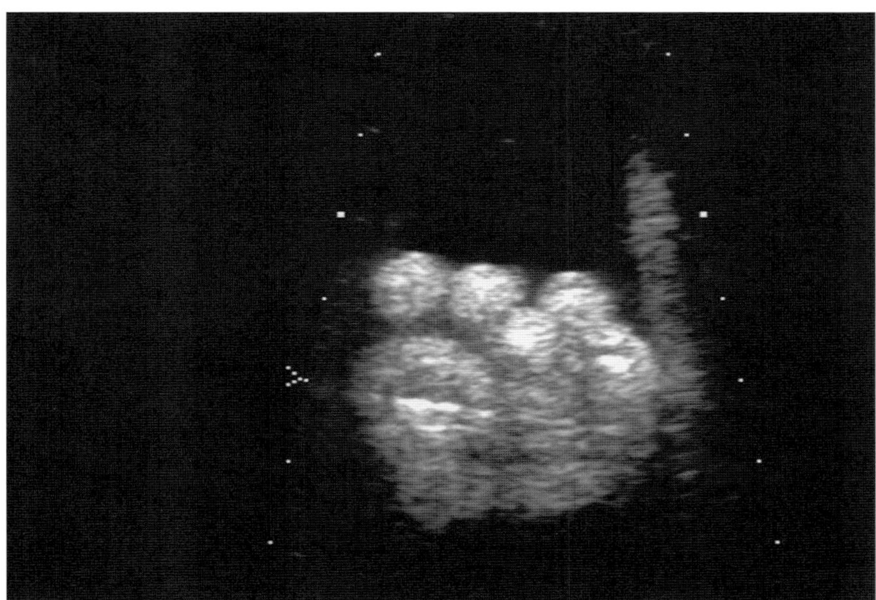

Fig. 9.**40** **Trisomy 18.** Fetal foot showing deformation of the toes at 40 + 1 weeks.

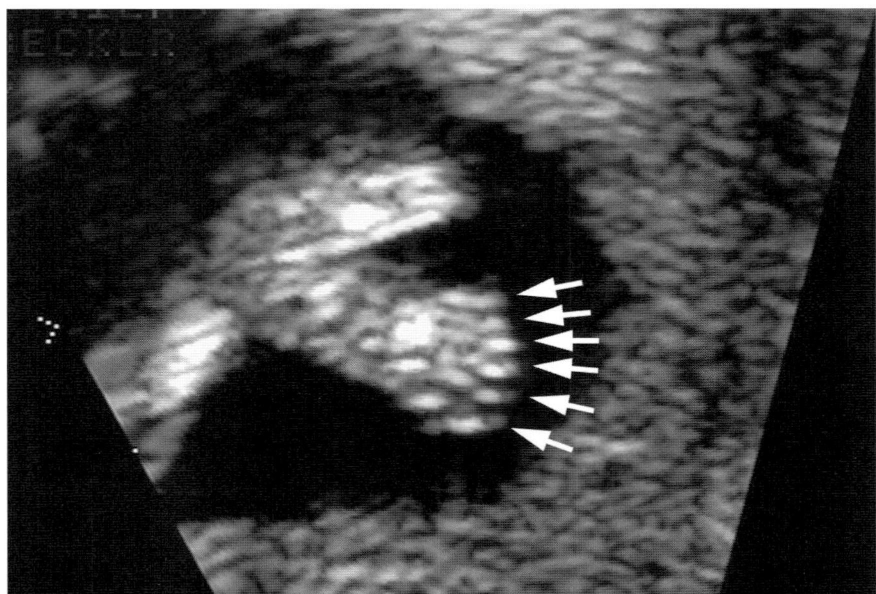

Fig. 9.**41** **Trisomy 18.** Fetal foot with hexadactyly at 12 + 3 weeks.

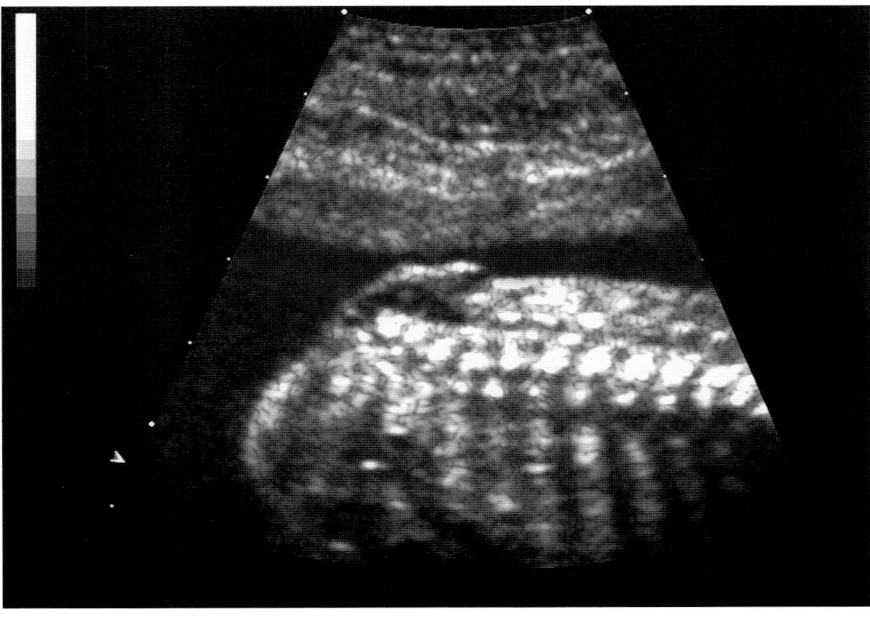

Fig. 9.**42** **Trisomy 18.** Spina bifida at 21 weeks.

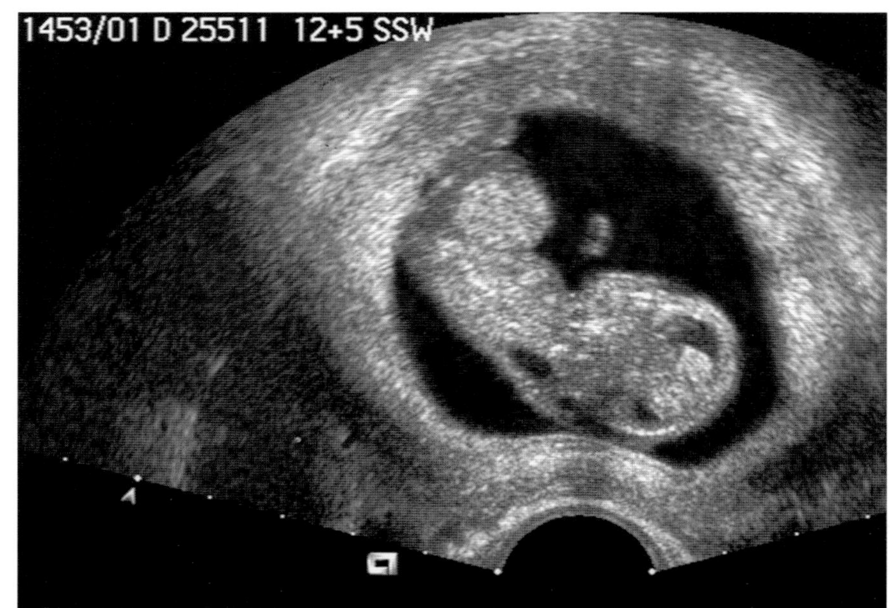

Fig. 9.**43** **Trisomy 18.** Hygroma colli as well as a large omphalocele at 12 + 5 weeks.

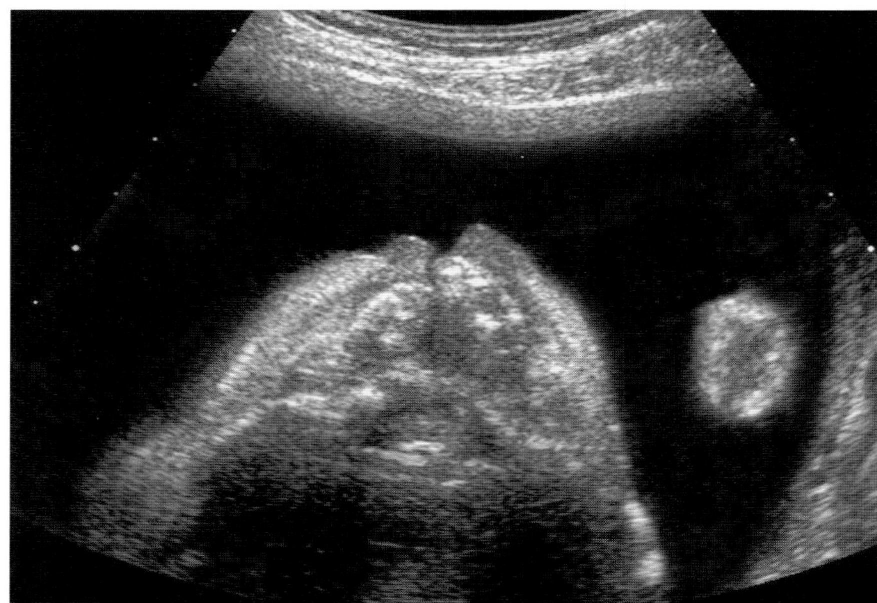

Fig. 9.**44** **Trisomy 18.** Unilateral cleft lip and cleft palate at 30 + 3 weeks.

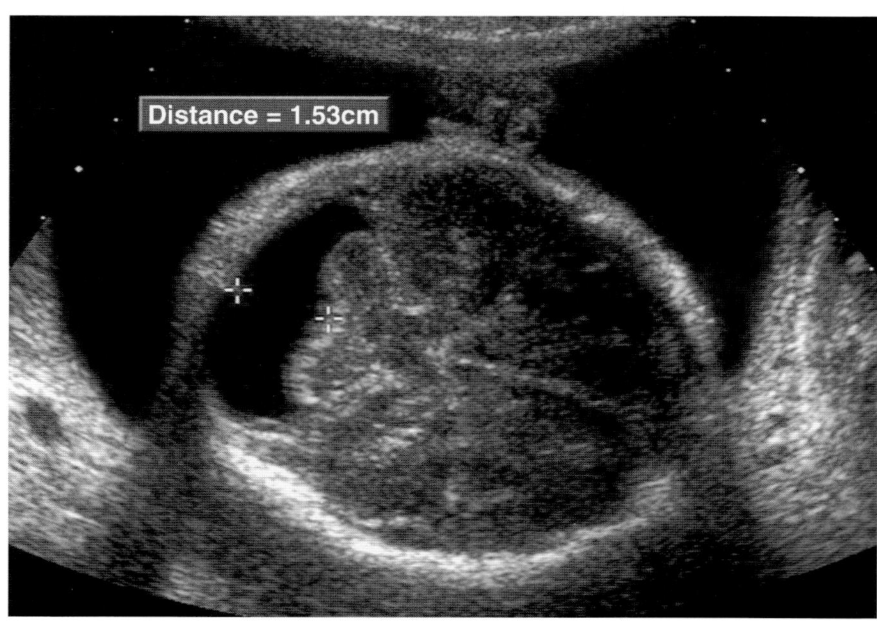

Fig. 9.**45** **Trisomy 18.** Same fetus as before. The cerebellomedullary cistern is dilated to 15.3 mm.

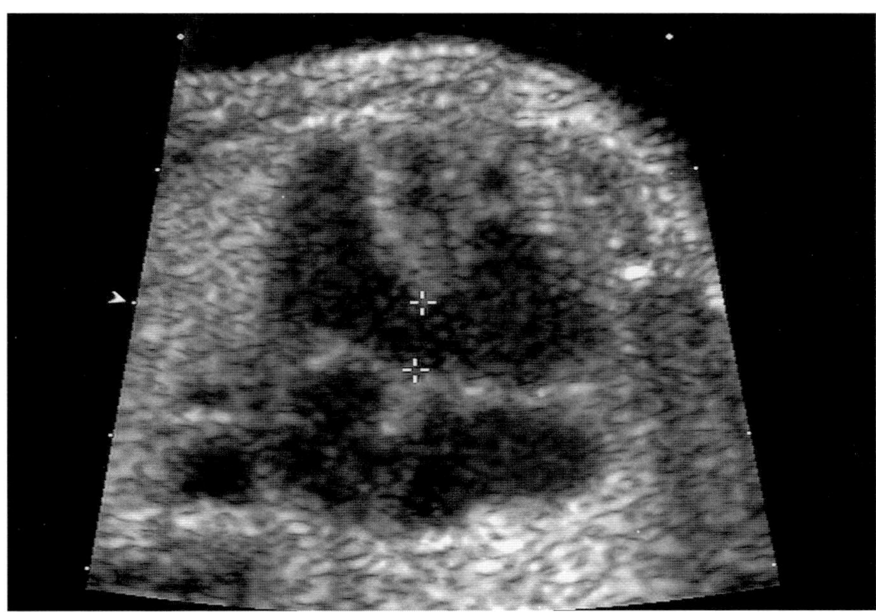

Fig. 9.**46** **Trisomy 18.** Same fetus. A membranous VSD is demonstrated in the apical four-chamber view.

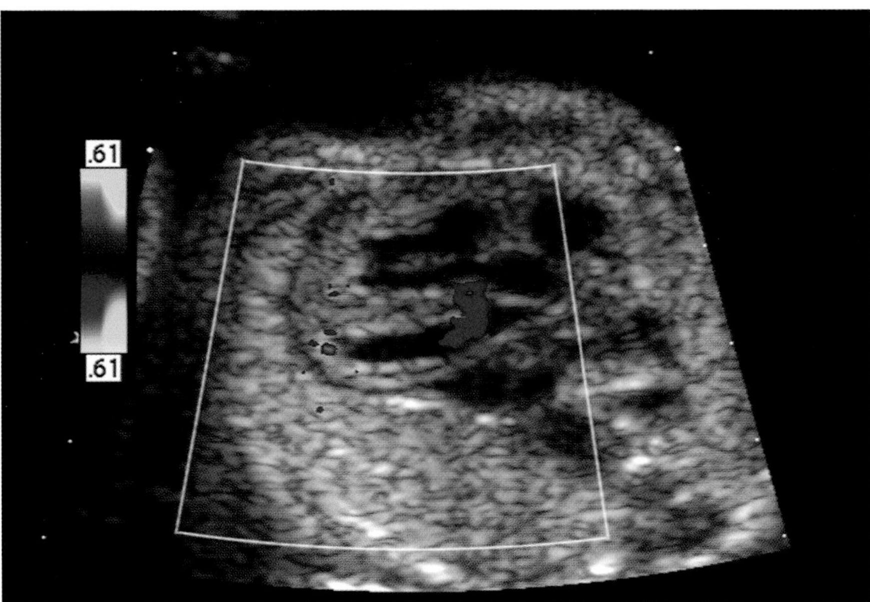

Fig. 9.**47** **Trisomy 18.** Same fetus. A membranous VSD as seen using Doppler color mapping.

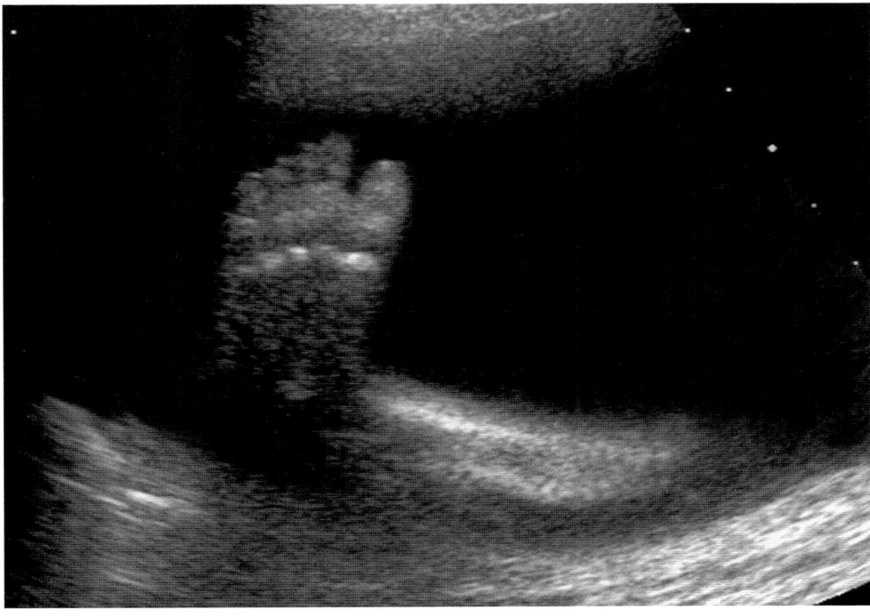

Fig. 9.**48** **Trisomy 18.** Same fetus, showing club foot.

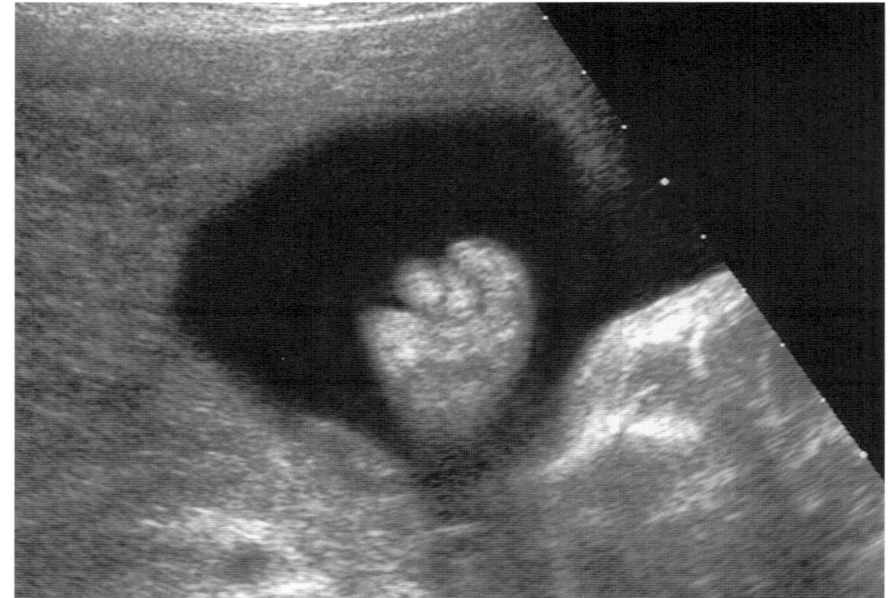

Fig. 9.**49** **Trisomy 18.** Same fetus. Overlapping of fingers (clinodactyly).

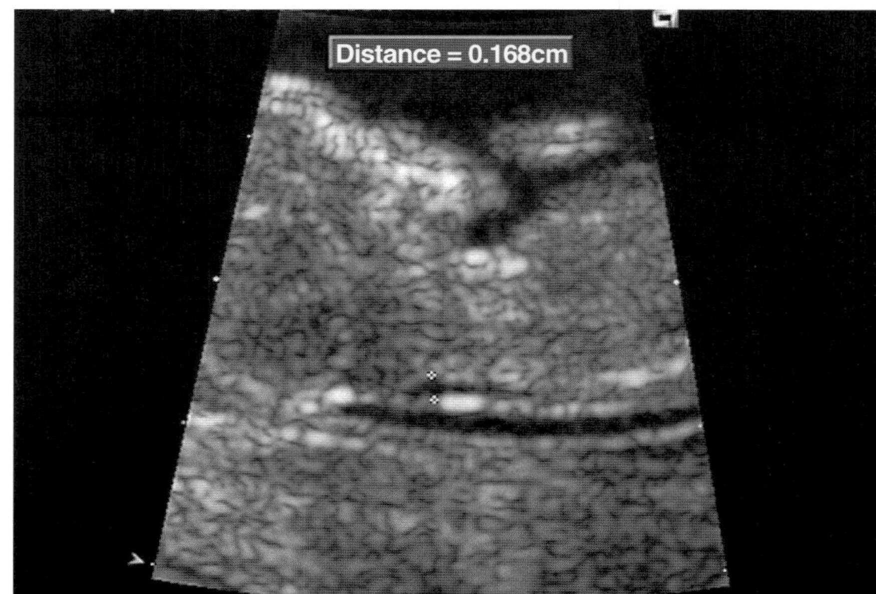

Fig. 9.**50** **Trisomy 18.** Fetal neck at 12 + 1 weeks, showing a normal value for nuchal translucency (1.7 mm).

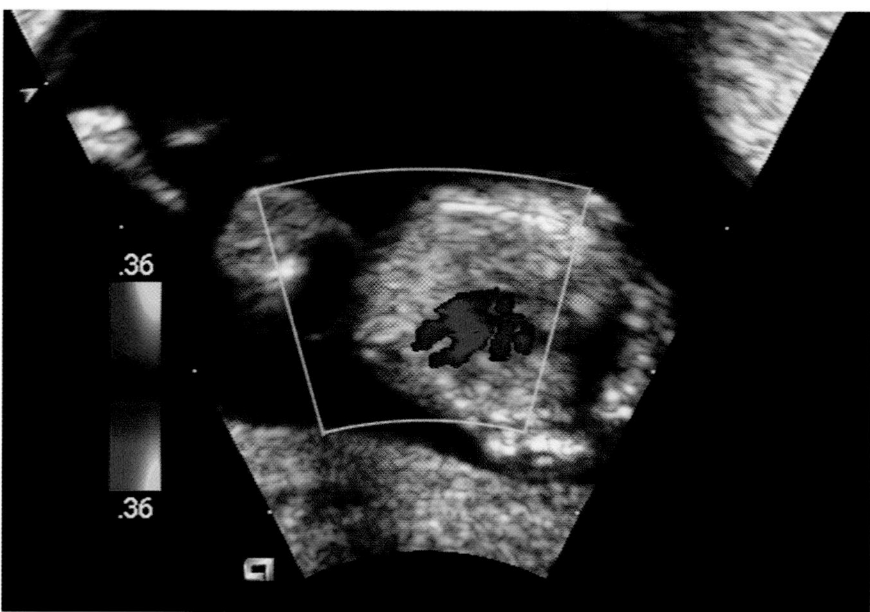

Fig. 9.**51** **Trisomy 18.** Same fetus. Doppler color mapping demonstrates an AV canal in the fetal heart.

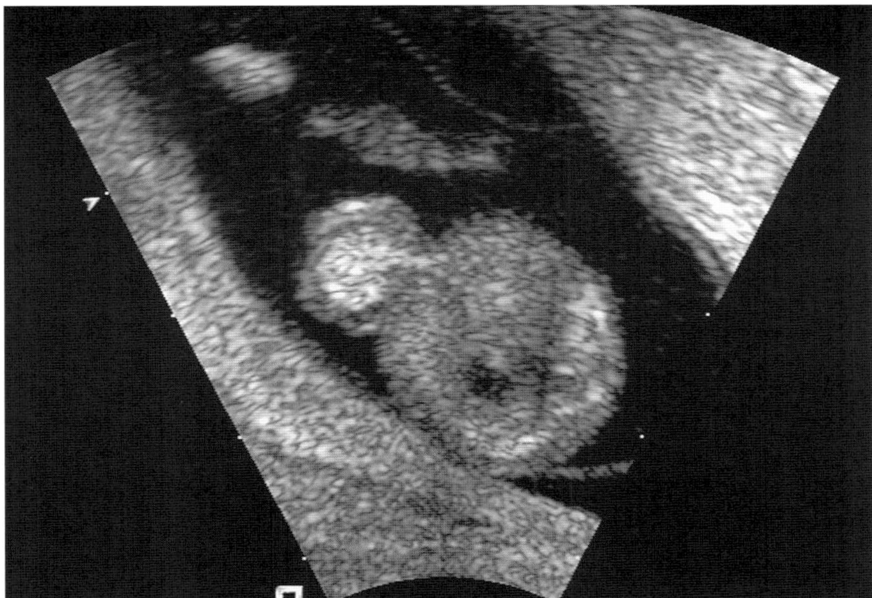

Fig. 9.**52** **Trisomy 18.** Same fetus, showing an omphalocele.

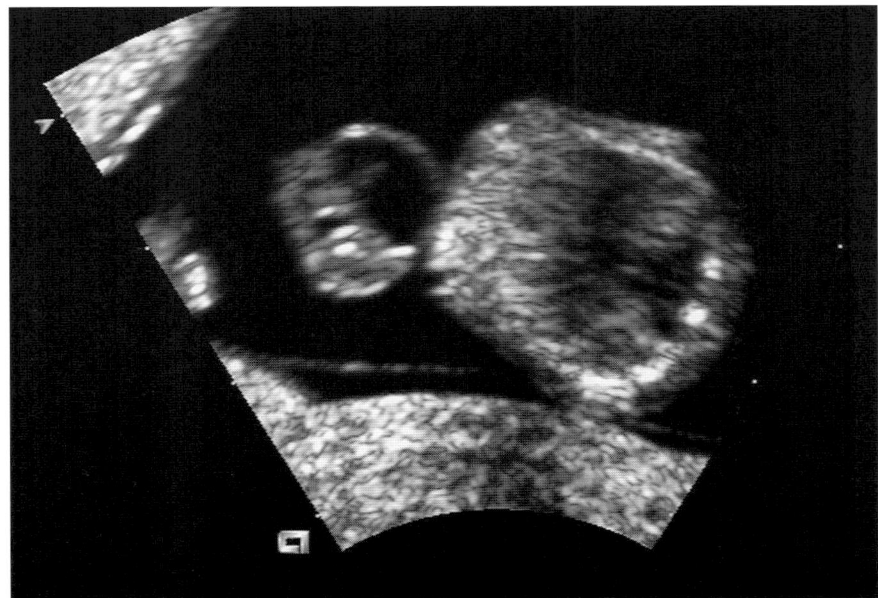

Fig. 9.**53** **Trisomy 18.** Same fetus. A cyst in the umbilical cord is detected next to the omphalocele.

References

Bakos O, Moen KS, Hansson S. Prenatal karyotyping of choroid plexus cysts. Eur J Ultrasound 1998; 8: 79–83.

Benacerraf BR, Miller WA, Frigoletto FDJ. Sonographic detection of fetuses with trisomies 13 and 18: accuracy and limitations. Am J Obstet Gynecol 1988; 158: 404–9.

Brewer CM, Holloway SH, Stone DH, Carothers AD, FitzPatrick DR. Survival in trisomy 13 and trisomy 18 cases ascertained from population based registers. J Med Genet 2002; 39: e54.

De Biasio P, Canini S, Prefumo F, Venturini PL. Trisomy 18 in a fetus with normal NT and abnormal maternal serum biochemistry. Prenat Diagn 2002; 22: 492–3.

McCaffrey F. Around PediHeart: trisomy 18, an ethical dilemma. Pediatr Cardiol 2002; 23: 181.

Nyberg DA, Kramer D, Resta RG, et al. Prenatal sonographic findings of trisomy 18: review of 47 cases. J Ultrasound Med 1993; 12: 103–13.

Pearce JM, Griffin D, Campbell S. Cystic hygromata in trisomy 18 and 21. Prenat Diagn 1984; 4: 371–5.

Quintero RA, Johnson MP, Mendoza G, Evans MI. Ontogeny of clenched-hand development in trisomy 18 fetuses: a serial transabdominal fetoscopic observation. Fetal Diagn Ther 1999; 14: 68–70.

Sepulveda W Treadwell MC, Fisk NM. Prenatal detection of preaxial upper limb reduction in trisomy 18. Obstet Gynecol 1995; 85: 847–50.

Sherod C, Sebire NJ, Soares W Snijders RJ, Nicolaides M. Prenatal diagnosis of trisomy 18 at the 10–14-week ultrasound scan. Ultrasound Obstet Gynecol 1997; 10: 387–90.

Shields LE, Carpenter LA, Smith KM, Nghiem HV. Ultrasonographic diagnosis of trisomy 18: is it practical in the early second trimester? J Ultrasound Med 1998; 17: 327–31.

Steiger RM, Porto M, Lagrew DC, Randall R. Biometry of the fetal cisterna magna: estimates of the ability to detect trisomy 18. Ultrasound Obstet Gynecol 1995; 5: 384–90.

Trisomy 21 (Down Syndrome)

Definition: Numerical chromosomal aberration, with an extra chromosome 21. This is the most common trisomy in live-born neonates. The phenotype (*Down syndrome*) is characterized by severe malformations and developmental disorder. Cardiac anomalies and mental impairment are the commonest features.

Incidence: One in 700–800 births.

Sex ratio: M : F = 1 : 1.

Clinical history/genetics: The incidence of Down syndrome correlates with maternal age. As in trisomy 13, three forms of chromosomal aberrations are found in trisomy 21: *free trisomy,* found in about 95% of patients with Down syndrome; *translocation trisomy 21,* affecting about 3%; and *trisomy 21 mosaic,* affecting 2% of patients.

In free trisomy 21, the recurrence risk lies 1% above that for the maternal age. Only 30% of trisomy 21 cases would be diagnosed if all mothers over the age of 35 had chromosomal analysis carried out during prenatal screening. Using the triple test, prenatal diagnosis can be

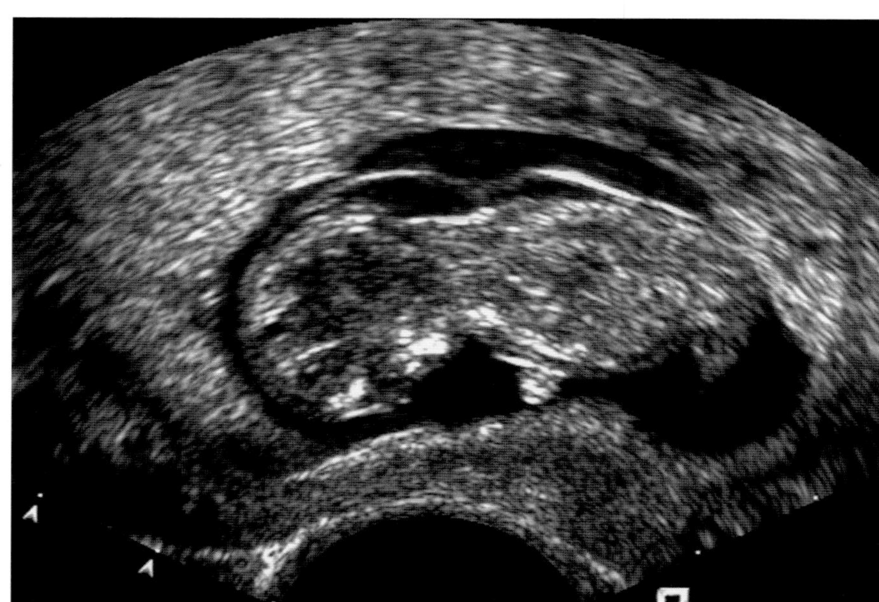

Fig. 9.**54** **Trisomy 21.** Longitudinal section at 11 + 1 weeks, showing hygroma colli.

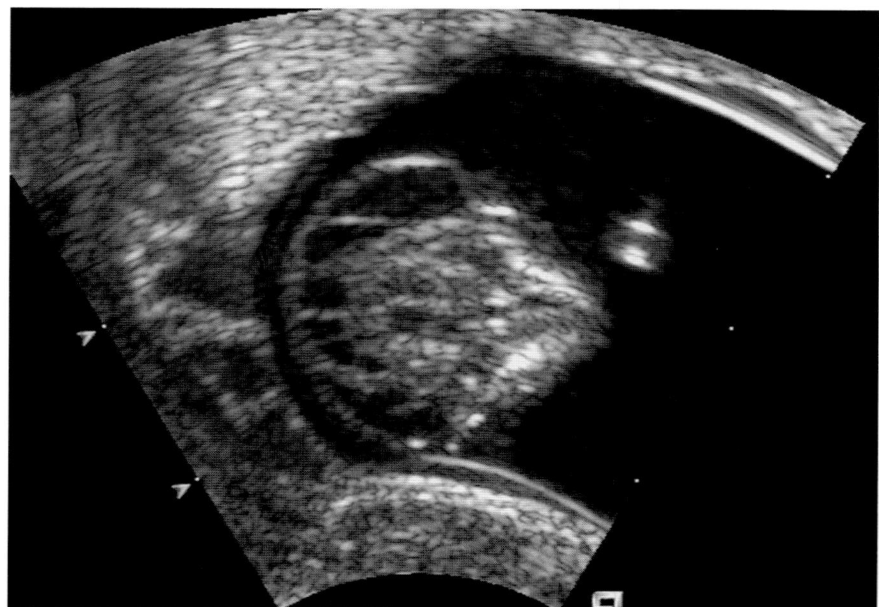

Fig. 9.**55** **Trisomy 21.** Same fetus as before. A cross-sectional view demonstrates the presence of septa within the hygroma.

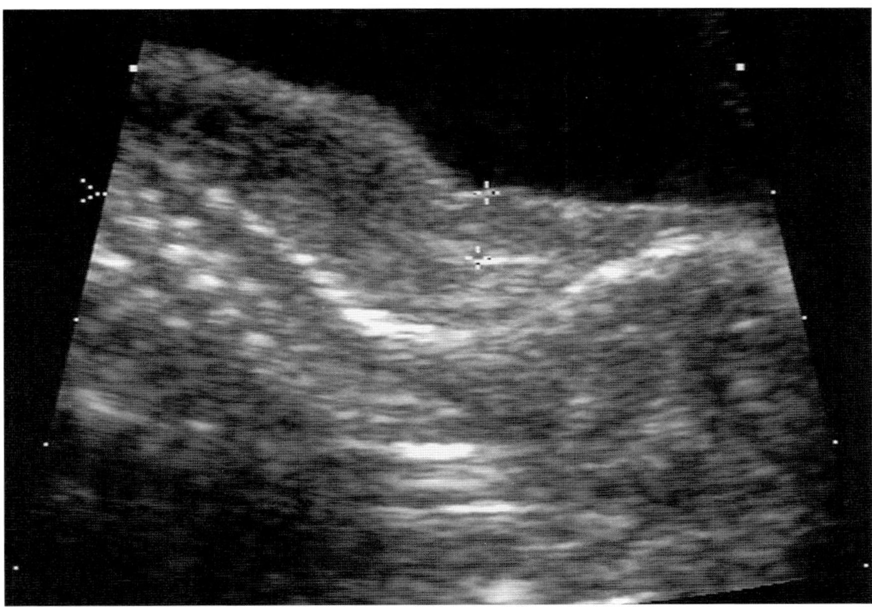

Fig. 9.**56** **Trisomy 21.** Nuchal translucency at 17 + 6 weeks.

achieved in 60%. Using a combination of maternal age, measurement of nuchal translucency (11–13 weeks) and determination of PAPP-A and free β-HCG in maternal serum, diagnosis can be achieved in 90% (cut-off level 1 : 350).

Teratogens: Not known.

Etiology: Chromosome 21 is found twice in the ovum or the sperm, as a result of incorrect division during germ-cell development (meiotic nondisjunction). This process of meiotic nondisjunction occurs in 95% of cases in maternal germ-cell development; the paternal germ cells are responsible in only 5% of cases.

Ultrasound findings: Nuchal translucency screening at 11–13 weeks detects a *thickening of the nuchal fold* in 70–80% of affected fetuses. The upper limit for this measurement (mostly > 2.5 mm) depends on the maternal age and fetal crown–rump length. A nuchal fold measurement of above 6 mm at about 18 weeks of gestation may also be suspicious for Down syndrome, but the sensitivity is low at this gestational age. *Other ultrasound findings are:* nonimmune fetal hydrops, isolated hydrothorax, mild ventriculomegaly, brachycephaly, flat facial profile with a small nose, urethral valve syndrome with megacystis, intestines with a strong echo (the echo from the small bowel resembles that from the bones), duodenal stenosis ("double bubble", seen after 24 weeks), omphalocele, mild dilation of the renal pelvis (> 4–5 mm at 21 weeks), clinodactyly, hypoplasia of the middle phalanx of the fifth finger (difficult to reproduce), short femur and humerus (frequently false-positive), general growth restriction, sandal gap between the big and the second toes. In 40–50% of cases, *cardiac anomalies* such as AV canal, membranous inlet VSD, hypoplasia of the left heart, and tetralogy of Fallot.

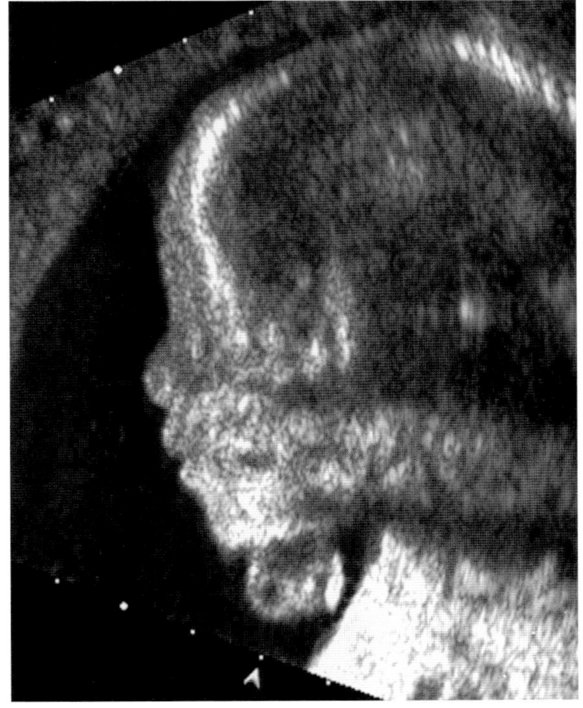

Fig. 9.**57** **Trisomy 21.** Slightly abnormal facial profile at 23 weeks, with flattening of the nose.

Differential diagnosis: Depending on the ultrasound findings, various syndromes can be considered, for example: Cornelia de Lange syndrome, Noonan syndrome, Roberts syndrome, Smith–Lemli–Opitz syndrome, hypoplasia of the

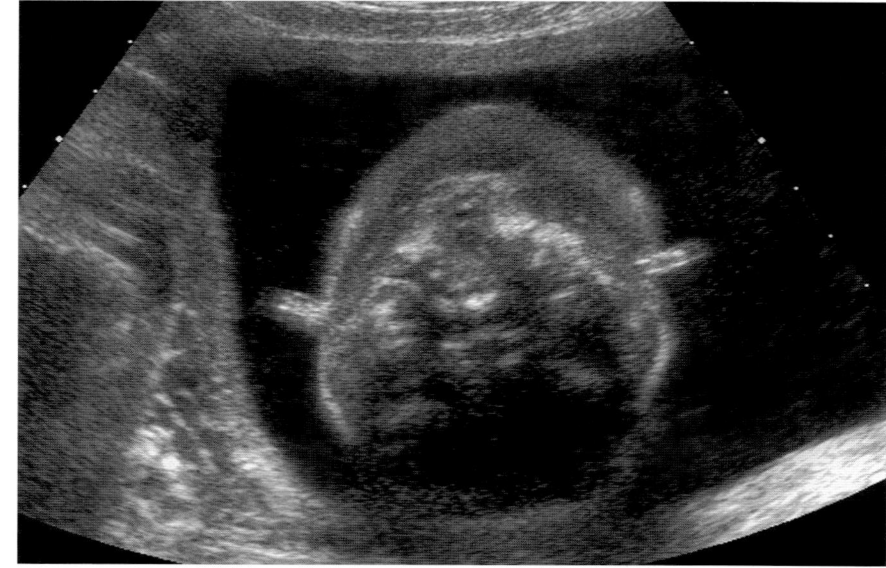

Fig. 9.**58** **Trisomy 21.** Fetal neck at 21 + 3 weeks. In addition to swelling of the neck, dysplasia of the fetal ears is seen.

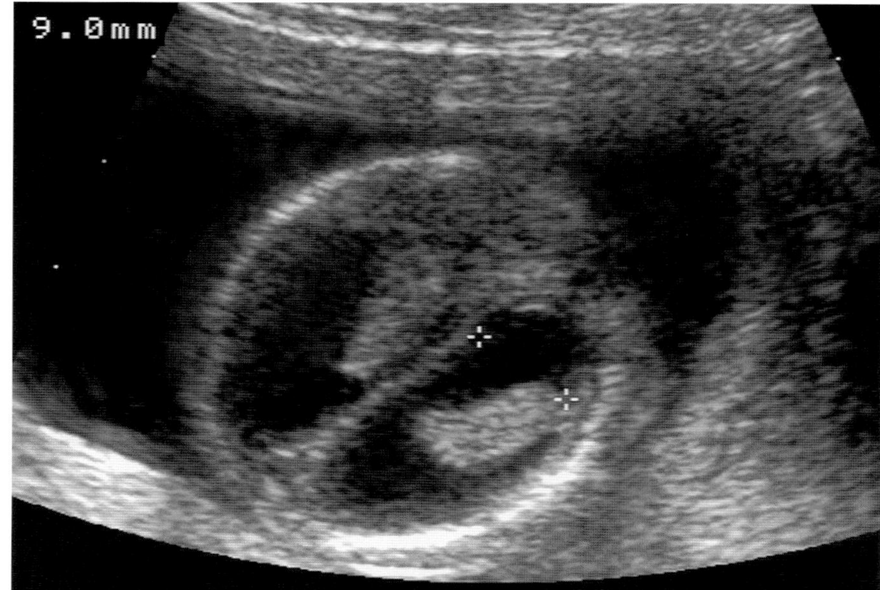

Fig. 9.**59** **Trisomy 21.** The lateral ventricle is widened, measuring 9 mm at 15 + 5 weeks.

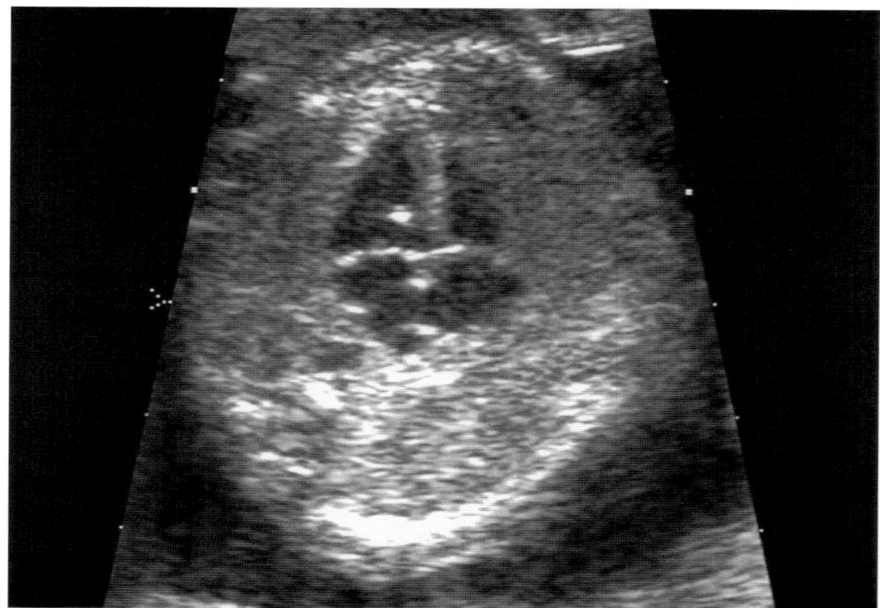

Fig. 9.**60** **Trisomy 21.** Fetal heart at 21 + 3 weeks, demonstrating a "white spot" within the left ventricle.

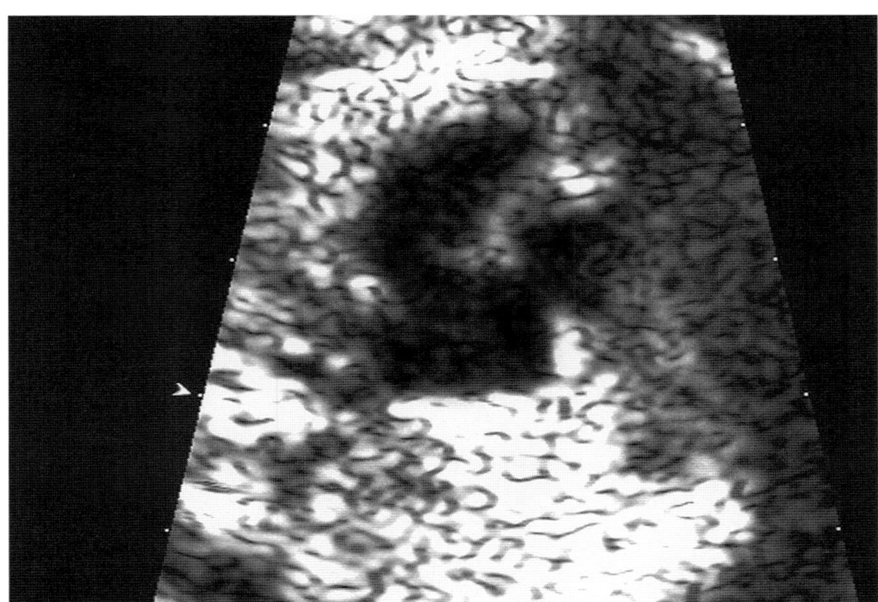

Fig. 9.**61** **Trisomy 21.** AV canal, 21 + 6 weeks.

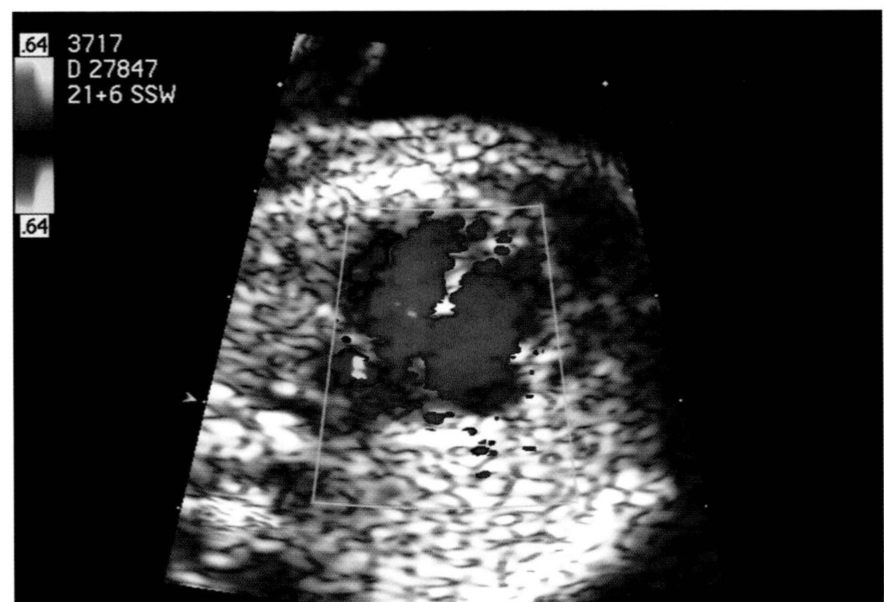

Fig. 9.**62** **Trisomy 21.** Same situation, showing blood flow in the diastolic phase using Doppler color mapping.

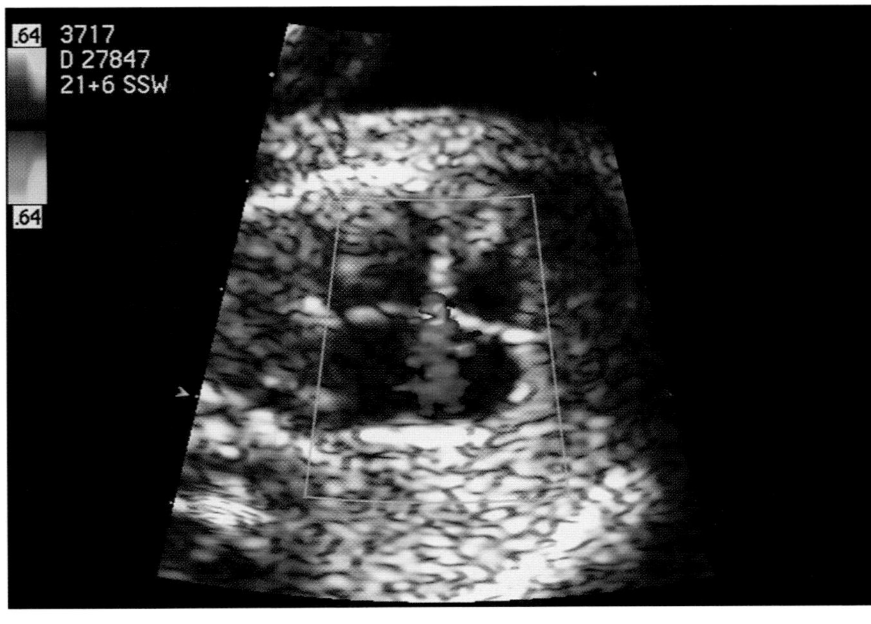

Fig. 9.**63** **Trisomy 21.** Same fetus as before. The fused AV valve is causing incompetence, showing a systolic jet on Doppler color mapping.

3

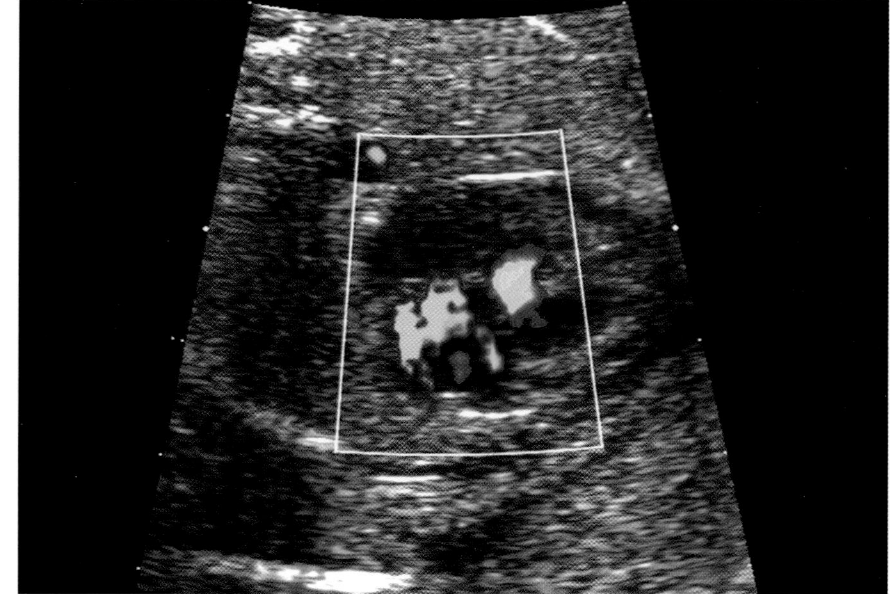

Fig. 9.**64** **Trisomy 21.** Membranous ventricular septal defect: a right–left shunt in the systolic phase is demonstrated using Doppler color mapping.

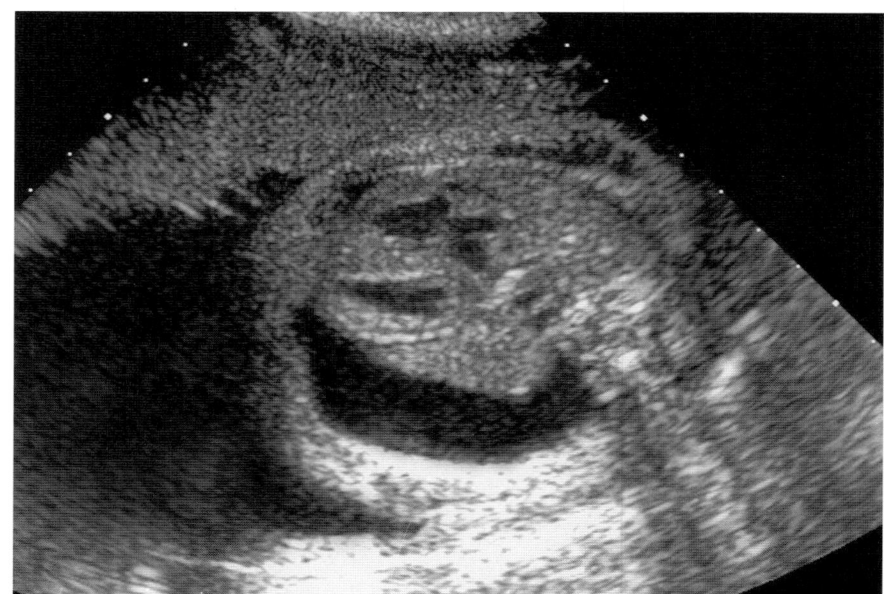

Fig. 9.**65** **Trisomy 21.** Unilateral hydrothorax at 29 + 2 weeks. An earlier scan at 22 weeks was normal.

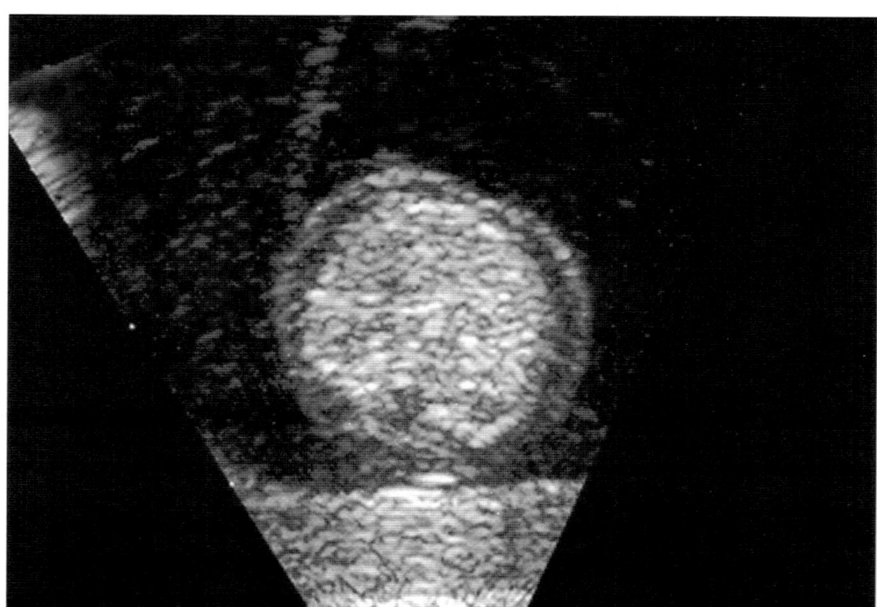

Fig. 9.**66** **Trisomy 21.** Nonimmune fetal hydrops at 12 weeks. The abdomen is seen in cross-section; anasarca.

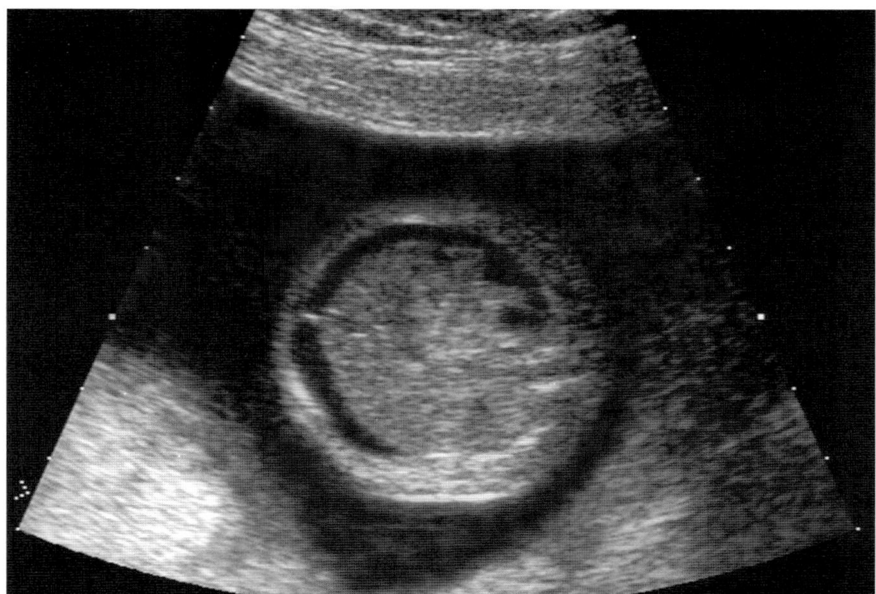

Fig. 9.**67** **Trisomy 21.** Cross-section of the fetal abdomen at 15 + 5 weeks, showing fetal ascites.

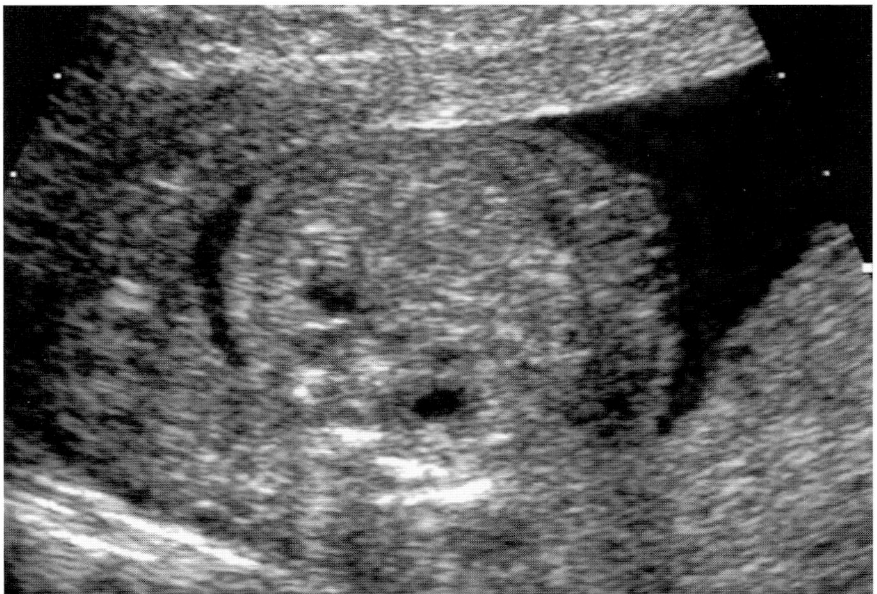

Fig. 9.**68** **Trisomy 21.** Discrete bilateral dilation of the renal pelvis at 17 + 2 weeks.

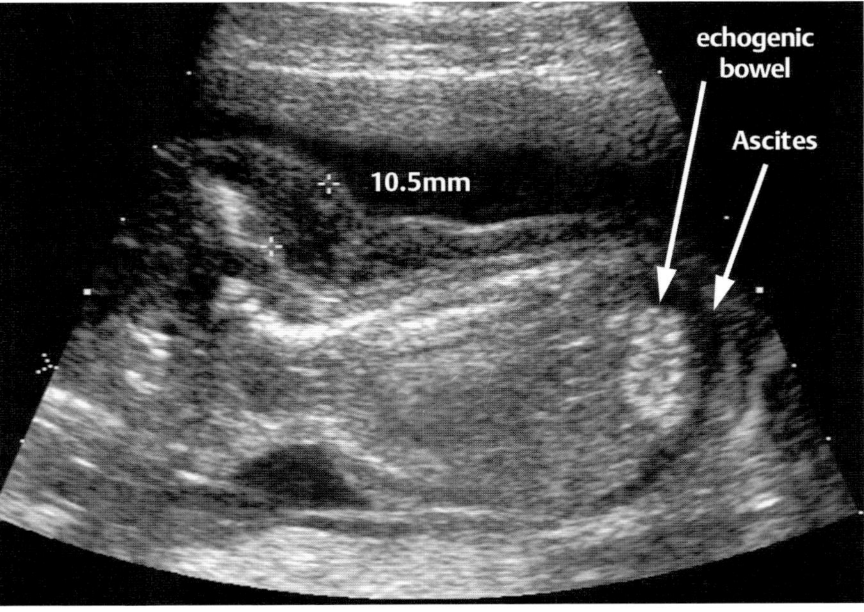

Fig. 9.**69** **Trisomy 21.** Fetus at 15 + 5 weeks. Nuchal translucency 10.5 mm, ascites, and echogenic bowel (intestines).

femur, unusual facial syndrome, hypochondroplasia, thorax dysplasia Jeune, spondyloepiphyseal dysplasia, Turner syndrome.

Clinical management: Karyotyping, as well as further ultrasound screening, including fetal echocardiography. The option of terminating the pregnancy may be discussed with the parents, depending on their religious and ethical views. If the parents are willing to accept a child with Down syndrome, then the pregnancy should be managed as a high-risk pregnancy, to avoid secondary complications. The prognosis depends on the extent of the cardiac lesion. The severity of mental impairment is not predictable at the prenatal stage. Duodenal atresia can cause hydramnios and lead to premature labor. Fetal monitoring during labor is carried out, and obstetric measures taken as necessary. It is advisable to deliver the mother in a perinatal center where a pediatrician can be present at the time of birth. He or she should be informed of the anomalies to be expected, as diagnosed with ultrasound screening.

Procedure after birth: Therapeutic measures are needed soon after birth. Surgical intervention is needed earliest for intestinal anomalies. Cardiac lesions rarely cause symptoms requiring surgical treatment in the immediate neonatal stage.

Prognosis: Cardiac anomalies are mainly responsible for the high rate of neonatal mortality. The rate of mortality remains there after relatively stable until 40 years, and increases rapidly due to premature ageing. The intelligence quotient lies between 50 and 80 in childhood, but decreases as the patient gets older.

Recommendation for the mother: In sporadic cases, the recurrence risk lies 1% above the risk for the maternal age, but for translocation trisomy 21, the risk is considerably higher. Genetic counseling is recommended. In the subsequent pregnancy, diagnosis of trisomy can be excluded at 11 to 12 weeks by chorionic villus sampling. Using nuchal translucency measurements (11–13 weeks), an effective screening program can also be offered to younger women. However, diagnosis of Down syndrome with absolute certainty is only possible using invasive prenatal diagnostic procedures. Self-help organizations provide very good support for the affected parents.

Self-Help Organization

Title: National Down Syndrome Congress

Description: Support, information and advocacy for families affected by Down syndrome. Promotes research and public awareness. Serves as a clearing-house and network for parent groups. Newsletter ($25/y). Annual convention, phone support, chapter development guidelines.

Scope: National

Number of groups: 600+ parent group networks

Founded: 1974

Address: 7000 Peachtree-Dunwoody Rd., Atlanta, GA 30328, United States

Telephone: 1-800-232-NDSC or 770-604-9500

Fax: 770-604-9898

E-mail: NDSCcenter@aol.com

Web: http://www.NDSCcenter.org

References

ACOG Practice Bulletin. Clinical management guidelines for obstetrician-gynecologists: prenatal diagnosis of fetal chromosomal abnormalities. Obstet Gynecol 2001; 97: 1–12.

Gekas J, Gondry J, Mazur S, Cesbron P, Thepot F. Informed consent to serum screening for Down syndrome: are women given adequate information. Prenat Diagn 1999; 19: 1–7.

Graupe MH, Naylor CS, Greene NH, Carlson DE, Platt L. Trisomy 21: second-trimester ultrasound. Clin Perinatol 2001; 28: 303–19.

Jenderny J, Schmidt W, Hecher K, et al. Increased nuchal translucency, hydrops fetalis or hygroma colli: a new test strategy for early fetal aneuploidy detection. Fetal Diagn Ther 2001; 16: 211–4.

Lai FM, Woo BH, Tan KH, et al. Birth prevalence of Down syndrome in Singapore from 1993 to 1998. Singapore Med J 2002; 43: 70–6.

Nyberg DA. Ultrasound markers of fetal Down syndrome. JAMA 2001; 285: 2856.

Rosati P, Guariglia L. Early transvaginal measurement of cephalic index for the detection of Down syndrome fetuses. Fetal Diagn Ther 1999; 14: 38–40.

Souter VL, Nyberg DA, El-Bastawissi A, Zebelman A, Luthhardt F, Luthy DA. Correlation of ultrasound findings and biochemical markers in the second trimester of pregnancy in fetuses with trisomy 21. Prenat Diagn 2002; 22: 175–82.

Turner Syndrome

Definition: Complete or partial absence of an X chromosome.

Incidence: One in 5000 births.

Clinical history/genetics: Sporadic occurrence; maternal age does not influence the risk of having an affected child. Laboratory findings may give useful hints: the concentration of alpha fetoprotein is increased in maternal serum, in association with hygroma colli and fetal hydrops. Meiotic nondisjunction is found in 60% of cases, leading to a complete 45,X0 karyotype. In 40% of cases, mosaicism or structural aberrations are found. Spontaneous demise occurs in 93% of 45,X0 zygotes.

Teratogens: Not known.

Ultrasound findings: *Cystic hygroma colli* is a typical finding in severe forms of Turner syndrome, developing between the first and second trimester. At a later stage, *isolated hydrothorax, ascites,* or generalized hydrops may develop. One of the commonest cardiac anomalies in Turner syndrome is *stenosis of the aortic isthmus.* This may be difficult to detect in prenatal scan, as narrowing of the aortic isthmus usually manifests after the closure of Botallo 's duct. The main symptoms due to this stenosis are asymmetry of the ventricles, the right heart chamber being larger than the left. Some *renal anomalies* are also seen typically in Turner syndrome: unilateral renal agenesis, horseshoe kidney, pelvic kidney. Oligohydramnios is found in some cases. Shortening of the femur may also be present.

Differential diagnosis: Trisomy 21, trisomy 18, Noonan syndrome, multiple pterygium syndrome, achondrogenesis, Apert syndrome, Cornelia de Lange syndrome, EEC syndrome, Fryns syndrome, Joubert syndrome, Kniest syndrome, Roberts syndrome, Smith–Lemli–Opitz syndrome.

Clinical management: Karyotyping, as well as further ultrasound screening, including fetal echocardiography. Further management depends on how the parents feel. Parents should be informed that there is a high rate of spontaneous demise in these pregnancies. They should also be told that normal mental development can be expected in these children and that of all the chromosomal disorders, this one has the fewest severe anomalies. If parents accept this and decide to continue with the pregnancy, then the further management does not differ from that in a normal pregnancy. If a cardiac anomaly is present, then the delivery should take place in a perinatal center.

Procedure after birth: A pediatrician should care for the neonate immediately after birth. The cardiac anomaly should be differentiated between

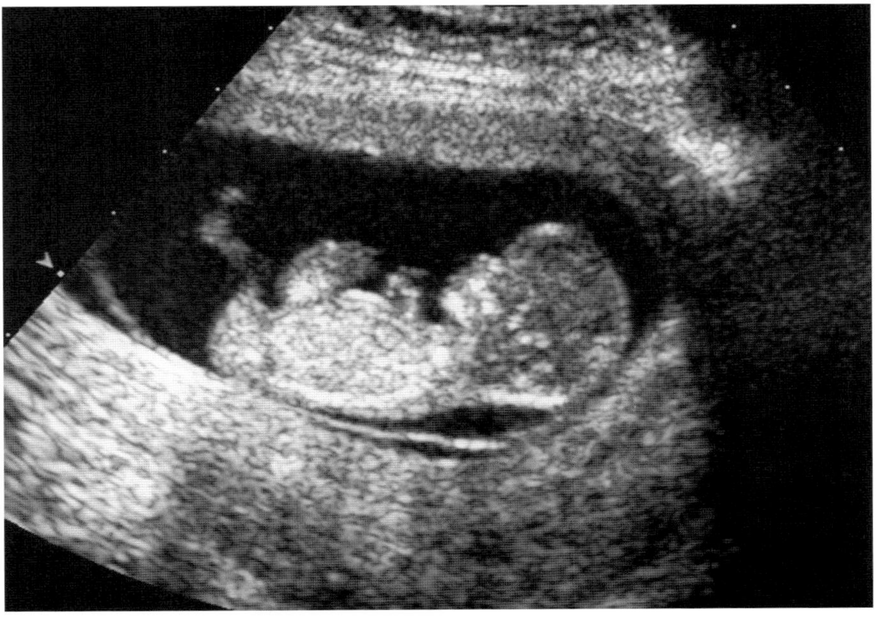

Fig. 9.**70** **Turner syndrome.** Fetus at 11 + 1 weeks. Crown–rump length 53 mm, nuchal translucency 4.4 mm. Chorionic villus sampling confirmed Turner syndrome.

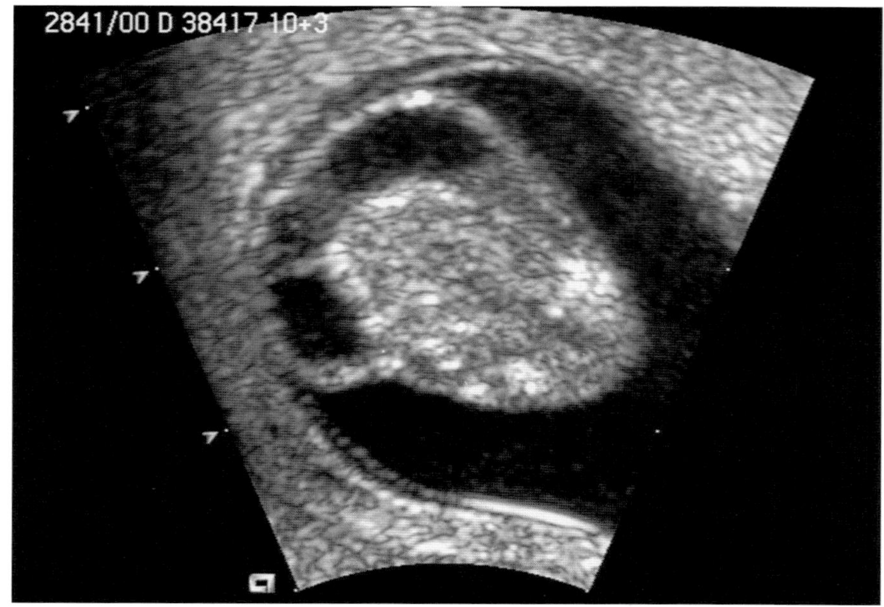

Fig. 9.**71** **Turner syndrome.** Cross-section of fetal neck in Turner syndrome at 10 + 3 weeks (crown–rump length 36 mm). Hygroma colli of 4.4 mm, with septa.

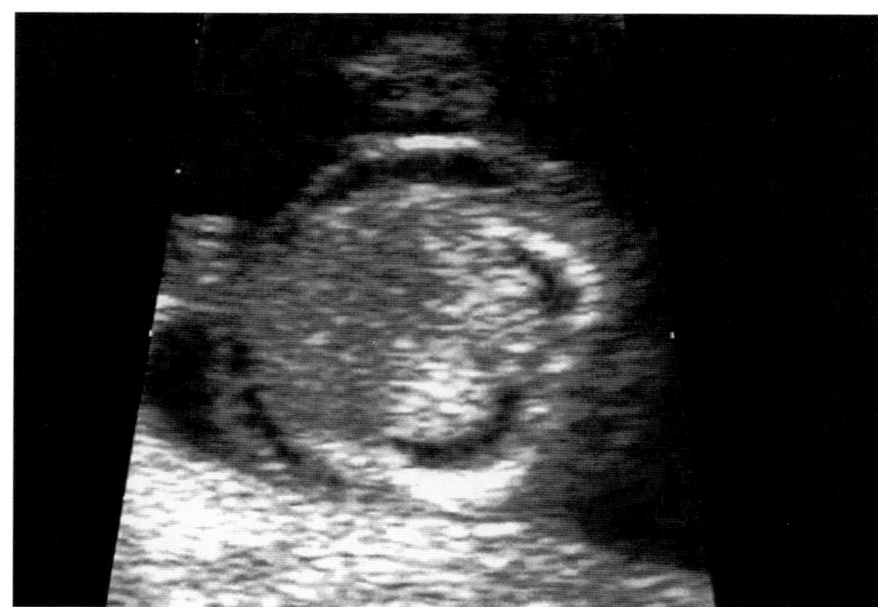

Fig. 9.**72** **Turner syndrome.** Cross-section of fetal thorax at 13 + 0 weeks; anasarca and bilateral pleural effusions.

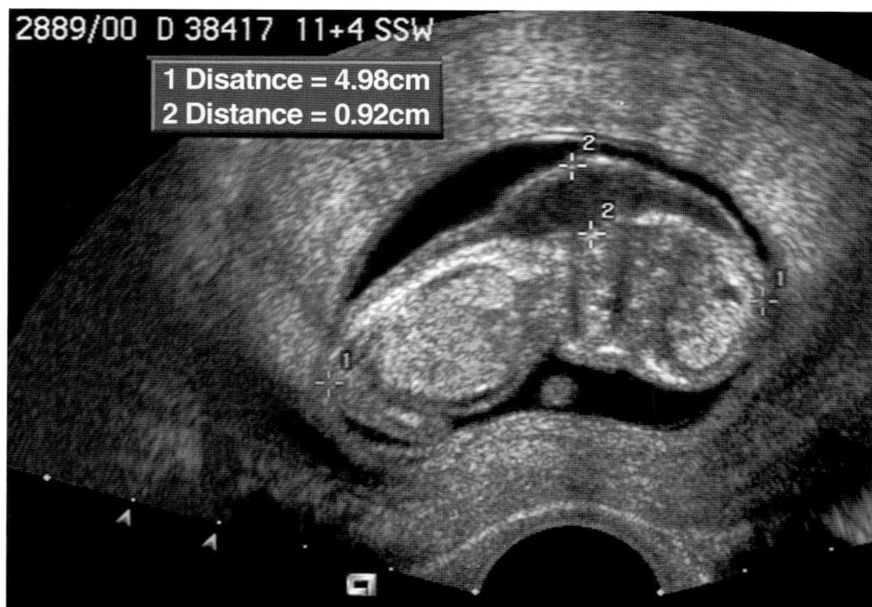

Fig. 9.**73** **Turner syndrome.** Fetus of 50 mm at 11 + 4 weeks; severe nuchal translucency of 8.2 mm.

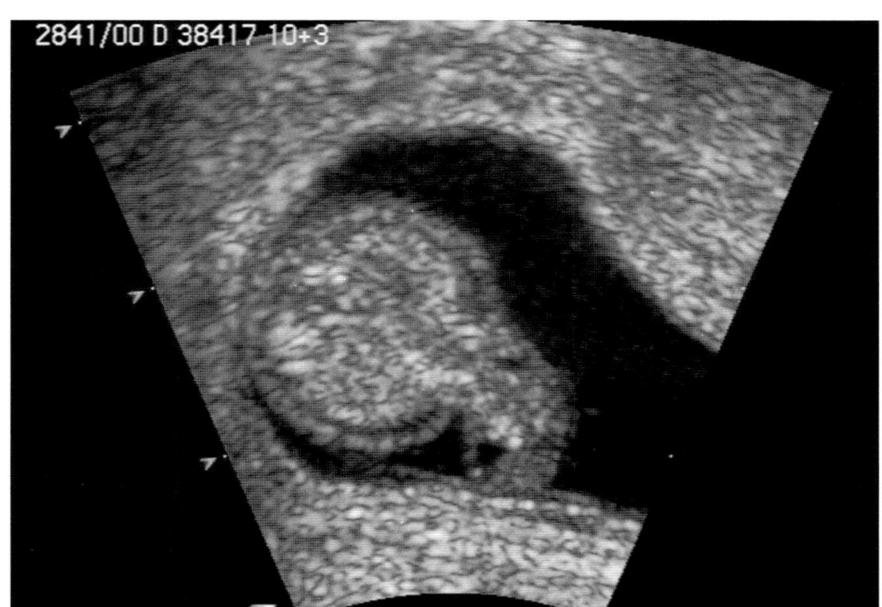

Fig. 9.**74** **Turner syndrome.** Fetal ascites and omphalocele (possibly physiological) at 10 + 3 weeks.

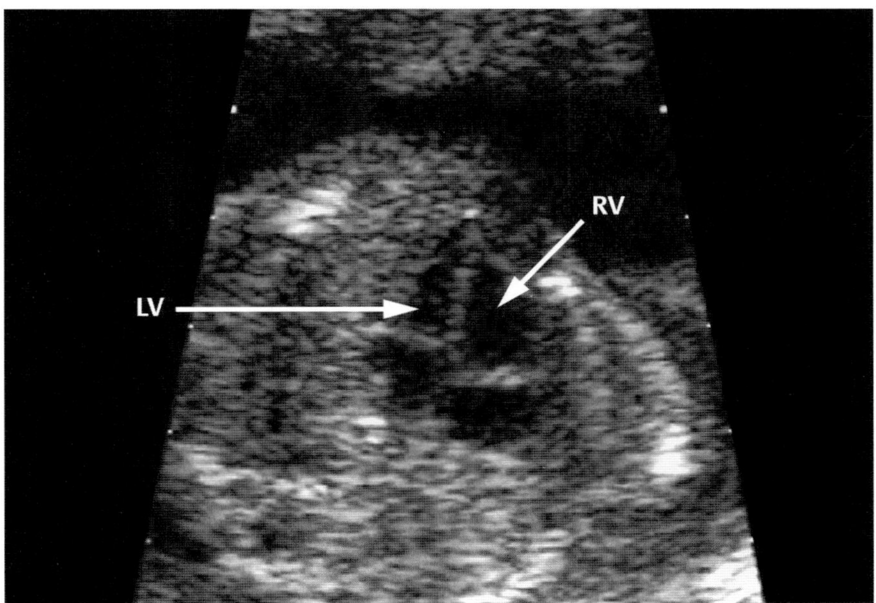

Fig. 9.**75** **Turner syndrome.** Fetal heart at 20 + 4 weeks in an apical four-chamber view: the left ventricle (LV) appears somewhat smaller than the right ventricle (RV), the mitral valve is displaced towards the apex of the heart. Diagnosis: Turner syndrome.

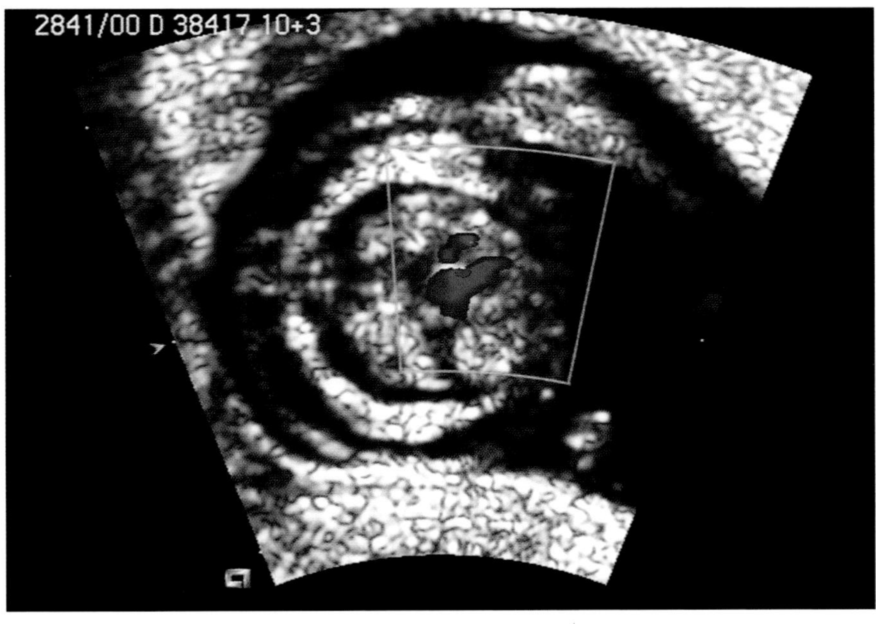

Fig. 9.**76** **Turner syndrome.** Cross-section of fetal thorax at 10 + 3 weeks, at the level of the heart in a case of Turner syndrome. Subcutaneous edema (anasarca), bilateral pleural effusion and both the cardiac ventricles (Doppler color mapping) are demonstrated.

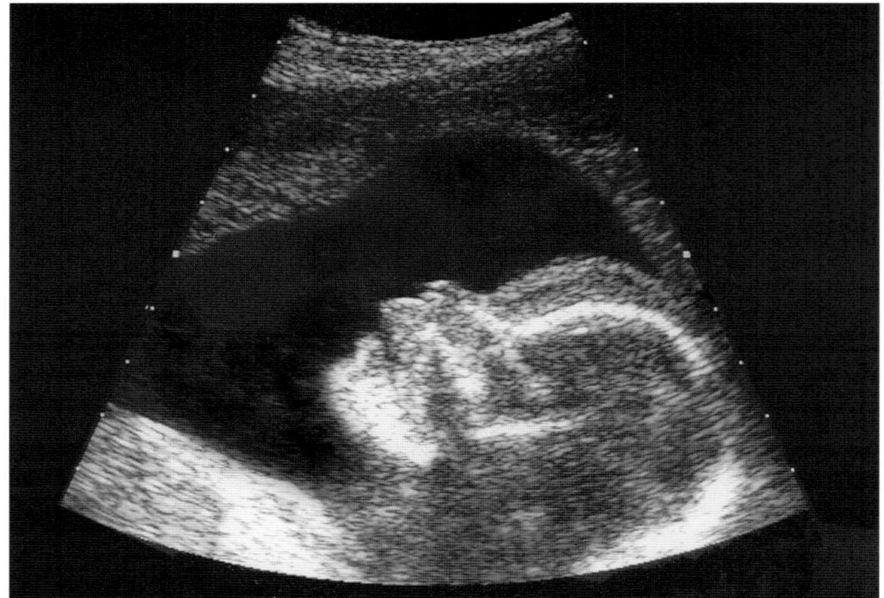

Fig. 9.**77** **Turner syndrome.** Facial profile at 21 + 5 weeks showing edema in the region of the forehead.

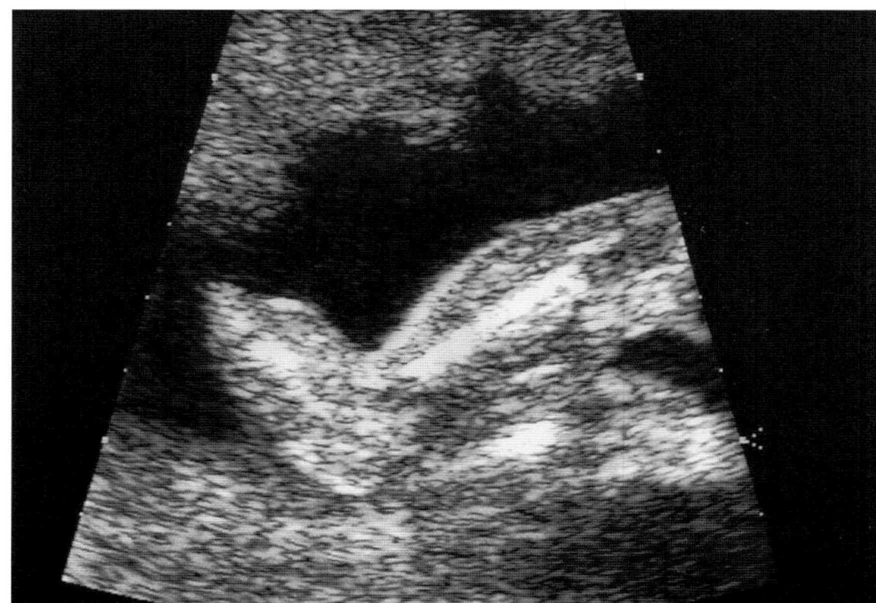

Fig. 9.**78** **Turner syndrome.** Edema at the back of the foot at 21 + 5 weeks.

aortic isthmus stenosis and persistent ductus arteriosus, to avoid administration of a high percentage of oxygen. If generalized fetal hydrops is present, intrauterine fetal death is the usual outcome. An isolated finding of cystic hygroma colli may regress spontaneously in the course of the pregnancy. Cardiac anomalies present a higher risk for the newborn. Intensive care of the infant and cardiac surgery reduce the mortality rate considerably. In the absence of mosaicism, the affected individual has reduced growth and is infertile (gonadal dysgenesis). Hearing impairment is detected in 50% of children. Administration of hormones is necessary at puberty for further development. The affected individual is usually of normal intelligence.

Information for the mother: All cases are sporadic, without exception. The risk of recurrence is not increased. The development of affected children depends on the medical care they receive (cardiac defect, growth, hormone substitution). Self-help organizations may give useful hints.

Self-Help Organizations

Title: Turner Syndrome Society of the United States

Description: Self-help for women, girls, and their families affected by Turner's syndrome. Increases public awareness about the disorder. Quarterly newsletter, chapter development assistance, annual conference.

Scope: National

Number of groups: 32 chapters

Founded: 1988

Address: 14450 TC Jester, Suite 260, Houston, TX 77014, United States

Telephone: 832–249–9988 or 1–800–365–9944

Fax: 832–249–9987

E-mail: tssus@turner-syndrome-us.org

Web: http://www.turner-syndrome-us.org

Title: Turner Syndrome Support Network

Description: Network and exchange of information for parents of children with Turner's syndrome. Information and referrals, phone support, pen pals, conferences, literature. Annual convention. Newsletter ($25/year).

Scope: National

Founded: 1989

Address: c/o MAGIC Foundation, 1327 N. Harlem, Oak Park, IL 60302, United States

Telephone: 1–800–3-MAGIC-3 or 708–383–0808

Fax: 709–383–0899

E-mail: pam@magicfoundation.org

Web: http://www.magicfoundation.org

References

Abir R, Fisch B, Nahum R, Orvieto R, Nitke S, Ben Rafael Z. Turner's syndrome and fertility: current status and possible putative prospects [review]. Hum Reprod Update 2001; 7: 603–10.

Gilbert B, Yardin C, Briault S, et al. Prenatal diagnosis of female monozygotic twins discordant for Turner syndrome: implications for prenatal genetic counselling. Prenat Diagn 2002; 22: 697–702.

Hall GH, Weston MJ, Campbell DJ. Transitory unilateral pleural effusion associated with mosaic Turner's syndrome. Prenat Diagn 2001; 21: 421–2.

Hartling UB, Hansen BF, Keeling JW, Skovgaard LT, Kjaer I. Short bi-iliac distance in prenatal Ullrich–Turner syndrome. Am J Med Genet 2002; 108: 290–4.

Henrion R, Aubry MC, Aubry JP, Emmanuelli CN, Dumez Y, Oury JR. The antenatal diagnosis of Bonnevie–Ullrich's syndrome: the role of ultrasound. J Gynecol Obstet Biol Reprod (Paris) 1981; 10: 831–7.

Hsu LY. Phenotype/karyotype correlations of Y chromosome aneuploidy with emphasis on structural aberrations in postnatally diagnosed cases. Am J Med Genet 1994; 53: 108–40.

Kohn G, Yarkoni S, Cohen MM. Two conceptions in a 45,X woman. Am J Med Genet 1980; 5: 339–43.

Lustig L, Clarke S, Cunningham G, Schonberg R, Tompkinson G. California's experience with low MS-AFP results. Am J Med Genet 1988; 31: 211–22.

Schröder W. [Hygroma colli in the ultrasound image as an early indication of fetal Ullrich–Turner syndrome; in German.] Z Geburtshilfe Perinatol 1990; 194: 283–5.

Tanriverdi HA, Hendrik HJ, Ertan AK, Axt R, Schmidt W. Hygroma colli cysticum: prenatal diagnosis and prognosis. Am J Perinatol 2001; 18: 415–20.

Varela M, Shapira E, Hyman DB. Ullrich–Turner syndrome in mother and daughter: prenatal diagnosis of a 46,X,de1(X)(p21) offspring from a 45,X mother with low-level mosaicism for the del(X)(p21) in one ovary. Am J Med Genet 1991; 39: 411–2

Weisner D, Fiestas HA, Grote W. [An enlarged neck fold: a sonographic marker of Down's syndrome; in German]. Z Geburtshilfe Perinatol 1988; 192: 142–4.

Wolf–Hirschhorn Syndrome (Chromosome 4 p Syndrome)

Definition: A chromosomal aberration characterized by growth restriction, microcephaly, iris coloboma, cardiac malformation, restriction of psychomotor development, and craniofacial dysmorphism.

Incidence: Rare; only about 150 cases have been described.

Etiology/genetics: Deletion of part of the short arm of chromosome 4 p (4 p16.3), mostly of paternal origin. Cytogenetic examination actually shows a normal chromosomal finding; a molecular-genetic test is needed to detect the deletion. A balanced translocation is present in 10% of parents. If parental chromosomes are normal, there is no elevated risk of recurrence.

Ultrasound findings: Characteristic findings in the *head and face* are: microcephaly, agenesis of the corpus callosum, asymmetry of the cranium, hypertelorism, squint, ptosis of the eyelid, iris coloboma, (in 30%), small, deep-set ears, narrow external auditory canal, preauricular skin tags, flat hooked nose, short upper lip ridge, fish mouth. Intrauterine growth restriction is usually present. In addition, following anomalies may also be detected: club feet, cardiac defect, cere-

3

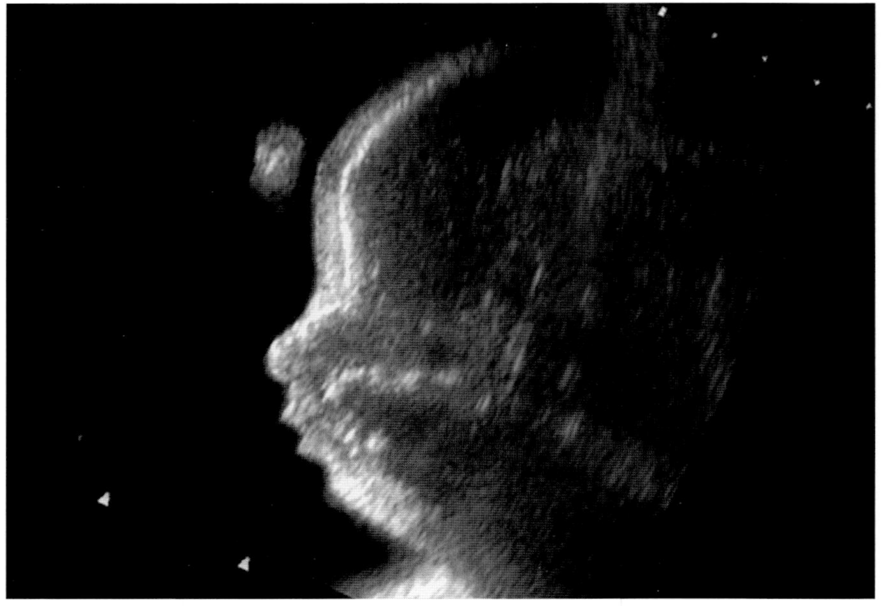

Fig. 9.**79** **Wolf–Hirschhorn syndrome.** Fetal profile at 32 weeks showing a small nose and mild retrognathia (courtesy of Dr. Lebek).

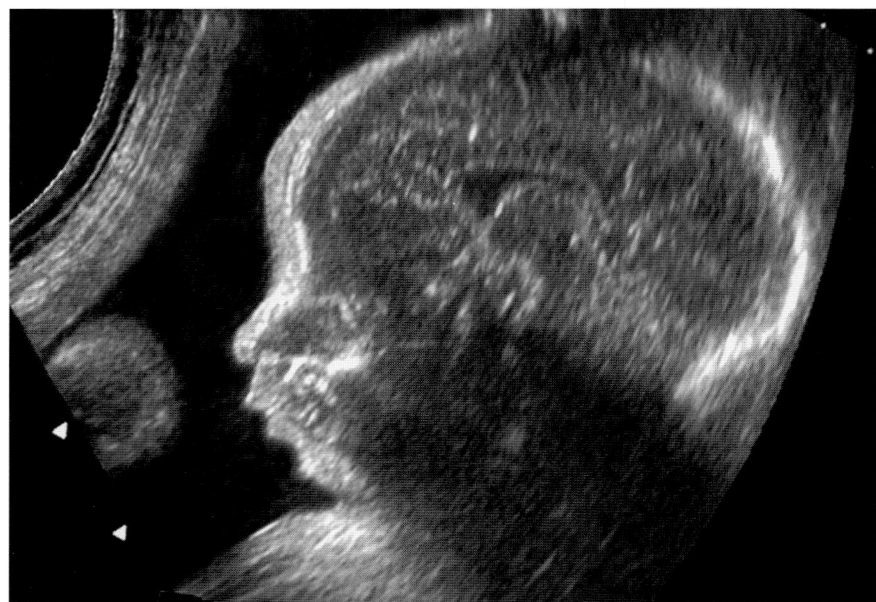

Fig. 9.**80** **Wolf–Hirschhorn syndrome.** Fetal profile at 32 weeks, showing a small nose and mild retrognathia. The corpus callosum is not evident (courtesy of Dr. Lebek).

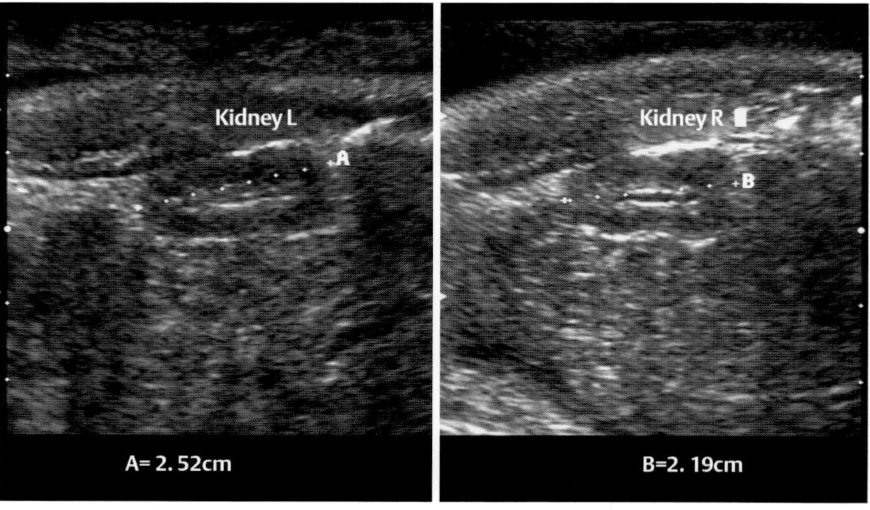

Fig. 9.**81** **Wolf–Hirschhorn syndrome.** Longitudinal section of both kidneys at 32 weeks, showing bilateral renal hypoplasia (courtesy of Dr. Lebek).

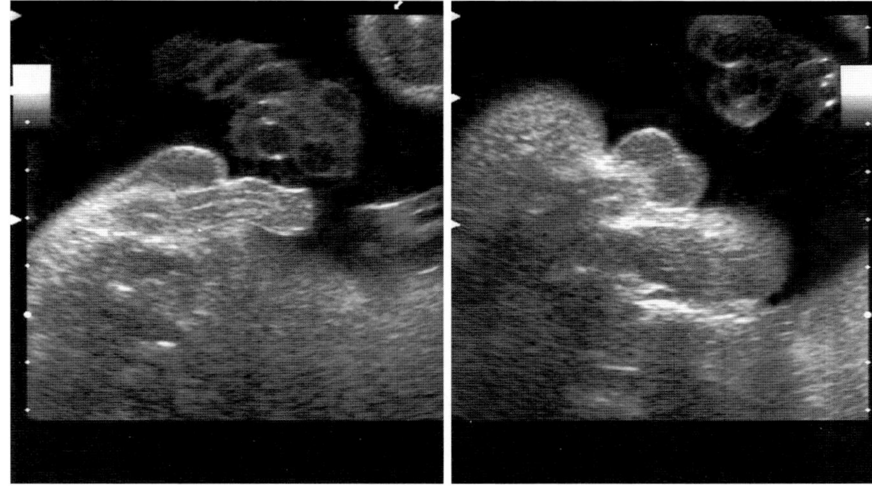

Fig. 9.**82** **Wolf–Hirschhorn syndrome.** Fetal male genitalia at 32 weeks; both testes are undescended, and the penis has an atypical shape due to hypospadias (courtesy of Dr. Lebek).

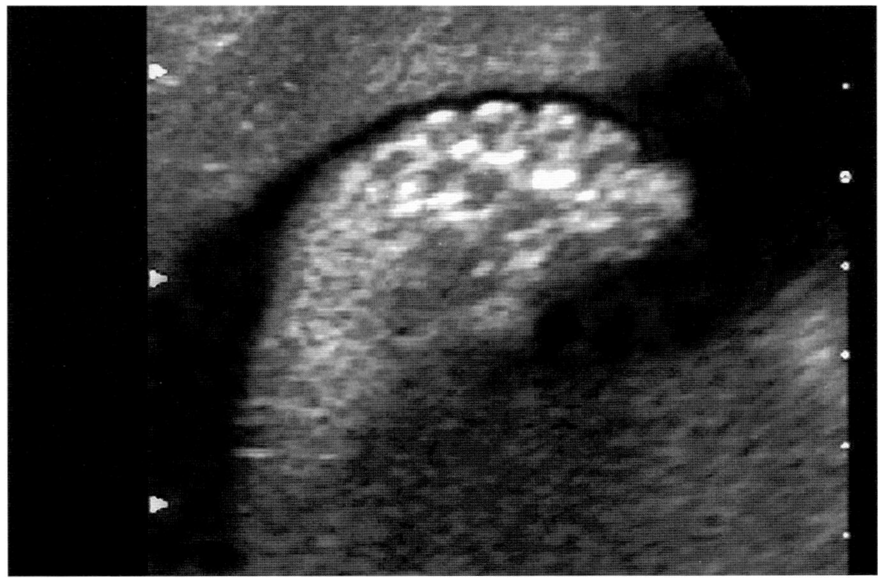

Fig. 9.**83** **Wolf–Hirschhorn syndrome.** Atypical shape of the fetal foot at 32 weeks (courtesy of Dr. Lebek).

bellar hypoplasia, cleft lip and palate, microgenia, diaphragmatic hernia, renal anomalies, cryptorchism, hypospadias.

Differential diagnosis: Cri-du-chat syndrome, Fryns syndrome, Jacobsen syndrome, triploidy, trisomy 9, trisomy 18.

Prognosis: The outcome is poor; one-third of the infants die within the first year of life. Eighty percent suffer from fits, and in most cases there is severe restriction in psychomotor development. The oldest patient was 24 years of age. Girls are affected in two-thirds of cases.

Self-Help Organization

Title: 4 p Parent Contact Group

Description: Provides support and information to families only of children with Wolf–Hirschhorn syndrome. Offers phone support, biographies of other children with this syndrome. Newsletter.

Scope: National

Number of groups: One group in the United Kingdom

Founded: 1984

Address: 1874 NW 108th Ave, Plantation, FL 33322, United States

Telephone: 954–476–9345

E-mail: bbr@juno.com

Web: www.4 p-supportgroup.org

References

De Keersmaecker B, Albert M, Hillion Y, Ville Y. Prenatal diagnosis of brain abnormalities in Wolf-Hirschhorn (4 p–) syndrome. Prenat Diagn 2002; 22: 366–70.

Eiben B, Leipoldt M, Schubbe I, Ulbrich R, Hansmann I. Partial deletion of 4 p in fetal cells not present in chorionic villi. Clin Genet 1988; 33: 49–52.

Shannon NL, Maltby EL, Rigby AS, Quarrell OW. An epidemiological study of Wolf–Hirschhorn syndrome: life expectancy and cause of mortality. J Med Genet 2001; 38: 674–9.

Tachdjian G, Fondacci C, Tapia S, Huten Y, Blot P, Nessmann C. The Wolf–Hirschhorn syndrome in fetuses. Clin Genet 1992; 42: 281–7.

Witters I, Van Schoubroeck D, Fryns JP. Choroid plexus cysts and oligohydramnios: presenting echographic signs in a female fetus with deletion of the Wolf–Hirschhorn syndrome region (4 p16.3). Genet Couns 2001; 12: 387–8.

10 Soft Markers of Chromosomal Aberrations

Abnormal Shape of the Head

Definition: Brachycephaly: the head ratio (biparietal diameter/frontal occipital diameter, BPD/FOD) is above the 95th percentile; for example, head ratio >0.88, depending on the method of measurement.

Incidence: As defined above, this applies to about 5% of all fetuses.

Ultrasound findings: The horizontal cross-section shows a *round shape*, with the BPD being relatively large compared to the FOD.

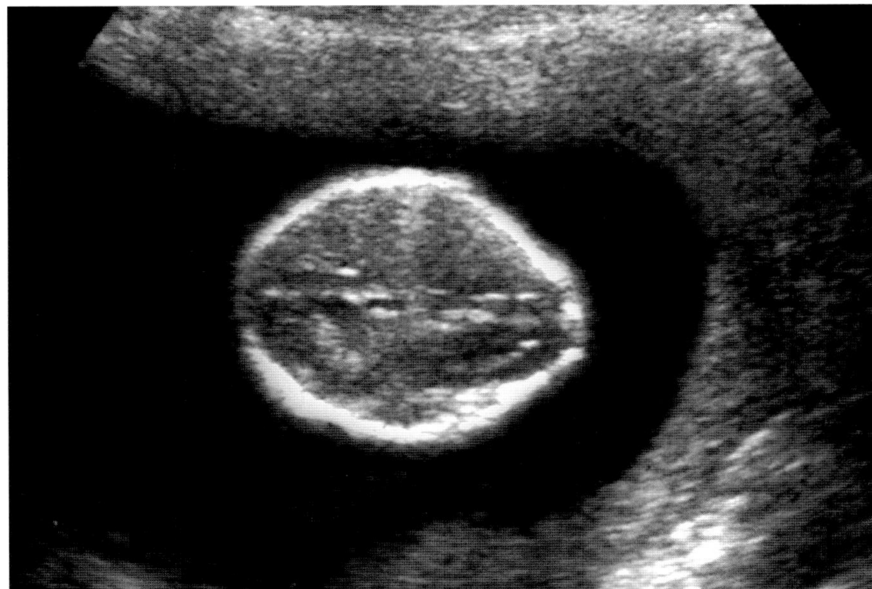

Fig. 10.1 **Strawberry sign,** in a case of trisomy 18 at 19 + 1 weeks.

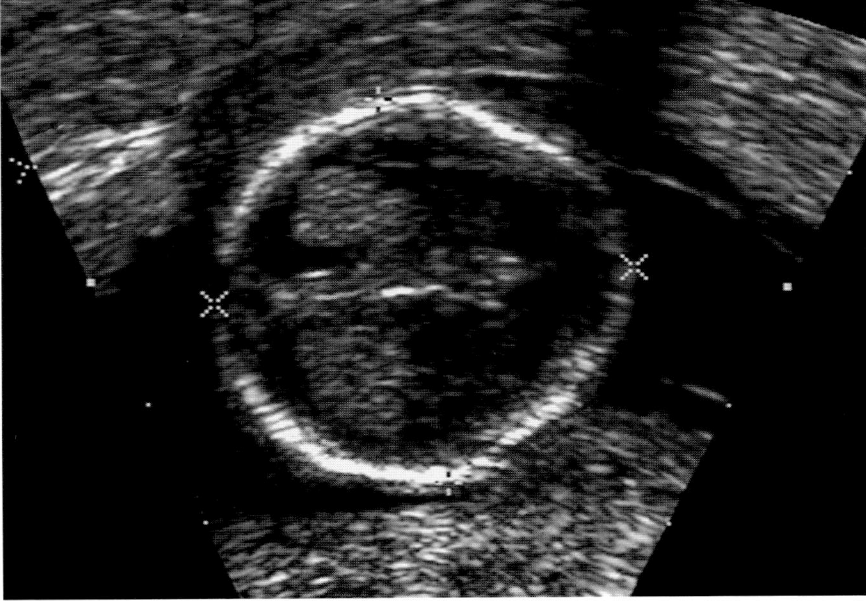

Fig. 10.2 **Brachycephaly.** Rounded head at 14 + 1 weeks in trisomy 13.

3

Caution: Following some initial euphoria regarding the use of this ratio to detect Down syndrome, large studies have since shown that there is a normal biological variation in head size and that potential measurement inaccuracies may lead to incorrect conclusions. The ratio has therefore lost its importance as a soft marker for detecting chromosomal disorders. When brachycephaly is found, the examiner should be alerted to other possible malformations. The head ratio should not be commented on in relation to chromosomal disorders, as this may cause unnecessary anxiety for the parents.

References

Becker R, Brinnef C, Arabin B. Der Kopfindex—ein vernachlässigter Parameter der fetalen Standardbiometrie. Ultraschall Med 1992; 13: 2–6.
Borrell A, Costa D, Martinez JM, et al. Brachycephaly is ineffective for detection of Down syndrome in early midtrimester fetuses. Early Hum Dev 1997; 4: 57–61.
Buttery B. Occipitofrontal-biparietal diameter ratio: an ultrasonic parameter for the antenatal evaluation of Down's syndrome. Med J Aust 1979; 2: 662–4.
Stempfle N, Huten Y, Fredouille C, Brisse H, Nessmann C. Skeletal abnormalities in fetuses with Down's syndrome: a radiographic post-mortem study. Pediatr Radiol 1999; 29: 682–8.

Dandy–Walker Variant (Open Cerebellar Vermis)

Definition: A connection between the fourth ventricle and the cisterna magna is a normal finding up to 18 weeks of gestation; thereafter, this diagnosis is applicable. It is advisable to determine the chromosome set, as an association with a chromosomal disorder is frequent. Detailed ultrasound screening should also be carried out to detect other malformations. The boundary to Dandy–Walker syndrome is hazy.

Associated syndromes: Smith–Lemli–Opitz syndrome, Joubert syndrome, Meckel–Gruber syndrome, Neu–Laxova syndrome, Walker–Warburg syndrome, Ellis–van Creveld syndrome, Majewski syndrome, TAR syndrome, tetrasomy 12 p, triploidy, trisomy 9, trisomy 18, arthrogryposis, CHARGE association, Fryns syndrome, MURCS association.

Ultrasound findings: A *small, slit-like connection* is detected between *the fourth ventricle and the cisterna magna, without widening of the latter.* This finding distinguishes the Dandy–Walker variant from the Dandy–Walker syndrome. False-positive as well as false-negative findings can be produced by inaccurate ultrasound scanning in the wrong plane.

Caution: At 13 weeks of gestation, Dandy–Walker variant is almost always detectable, and is considered to be a normal finding up to 18 weeks.

Prognosis: This may be a harmless finding with a good prognosis, or may be associated with other syndromes with a poor prognosis.

References

Blaicher W, Ulm B, Ulm MR, Hengstschlager M, Deutinger J, Bernaschek G. Dandy–Walker malformation as sonographic marker for fetal triploidy. Ultraschall Med 2002; 23: 129–33.
Bromley B, Nadel AS, Pauker S, Estroff JA, Benacerraf BR. Closure of the cerebellar vermis: evaluation with second trimester US. Radiology 1994; 193: 761–3.
Ecker JL, Shipp TD, Bromley B, Benacerraf B. The sonographic diagnosis of Dandy–Walker and Dandy–Walker variant: associated findings and outcomes. Prenat Diagn 2000; 20: 328–32.
Laing FC, Frates MC, Brown DL, Benson CB, Di Salvo DN, Doubilet PM. Sonography of the fetal posterior fossa: false appearance of mega-cisterna magna and Dandy–Walker variant. Radiology 1994; 192: 247–51.

Echogenic Bowel

Definition: Increased echogenicity of the bowel in the second trimester, such that it is equal to that of surrounding fetal bone. The most frequent cause is intra-amniotic bleeding. The echogenicity is a soft marker for chromosomal anomaly, especially for Down syndrome. In the third trimester, bowel containing echogenic meconium is a normal finding.

Incidence: 0.6% of all fetuses in the second trimester.

Ultrasound findings: Loops of the bowel show a strong echogenic content. Weak echo can be excluded by reducing the overall density of the ultrasound picture. At the lowest level of reduction, only the bones and the echogenic bowel can be demonstrated if their echogenicity is similar.

Differential diagnosis: The differential diagnosis in these findings can be clarified from the study by Yaron et al., who investigated 79 cases of echogenic bowel. No cause was found in 30 cases (38%); intra-amniotic bleeding was the cause in 19% (n = 15); other anomalies were associated in

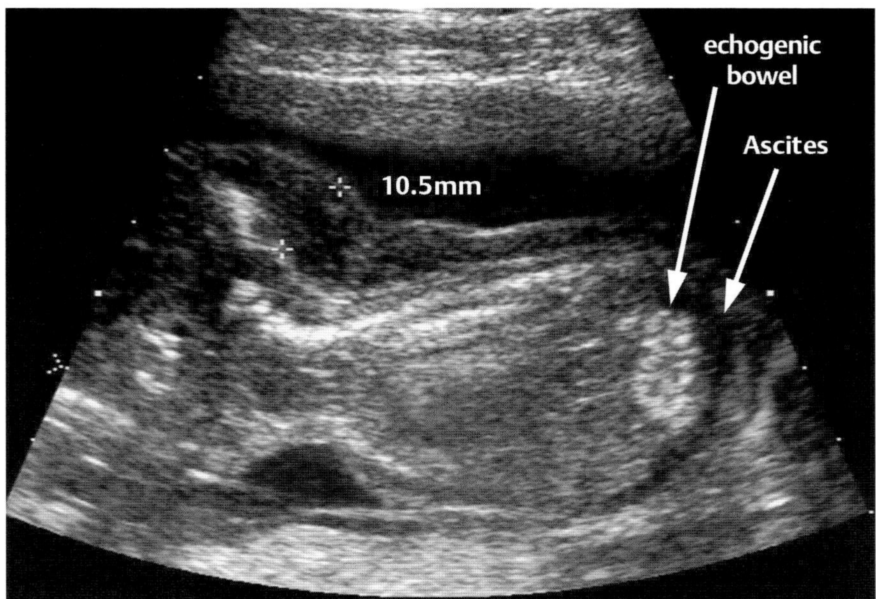

Fig. 10.3 **Echogenic bowel.** The scan shows echogenic bowel as well as ascites and hygroma colli in a fetus with trisomy 21.

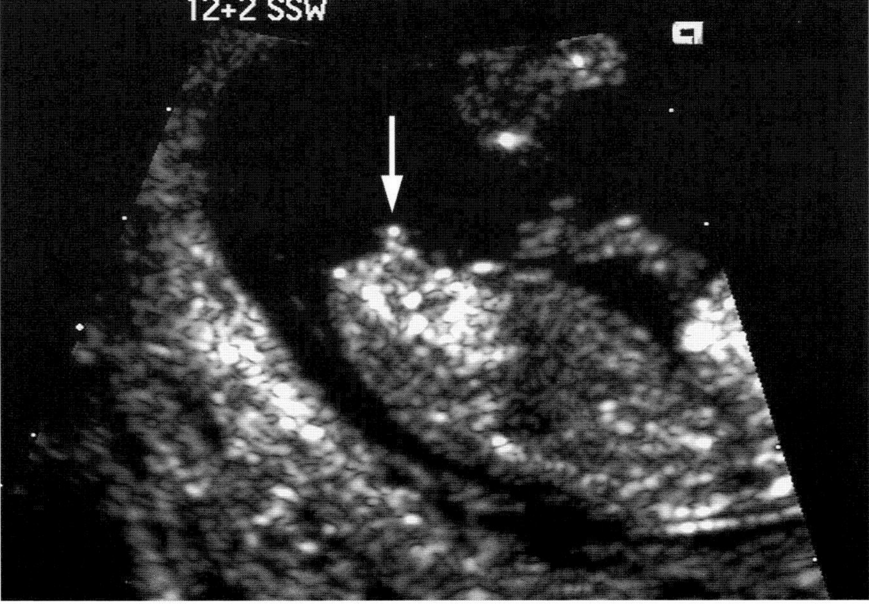

Fig. 10.4 **Echogenic bowel.** Longitudinal section of a male fetus (arrow: penis) at 12 + 2 weeks.

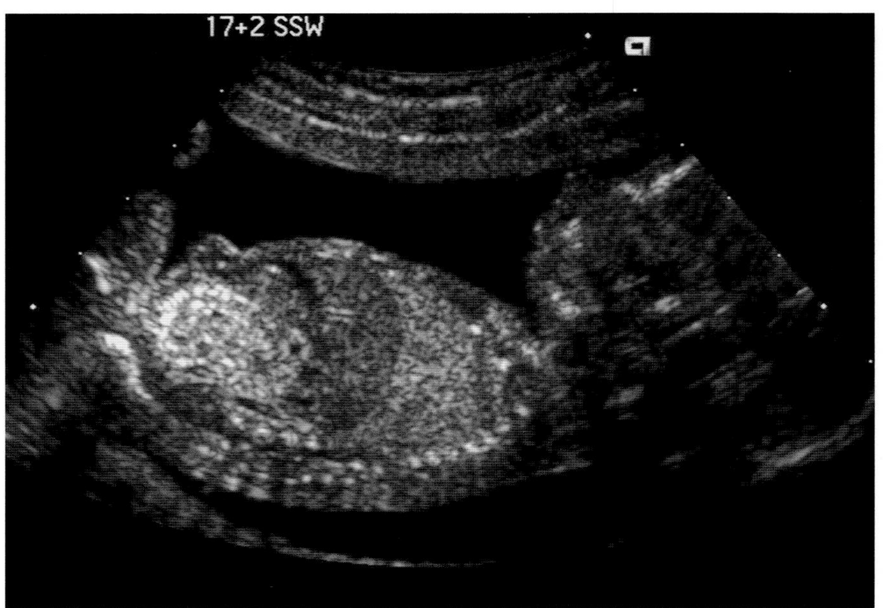

Fig. 10.5 **Echogenic bowel.** Fetus at 17 + 2 weeks.

8% (n = 7); seven fetuses were affected in multiple pregnancies; and five (6.3%) showed bowel obstruction without cystic fibrosis. Chromosomal aberrations were found in five cases, and in a further five cases, intrauterine infection was the cause. Cystic fibrosis was diagnosed in only two cases (2.5%). Three fetuses (3.8%) were stillborn without any obvious cause. Hogge et al. reported two cases of cystic fibrosis in four detected cases.

Clinical management: Further ultrasound screening, including fetal echocardiography, karyotyping, TORCH serology, exclusion of cystic fibrosis (frequency 2–3%). Pregnancy should be followed up closely, using Doppler monitoring, as there is a high risk of stillbirth.

Prognosis: Benacerraf found Down syndrome in 16% of cases of echogenic bowel; the findings were isolated, with no other anomaly, in only 1.4% of cases of echogenic bowel. Sipes et al. observed spontaneous disappearance of echogenic bowel in five of seven cases during the course of pregnancy; in the other two cases, the infants did not show any anomalies after birth. Nicolaides reports that there is a fivefold increase in the incidence of Down syndrome in fetuses with echogenic bowel.

References

Al-Kouatly HB, Chasen ST, Streltzoff J, Chervenak FA. The clinical significance of fetal echogenic bowel. Am J Obstet Gynecol 2001; 185: 1035–8.

Dunne M, Haney P, Sun CC. Sonographic features of bowel perforation and calcific meconium peritonitis in utero. Pediatr Radiol 1983; 13: 231–3.

Font GE, Solari M. Prenatal diagnosis of bowel obstruction initially manifested as isolated hyperechoic bowel. J Ultrasound Med 1998; 17: 721–3.

Hogge WA, Hogge JS, Boehm CD, Sanders RC. Increased echogenicity in the fetal abdomen: use of DNA analysis to establish a diagnosis of cystic fibrosis. J Ultrasound Med 1993; 12: 451–4.

Nyberg DA, Souter VL, El-Bastawissi A, Young S, Luthhardt F, Luthy DA. Isolated sonographic markers for detection of fetal Down syndrome in the second trimester of pregnancy. J Ultrasound Med 2001; 20: 1053–63.

Sipes SL, Weiner CP, Wenstrom KD, Williamson RA, Grant SS, Mueller GM. Fetal echogenic bowel on ultrasound: is there clinical significance? Fetal Diagn Ther 1994; 9: 38–43.

Smith-Bindman R, Hosmer W, Feldstein VA, Deeks JJ, Goldberg JD. Second-trimester ultrasound to detect fetuses with Down syndrome: a meta-analysis. JAMA 2001; 285: 1044–55.

Souter VL, Nyberg DA, El-Bastawissi A, Zebelman A, Luthhardt F, Luthy DA. Correlation of ultrasound findings and biochemical markers in the second trimester of pregnancy in fetuses with trisomy 21. Prenat Diagn 2002; 22: 175–82.

Yaron Y, Hassan S, Geva E, Kupferminc MJ, Yavetz H, Evans MI. Evaluation of fetal echogenic bowel in the second trimester. Fetal Diagn Ther 1999; 14: 176–80.

Echogenic Kidneys

Definition and clinical significance: The kidneys are more echogenic than the liver. This may be a normal finding, or may be the first sign of nephrotic syndrome or other renal anomalies. A case associated with cytomegalovirus infection has been reported. Benacerraf published 19 cases, in which there was a normal postnatal outcome in only four (21%). Five (26%) died and had either infantile polycystic kidneys or multicystic renal dysplasia. In two cases, oligohydramnios only developed after 24 weeks; in one case, partial trisomy 10 was found.

Associated syndromes: Infantile polycystic kidneys, Meckel–Gruber syndrome, trisomy 13, Perlman syndrome, cystic renal dysplasia, Beckwith–Wiedemann syndrome.

Ultrasound findings: The volume of the kidneys is increased (above the 95th percentile), with a high echogenicity. If the renal function is affected, oligohydramnios or anhydramnios are found and the bladder is hardly filled. In some cases, oligohydramnios may even be detected at 15 weeks.

Prognosis: The decisive prognostic criterion is renal function, determined by the extent of amniotic fluid. Cases of severe oligohydramnios have a poor outcome.

References

Carr MC, Benacerraf BR, Estroff JA, Mandell J. Prenatally diagnosed bilateral hyperechoic kidneys with normal amniotic fluid: postnatal outcome. J Urol 1995; 153: 442–4.

Choong KK, Gruenewald SM, Hodson EM. Echogenic fetal kidneys in cytomegalovirus infection. J Clin Ultrasound 1993; 21: 128–32.

Lilford RJ, Irving HC, Allibone EB. A tale of two prior probabilities: avoiding the false positive antenatal diagnosis of autosomal-recessive polycystic kidney disease. Br J Obstet Gynaecol 1992; 99: 216–9.

Nyberg DA, Hallesy D, Mahony BS, Hirsch JH, Luthy DA, Hickok D. Meckel–Gruber syndrome: importance of prenatal diagnosis. J Ultrasound Med 1990; 9: 691–6.

Vintzileos AM, Egan JF. Adjusting the risk for trisomy 21 on the basis of second-trimester ultrasonography [review]. Am J Obstet Gynecol 1995; 172: 837–44.

Wisser J, Hebisch G, Froster U, et al. Prenatal sonographic diagnosis of autosomal-recessive polycystic kidney disease (ARPKD) during the early second trimester. Prenat Diagn 1995; 15: 868–71.

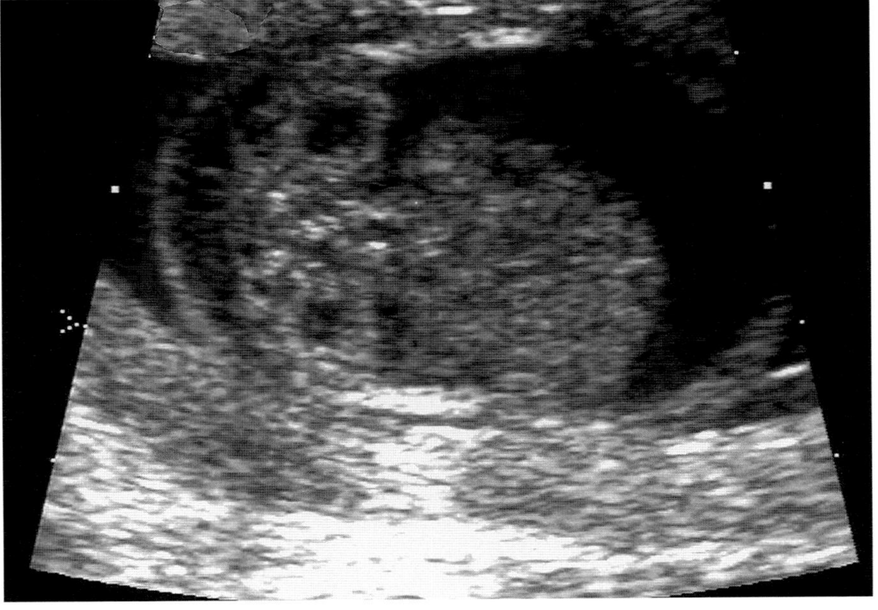

Fig. 10.6 **Echogenic kidneys.** Dilation of the renal pelvis and fetal ascites in a fetus with trisomy 9.

Mild Ventriculomegaly

Definition: The upper limit of the width of the posterior horn of lateral cerebral ventricle lies at 8–10 mm. Dilation of the posterior horn above 10 mm is definitely a pathological finding. Mild ventriculomegaly is regarded as a soft marker for chromosomal aberrations. It may be a harmless finding, or may be the earliest sign of a developing hydrocephalus.

Ultrasound findings: The posterior horns of the lateral ventricles (the first and second ventricles) can be well detected and measured behind the choroid plexus. As defined above, one differentiates between the marginal form (8–10 mm) and pathological form (> 10 mm) of ventriculomegaly. Asymmetrical dilation of the ventricles is a common finding. On scanning, the ventricle lying nearest to the transducer is difficult to measure, due to loss of scanning intensity immediately behind the skull bone. However, by changing the plane of the transducer and thus altering the angle, it is almost always possible to demonstrate it, especially in the second trimester.

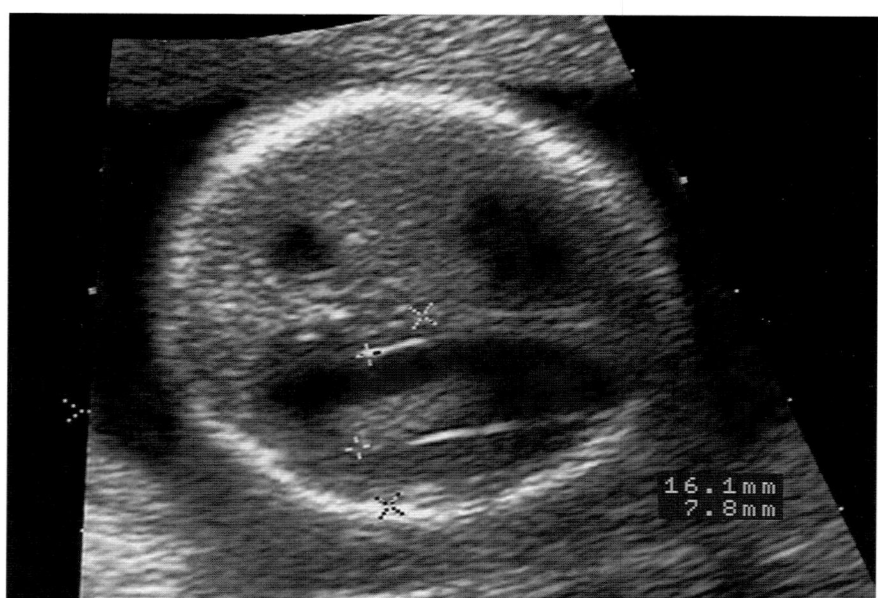

Fig. 10.**7** **Mild ventriculomegaly.** Marginal dilation of the cerebral ventricles: 7.8 mm at 15 + 6 weeks, in a fetus with trisomy 13.

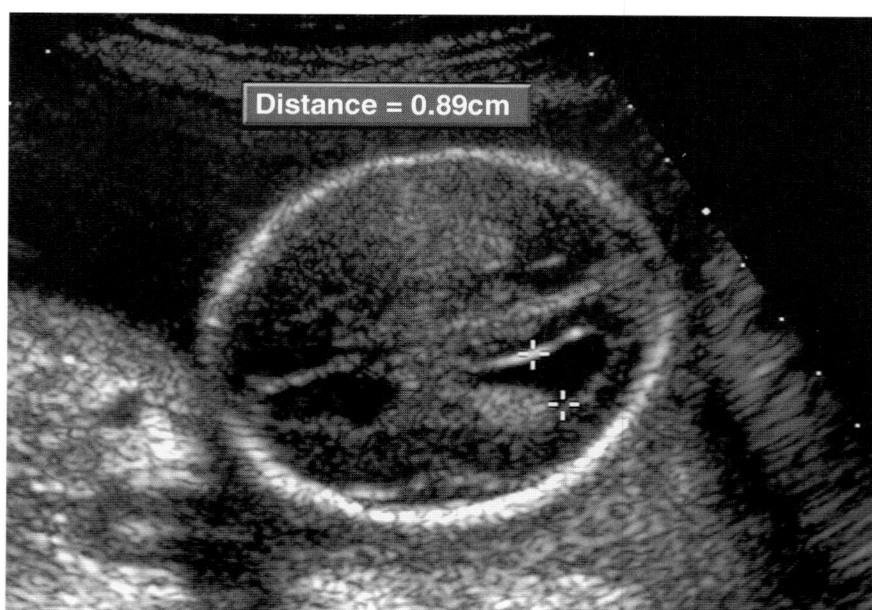

Fig. 10.**8** **Mild ventriculomegaly.** The width of the posterior horn of the left lateral ventricle is 8.9 mm, without pathology.

Associated syndromes: Goldenhar syndrome, Gorlin syndrome, hydrolethalus, Meckel–Gruber syndrome, Miller–Dieker syndrome, Neu–Laxova syndrome, Mohr syndrome, spinal dysraphism, Walker–Warburg syndrome, X-chromosome hydrocephalus, achondroplasia, camptomelic dysplasia, chondrodysplasia punctata, Fanconi anemia, metatrophic dysplasia, multiple pterygium syndrome, osteopetrosis, Roberts syndrome, Apert syndrome, Crouzon syndrome, Pfeiffer syndrome, 11 q deletion, triploidy, trisomy 9/13/18/21, arthrogryposis, CHARGE association, Fryns syndrome, renal agenesis.

Clinical management: Further ultrasound screening, including fetal echocardiography, TORCH serology (especially cytomegalovirus infection, toxoplasmoses). Karyotyping should be offered.

Procedure after birth: The finding should be confirmed by transfontanelle scanning of the neonate's skull. The plane of measurement used in prenatal scanning is not always reproducible after birth, so that confirmation of the diagnosis after birth is often difficult.

Prognosis: Studies regarding the clinical significance of mild ventriculomegaly are difficult to interpret, due to the small number of cases investigated. The prognosis is favorable if there are no other associated anomalies and a normal karyotype exists. Goldstein et al. reported only one death in nine cases without other anomalies. If other malformations were present, then nine of 16 affected infants died. Benacerraf examined 44 fetuses with ventricle measurements of 10–12 mm and found an abnormal karyotype in 12%. Seventy-two percent of the affected infants with a normal karyotype showed normal mental development. In cases of mild ventriculomegaly, 80% developed normally. Patel et al. reported that 75% of fetuses with a ventricle width of 10–11 mm were male. The sex was a decisive prognostic factor in this study: within the first year of life, 75% of male infants developed normally, in comparison to only 50% of affected females. Mild ventriculomegaly may normalize in course of the pregnancy, but the development of hydrocephalus has also been observed.

References

Abramowicz J, Jaffe R. Diagnosis and intrauterine management of enlargement of the cerebral ventricles. Perinat Med 1988; 16: 165–73.

Cardoza JD, Goldstein RB, Filly RA. Exclusion of fetal ventriculomegaly with a single measurement: the width of the lateral ventricular atrium. Radiology 1988; 169: 711–4.

Chervenak FA, Berkowitz RL, Tortora M, Chitkara U, Hobbins JC. Diagnosis of ventriculomegaly before fetal viability. Obstet Gynecol 1984; 64: 652–6.

Chervenak FA, Duncan C, Ment LIZ, et al. Outcome of fetal ventriculomegaly. Lancet 1984; ii: 179–81.

Glick PL, Harrison MR, Nakayama DK, et al. Management of ventriculomegaly in the fetus. J Pediatr 1984; 105: 97–105.

Goldstein RB, La Pidus AS, Filly RA, Cardoza J. Mild lateral cerebral ventricular dilatation in utero: clinical significance and prognosis. Radiology 1990; 176: 237–42.

Graham E, Duhl A, Ural S, Allen M, Blakemore K, Witter F. The degree of antenatal ventriculomegaly is related to pediatric neurological morbidity. J Matern Fetal Med 2001; 10: 258–63.

Greco P, Vimercati A, De Cosmo L, Laforgia N, Mautone A, Selvaggi L. Mild ventriculomegaly as a counselling challenge. Fetal Diagn Ther 2001; 16: 398–401.

Greco P, Vimercati A, Selvaggi L. Isolated mild fetal cerebral ventriculomegaly. Prenat Diagn 2002; 22: 162–3.

Kelly EN, Allen VM, Seaward G, Windrim R, Ryan G. Mild ventriculomegaly in the fetus: natural history, associated findings and outcome of isolated mild ventriculomegaly—a literature review. Prenat Diagn 2001; 21: 697–700.

Ko TM, Hwa HL, Tseng LH, Hsieh FJ, Huang SF, Lee TY. Prenatal diagnosis of X-linked hydrocephalus in a Chinese family with four successive affected pregnancies. Prenat Diagn 1994; 14: 57–60.

Lipitz S, Yagel S, Malinger G, Meizner I, Zalel Y, Achiron R. Outcome of fetuses with isolated borderline unilateral ventriculomegaly diagnosed at mid-gestation. Ultrasound Obstet Gynecol 1998; 12: 23–6.

Nicolaides KH, Berry S, Snijders RJ, Thorpe BJ, Gosden C. Fetal lateral cerebral ventriculomegaly: associated malformations and chromosomal defects. Fetal Diagn Ther 1990; 5: 5–14.

Patel MD, Filly AL, Hersh DR, Goldstein RB. Isolated mild fetal cerebral ventriculomegaly: clinical course and outcome. Radiology 1994; 192: 759–64.

Souter VL, Nyberg DA, El-Bastawissi A, Zebelman A, Luthhardt F, Luthy DA. Correlation of ultrasound findings and biochemical markers in the second trimester of pregnancy in fetuses with trisomy 21. Prenat Diagn 2002; 22: 175–82.

Stefanou EG, Hanna G, Foakes A, Crocker M, Fitchett M. Prenatal diagnosis of cri du chat (5 p–) syndrome in association with isolated moderate bilateral ventriculomegaly. Prenat Diagn 2002; 22: 64–6.

Toi A. Spontaneous resolution of fetal ventriculomegaly in a diabetic patient. J Ultrasound Med 1987; 6: 37–39.

Ulm B, Ulm MR, Deutinger J, Bernaschek G. Dandy–Walker malformation diagnosed before 21 weeks of gestation: associated malformations and chromosomal abnormalities. Ultrasound Obstet Gynecol 1997; 10: 167–70.

Mild Dilation of the Renal Pelvis

Definition and clinical significance: The normal width of the renal pelvis is dependent on the gestational age. A renal pelvic dilation of more than 4.5 mm in the anterior–posterior diameter in the second trimester is considered to be a marginal form. The finding is usually harmless and affects male and female fetuses. Repeated check-ups during the course of the pregnancy and after birth are advised. The significance of this finding as a soft marker for chromosomal aberrations, especially for Down syndrome, is disputed. Benacerraf found Down syndrome in 3.3% of fetuses with marginal pelvic distension, and 25% of fetuses with Down syndrome showed marginal pelvic distension. If other anomalies are not detected, then only one case of Down syndrome is to be expected in 340 cases of mild dilation of the renal pelvis. According to Nicolaides et al., the risk of Down syndrome is increased by a factor of 1.5 above that of age related risk.

Incidence: 2% of fetuses in the second trimester.

Ultrasound findings: The renal pelvis can be detected well as echo-free structures in the kidneys. Kidneys can be observed in all three planes. Measurement of the anteroposterior diameter is carried out on the axial plane of the abdomen. A horizontal level is selected, without deviating in the cranial or caudal direction. The upper limit lies at 4.5 mm at 22 weeks of gestation. If pelvic distension is diagnosed, then the kidneys should be scanned in all three planes.

Caution: The anteroposterior diameter has to be demonstrated exactly for accurate measurement. Slight tilting of the angle or use of the wrong plane tend to give higher values, even when there are normal kidneys.

Clinical management: Further ultrasound screening, including fetal echocardiography; karyotyping should be offered. Scan control in the third trimester. Renal scan after birth.

Procedure after birth: If the findings persist well into the third trimester, the kidneys should be scanned after birth.

Prognosis: In most cases, the finding is harmless and normalizes spontaneously. Rarely, pathological dilation of the renal pelvis may develop further on.

References

Dorin S, Dufour P, Valat AS, et al. Ultrasonographic signs of chromosome aberrations. J Gynecol Obstet Biol Reprod (Paris) 1998; 27: 290–7.

Feldman DM, DeCambre M, Kong E, et al. Evaluation and follow-up of fetal hydronephrosis. J Ultrasound Med 2001; 20: 1065–9.

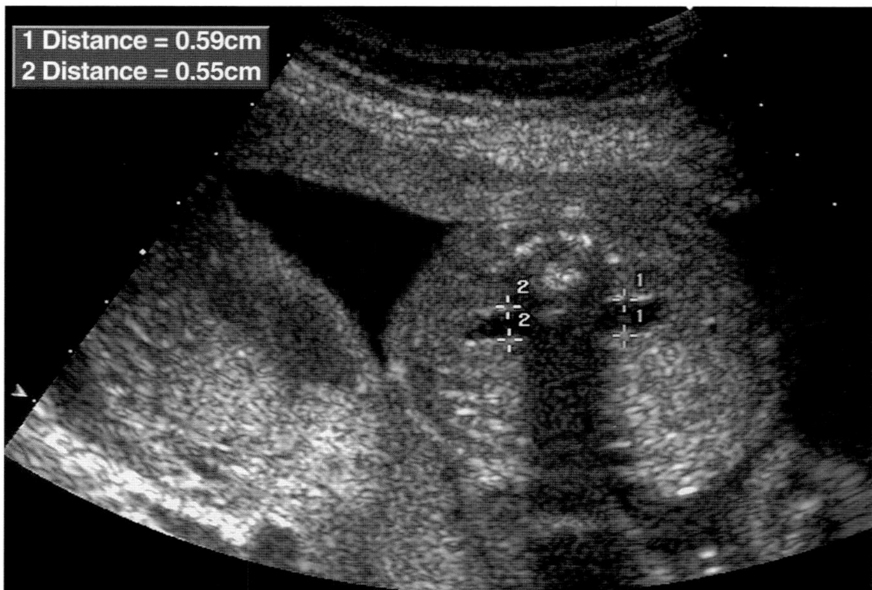

Fig. 10.**9** **Mild dilation of renal pelvis.** The renal pelves are marginally dilated—5.5 mm and 5.9 mm at 22 + 4 weeks. No other pathology was detected. Normal karyotype.

Nicolaides KH, Snijders RJ, Gosden CM, Berry C, Campbell S. Ultrasonographically detectable markers of fetal chromosomal abnormalities. Lancet 1992; 340: 704–7.

Sairam S, Al-Habib A, Sasson S, Thilaganathan B. Natural history of fetal hydronephrosis diagnosed on mid-trimester ultrasound. Ultrasound Obstet Gynecol 2001; 17: 191–6.

Snijders RJ, Sebire NJ, Faria M, Patel F, Nicolaides KH. Fetal mild hydronephrosis and chromosomal defects: relation to maternal age and gestation. Fetal Diagn Ther 1995; 10: 349–55.

Short Femur

Definition and clinical significance: This is defined as length of femur below the 5th percentile for the gestational age, or a ratio of BPD to femur that lies above the 95th percentile. In Down syndrome, short femur appears statistically more often than in the normal chromosomal set. In addition, shortened femur may be the first sign of skeletal dysplasia.

Incidence: According to the above definition, 5% of all fetuses.

Caution: The femur is not shortened significantly in all cases of chromosomal aberrations, especially in Down syndrome, in comparison with a healthy fetus. The biological range and possible inaccuracies in measurement are so extensive that shortening of the femur or a pathological BPD/femur ratio cannot be relied on as a marker for detecting chromosomal aberration. If the suspected finding is mentioned to the mother, it causes such uncertainty that reassurance is very difficult if karyotyping has not been done. The question is what value should be considered relevant for detecting Down syndrome. Very wide variations from the normal value should alert the physician to carry out detailed scanning of the other structures. Even then, for methodological reasons, chromosomal aberration cannot be definitively excluded. The parents should be counseled using computerized risk assessment (developed by Nicolaides) and risk for Down syndrome due to maternal age. Nyberg et al. reported shortening of the femur in only 14% of fetuses (seven of 49 cases) with Down syndrome, compared to 6% of fetuses (35 of 572) with normal chromosomes.

References

Ashkenazy M, Lurie S, Ben Itzhak I, Appelman Z, Caspi B. Unilateral congenital short femur: a case report. Prenat Diagn 1990; 10: 67–70.

Benacerraf BR, Gelman R, Frigoletto FDJ. Sonographic identification of second-trimester fetuses with Down's syndrome. N Engl J Med 1987; 317: 1371–6.

Campbell J, Henderson A, Campbell S. The fetal femur/foot length ratio: a new parameter to assess dysplastic limb reduction. Obstet Gynecol 1988; 72: 181–4.

Graham M. Congenital short femur: prenatal sonographic diagnosis. J Ultrasound Med 1985; 4: 361–3.

Keret D, Timor IE. Familial congenital short femur: intrauterine detection and follow-up by ultrasound: a case report. Orthop Rev 1988; 17: 500–4.

LaFollette L, Filly RA, Anderson R, Golbus MS. Fetal femur length to detect trisomy 21: a reappraisal. J Ultrasound Med 1989; 8: 657–60.

Makino Y, Inoue T Shirota K, Kubota S, Kobayashi H, Kawarabayashi T. A case of congenital familial short femur diagnosed prenatally. Fetal Diagn Ther 1998; 13: 206–8.

Nyberg DA, Resta RG, Hickok DE, Hollenbach KA, Luthy DA, Mahony BS. Femur length shortening in the detection of Down syndrome: is prenatal screening feasible? Am J Obstet Gynecol 1990; 162: 1247–52.

Pierce BT, Hancock EG, Kovac CM, Napolitano PG, Hume RF Jr, Calhoun BC. Influence of gestational age and maternal height on fetal femur length calculations. Obstet Gynecol 2001; 97: 742–6.

Ranzini AC, Guzman ER, Ananth CV, Day-Salvatore D, Fisher AJ, Vintzileos AM. Sonographic identification of fetuses with Down syndrome in the third trimester: a matched control study. Obstet Gynecol 1999; 93: 702–6.

Snijders RJ, Platt LD, Greene N, et al. Femur length and trisomy 21: impact of gestational age on screening efficiency. Ultrasound Obstet Gynecol 2000; 16: 142–5.

Sohl BD, Scioscia AL, Budorick NE, Moore TR. Utility of minor ultrasonographic markers in the prediction of abnormal fetal karyotype at a prenatal diagnostic center. Am J Obstet Gynecol 1999; 181: 898–903.

Twining P, Whalley DR, Lewin E, Foulkes K. Is a short femur length a useful ultrasound marker for Down's syndrome? Br J Radiol 1991; 64: 990–2.

Vintzileos AM, Egan JF, Smulian JC, Campbell WA, Guzman ER, Rodis JF. Adjusting the risk for trisomy 21 by a simple ultrasound method using fetal long-bone biometry. Obstet Gynecol 1996; 87: 953–8.

Nuchal Translucency

Definition and clinical significance: Measurement of nuchal fold (neck) thickness. Echo-free area ("black space") in neck region between skin and soft tissue. Evaluated according to the percentile curves published by the Fetal Medicine Foundation, taking into account the crown–rump length. For assessment of the risk of chromosomal abnormalities, gestational age and maternal age are taken into account. The upper value lies at 2.5–3.0 mm when all the above-mentioned parameters are considered. If the measured value lies higher than this, the risk for Down syndrome and other chromosomal disorders is increased. The risk is stated as a ratio—1 : 100 or 1 : 1000. Measurements are carried out between 11 and 13 weeks.

Incidence: According to the stated definition, about 5% of fetuses demonstrate increased nuchal translucency (above the 95th percentile).

Embryology: The thickened nuchal fold (neck area) of the fetus is believed to be due to collection of lymph. Dilation of the lymph vessels can be demonstrated in histological sections. Detection of septa within this area is highly suspicious of chromosomal anomaly.

Associated malformations: Fetuses with a normal karyotype and a pathological value for nuchal translucency have an increased risk of cardiac defects (especially aortic isthmus stenosis, VSD). In addition, other syndromes and skeletal anomalies are associated.

Associated syndromes: Cornelia de Lange syndrome, Noonan syndrome, Smith–Lemli–Opitz syndrome, Joubert syndrome, achondrogenesis, ectrodactyly–ectodermal dysplasia–clefting syndrome (EEC), multiple pterygium syndrome, Roberts syndrome, Apert syndrome, tetrasomy 12 p, triploidy, trisomy 10/13/18/21/22, Turner syndrome, Fryns syndrome, thanatophoric dysplasia.

Ultrasound findings: The following measures are advised for standardized assessment: the fetus should be viewed in the sagittal plane. The magnification should be such that the fetus fills the whole screen. The vertebral column should be positioned at the bottom, if possible. The head should be neither flexed nor overextended. The gestational age should be between 11 + 3 and 13 + 6 weeks, the crown–rump length measuring 47–84 mm. With these criteria, it is possible to detect 70–80% of fetuses with trisomy. The rate of false-negative findings is 4.1%. Spontaneous regression of abnormal nuchal translucency after 14 weeks does not necessarily mean a normal karyotype.

Caution: The amnion can be mistaken for neck skin, leading to false-positive measurements of increased nuchal translucency.

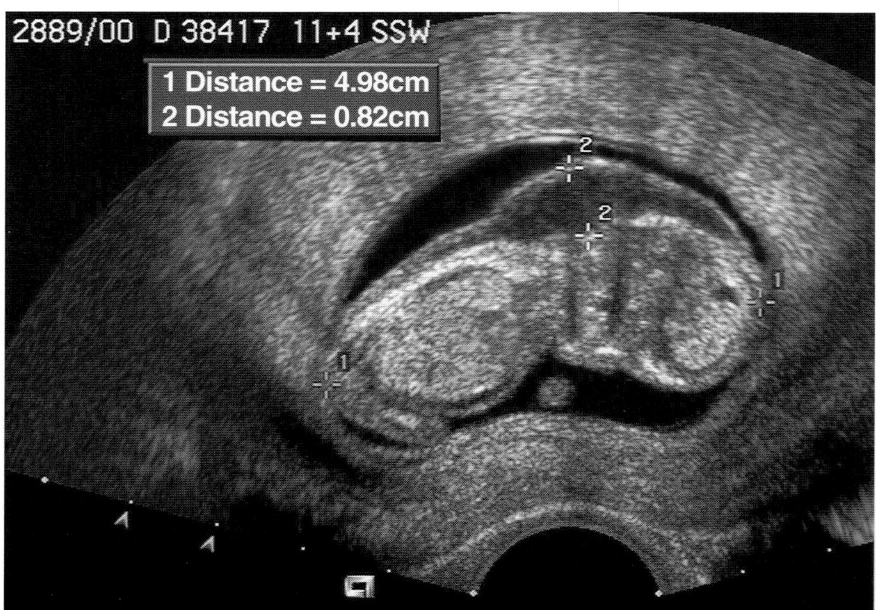

Fig. 10.**10** **Nuchal translucency.** Hygroma colli of 8 mm in fetal Turner syndrome.

Clinical management: When there are pathological findings, karyotyping should be offered (chorionic villus sampling), and careful ultrasound scanning of other organs, including echocardiography, should be performed.

Prognosis: If no other anomalies are associated, then the regression of nuchal edema is spontaneous and the prognosis is good.

Further information: Internet www.fetalmedicine.com

References

Areias JC, Matias A, Montenegro N, Brandao O. Early antenatal diagnosis of cardiac defects using transvaginal Doppler ultrasound: new perspectives? Fetal Diagn Ther 1998; 13: 111–4.

Benattar C, Audibert F, Taieb J, et al. Efficiency of ultrasound and biochemical markers for Down's syndrome risk screening: a prospective study. Fetal Diagn Ther 1999; 14: 112–7.

Biagiotti R, Brizzi L, Periti E, dAgata A, Vanzi E, Cariati E. First trimester screening for Down's syndrome using maternal serum PAPP-A and free beta-hCG in combination with fetal nuchal translucency thickness. Br J Obstet Gynaecol 1998; 105: 917–20.

Bindra R, Heath V, Liao A, Spencer K, Nicolaides KH. One-stop clinic for assessment of risk for trisomy 21 at 11–14 weeks: a prospective study of 15 030 pregnancies. Ultrasound Obstet Gynecol 2002; 20: 219–25.

Carvalho JS, Mavrides E, Shinebourne EA, Campbell S, Thilaganathan B. Improving the effectiveness of routine prenatal screening for major congenital heart defects. Heart 2002; 88: 387–91.

Gasiorek-Wiens A, Tercanli S, Kozlowski P, et al. Screening for trisomy 21 by fetal nuchal translucency and maternal age: a multicenter project in Germany, Austria and Switzerland. Ultrasound Obstet Gynecol 2001; 18: 645–8.

Hyett JA, Perdu M, Sharland GK, Snijders RS, Nicolaides KH. Increased nuchal translucency at 10–14 weeks of gestation as a marker for major cardiac defects. Ultrasound Obstet Gynecol 1997; 10: 242–6.

Jackson M, Rose NC. Diagnosis and management of fetal nuchal translucency. Semin Roentgenol 1998; 33: 333–8.

Josefsson A, Molander E, Selbing A. Nuchal translucency as a screening test for chromosomal abnormalities in a routine first trimester ultrasound examination. Acta Obstet Gynecol Scand 1998; 77: 497–9.

Kornman LH, Morssink LP, Beekhuis JR, De Wolf BT, Heringa MP, Mantingh A. Nuchal translucency cannot be used as a screening test for chromosomal abnormalities in the first trimester of pregnancy in a routine ultrasound practice. Prenat Diagn 1996; 16: 797–805.

Maymon R, Padoa A, Dreazen E, Herman A. Nuchal translucency measurements in consecutive normal pregnancies: is there a predisposition to increased levels? Prenat Diagn 2002; 22: 759–62.

Pajkrt E, Bilardo CM, van Lith JM, Mol BW, Bleker OP. Nuchal translucency measurement in normal fetuses. Obstet Gynecol 1995; 86: 994–7.

Salomon LJ, Bernard JP, Taupin P, Benard C, Ville Y. Relationship between nuchal translucency at 11–14 weeks and nuchal fold at 20–24 weeks of gestation. Ultrasound Obstet Gynecol 2001; 18: 636–7.

Spencer K, Souter V, Tul N, Snijders R, Nicolaides KH. A screening program for trisomy 21 at 10–14 weeks using fetal nuchal translucency, maternal serum free beta-human chorionic gonadotropin and pregnancy-associated plasma protein-A. Ultrasound Obstet Gynecol 1999; 13: 231–7.

Choroid Plexus Cysts

Definition and clinical significance: Unilateral or bilateral cystic structures in the choroid plexus. Commonly seen only in the second trimester; later, spontaneous regression. Most frequent finding in trisomy 18 (choroid plexus cysts are detectable before 23 weeks in 43% of fetuses with trisomy 18).

Incidence: 1–2% of all fetuses in the second trimester.

Ultrasound findings: A *round or oval-shaped cystic structure* is found in the choroid plexus situated in the lateral ventricle. The finding may be unilateral or bilateral. The cystic structures may be unilocular or multilocular and vary in size from a few millimeters to 2 cm.

Caution: The posterior horn of the lateral ventricle can be mistaken for a cyst of the choroid plexus. Between 15 and 19 weeks, small plexus cysts are commonly found. After 19 weeks, they are rare.

Clinical management: Further ultrasound screening, including fetal echocardiography; karyotyping if necessary. The risk of a genetic disorder increases if other anomalies are found, such as slight limb anomalies. The plexus cysts alone do not disturb further cerebral development, and disappear spontaneously by about 25–29 weeks. Rarely, some cases of plexus cyst of the third ventricle may present after birth with internal hydrocephalus, due to obstruction of cerebrospinal fluid circulation. There are no prenatal observations regarding this finding.

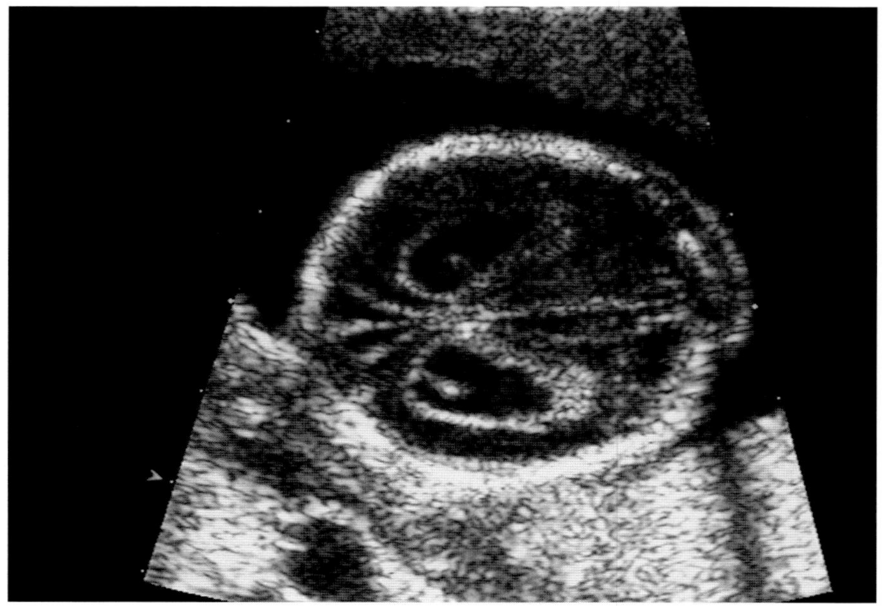

Fig. 10.**11** **Bilateral cystic lesions of the choroid plexus,** at 16 + 2 weeks. Normal karyotype. A healthy infant was born at the due date.

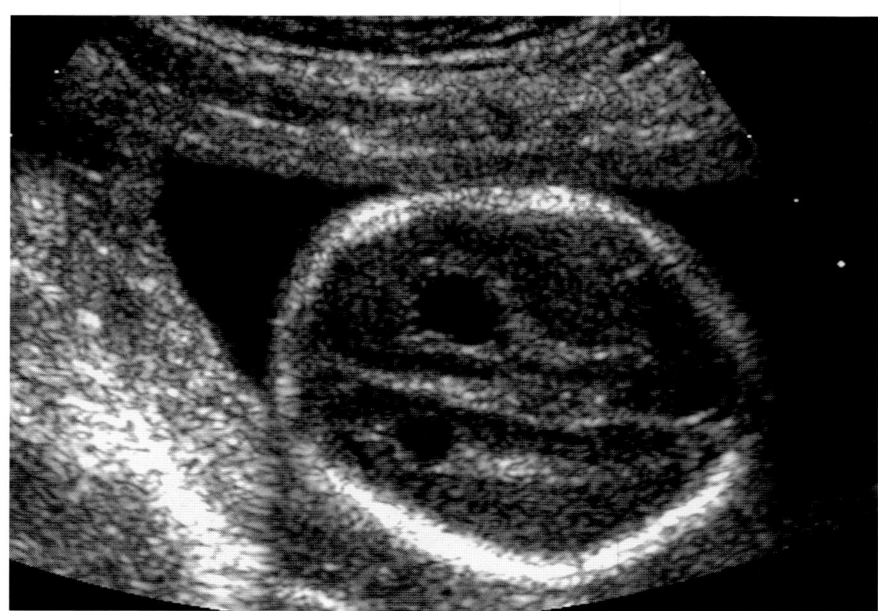

Fig. 10.**12** **Bilateral cysts of the choroid plexus.** Fetus with trisomy 18 at 22 + 5 weeks.

1 2 3 4 5

Procedure after birth: Ultrasound examination of the skull is advisable, to demonstrate normal findings and reassure the parents.

Prognosis: In the absence of other anomalies, the rate of chromosomal aberrations lies between one in 150 and one in 400. It is unimportant, whether the cysts are unilateral or bilateral. In the presence of associated anomalies, the rate of chromosomal disorders increases considerably. Isolated plexus cysts do not interfere with the infant's further development in any way.

References

Bakos O, Moen KS, Hansson S. Prenatal karyotyping of choroid plexus cysts. Eur J Ultrasound 1998; 8: 79–83.

Benacerraf BR. Asymptomatic cysts of the fetal choroid plexus in the second trimester. J Ultrasound Med 1987; 6: 475–8.

Bollmann R, Chaoui R, Zienert A, Körner H. Choroid plexus cysts in the 2nd trimester: an indication for trisomy 18. Zentralbl Gynäkol 1992; 114: 171–4.

Chudleigh P, Pearce JM, Campbell S. The prenatal diagnosis of transient cysts of the fetal choroid plexus. Prenat Diagn 1984; 4: 135–7.

Ghidini A, Strobelt N, Locatelli A, Mariani E, Piccoli MG, Vergani P. Isolated fetal choroid plexus cysts: role of ultrasonography in establishment of the risk of trisomy 18. Am J Obstet Gynecol 2000; 182: 972–7.

Gucer F, Yuce MA, Karasalihoglu S, Cakir B, Yardim T. Persistent large choroid plexus cyst: a case report. J Reprod Med 2001; 46: 256–8.

Howard RJ, Tuck SM, Long J, Thomas VA. The significance of choroid plexus cysts in fetuses at 18–20 weeks: an indication for amniocentesis? Prenat Diagn 1992; 12: 685–8.
Lodeiro JG, Feinstein SJ, Lodeiro SB. Late disappearance of fetal choroid plexus cyst: case report and review of the literature. Am J Perinatol 1989; 6: 450–2.
Sepulveda W, Lopez-Tenorio J. The value of minor ultrasound markers for fetal aneuploidy [review]. Curr Opin Obstet Gynecol 2001; 13: 183–91.
Sohn C, Gast AS, Krapfl E. Isolated fetal choroid plexus cysts: not an indication for genetic diagnosis? Fetal Diagn Ther 1997; 12: 255–9.
Viora E, Errante G, Bastonero S, Sciarrone A, Campogrande M. Minor sonographic signs of trisomy 21 at 15–20 weeks' gestation in fetuses born without malformations: a prospective study. Prenat Diagn 2001; 21: 1163–6.
Walkinshaw SA. Fetal choroid plexus cysts: are we there yet? Prenat Diagn 2000; 20: 657–62.

Single Umbilical Artery (SUA)

Definition: Only two vessels are found in the umbilical cord—one umbilical vein and one umbilical artery, instead of two umbilical arteries.

Incidence: 1 % of pregnancies.

Clinical history: Increased incidence in twin pregnancies and in diabetes mellitus.

Associated malformations: Other anomalies are found in 20% of cases, especially those affecting the heart and the urogenital system. Renal malformations or renal agenesis are found, usually on the side on which the artery is missing. Chromosomal aberrations are more frequently associated. Intrauterine growth restriction in the third trimester is expected more often than usual in isolated finding of SUA, leading to a higher perinatal mortality.

Ultrasound findings: A cross-section of the umbilical cord shows only two vessels. If ultrasound conditions are unfavorable, it is difficult to detect cord vessels in free-floating cord. Using the Doppler color mapping, the umbilical arteries can almost always be demonstrated in early pregnancy, running on either side of the fetal urinary bladder. This makes it possible to diagnose the side on which the artery is missing.

Caution: It may be very difficult to detect SUA in a coil of umbilical cord without the help of Doppler color mapping. When the color Doppler settings are highly sensitive, a signal may be picked up from the femoral artery on the side of the fetal urinary bladder, leading to false interpretation of the findings.

Clinical management: Further ultrasound screening, including fetal echocardiography; karyotyping if necessary. Doppler ultrasound at 30 and 36 weeks to exclude possible placental insufficiency.

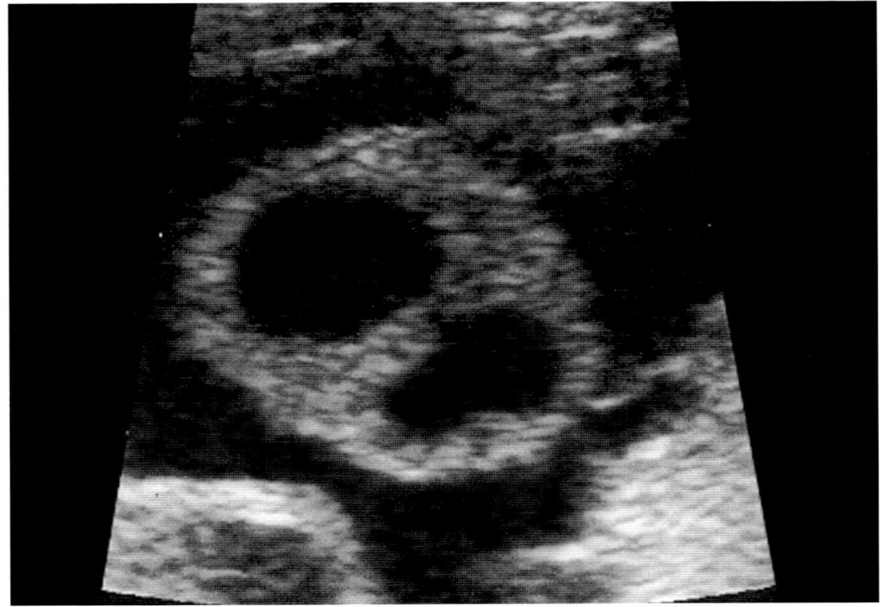

Fig. 10.**13** **Single umbilical artery.** Cross-section of the umbilical cord at 31 + 3 weeks.

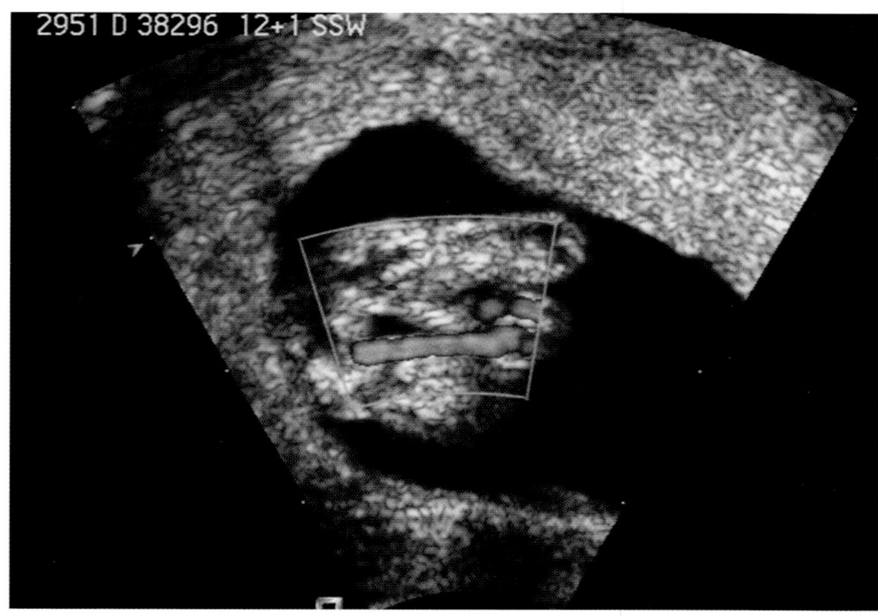

Fig. 10.**14** **Single umbilical artery.** A single umbilical artery is seen running on one side of the fetal urinary bladder; there is aplasia of the contralateral artery.

References

Aoki S, Hata T, Ariyuki Y, Makihara K, Hata K, Kitao M. Antenatal diagnosis of aberrant umbilical vessels. Gynecol Obstet Invest 1997; 43: 232–5.

Barr M Jr. Organ asymmetries as correlates of other anomalies. Am J Med Genet 2001; 101: 328–33.

Budorick NE, Kelly TF, Dunn JA, Scioscia AL. The single umbilical artery in a high-risk patient population: what should be offered? J Ultrasound Med 2001; 20: 619–27.

Catanzarite VA, Hendricks SK, Maida C, Westbrook C, Cousins L, Schrimmer D. Prenatal diagnosis of the two-vessel cord: implications for patient counselling and obstetric management. Ultrasound Obstet Gynecol 1995; 5: 98–105.

Goldkrand JW, Pettigrew C, Lentz SU, Clements SP, Bryant JL, Hodges J. Volumetric umbilical artery blood flow: comparison of the normal versus the single umbilical artery cord. J Matern Fetal Med 2001; 10: 116–21.

Jassani MN, Brennan JN, Merkatz IR. Prenatal diagnosis of single umbilical artery by ultrasound. JCU J Clin Ultrasound 1980; 8: 447–8.

Nyberg DA, Shepard T, Mack LA, Hirsch J, Luthy D, Fitzsimmons J. Significance of a single umbilical artery in fetuses with central nervous system malformations. J Ultrasound Med 1988; 7: 265–73.

Persutte WH, Hobbins J. Single umbilical artery: a clinical enigma in modern prenatal diagnosis. Ultrasound Obstet Gynecol 1995; 6: 216–29.

Pierce BT, Dance VD, Wagner RK, Apodaca CC, Nielsen PE, Calhoun BC. Perinatal outcome following fetal single umbilical artery diagnosis. J Matern Fetal Med 2001; 10: 59–63.

Raio L, Saile G, Bruhwiler H. Discordant umbilical cord arteries: prenatal diagnosis and significance. Ultraschall Med 1997; 18: 229–32.

Sepulveda WH. Antenatal sonographic detection of single umbilical artery. J Perinat Med 1991; 19: 391–5.

Wu MH, Chang FM, Shen MR, et al. Prenatal sonographic diagnosis of single umbilical artery. J Clin Ultrasound 1997; 25: 425–30.

White Spot (Echogenic Focus within the Heart)

Definition and clinical significance: Echogenic focus in the right ventricle, left ventricle, or both, appearing as an isolated focus or as a group of foci. These white spots have no functional significance and usually disappear in the third trimester. According to reports, these spots are considered to be a marker for chromosomal aberration, raising the risk slightly for Down syndrome and other genetic disorders.

Incidence: 2.0–7.4% of fetuses in the second trimester.

Embryology: These white spots represent microcalcifications in the papillary muscles and in the chordae tendineae at the mitral and tricuspid valves. In the course of the pregnancy, they usually disappear spontaneously.

Ultrasound findings: *Echogenic areas are seen in the right or the left cardiac ventricles.* They may be isolated or grouped findings. Detection depends on the level of contrast and the general sensitivity of the ultrasound apparatus. The echogenicity is as high as that of bone, and the

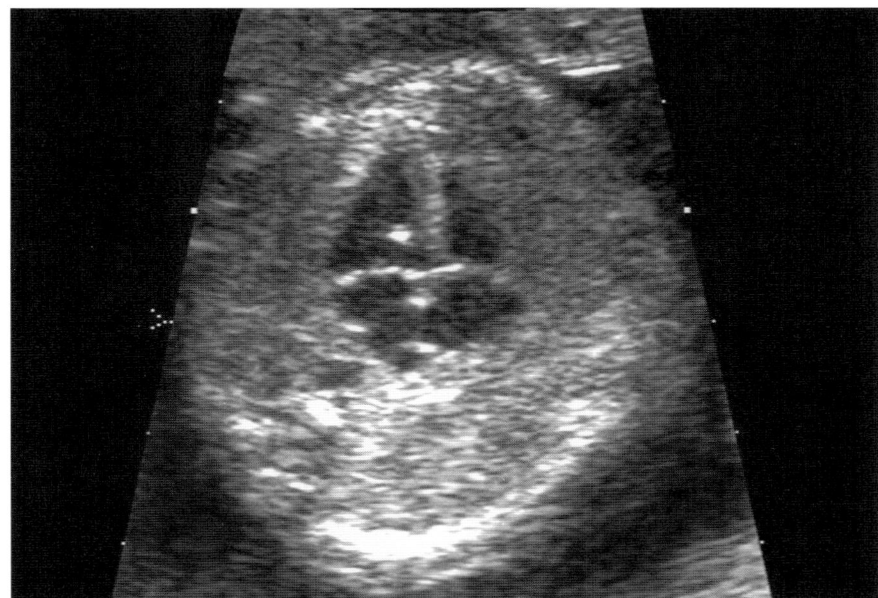

Fig. 10.**15** **White spot.** There is an echogenic focus in the left ventricle.

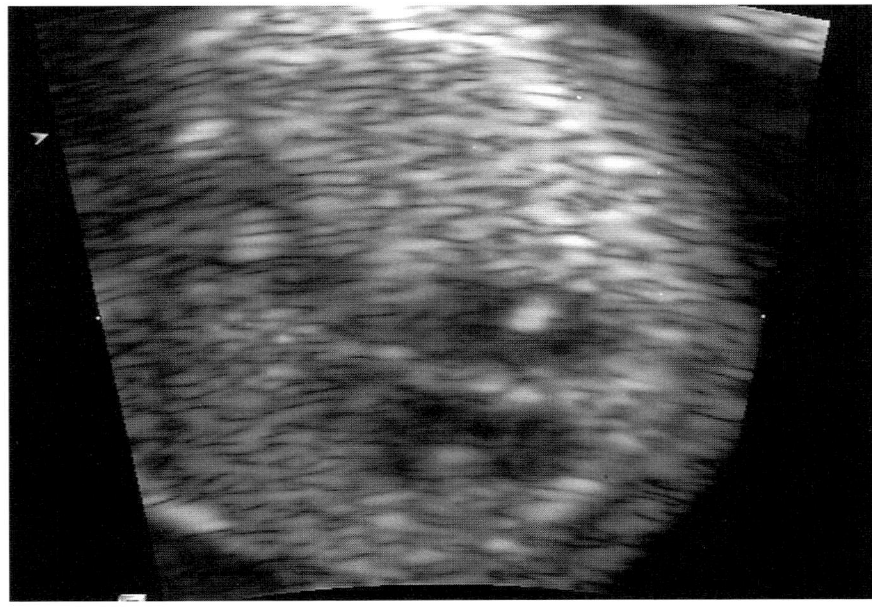

Fig. 10.**16** **White spot.** An echogenic focus seen in both ventricles at 12 + 5 weeks.

echogenicity of a vertebral body is used as a reference measurement. The findings are more frequent before 20 weeks of gestation rather than in late pregnancy.

Clinical management: Further ultrasound screening, including fetal echocardiography; possibly karyotyping.

Prognosis: Studies on this subject are controversial. Some reports do not describe any increase in the risk of chromosomal disorders; the majority, however, postulate a twofold to fourfold increase in the risk of Down syndrome. The risk is especially high if a complex pattern of white spots is present, or if the right ventricle is involved. Benacerraf found that, in 14 fetuses with Down syndrome, only one showed an isolated white spot without evidence of other anomalies; the maternal age in this case was 40 years.

References

Degani S, Leibovitz Z, Shapiro I, Gonen R, Ohel G. Cardiac function in fetuses with intracardiac echogenic foci. Ultrasound Obstet Gynecol 2001; 18: 131–4.

Petrikovsky B, Challenger M, Gross B. Unusual appearances of echogenic foci within the fetal heart: are they benign? Ultrasound Obstet Gynecol 1996; 8: 229–31.

Petrikovsky B, Klein V, Herrera M. Prenatal diagnosis of intra-atrial cardiac echogenic foci. Prenat Diagn 1998; 18: 968–70.

3

Prefumo F, Presti F, Mavrides E, et al. Isolated echogenic foci in the fetal heart: do they increase the risk of trisomy 21 in a population previously screened by nuchal translucency? Ultrasound Obstet Gynecol 2001; 18: 126–30.

Ranzini AC, McLean DA, Sharma S, Vintzileos AM. Fetal intracardiac echogenic foci: visualization depends on the orientation of the 4-chamber view. J Ultrasound Med 2001; 20: 763–6.

Schechter AG, Fakhry J, Shapiro LIZ, Gewitz MH. In utero thickening of the chordae tendineae: a cause of intracardiac echogenic foci. J Ultrasound Med 1987; 6: 691–5.

Wax JR, Royer D, Mather J, et al. A preliminary study of sonographic grading of fetal intracardiac echogenic foci: feasibility, reliability and association with aneuploidy. Ultrasound Obstet Gynecol 2000; 16: 123–7.

Selected Syndromes and Associations

11 Selected Syndromes and Associations

Apert Syndrome

Definition: Also known as acrocephalic syndactyly syndrome. It is characterized by a "tower-shaped" head, facial dysmorphism, and symmetrical syndactyly of the fingers and toes.

Incidence: about one in 100 000 births.

First described in 1906 by Apert.

Etiology/genetics: Partly autosomal-dominant inheritance, but frequently sporadic occurrence (new mutation). Advanced paternal age is a factor favoring its occurrence. Gene defect in the fibroblast growth factor receptor-2 gene (*FGFR2*), gene locus: 10 q26.

Clinical features: "Tower-shaped" head, early closure of cranial sutures, anomalies of the cervical vertebral column. Facial anomalies: denting of the forehead in the supraorbital region, hypertelorism, flat orbital bone, exophthalmos, squint, deep-set ears, small, beak-shaped nose, syndactyly (as extreme as "spoon hands"), fusion of the bony parts of fingers II–IV, short fingers, possibly short upper extremities. Mental impairment is not obligatory; in 80% of cases, the intelligence quotient lies above 50–70, and often it is normal. Other anomalies of the cardiac, renal, and gastrointestinal systems may also be present.

Ultrasound findings: The earliest prenatal diagnosis was possible at 12 weeks of gestation with *nuchal translucency* measurements. *Syndactyly* could also be detected at this stage. At a later stage, an unusual shape of the head resulting from premature closure of the cranial sutures (*tower-shaped head)* and facial dysmorphism (*hypoplasia of the midfacial region*) are characteristic features. Detailed scanning may also reveal deep-set ears, unusual shape of the nose, exophthalmos, and hypertelorism.

Differential diagnosis: Carpenter syndrome, Crouzon syndrome, cloverleaf skull anomaly, Pfeiffer syndrome, thanatophoric dysplasia, achondrogenesis, Cornelia de Lange syndrome, EEC syndrome, Fryns syndrome, Joubert syndrome, multiple pterygium syndrome, Noonan syndrome, Roberts syndrome, Smith–Lemli–Opitz syndrome, trisomy 21.

Clinical management: Further ultrasound screening including fetal echocardiography.

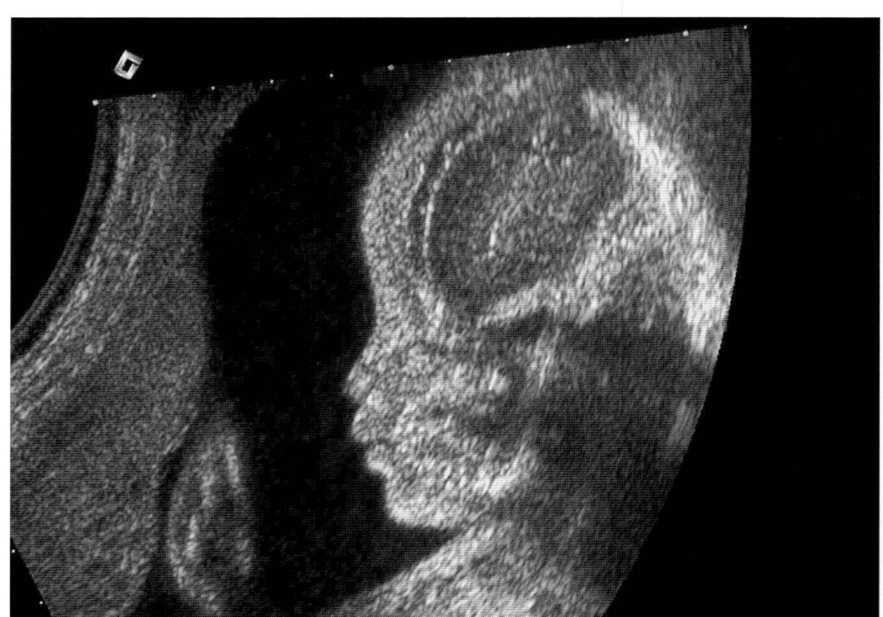

Fig. 11.**1** **Apert syndrome.** Fetal profile at 22 + 6 weeks. The striking feature is the high and prominent forehead.

Karyotyping (differential diagnosis), molecular-genetic evidence of the defective gene.

Prognosis: This depends on the extent of mental impairment and the associated organ anomalies. The mortality is increased in the first year of life.

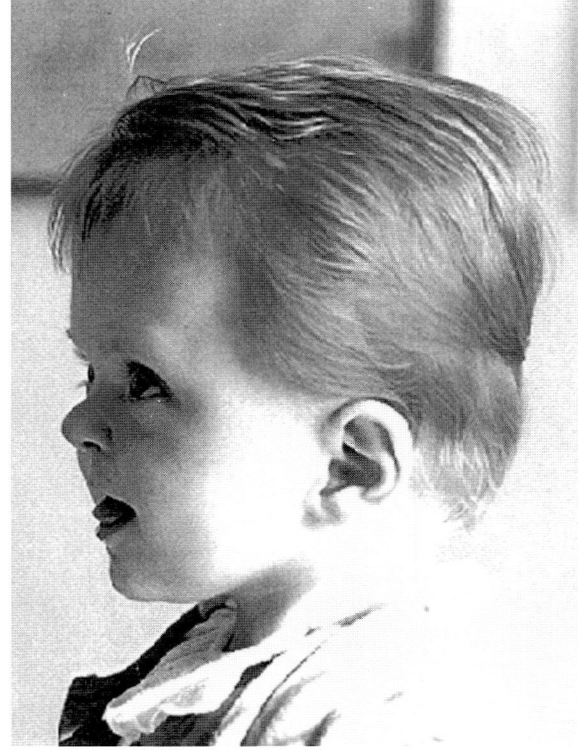

Fig. 11.2 **Apert syndrome.** Profile of a child with Apert syndrome.

Self-Help Organization

Title: Apert Syndrome Pen Pals

Description: Group correspondence program for persons with Apert syndrome to share experience. Information and referrals, pen pals, phone help.

Scope: National network

Founded: 1992

Address: P.O. Box 115, Providence, RI 02901, United States

Telephone: 401–454–0704 (after 4: 30 p.m.)

Title: Apert Support and Information Network

Description: Provides information and support to families and individuals facing the challenge of Apert syndrome. Provides information and referrals, newsletter, phone support network, pen pals, and annual family get-togethers.

Scope: International network

Founded: 1995

Address: P.O. Box 1184, Fair Oaks, CA 95628, United States

Telephone: 916–961–1092

Fax: 916–961–1092

E-mail: apertnet@ix.netcom.com

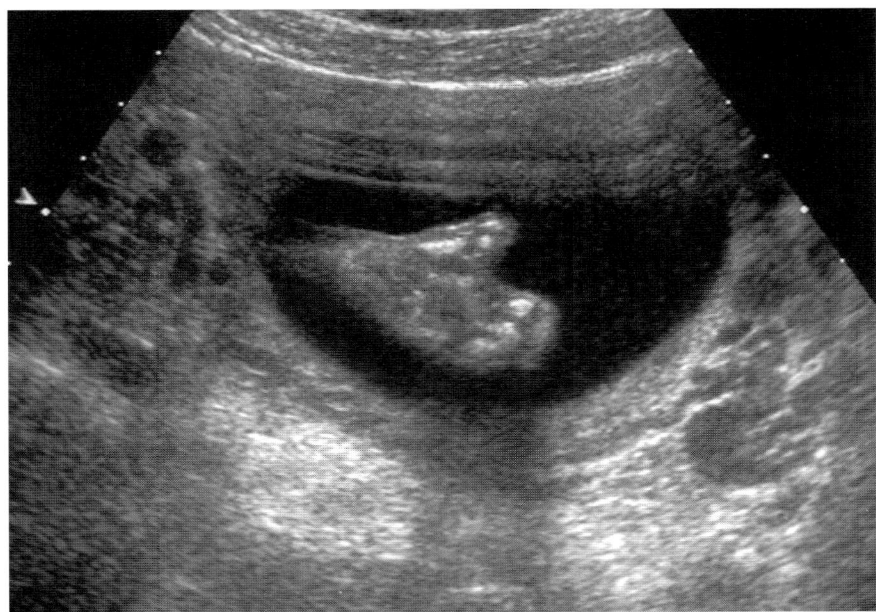

Fig. 11.3 **Apert syndrome.** Syndactyly of the hand, seen at 22 + 6 weeks.

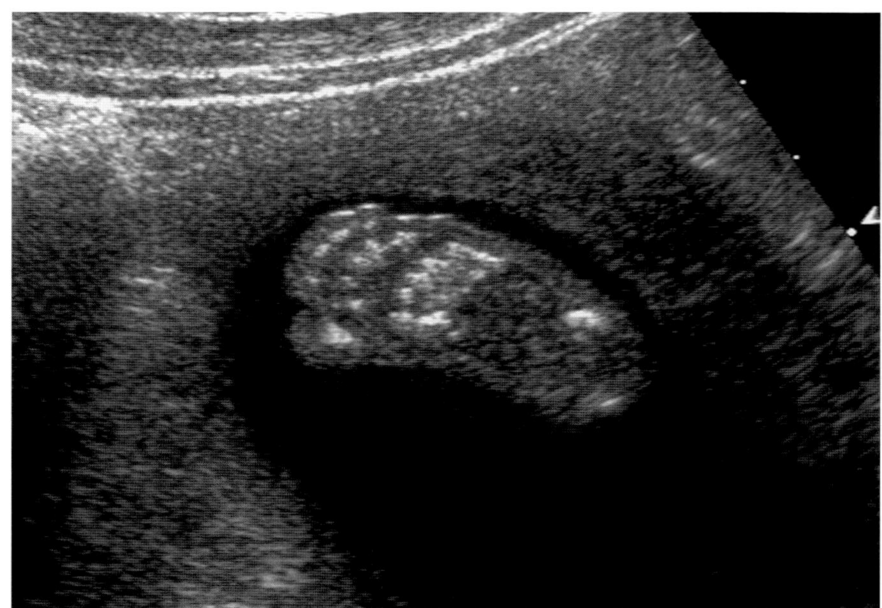

Fig. 11.4 **Apert syndrome.** Syndactyly of the foot at 22 + 6 weeks.

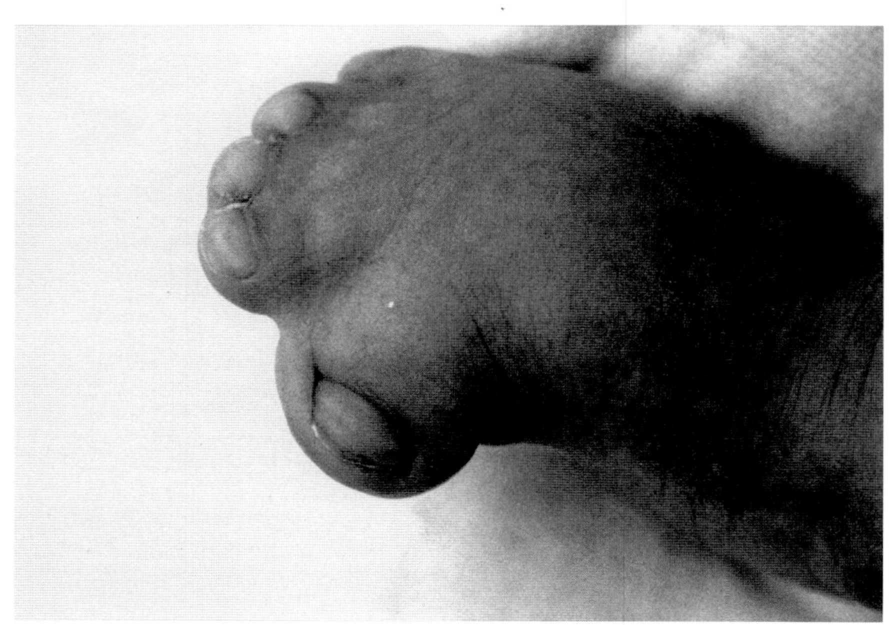

Fig. 11.5 **Apert syndrome.** Foot of a newborn infant with Apert syndrome.

1

2

3

4

5

References

Ferreira JC, Carter SM, Bernstein PS, et al. Second-trimester molecular prenatal diagnosis of sporadic Apert syndrome following suspicious ultrasound findings. Ultrasound Obstet Gynecol 1999; 14: 426–30.

Filkins K, Russo IF, Boehmer S, et al. Prenatal ultrasonographic and molecular diagnosis of Apert syndrome. Prenat Diagn 1997; 17: 1081–4.

Hafner E, Sterniste W, Scholler J, Schuchter K, Philipp K. Prenatal diagnosis of facial malformations. Prenat Diagn 1997; 17: 51–8.

Hill LM, Thomas ML, Peterson CS. The ultrasonic detection of Apert syndrome. J Ultrasound Med 1987; 6: 601–4.

Kaufmann K, Baldinger S, Pratt L. Ultrasound detection of Apert syndrome: a case report and literature review. Am J Perinatol 1997; 14: 427–30.

Lyu KJ, Ko TM. Prenatal diagnosis of Apert syndrome with widely separated cranial sutures. Prenat Diagn 2000; 20: 254–6.

Mahieu-Caputo D, Sonigo P, Amiel J, et al. Prenatal diagnosis of sporadic Apert syndrome: a sequential diagnostic approach combining three-dimensional computed tomography and molecular biology. Fetal Diagn Ther 2001; 16: 10–2.

Narayan H, Scott IV. Prenatal ultrasound diagnosis of Apert's syndrome. Prenat Diagn 1991; 11: 187–92.

Witters I, Devriendt K, Moerman P, van Hole C, Fryns JP. Diaphragmatic hernia as the first echographic sign in Apert syndrome. Prenat Diagn 2000; 20: 404–6.

Beckwith–Wiedemann Syndrome

Definition: This is a metabolic dysplasia syndrome with omphalocele, macroglossia, enlargement of organs, giantism, ear malformation, and hypoglycemia in the postnatal stage. There is an increased incidence of blastoma in childhood, especially Wilms tumor and adrenocortical cancers.

Incidence: One in 12 000–50 000 births.

First described in 1965 by Beckwith and Wiedemann.

Clinical history/genetics: Heterogeneous syndrome. Gene locus: 11 p15.5. The cause is dysregulation of a parental gene (genomic imprinting), which affects growth. Eighty-five percent of cases are sporadic, and 15% are of autosomal-dominant inheritance. In some cases of dominant inheritance, mutation of the cyclin-dependent kinase inhibitor 1 C (p57, Kip2) gene (*CDKN1 C*) is present. In the sporadic form, chromosomal aberrations are present in 1% of cases. Another 10–20% show paternal disomy 11; this means that the 11 p15 region of both chromosomes originates from the father and that maternal alleles are not present. Some patients demonstrate mutation of the *KVLQT1* gene and, as in the case of dominant inheritance, of the *CDKN1 C* gene. In 50% of cases, an imprinting mutation is seen in which expression of the insulin-like growth factor-2 gene (*IGF2*) is also determined by a maternal allele.

Ultrasound findings: Macrosomia is evident in the later stages of the second trimester. Other features are: hydramnios, anomalies of the placenta such as partial molar degeneration, macroglossia, hypertrophy of organs, especially large and echogenic kidneys, cardiomyopathy and cardiomegaly, and omphalocele. In addition, cryptorchism and hypospadias may also be evident. Detection has been reported as early as at 12 weeks of gestation.

Differential diagnosis: Diabetic fetopathy, Perlman syndrome, Simpson–Golabi–Behmel syndrome, Marfan syndrome, Marshall–Smith syndrome, Sotos syndrome, Weaver syndrome.

Prognosis: The perinatal fatality is about 20% and is due to macrosomia, omphalocele, hypoglycemia, fits, and cardiac failure. Mental development may be adequate as long as damage to the brain tissue due to hypoglycemia can be avoided (the tendency to hypoglycemia can continue into the first years of life). Hypertrophy of the viscera regresses in the course of development. Body size may be normal. Regular checks are necessary in the first 6 years of life for early detection of blastomas.

Self-Help Organization

Title: Beckwith–Wiedemann Support Network

Description: Support and information for parents of children with Beckwith–Wiedemann syndrome or isolated hemihypertrophy, and interested medical professionals. Newsletter, parent directory, information and referrals, phone support. Aims to increase public awareness and encourages research.

Scope: International network

Founded: 1989

Address: 2711 Colony Rd., Ann Arbor, MI 48 104, United States

Telephone: 734–973–0263; parents' toll-free number 1–800–837–2976

Fax: 734–973–9721

E-mail: a800 bwsn@aol.com

Web: http://www.beckwith-wiedemann.org

References

Cobellis G, Iannoto P, Stabile M, et al. Prenatal ultrasound diagnosis of macroglossia in the Wiedemann–Beckwith syndrome. Prenat Diagn 1988; 8: 79–81.

Fert-Ferrer S, Guichet A, Tantau J, et al. Subtle familial unbalanced translocation t(8; 11)(p23.2;p15.5) in two fetuses with Beckwith–Wiedemann features. Prenat Diagn 2000; 20: 511–5.

Fremond B, Poulain P, Odent S, Milon J, Treguier C, Babut JM. Prenatal detection of a congenital pancreatic cyst and Beckwith–Wiedemann syndrome. Prenat Diagn 1997; 17: 276–80.

Hamada H, Fujiki Y, Obata-Yasuoka M, Watanabe H, Yamada N, Kubo T. Prenatal sonographic diagnosis of Beckwith–Wiedemann syndrome in association with a single umbilical artery. J Clin Ultrasound 2001; 29: 535–8.

Hewitt B, Bankier A. Prenatal ultrasound diagnosis of Beckwith–Wiedemann syndrome. Aust N Z J Obstet Gynaecol 1994; 34: 488–90.

Koontz WL, Shaw LA, Lavery JP. Antenatal sonographic appearance of Beckwith–Wiedemann syndrome. JCU J Clin Ultrasound 1986; 14: 57–9.
Nowotny T, Bollmann R, Pfeifer L, Windt E. Beckwith–Wiedemann syndrome: difficulties with prenatal diagnosis. Fetal Diagn Ther 1994; 9: 256–60.
Reish O, Lerer I, Amiel A, et al. Wiedemann–Beckwith syndrome: further prenatal characterization of the condition [review]. Am J Med Genet 2002; 107: 209–13.
Shah YG, Metlay L. Prenatal ultrasound diagnosis of Beckwith–Wiedemann syndrome. J Clin Ultrasound 1990; 18: 597–600.
Viljoen DL, Jaquire Z, Woods DL. Prenatal diagnosis in autosomal-dominant Beckwith–Wiedemann syndrome. Prenat Diagn 1991; 11: 167–75.
Whisson CC, Whyte A, Ziesing P Beckwith–Wiedemann syndrome: antenatal diagnosis. Australas Radiol 1994; 38: 130–1.
Winter SC, Curry CJ, Smith JC, Kassel S, Miller L, Andrea J. Prenatal diagnosis of the Beckwith–Wiedemann syndrome. Am J Med Genet 1986; 24: 137–41.

Body Stalk Anomaly

Definition: A fatal malformation, probably resulting from early rupture of the amnion. At least two of three malformations must be present as diagnostic criteria: myelomeningocele or caudal regression syndrome, thoraco-abdominoschisis or abdominoschisis, anomalies of the extremities.

Incidence: One in 14 000 births.

Clinical history: Sporadic occurrence.

Teratogen: Not known.

Origin: Early developmental disturbances in the embryonic stage due to early amnion rupture have been discussed as a possible cause. Part of the embryo may be found in the celom.

Ultrasound findings: Following are characteristic findings: large *abdominal wall defects*, severe *neural tube defects*, extreme *kyphoscoliosis* with shortening of the vertebral column and caudal regression syndrome. A typical feature is an *absence* of one or more *extremities. Club foot* may also be present. *Meningomyelocele* may be associated with Arnold–Chiari malformation and development of hydrocephalus. *Ectopia cordis* may result from thoraco-abdominoschisis. In addition, *facial clefts* are observed. In extreme cases, the umbilical cord may even be absent, the fetus being joined directly to the placenta. *Increased nuchal translucency* is also a typical feature.

Clinical management: Karyotyping to evaluate the risk of recurrence (translocation?). Determination of the extent of malformations for further prognosis. Termination of pregnancy is justified

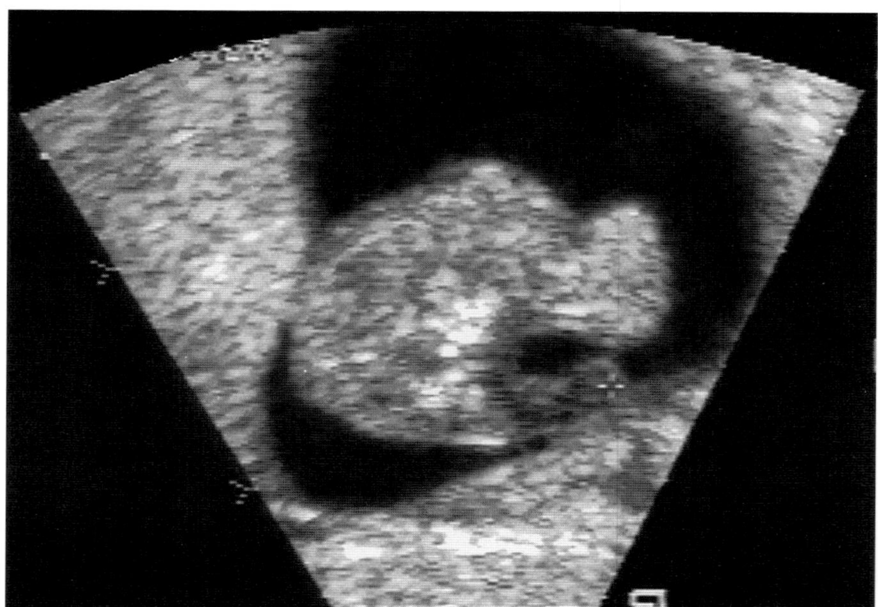

Fig. 11.6 **Body stalk anomaly.** Longitudinal section of the lower torso at 9 + 3 weeks, with an extensive omphalocele-like structure.

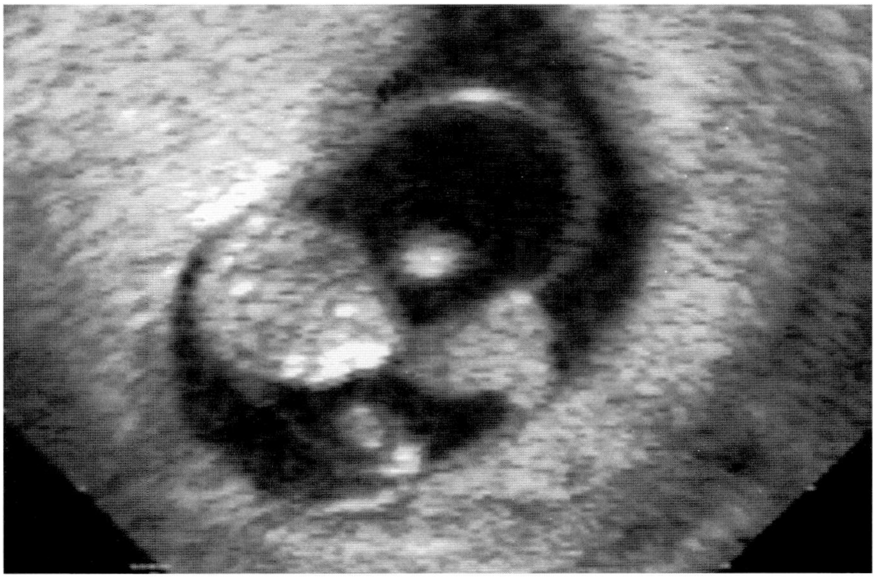

Fig. 11.7 **Body stalk anomaly.** Demonstration of the fetal head within the amnion as well as an omphalocele-like structure outside the amnion in the extraembryonic celom, in a case of body stalk anomaly at 9 + 3 weeks.

in most cases. Obstetric intervention due to fetal distress should be avoided.

Procedure after birth: Intensive medical treatment of the neonate should be avoided.

Prognosis: In case of full expression of the anomaly, the outcome is fatal. Only mildly affected individuals may survive. See also the section (8.4 above) on amniotic band syndrome.

References

Becker R, Runkel S, Entezami M. Prenatal diagnosis of body stalk anomaly at 9 weeks of gestation. Fetal diagnosis and therapy 2000; 15: 301–3.

Chan Y, Silverman N, Jackson L, Wapner R, Wallerstein R. Maternal uniparental disomy of chromosome 16 and body stalk anomaly. Am J Med Genet 2000; 94: 284–6.

Ginsberg NE, Cadkin A, Strom C. Prenatal diagnosis of body stalk anomaly in the first trimester of pregnancy. Ultrasound Obstet Gynecol 1997; 10: 419–21.

Hiett AK, Devoe LD, Falls DG, Martin SA. Ultrasound diagnosis of a twin gestation with concordant body stalk anomaly: a case report. J Reprod Med 1992; 37: 944–6.

Jauniaux E, Vyas S, Finlayson C, Moscoso G, Driver M, Campbell S. Early sonographic diagnosis of body stalk anomaly. Prenat Diagn 1990; 10: 127–32.

Martinez JM, Fortuny A, Comas C, et al. Body stalk anomaly associated with maternal cocaine abuse. Prenat Diagn 1994; 14: 669–72.

Paul C, Zosmer N, Jurkovic D, Nicolaides K. A case of body stalk anomaly at 10 weeks of gestation. Ultrasound Obstet Gynecol 2001; 17: 157–9.

Shalev E, Eliyahu S, Battino S, Weiner E. First trimester transvaginal sonographic diagnosis of body stalk anomaly [correction of anatomy]. J Ultrasound Med 1995; 14: 641–2.

CHARGE Association

Definition: CHARGE is the acronym for *c*oloboma, *h*eart disease, *a*tresia of choanae, *r*etarded mental development, *g*enital hypoplasia, *e*ar anomalies and deafness.

Incidence: Rare; only 200 cases have been described.

Origins/genetics: Mostly sporadic occurrence (multifactorial inheritance), occasionally autosomal-dominant. The cause appears to be a disturbance in differentiation at the embryonic stage between the 35th and 45th day after conception. In sporadic forms, the risk of recurrence is 1%.

Clinical features: Mental impairment, ocular coloboma; rarely, microphthalmia and anophthalmia are present. The choanal atresia is usually bilateral. Dysplasia of the auricles, hearing impairment, and deafness may also be detected. Typical cardiac anomalies consist of persistent Botallo's duct, ASD, VSD, tetralogy of Fallot, and AV canal. Seventy-four percent of cases show hypoplasia of the genitals. In addition, growth retardation, facial clefts, atresia of the esophagus,

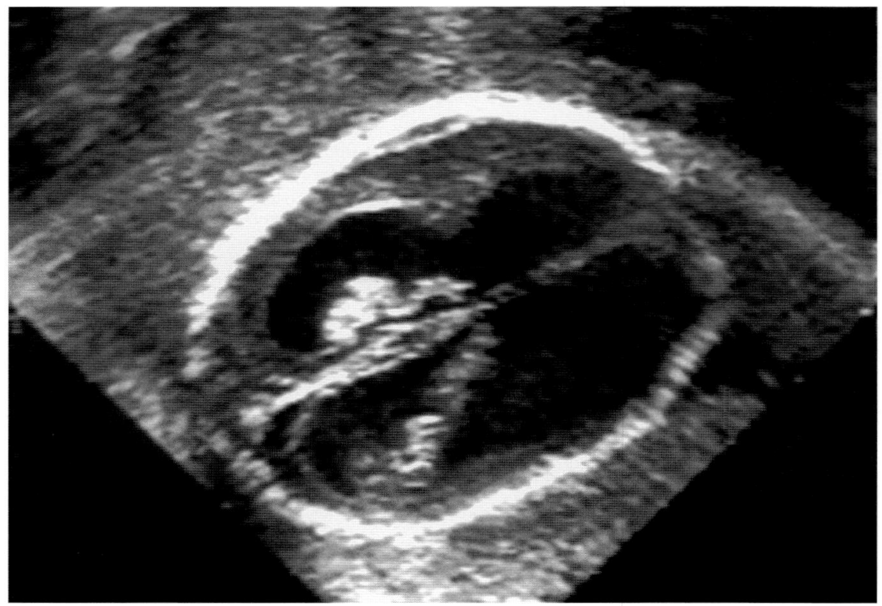

Fig. 11.8 **CHARGE association.** Cross-section of fetal head at 18 + 1 weeks: widening of both the lateral ventricles, underdeveloped and coil-shaped choroid plexus.

renal malformations, microgenia, hemivertebrae, syndactyly, scoliosis, facial pareses, central nervous system anomalies, and anal atresia may also be detected.

Ultrasound findings: Accurate classification of this syndrome at the prenatal stage is often difficult. The diagnosis is confirmed if the following combination of anomalies is detected: severe hydramnios, enlargement of cerebral ventricles, Dandy–Walker variant, genital hypoplasia, small stomach and cardiac anomaly, possibly dysplasia of the ear. Suspicion of choanal atresia can be verified using color-coded Doppler imaging.

Differential diagnosis: Wolf–Hirschhorn syndrome, trisomy 13, trisomy 18, Noonan syndrome, Pena–Shokeir syndrome, Smith–Lemli–Opitz syndrome, Treacher–Collins syndrome, VACTERL association.

Prognosis: This depends on the extent of the malformations. In severe cases, death results soon after birth, due either to respiratory failure, treatment-resistant hypocalcemia, or heart failure. Mental impairment can be expected in survivors.

Self-Help Organization

Title: CHARGE Syndrome Foundation, Inc.

Description: Networking of families affected by CHARGE syndrome. Offers an organization manual for parents, newsletter, information, and parent-to-parent support. Biannual international conference. Newsletter.

Scope: National network

Founded: 1993

Address: 2004 Parkade, Columbia, MO 65 202, United States

Telephone: 573–499–4694. Families only call 1–800–442–7604

Fax: 573–499–4694

E-mail: marion@chargesyndrome.org

Web: http://www.chargesyndrome.org

References

Becker R, Stiemer B, Neumann L, Entezami M. Mild ventriculomegaly, mild cerebellar hypoplasia and dysplastic choroid plexus as early prenatal signs of CHARGE association. Fetal Diagn Ther 2001; 16: 280–3.

Hertzberg BS, Kliewer MA, Lile RL. Antenatal ultrasonographic findings in the CHARGE association. J Ultrasound Med 1994; 13: 238–42.

Cornelia de Lange Syndrome (Brachmann–de Lange Syndrome)

Definition: This syndrome consists of malformations of the face and the extremities, growth retardation, microcephaly, and mental impairment.

Incidence: On the whole, relatively rare; 300 cases have been described.

First described by Brachmann in 1916 and de Lange in 1933.

Origin/genetics: Isolated autosomal-dominant or autosomal-recessive inheritance, with variable expression. Gene locus: 3 q26.3; mostly sporadic occurrence.

Ultrasound findings: An *abnormal nuchal translucency* is detected in the first trimester. *Growth restriction* is first evident at 20–25 weeks. In addition, *brachycephaly, microcephaly, and microgenia* are diagnosed. Cardiac anomalies such as VSD and ASD are common. Further anomalies include hypospadias, cryptorchism, micromelia, syndactyly, dysplasia of ulna, oligodactyly. The earliest diagnosis was made at 12 weeks on the basis of a nuchal edema.

Differential diagnosis: Apert syndrome, chromosomal aberrations, Fanconi anemia, Holt–Oram syndrome, multiple pterygium syndrome, Roberts syndrome, Smith–Lemli–Opitz syndrome, TAR syndrome.

Clinical management: Further ultrasound screening, including fetal echocardiography, karyotyping (normal finding). A low level of alpha fetoprotein in maternal serum has been reported in association with Cornelia de Lange syndrome.

Prognosis: The perinatal mortality is increased. Survivors show mental impairment and growth restriction.

Self-Help Organization

Title: Cornelia de Lange Syndrome Foundation, Inc.

Description: Provides support and education to families affected by Cornelia de Lange syndrome. Supports research. Newsletter. Family album available for networking and mutual support. Annual convention. Professional network. Assistance in starting groups.

Scope: International

Number of groups: 2500 + member families

Founded: 1981

Address: 302 West Main St., Suite 100, Avon, CT 6001, United States

Telephone: 1–800–223–8355 or 860–676–8166

Fax: 860–676–8337

E-mail: CDLSintl@iconn.net

Web: http://cdlsoutreach.org

References

Boog G, Sagot F, Winer N, David A, Nomballais MF. Brachmann–de Lange syndrome: a cause of early symmetric fetal growth delay. Eur J Obstet Gynecol Reprod Biol 1999; 85: 173–7.

Bruner JP, Hsia YE. Prenatal findings in Brachmann–de Lange syndrome. Obstet Gynecol 1990; 76: 966–8.

Huang WH, Porto M. Abnormal first-trimester fetal nuchal translucency and Cornelia de Lange syndrome. Obstet Gynecol 2002; 99: 956–8.

Kliewer MA, Kahler SG, Hertzberg BS, Bowie JD. Fetal biometry in the Brachmann–de Lange syndrome. Am J Med Genet 1993; 47: 1035–41.

Marino T, Wheeler PG, Simpson LL, Craigo SD, Bianchi DW. Fetal diaphragmatic hernia and upper limb anomalies suggest Brachmann–de Lange syndrome. Prenat Diagn 2002; 22: 144–7.

Sekimoto H, Osada H, Kimura H, Kamiyama M, Arai K, Sekiya S. Prenatal findings in Brachmann–de Lange syndrome. Arch Gynecol Obstet 2000; 263: 182–4.

Urban M, Hartung J. Ultrasonographic and clinical appearance of a 22-week-old fetus with Brachmann–de Lange syndrome. Am J Med Genet 2001; 102: 73–5.

Crouzon Syndrome (Craniofacial Dysostosis Type I)

Definition: Premature closure of the cranial sutures, causing characteristic anomalies of the head and face. The coronal, lambdoid, and sagittal sutures are mainly affected. The resulting dysmorphisms include a clover-shaped or tower-shaped skull, hypoplasia of the midfacial region, and exophthalmos.

First described in 1912 by Crouzon.

Origin/genetics: Autosomal-dominant inheritance. Mutation of the fibroblast growth factor receptor-2 gene. Gene locus: 10q25–q26. New mutations are observed in about 25% of cases.

Ultrasound findings: These include an abnormally shaped skull, in severe cases *clover-shaped skull* (which is a special form of tower-shaped head), hypertelorism, beaked nose, micrognathia, progenia, exophthalmos, possibly combined with widening of the cerebral ventricles, agenesis of the corpus callosum, and cleft lip and palate. If there is a positive family history, it is possible to diagnose this disorder in the second trimester on finding widening of the interorbital distance.

Differential diagnosis: Apert syndrome, Carpenter syndrome, clover-shaped skull, Pfeiffer syndrome, thanatophoric dysplasia.

Procedure after birth: Surgery is necessary due to closure of the sutures. Some of the skull deformities can be corrected in this way. Mental development is improved after neurosurgical interventions to reduce intracranial pressure.

Prognosis: Atrophy of the optical nerve may cause blindness. Respiratory obstruction is also possible. Fits and mental impairment are rarely seen.

Self-Help Organization

Title: Craniosynostosis and Parents Support, Inc.

Description: Dedicated to helping families find support and information to help deal with craniosynostosis. The aim is to raise awareness through public and professional education. Provides a newsletter, literature, hospital care packages, pen pals, and phone support. Advocacy, information and referrals. Supports research.

Scope: International network

Founded: 1999

Address: 1136 Iris Lane, Beaufort, SC 29906, United States

Telephone: 1–877–686-CAPS

Fax: 843–846–0779

E-mail: CAPS2000@gosiggy.com

Web: http://www.caps2000.org

References

Kjaer I, Hansen BF, Kjaer KW, Skovby F. Abnormal timing in the prenatal ossification of vertebral column and hand in Crouzon syndrome. Am J Med Genet 2000; 90: 386–9.

Leo MV, Suslak L, Ganesh VL, Adhate A, Apuzzio JJ. Crouzon syndrome: prenatal ultrasound diagnosis by binocular diameters. Obstet Gynecol 1991; 78: 906–8.

Martinelli P, Russo R, Agangi A, Paladini D. Prenatal ultrasound diagnosis of frontonasal dysplasia. Prenat Diagn 2002; 22: 375–9.

Miller C, Losken HW, Towbin R, et al. Ultrasound diagnosis of craniosynostosis. Cleft Palate Craniofac J 2002; 39: 73–80.

Ellis–van Creveld Syndrome

Definition: Short-limb dwarfism with hexadactyly, hypoplasia of the nails, abnormal connection of the mucous membranes between the upper lip and upper gum.

Incidence: Rare; about 250 cases have been reported; there is an incidence of one in 200 in the Amish population (Lancaster County, Pennsylvania, USA).

First described in 1940.

Origin/genetics: Autosomal-recessive inheritance with variable expression. Mutations in the Ellis–van Creveld gene, gene locus: 4 p16.

Ultrasound findings: *Disproportionate short-limb dwarfism*, with shortening of the limbs increasing distally. Hexadactyly of the hands, occasionally of the feet. Short femur, club feet, Dandy–Walker malformation, sometimes genital anomalies. Cardiac anomalies are found in 50% of cases, most frequently ASD.

Differential diagnosis: At the neonatal stage, short rib–polydactyly syndrome has to be differentiated from this. Definitive diagnosis is possible at a later stage.

Clinical management: If there is a positive family history, chorionic villus sampling and DNA analysis is recommended.

Prognosis: There is an increased neonatal mortality due to respiratory complications resulting from short ribs (30–50% of affected infants). In addition, the prognosis also depends on the associated cardiac anomaly. The adult height varies considerably, between 105 and 160 cm. Affected individuals have normal intelligence.

References

Arya L, Mendiratta V, Sharma RC, Solanki RS. Ellis–van Creveld Syndrome: a report of two cases. Pediatr Dermatol 2001; 18: 485–9.

Berardi JC, Moulis M, Laloux V, Godard J, Wipff P, Botto C. Ellis–van Creveld syndrome: contribution of echography to prenatal diagnosis—apropos of a case. J Gynecol Obstet Biol Reprod (Paris) 1985; 14: 43–7.

Dugoff L, Thieme G, Hobbins JC. First trimester prenatal diagnosis of chondroectodermal dysplasia (Ellis–van Creveld syndrome) with ultrasound. Ultrasound Obstet Gynecol 2001; 17: 86–8.

Guschmann M, Horn D, Gasiorek-Wiens A, Urban M, Kunze J, Vogel M. Ellis–van Creveld syndrome: examination at 15 weeks' gestation. Prenat Diagn 1999; 19: 879–83.

Meinel K, Himmel D. Status of ultrasound and roentgen diagnosis in prenatal detection of osteochondrodysplasias. Zentralbl Gynäkol 1987; 109: 1303–3.

Sergi C, Voigtlander T, Zoubaa S, et al. Ellis–van Creveld syndrome: a generalized dysplasia of enchondral ossification. Pediatr Radiol 2001; 31: 289–93.

Tongsong T, Chanprapaph P. Prenatal sonographic diagnosis of Ellis–van Creveld syndrome. J Clin Ultrasound 2000; 28: 38–41.

Torrente I, Mangino M, De Luca A, et al. First-trimester prenatal diagnosis of Ellis–van Creveld syndrome using linked microsatellite markers. Prenat Diagn 1998; 18: 504–6.

Zimmer EZ, Weinraub Z, Raijman A, Pery M, Peretz BA. Antenatal diagnosis of a fetus with an extremely narrow thorax and short limb dwarfism. JCU J Clin Ultrasound 1984; 12: 112–4.

Freeman–Sheldon Syndrome (Whistling Face)

Definition: This is a syndrome with a characteristic facial expression of "whistling face," hypoplasia of the nostrils, ulnar deviation of the hands, bent fingers and club feet.

Incidence: Generally rare; only 100 cases have been reported.

Origin/genetics: Autosomal-dominant inheritance is the frequent form, although autosomal-recessive and sporadic forms have also been described.

Clinical features: A rounded, chubby, mask-like face without expression; the small mouth appears to be "whistling."

Ultrasound findings: Hypertelorism, deep-set nasal bridge, small nose, hypoplasia of the nostrils, long median ridge in the upper lip, ulnar deviation of the hands, contracted bent fingers, especially the thumb, and club feet with contractures of the toes. Raised palate, possibly cleft palate. Short neck with pterygium. Dwarfism, scoliosis, microcephaly. In a case with a positive family history, the diagnosis was made at 21 weeks due to club feet and facial anomalies.

Differential diagnosis: Arthrogryposis, Schwartz–Jampel syndrome, amniotic band sequence, Cornelia de Lange syndrome, multiple pterygium syndrome, Pena–Shokeir syndrome, Seckel syndrome, Smith–Lemli–Opitz syndrome, trisomy 18.

Prognosis: Life expectancy is normal, usually with no mental impairment. However, cases of mental impairment and fits have also been described.

Self-Help Organization

Title: Freeman–Sheldon Parent Support Group

Description: Emotional support for parents of children with Freeman–Sheldon and for adults with this syndrome. Sharing of helpful medical literature library. Information on growth and development of individuals affected. Participates in research projects. Members network by phone and mail. Newsletter.

Scope: International network

Founded: 1982

Address: 509 E. Northmont Way, Salt Lake City, UT 84 103, United States

Telephone: 801–364–7060

E-mail: fspsg@aol.com

Web: http://www.fspsg.org

References

Cruickshanks GF, Brown S, Chitayat D. Anesthesia for Freeman–Sheldon syndrome using a laryngeal mask airway. Can J Anaesth 1999; 46: 783–7.

Krakowiak PA, O'Quinn JR, Bohnsack JF, et al A variant of Freeman–Sheldon syndrome maps to 11 p15.5-pter. Am J Hum Genet 1997; 60: 426–32.

Krakowiak PA, Bohnsack JF, Carey JC, Bamshad M. Clinical analysis of a variant of Freeman–Sheldon syndrome (DA2 B). Am J Med Genet 1998; 76: 93–8.

Manji KP, Mbise RL. Generalized muscle hypertonia with mask-like face (Freeman–Sheldon syndrome) in a Tanzanian girl. Clin Genet 1998; 54: 252–3.

Robbins-Furman P, Hecht JT, Rocklin M, Maklad N, Greenhaw G, Wilkins I. Prenatal diagnosis of Freeman–Sheldon syndrome (whistling face). Prenat Diagn 1995; 15: 179–82.

Robinson PJ. Freeman–Sheldon syndrome: severe upper airway obstruction requiring neonatal tracheostomy [review]. Pediatr Pulmonol 1997; 23: 457–9.

Schefels J, Wenzl TG, Merz U, et al. Functional upper airway obstruction in a child with Freeman–Sheldon syndrome. ORL J Otorhinolaryngol Relat Spec 2002; 64: 53–6.

Schrander-Stumpel C, Fryns JP, Beemer FA, Rive FA. Association of distal arthrogryposis, mental retardation, whistling face, and Pierre Robin sequence: evidence for nosologic heterogeneity. Am J Med Genet 1991; 38: 557–61.

Fryns Syndrome

Definition: This syndrome combines facial dysmorphism, anomalies of the distal extremities, and diaphragmatic hernia.

First described in 1979 by Fryns.

Incidence: About one in 15 000 births.

Origin/genetics: Autosomal-recessive inheritance.

Ultrasound findings: Thickening of the neck region in the form of *hygroma colli* is evident in the first trimester. Later on, *hydramnios* and *fetal hydrops* develop. *Craniofacial dysmorphism* is characterized by coarse facial features, a prominent glabella, flat nasal bridge, large nose with anteverted nostrils, short upper lip, macrostomia, cleft lip and palate, retrogenia, and dysplasia of the auricles. A characteristic feature is diaphragmatic hernia, the posterolateral part being absent. Malformations of the limbs are also present: brachytelephalangia (hypoplasia of the distal phalanges) of the fingers and toes. In addition, microphthalmia, clouded cornea, retinal dysplasia, short neck, pterygium, cystic renal dysplasia, Dandy–Walker malformation, widening of the cranial ventricles, club feet, cardiac defects such as VSD, and anal atresia may also be detected. Diagnosis is possible at the earliest at 13 weeks due to severe hygroma colli.

Differential diagnosis: Hydrolethalus, Schinzel–Giedion syndrome, Rüdiger syndrome, Wolf–Hirschhorn syndrome, tetrasomy 12 p, trisomy 18 and 21, Walker–Warburg syndrome, achondrogenesis, Apert syndrome, Cornelia de Lange syndrome, Kniest syndrome, multiple pterygium syndrome, Noonan syndrome, Roberts syndrome, Smith–Lemli–Opitz syndrome.

Prognosis: There is a high mortality rate due to respiratory failure (pulmonary hypoplasia) secondary to diaphragmatic hernia. In the absence of the above, infants may survive, but mental impairment can be expected.

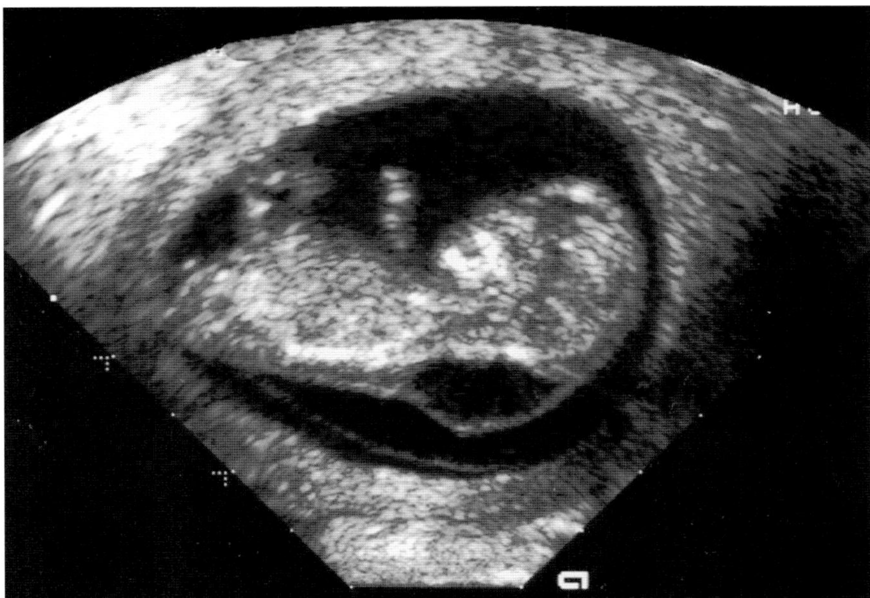

Fig. 11.**9** **Fryns syndrome.** Fetus at 12 + 3 weeks with severe cystic hygroma, nuchal thickness measuring 8 mm. Chorionic villus sampling showed a normal karyotype.

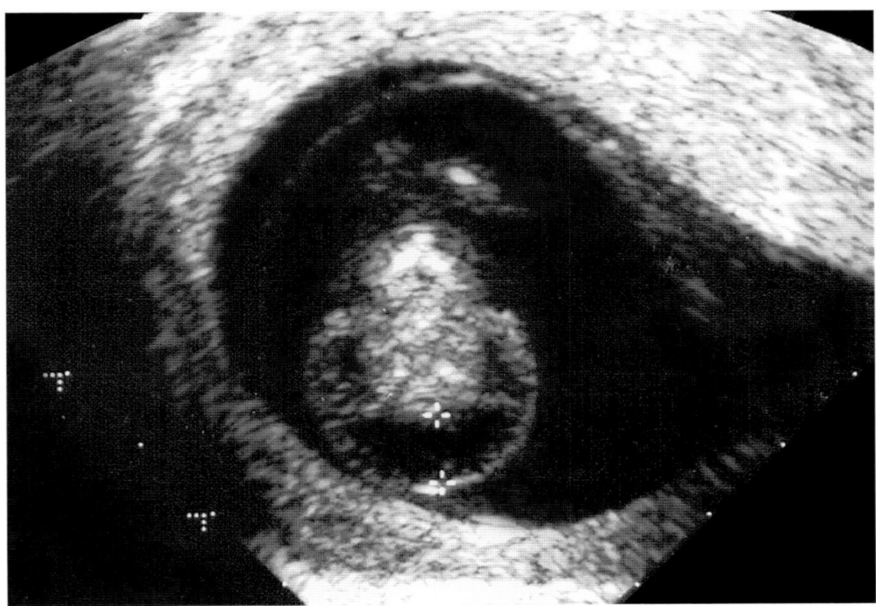

Fig. 11.**10** **Fryns syndrome.** Same fetus. Cross-section of the fetal neck. Further clinical progress: normal fetal echocardiography, regression of hygroma.

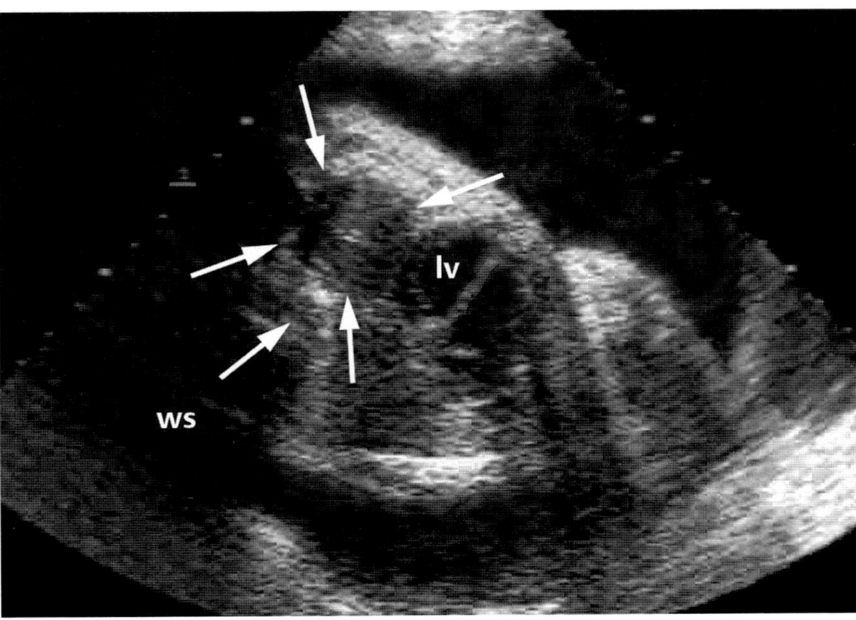

Fig. 11.**11** **Fryns syndrome.** Same fetus seen at 36 + 3 weeks : for the first time, the heart is seen displaced to the right (lv: left ventricle), due to the left kidney (arrows) being pushed up into the thoracic cavity: fetal diaphragmatic hernia. Fryns syndrome was diagnosed after birth.

References

Dix U, Beudt U, Langenbeck U. Fryns syndrome: pre- and postnatal diagnosis. Z Geburtshilfe Perinatol 1991; 195: 280–4.

Enns GM, Cox VA, Goldstein RB, Gibbs DL, Harrison MR, Golabi M. Congenital diaphragmatic defects and associated syndromes, malformations, and chromosome anomalies: a retrospective study of 60 patients and literature review. Am J Med Genet 1998; 79: 215–25.

Hösli IM, Tercanli S, Rehder H, Holzgreve W. Cystic hygroma as an early first-trimester ultrasound marker for recurrent Fryns' syndrome. Ultrasound Obstet Gynecol 1997; 10: 422–4.

Meinecke P, Fryns JP. The Fryns syndrome: diaphragmatic defects, craniofacial dysmorphism, and distal digital hypoplasia: further evidence for autosomal-recessive inheritance. Clin Genet 1985; 28: 516–20.

Ramsing M, Gillessen-Kaesbach G, Holzgreve W, Fritz B, Rehder H. Variability in the phenotypic expression of Fryns syndrome: a report of two sibships. Am J Med Genet 2000; 95: 415–24.

Sheffield JS, Twickler DM, Timmons C, Land K, Harrod MJ, Ramus RM. Fryns syndrome: prenatal diagnosis and pathologic correlation. J Ultrasound Med 1998; 17: 585–9.

Van Wymersch D, Favre R, Gasser B. Use of three-dimensional ultrasound to establish the prenatal diagnosis of Fryns syndrome. Fetal Diagn Ther 1996; 11: 335–40.

Goldenhar Syndrome

Definition: This is a group of malformations consisting of facial asymmetry, anomalies of the eyes, ears and cheeks. It may also be combined with defects in the vertebral column.

Incidence: One in 3000–5000 births.

Origin/genetics: This is a heterogeneous and complex malformation syndrome. The occurrence is mostly sporadic—for example, due to restricted placenta perfusion at a sensitive stage of development. There is a disturbance in the development of the first and second branchial arches. Rarely, autosomal-dominant or autosomal-recessive inheritance has been observed. Males are more often affected. With one affected child, there is a 3% risk of recurrence; if two siblings are affected, the risk rises to 6%.

Clinical features and ultrasound findings: *Asymmetrical face* resulting from unilateral hypoplasia of bone and soft tissue, frontal bossing, hypoplasia of zygomatic arch and mandibular bone, retrogenia. *Malformations of the eye*: epibulbar dermoid or lipodermoid at the junction of the sclera and cornea, coloboma of the upper lid. *Malformations of the ear*: preauricular tags, small ears, anomalies of the external ear. Further anomalies include: unilateral microstomia, cleft jaw, partial vertebral scoliosis. Development of *hydramnios* is frequent. In addition, cardiac defects, renal anomalies and widening of the cranial ventricles are also detected. The *main finding* is slight facial dysmorphism and hydramnios. The earliest diagnosis was reported at 16 weeks on the basis of maxillary clefts and unilateral microphthalmia.

Associated syndromes: Mandibulofacial dysostosis, hemifacial microsomia, Wildervanck syndrome, Frase syndrome, Fryns syndrome, Klippel–Pfeil sequence, Nager syndrome, Treacher–Collins syndrome, trisomy 13 and 18.

Prognosis: This is usually favorable, with normal mental development and intelligence. Cosmetic surgery is needed to correct the facial anomalies. Physical handicap may result due to deafness and microphthalmia.

Self-Help Organization

Title: Goldenhar Syndrome Support Network

Description: Support and information for families affected by Goldenhar syndrome (hemifacial microsomia). Information and referrals, newsletter, literature, pen pals, and advocacy. Online mailing list.

Scope: International network

Founded: 1998

Address: 9325 163 Street, Edmonton, Alberta T5 R 2 P4, Canada

E-mail: bbds.page@i.am

Web: http://www.goldenharsyndrome.org

References

De Catte L, Laubach M, Legein J, Goossens A. Early prenatal diagnosis of oculoauriculovertebral dysplasia or the Goldenhar syndrome. Ultrasound Obstet Gynecol 1996; 8: 422–4.

Dillon E, Renwick M, Wright C. Congenital diaphragmatic herniation: antenatal detection and outcome. Br J Radiol 2000; 73: 360–5.
Tamas DE, Mahony BS, Bowie JD, Woodruff WW HH. Prenatal sonographic diagnosis of hemifacial microsomia (Goldenhar–Gorlin syndrome). J Ultrasound Med 1986; 5: 461–3.
Witters I, Schreurs J, Van Wing J, Wouters W, Fryns JP. Prenatal diagnosis of facial clefting as part of the oculo-auriculo-vertebral spectrum. Prenat Diagn 2001; 21: 62–4.

Holt–Oram Syndrome

Definition: This syndrome consists of anomalies of the heart and upper limbs.

Incidence: Rare, although over a hundred cases have been reported.

First described in 1960 by Holt and Oram.

Origin/genetics: Autosomal-dominant inheritance with full penetrance and variable expression. New mutations are found in 50–80%. Gene locus: 12 q24.1. Girls are more severely affected than boys.

Ultrasound findings: *Cardiac anomalies* (85%): ASD II (partially combined with cardiac arrhythmia); rarely VSD. *Malformations of the upper extremities*: three digits or hypoplasia or aplasia of the thumb, dysplasia or aplasia of the radius, and anomalies of the small finger, elbow, and shoulder joint. Occasionally, radioulnar synostosis, hypoplasia of the humerus, and phocomelia have also been observed. Diagnosis is possible in the second trimester after careful scanning of the lower arm and thumb.

Differential diagnosis: TAR syndrome, Fanconi anemia, thalidomide syndrome, Tabatznik syndrome, Rogers syndrome, Cornelia de Lange syndrome, Nager syndrome, trisomy 13 and 18, VACTERL association.

Prognosis: This depends on the type of cardiac anomaly present; normal mental development can be expected.

References

Brons JT, van Geijn HP, Wladimiroff JW, et al. Prenatal ultrasound diagnosis of the Holt–Oram syndrome. Prenat Diagn 1988; 8: 175–81.
Lehner R, Wenzl R, Vanura H, Frank W Safar P, Husslein P. Diagnosis of familial Holt–Oram syndrome. Z Geburtshilfe Perinatol 1994; 198: 143–9.
Muller LM, De Jong G, Van Heerden KM. The antenatal ultrasonographic detection of the Holt–Oram syndrome. S Afr Med J 1985; 68: 313–5.
Tongsong T, Chanprapaph P. Prenatal sonographic diagnosis of Holt–Oram syndrome. J Clin Ultrasound 2000; 28: 98–100.

Hydrolethalus

Definition: This is a fatal complex of malformations, with hydrocephalus and other cranial anomalies, facial dysmorphism, including facial clefts, polydactyly of the hands and feet, and pulmonary hypoplasia.

Incidence: In Finland, one in 20 000 births. Incidences in African and Arabic families has also been reported. About 60 cases have been described.

First description: 28 cases were reported in Finland in 1981.

Genetics: Autosomal-recessive inheritance.

Ultrasound findings: Growth restriction, hydramnios (obligatory finding). *Head and face*: hydrocephalus (93%), agenesis of the corpus callosum, absence of the septum pellucidum, Dandy–Walker malformation; cleft palate, cleft lip (56%), microgenia (84%), small tongue, which may even be absent. *Thorax:* tracheobronchial malformations (65%), abnormal pulmonary lobes; cardiac defects (58%): VSD, AV canal. *Extremities:* polydactyly (88%), club feet. Diagnosis is possible as early as at 13 weeks (central nervous system anomalies with limb defects).

Hydramnios and severe obstructive hydrocephalus develop at a later stage. In contrast to Meckel– Gruber syndrome, cystic kidneys and encephalocele are absent.

Differential diagnosis: Meckel–Gruber syndrome, septooptic dysplasia, Walker–Warburg syndrome, Goldenhar syndrome, Fryns syndrome, Ivemark syndrome, Smith–Lemli–Opitz syndrome, trisomy 13, Apert syndrome, Fanconi anemia, Mohr syndrome, Pfeiffer syndrome, camptomelic dysplasia, Crouzon syndrome, Gorlin syndrome, multiple pterygium syndrome, Neu–Laxova syndrome, Roberts syndrome.

Prognosis: The outcome is always fatal, usually in the neonatal stage.

Caudal Regression Syndrome

Definition: The caudal aplasia–dysplasia sequence is caused by a partial or total absence of the distal part of the neural tube. This results in anomalies of the lower limb and of the gastrointestinal and urogenital tracts.

Incidence: One in 20 000–100 000 births.

Clinical history/genetics: Mostly sporadic occurrence, genetically heterogeneous. Autosomal or X-chromosome-dominant inheritance has rarely been described.

Teratogen: Diabetes mellitus.

Embryology: The lower segment of the spinal canal develops until 7 weeks after conception. Primary absence of this segment, rather than secondary regression of an already formed segment, is the most probable cause of the caudal regression syndrome. It is not yet clear whether *sirenomelia* represents the most severe form of caudal regression syndrome or whether it is a distinct entity. An early insult to the developing lower spinal column results in aplasia or dysplasia of the sacrum.

Ultrasound findings: Absence of the sacrum, abnormal lumbar vertebrae, deformation of the pelvis, hypoplasia of the femur, club feet, contractures of the lower limbs, decreased movements of the lower limbs. In addition, the following anomalies may be detected: renal agenesis, cardiac defects, pulmonary hypoplasia, neural tube defects, anal atresia, facial clefts. In sirenomelia, the lower limbs are joined together, or only one combined lower limb is found. The earliest prenatal diagnosis is possible at 10 weeks; a short crown–rump length and anomalies of the yolk sac raise the initial suspicion. Protrusion of the caudal region develops at a later stage.

Associated malformations: Cardiac anomalies are common. In case of sirenomelia, renal anomalies are further evident. Hydrocephalus may also develop.

Differential diagnosis: In sirenomelia, the lower extremities are fused together and the accompanying renal anomalies dominate the finding. Otherwise, Fraser syndrome, MURCS association, and VACTERL association should be considered.

Clinical management: Further ultrasound scanning, including fetal echocardiography and karyotyping. Maternal diabetes should be excluded. If the pregnancy is continued, normal antenatal care should be provided. Breech presentation is common, and a cesarean section may be necessary if there is severe fetal abdominocranial disproportion.

Procedure after birth: Multidisciplinary care at a perinatal center.

Prognosis: This is similar to that with myelomeningocele situated at a higher lumbar level. Impaired lower limb function and fecal and urinal incontinence is to be expected.

Advice to the mother: In the presence of diabetes mellitus, blood sugar levels should be strictly controlled before conception, reducing the risk of malformations considerably during the subsequent pregnancy.

References

Aslan H, Yanik H, Celikaslan N, Yildirim G, Ceylan Y. Prenatal diagnosis of caudal regression syndrome: a case report. BMC Pregnancy Childbirth 2001; 1: 8.

Baxi L, Warren W, Collins MH, Timor TI. Early detection of caudal regression syndrome with transvaginal scanning. Obstet Gynecol 1990; 75: 486–9.
Das BB, Rajegowda BK, Bainbridge R, Giampietro PF. Caudal regression syndrome versus sirenomelia: a case report. J Perinatol 2002; 22: 168–70.
Fukada Y, Yasumizu T, Tsurugi Y, Ohta S, Hoshi K. Caudal regression syndrome detected in a fetus with increased nuchal translucency. Acta Obstet Gynecol Scand 1999; 78: 655–6.
Houfflin V, Subtil D, Cosson M, et al. Prenatal diagnosis of three caudal regression syndromes associated with maternal diabetes. J Gynecol Obstet Biol Reprod (Paris) 1996; 25: 389–95.
Loewy JA, Richards DG, Toi A. In-utero diagnosis of the caudal regression syndrome: report of three cases. JCU J Clin Ultrasound 1987; 15: 469–74.
Twickler D, Budorick N, Pretorius D, Grafe M, Currarino G. Caudal regression versus sirenomelia: sonographic clues. J Ultrasound Med 1993; 12: 323–30.
Valenzano M, Paoletti R, Rossi A, Farinini D, Garlaschi G, Fulcheri E. Sirenomelia: pathological features, antenatal ultrasonographic clues, and a review of current embryogenic theories. Hum Reprod Update 1999; 5: 82–6.
Zaw W, Stone DG. Caudal regression syndrome in twin pregnancy with type II diabetes. J Perinatol 2002; 22: 171–4.

Klippel–Trénaunay–Weber Syndrome

Definition: This is a complex malformation involving the blood vessels; it consists of arteriovenous malformations, cutaneous hemangiomas or lymphangiomas, unilateral hypertrophy especially segmental gigantism of certain body parts (*angio-osteohypertrophic syndrome*).

Incidence: Rare.

Sex ratio: M : F = 1 : 1.

Clinical history/genetics: Sporadic occurrence.

Teratogen: Not known.

Ultrasound findings: Localized *enlargement* of one or more extremities, or of the torso. The long bones are *asymmetrical.* Cystic lesions on the body surface (lymphangiomas) are occasionally found. Severe arteriovenous anastomoses lead to cardiac failure and fetal hydrops due to high volume overload. Associated anomalies include hemangiomas of the gastrointestinal tract or of the retroperitoneal region and asymmetrical facial hypertrophy. The earliest diagnosis was made at 15 weeks, after detection of a tumor on the thoracic wall.

Differential diagnosis: Cystic hygroma, disseminated hemangioma syndrome, Maffucci syndrome, Proteus syndrome, sacrococcygeal teratoma, Turner syndrome.

Clinical management: Karyotyping is essential. Further ultrasound scanning, including fetal echocardiography. Magnetic resonance imaging can confirm the diagnosis in difficult cases. If signs of cardiac insufficiency develop in the

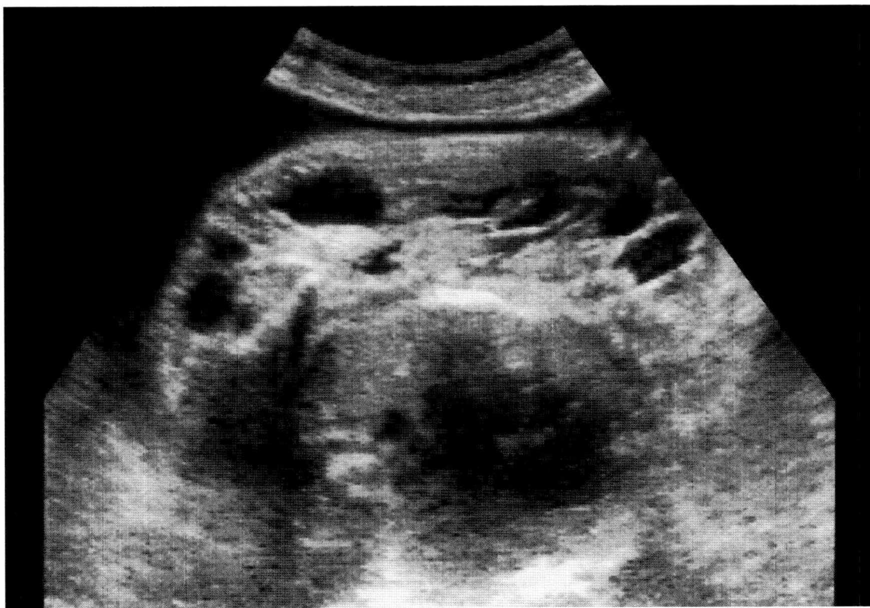

Fig. 11.**12** **Klippel–Trénaunay–Weber syndrome.** Cross-section of the fetal thorax at 32 weeks. Severe multicystic lesions are demonstrated in the subcutaneous tissue.

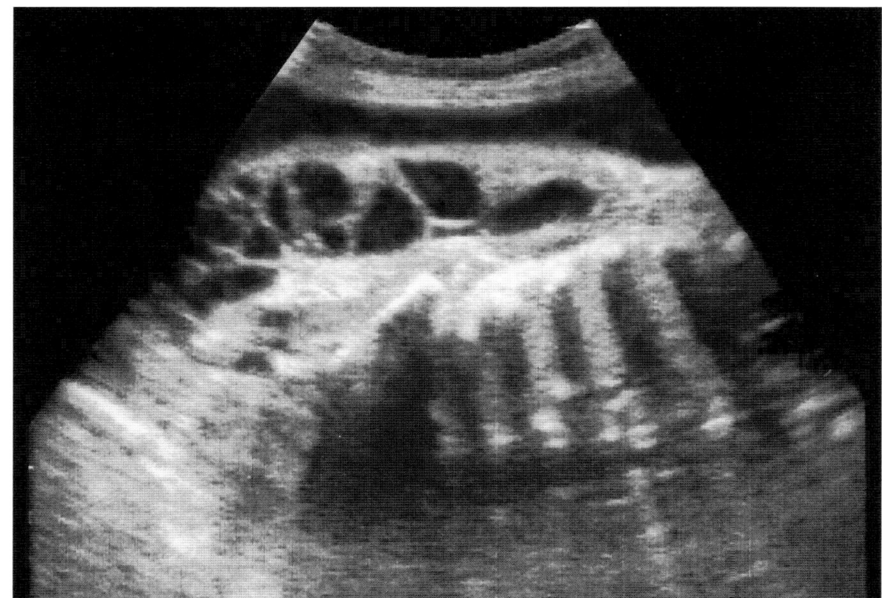

Fig. 11.13 **Klippel–Trénaunay–Weber syndrome.** Longitudinal section of the fetal thorax in a fetus with Klippel–Trénaunay–Weber syndrome.

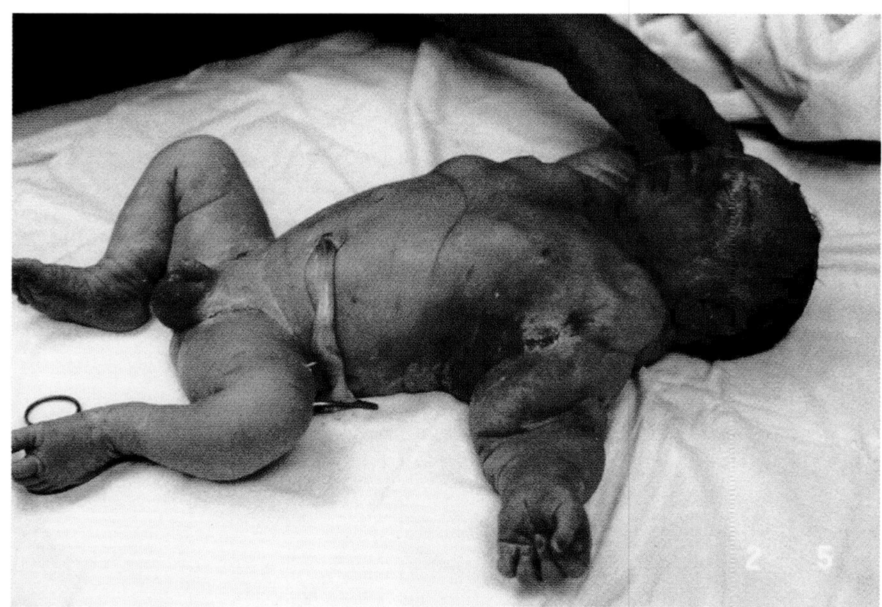

Fig. 11.14 **Klippel–Trénaunay–Weber syndrome.** The neonate seen immediately after birth. Successful surgical correction was carried out at a later stage.

fetus, then the fetus should be treated by administration of digitalis to the mother. In such cases, the delivery should be planned at 32 weeks. Cesarean section may be necessary in case of extensive hemangioma and the associated macrosomia.

Procedure after birth: Except in cases of fetal hydrops, no special management is necessary. Surgical correction or local compression may be required, depending on the lesions found.

Prognosis: This depends on the extent of malformations. Skin anomalies are well corrected by surgery, so that hypertrophy of certain parts can be avoided. In other cases, functional disability and cosmetic changes persist.

References

Becker R, Hoffbauer H, Entezami M, Waldschmidt J, Weitzel HK. Thorakale Manifestation eines Klippel–Trénaunay-Syndroms. Fallbericht und kurze Literaturübersicht. Ultraschall Med 1994; 15: 45–8.

Christenson L, Yankowitz J, Robinson R. Prenatal diagnosis of Klippel–Trénaunay–Weber syndrome as a cause for in utero heart failure and severe postnatal sequelae. Prenat Diagn 1997; 17: 1176–80.

Entezami M, Becker R, Vollert W, Arabin B, Weitzel HK. Fetale Makrosomie and Hydramnion. Intrauterine Symptome einer Kombination von Sturge–Weber–Krabbe und Klippel–Trénaunay-Syndrom. Ultraschall Med 1995; 16: 41–3.

Götze S, Weitzel H. Prenatal diagnosis and obstetric management of a case of Klippel–Trenaunay–Weber syndrome. Z Geburtshilfe Perinatol 1987; 191: 43–5.

Marler JJ, Fishman SJ, Upton J, et al. Prenatal diagnosis of vascular anomalies. J Pediatr Surg 2002; 37: 318–26.

Meholic AJ, Freimanis AK, Stucka J, LoPiccolo ML. Sonographic in utero diagnosis of Klippel–Trénaunay–Weber syndrome. J Ultrasound Med 1991; 10: 111–4.
Meizner I, Rosenak D, Nadjari M, Maor E. Sonographic diagnosis of Klippel–Trénaunay–Weber syndrome presenting as a sacrococcygeal mass at 14 to 15 weeks' gestation. J Ultrasound Med 1994; 13: 901–4.
Shalev E, Romano S, Nseir T, Zuckerman H. Klippel–Trénaunay syndrome: ultrasonic prenatal diagnosis. JCU J Clin Ultrasound 1988; 16: 268–70.
Yankowitz J, Slagel DD, Williamson R. Prenatal diagnosis of Klippel–Trénaunay–Weber syndrome by ultrasound. Prenat Diagn 1994; 14: 745–9.
Zoppi MA, Ibba RM, Floris M, Putzolu M, Crisponi G, Monni G. Prenatal sonographic diagnosis of Klippel–Trénaunay–Weber syndrome with cardiac failure. J Clin Ultrasound 2001; 29: 422–6.

Larsen Syndrome

Definition: Multiple congenital joint dislocations, facial dysmorphism, anomalies of the hand, finger and feet, and anomalies of the spinal column.

Incidence: Over a hundred cases have been described.

Origin/genetics: A collagen defect has been postulated. There are autosomal-dominant (gene locus: 3 p21.1 –p14.1) and autosomal-recessive forms of inheritance. Girls are more frequently affected than boys.

Ultrasound findings: Dislocation of the hip, knee and elbow joints is frequent. *Head and face:* flat, square shaped face; deep-set nasal bridge; frontal bossing, hypertelorism, cleft palate (50%). *Vertebral column and extremities*: scoliosis, spatula-like thumb, stubby fingers, short nails, short upper limbs, pedes equinovarus or valgus, short, stubby distal phalanges, short metacarpals. *Thorax:* occasionally cardiac defects, tracheomalacia. In a case with a positive family history, the diagnosis was made as early as at 16 weeks. The major finding here was *hyperextension of the knee joint.* A case has been reported in which the detection of anomalies on ultrasound scanning and diagnosis of the fetus led to confirmation of the diagnosis in the father.

Differential diagnosis: Otopalatodigital syndrome, Ehlers–Danlos syndrome, Marfan syndrome, arthrogryposis, diastrophic dysplasia, Pena–Shokeir syndrome, trisomy 18.

Prognosis: This is variable. Severe physical handicap may be present due to joint dislocations. Compression of the spinal cord is also possible. Mental development is normal.

References

Becker R, Wegner RD, Kunze J, Runkel S, Vogel M, Entezami M. Clinical variability of Larsen syndrome: diagnosis in a father after sonographic detection of a severely affected fetus. Clin Genet 2000; 57: 148–50.
Dören M, Rehder H, Holzgreve W. Prenatal diagnosis and obstetric management of Larsen's syndrome in a patient with an unrecognized family history of the disease. Gynecol Obstet Invest 1998; 46: 274–8.
Lewit N, Batino S, Groisman GM, Stark H, Bronshtein M. Early prenatal diagnosis of Larsen's syndrome by transvaginal sonography. J Ultrasound Med 1995; 14: 627–9.
Rochelson B, Petrikovsky B, Shmoys S. Prenatal diagnosis and obstetric management of Larsen syndrome. Obstet Gynecol 1993; 81: 845–7.
Tongsong T, Wanapirak C, Pongsatha S, Sudasana J. Prenatal sonographic diagnosis of Larsen syndrome. J Ultrasound Med 2000; 19: 419–21.

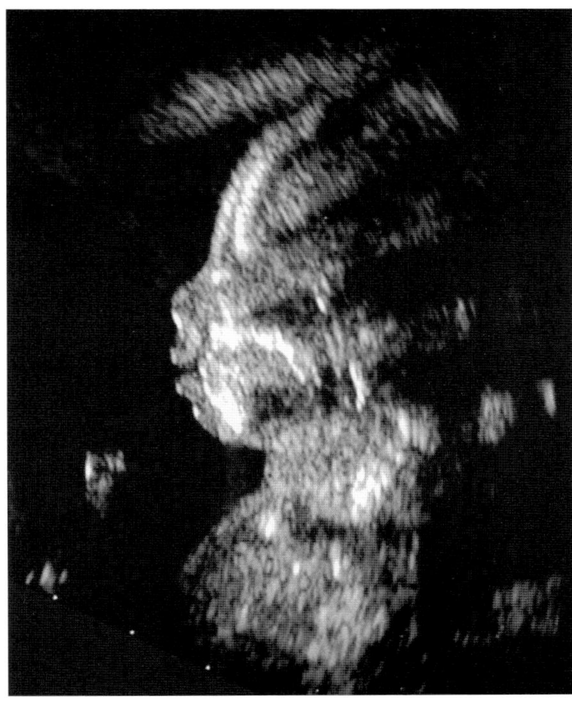

Fig. 11.**15** **Larsen syndrome.** Flattened fetal profile at 16 + 3 weeks.

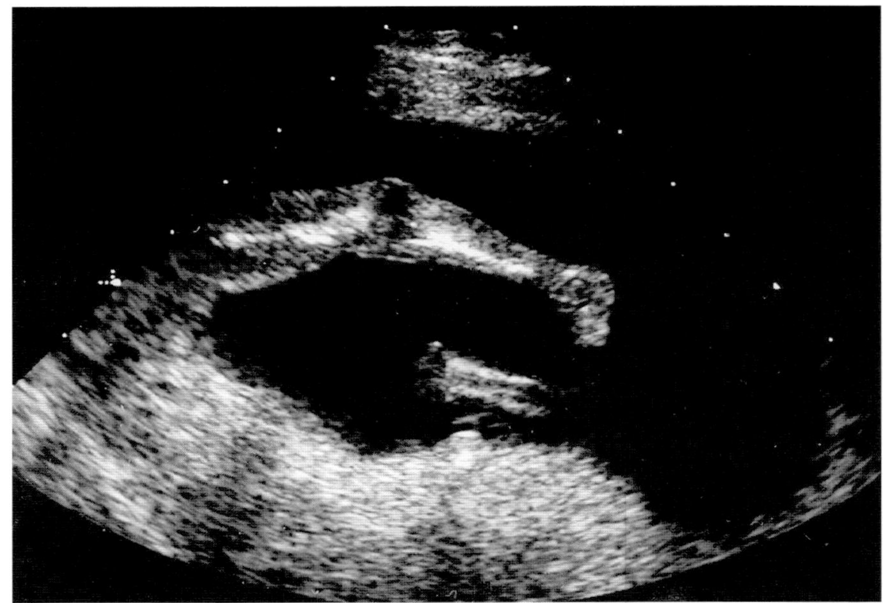

Fig. 11.**16** **Larsen syndrome.** Lower fetal limb at 16 + 3 weeks in Larsen syndrome. There is malpositioning of the knee joint.

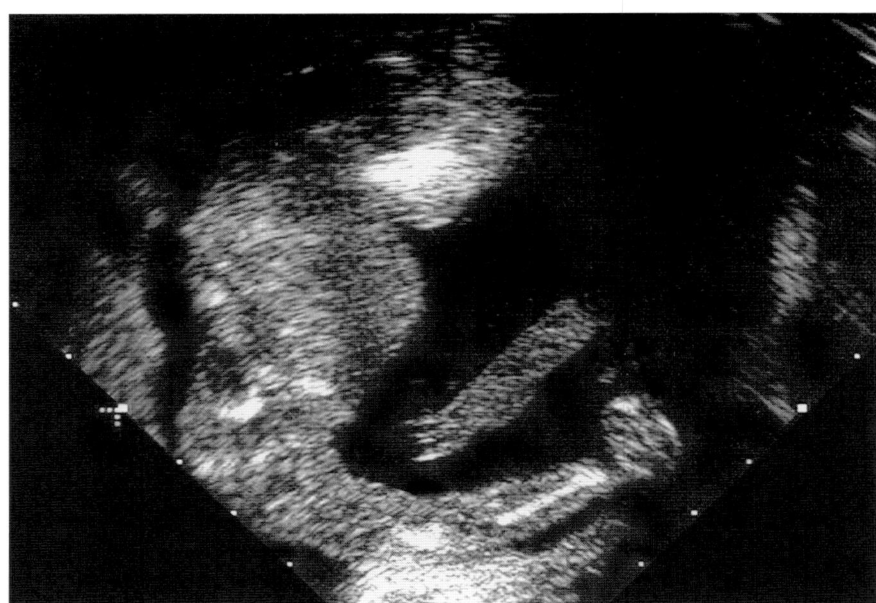

Fig. 11.**17** **Larsen syndrome.** Lower limb, showing nonphysiological overextension—genu recurvatum.

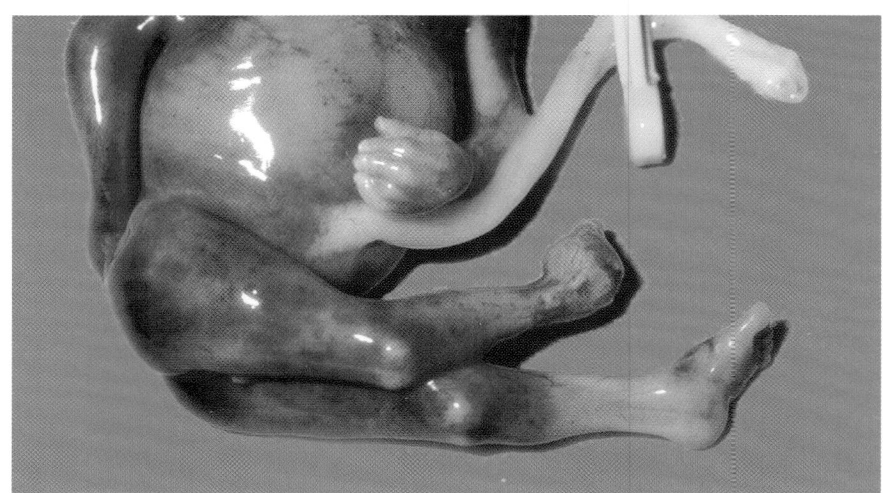

Fig. 11.**18** **Larsen syndrome.** Same fetus after termination of the pregnancy, showing severe genua recurvata.

Meckel–Gruber Syndrome (Dysencephalia Splanchnocystica)

Definition: This syndrome consists of encephalocele, postaxial hexadactyly, and cystic renal dysplasia.

Incidence: This varies according to ethnic origins. In the United Kingdom, it is one in 140 000; among Ashkenazi Jews, one in 50 000; in Finland, one in 8500; in Massachusetts, one in 13 250; in Belgium, one in 3000; in Gujarat, India, one in 1300.

Genetics: Autosomal-recessive inheritance, genetically heterogeneous. Gene locus: 17 q21–24, 11 q13.

Ultrasound findings: Due to reduced renal function, oligohydramnios or anhydramnios are common. Encephalocele (80%), microcephaly or anencephaly may also be present. Dandy–Walker malformation, agenesis of the corpus callosum, cerebellar hypoplasia, Arnold–Chiari malformation. *Cystic renal dysplasia (95%)*, anomalies of the ureter, cysts of the liver, *postaxial hexadactyly of hands and feet* (75%). In addi-

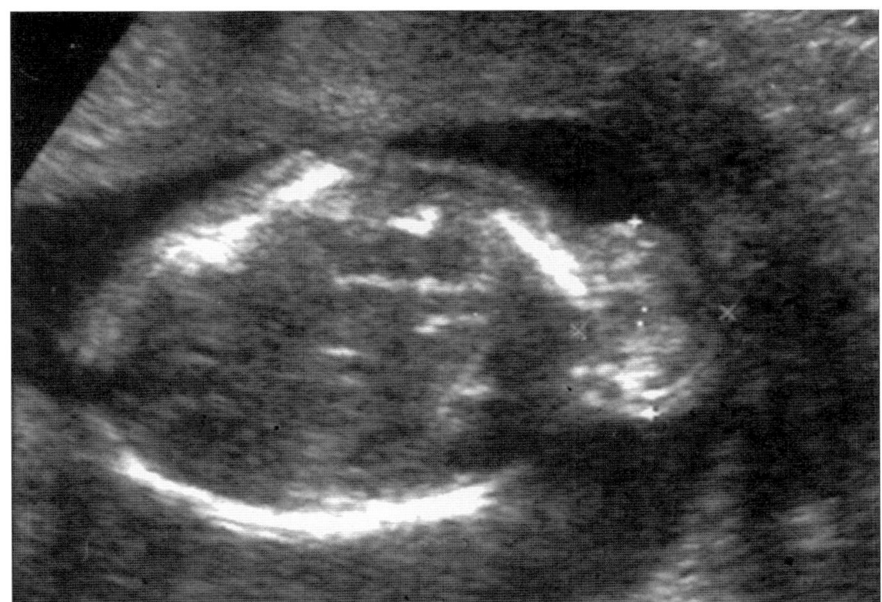

Fig. 11.**19** **Meckel–Gruber syndrome.** Cross-section of fetal head at 19 + 4 weeks showing occipital encephalocele. Scan after amnioinfusion.

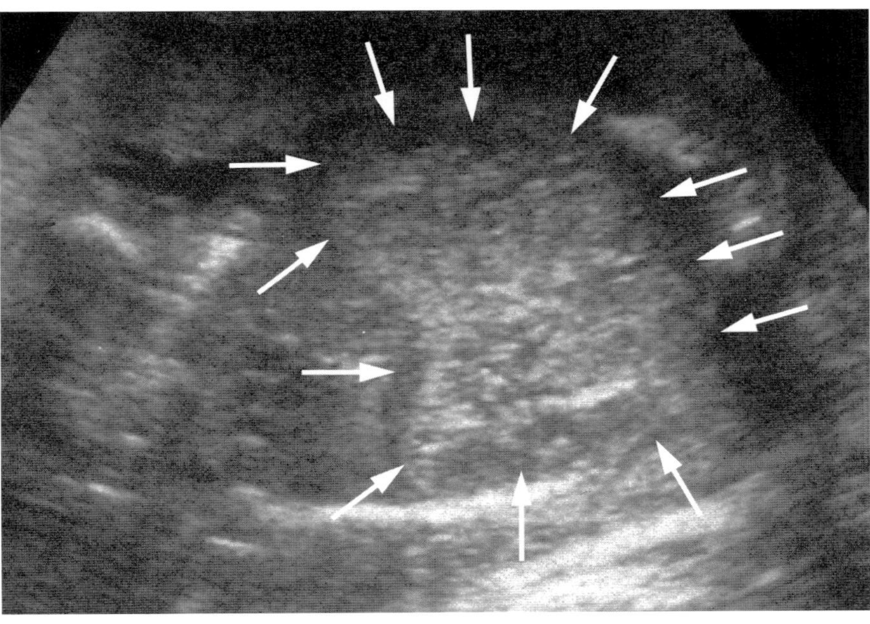

Fig. 11.**20** **Meckel–Gruber syndrome.** Frontal view of the fetal retroperitoneum in a case of Meckel–Gruber syndrome at 19 + 4 weeks. There is enlargement of both kidneys (arrows), which are also filled with small cysts. Demonstration was difficult due to anhydramnios.

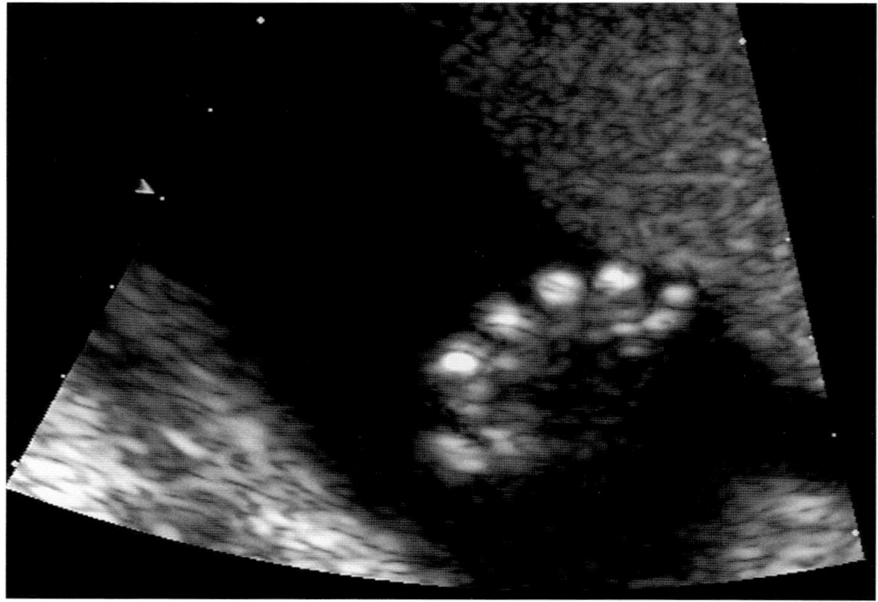

Fig. 11.**21** **Meckel–Gruber syndrome.** Hexadactyly of the foot in Meckel–Gruber syndrome at 12 + 6 weeks.

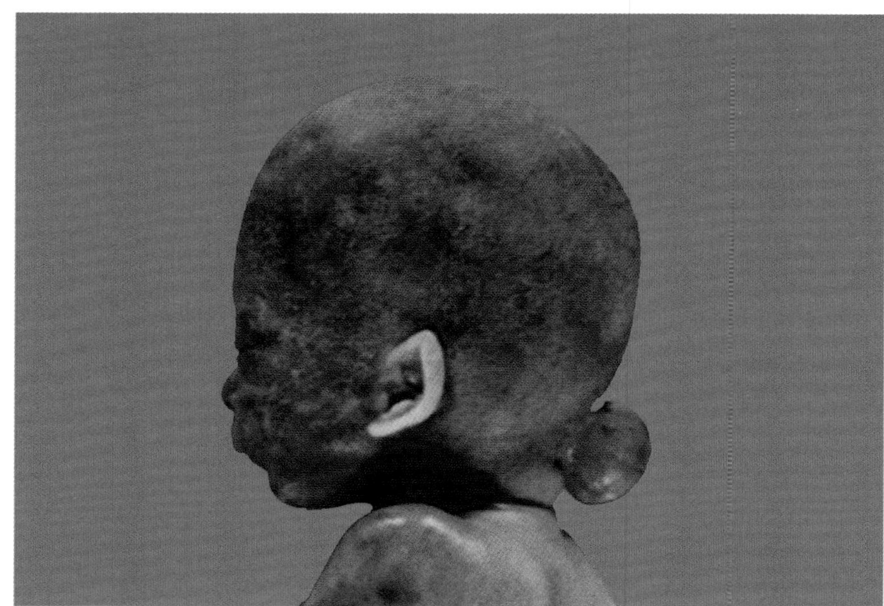

Fig. 11.**22** **Meckel–Gruber syndrome.** Fetus after termination of the pregnancy, showing occipital encephalocele.

tion, *facial dysmorphism* is also seen: cleft lip, cleft palate, microphthalmia, hypertelorism, macrostomia, anomaly of the tongue, narrow chin, deep-set ears, short neck. Cardiac and genital anomalies are also seen. Diagnosis has been possible at 11 weeks after detection of encephalocele and polydactyly.

Differential diagnosis: Potter sequence, trisomy 13, hydrolethalus, Smith–Lemli–Opitz syndrome, infantile polycystic kidney disease, Joubert syndrome, Mohr syndrome, short rib-polydactyly syndrome.

Prognosis: About one-third of the fetuses are stillborn. In almost all cases, death occurs within 3 h after birth.

References

Braithwaite JM, Economides DL. First-trimester diagnosis of Meckel–Gruber syndrome by transabdominal sonography in a low-risk case. Prenat Diagn 1995; 15: 1168–70.

Gallimore AP, Davies PF. Meckel syndrome: prenatal ultrasonographic diagnosis in two cases showing marked differences in phenotypic expression. Australas Radiol 1992; 36: 62–4.

Nyberg DA, Hallesy D, Mahony BS, Hirsch JH, Luthy DA, Hickok D. Meckel–Gruber syndrome: importance of prenatal diagnosis. J Ultrasound Med 1990; 9: 691–6.

Pachi A, Giancotti A, Torcia F, de Prosperi V, Maggi E. Meckel–Gruber syndrome: ultrasonographic diagnosis at 13 weeks' gestational age in an at-risk case. Prenat Diagn 1989; 9: 187–90.

Schmidt W, von Hoist T, Schroeder T, Kubli F. [Prenatal diagnosis of Meckel–Gruber's syndrome by ultrasound; in German]. Z Geburtshilfe. Perinatol 1981; 185: 67–71.

Tanriverdi HA, Hendrik HJ, Ertan K, Schmidt W. Meckel Gruber syndrome: a first trimester diagnosis of a recurrent case. Eur J Ultrasound 2002; 15: 69–72.

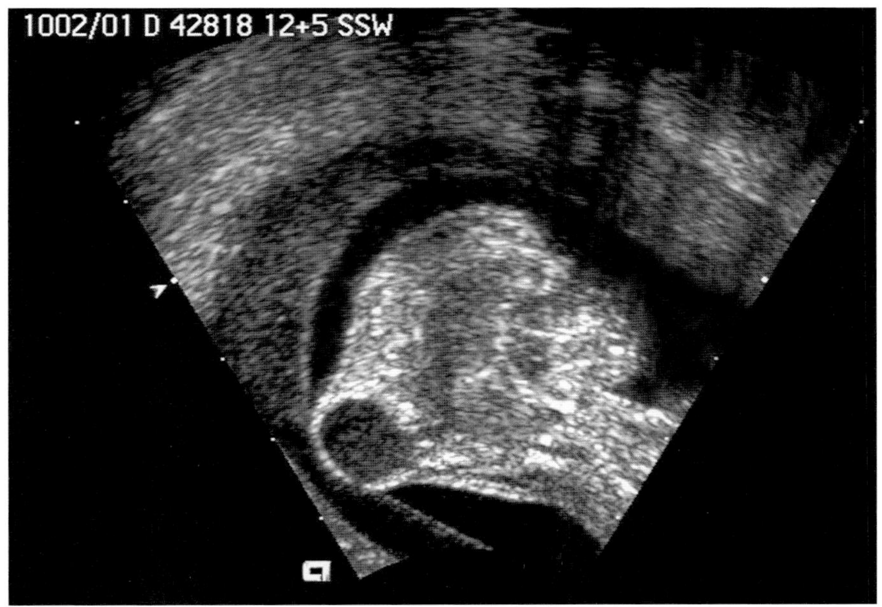

Fig. 11.**23** **Meckel–Gruber syndrome.** Transvaginal scan (10 MHz), demonstrating occipital encephalocele at 12 + 5 weeks in a fetus with Meckel–Gruber syndrome.

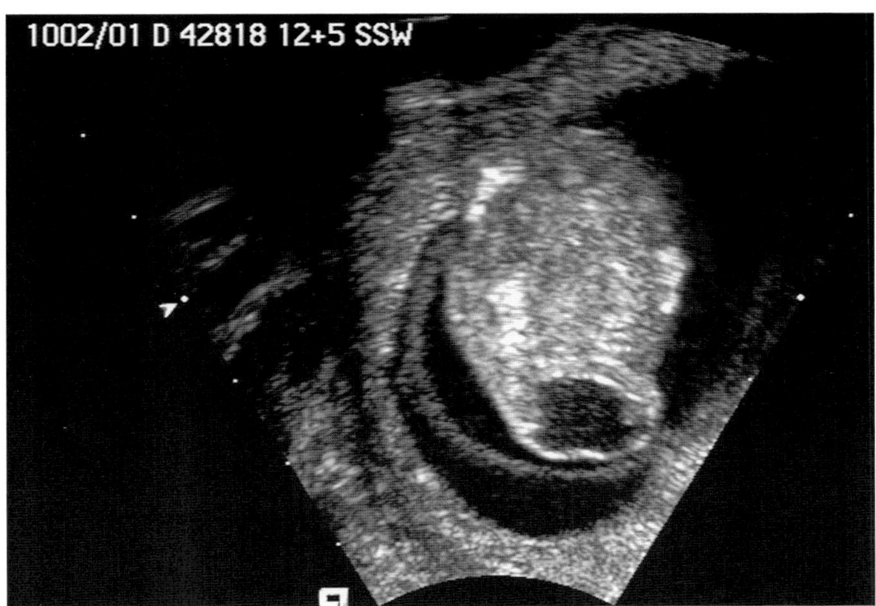

Fig. 11.**24** **Meckel–Gruber syndrome.** Same fetus. Cross-section of the fetal head, showing protrusion of brain tissue.

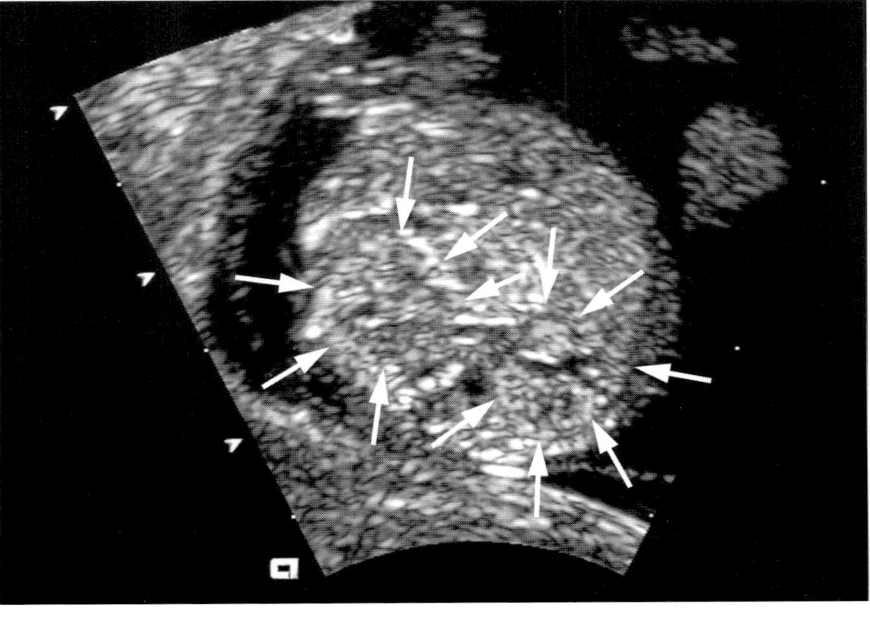

Fig. 11.**25** **Meckel–Gruber syndrome.** Same fetus. Cross-section of the abdomen, showing echogenic, enlarged kidneys.

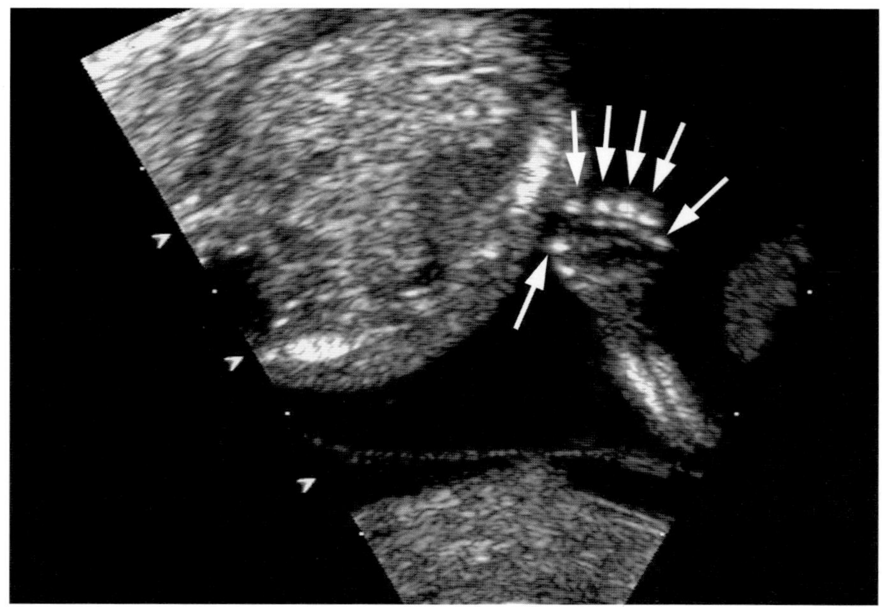

Fig. 11.**26** **Meckel–Gruber syndrome.** Same fetus. Demonstration of postaxial hexadactyly.

Miller–Dieker Syndrome (Lissencephaly Type I)

Definition: This is a structural chromosomal anomaly characterized by an almost complete absence of the cerebral gyri. It is combined with microcephaly, dysplasia of the ear, facial dysmorphisms such as flared nostrils, and mental impairment.

Incidence: Extremely rare; only 20 cases have been described.

Origin/genetics: Usually, a defect in chromosome 17 (17 p13.3) is found; there is partial loss of the short arm; translocation or a ring chromosome may also be present. The risk of recurrence is 25%, but in case of new mutation the recurrence risk is not increased. In familial translocation forms, diagnosis is possible during prenatal screening by chromosomal analysis (high-resolution banding).

Clinical features: *Head and face*: microcephaly, high forehead, prominent occipital region, bitemporal pitting, long upper lip median ridge, thin upper lip, lissencephaly or pachygyria, thickened skull, widening of cerebral ventricles, microgenia, dysplasia of the auricles, broad nasal bridge, flared nostrils. In addition, cardiac defects, cryptorchism, clouding of the cornea, neonatal fits, reduced muscle tone, severe mental impairment.

Ultrasound findings: The diagnosis can be made at 26 weeks at the earliest. *Microcephaly and agyria* are first evident at this stage. *Widening of the cerebral ventricles and abnormal shape of the head* are suspicious for lissencephaly. Additional findings are: hydramnios, growth restriction, microgenia, dysplasia of the auricles, broad nasal bridge, and flared nostrils. There is a reduction in fetal movement. Cardiac anomalies, renal malformations, cryptorchism, and duodenal atresia may not always be present.

Differential diagnosis: Walker–Warburg syndrome, Norman–Roberts syndrome, agenesis of the corpus callosum, Cornelia de Lange syndrome, Wolf–Hirschhorn syndrome, cri-du-chat syndrome, Jacobsen syndrome, Fanconi anemia, Freeman–Sheldon syndrome, Meckel–Gruber syndrome, multiple pterygium syndrome, Neu–Laxova syndrome, neural tube defects, Roberts syndrome, Seckel syndrome, Shprintzen syndrome, Smith–Lemli–Opitz syndrome, triploidy, trisomy 9, trisomy 13.

Clinical management: Magnetic resonance imaging at the prenatal stage is a useful method of examining the cerebrum and other intracranial structures. If the fetus is lying with a cephalic presentation, then a vaginal scan can also be used to examine intracranial structures.

Prognosis: This is generally unfavorable; severe mental impairment, growth restriction, and fits can be expected. About 50% of affected infants die within the first 6 months of life; the remainder die in early childhood.

Self-Help Organizations

Title: The Lissencephaly Network

Description: Support for families affected by lissencephaly or other neuronal migration disorders, and their families. Helps relieve the stress of caring for an ill child. Research updates, newsletter, database of affected children. Networking of parents.

Scope: International network

Founded: 1991

Address: 10408 Bitterroot Ct., Ft. Wayne, IN 46804, United States

Telephone: 219–432–4310

Fax: 219–432–4310

E-mail: DianneFitz@aol.com

Web: http://www.lissencephaly.org

Title: Foundation for Nager and Miller Syndromes

Description: Networking for families that are affected by Nager or Miller syndromes. Provides referrals, library of information, phone support, newsletter, brochures, scholarships for Camp About Face.

Scope: International

Founded: 1989

Address: 1827 Grove St., Glenview, IL 60025–2913, United States

Telephone: 1–800–507–3667

Fax: 847–724–6449

E-mail: fnms@interaccess.com

Web: http://www.fnms.net

References

Chitayat D, Toi A, Babul R, et al. Omphalocele in Miller–Dieker syndrome: expanding the phenotype. Am J Med Genet 1997; 69: 293–8.

Kingston HM, Ledbetter DH, Tomlin PI, Gaunt KL. Miller–Dieker syndrome resulting from rearrangement of a familial chromosome 17 inversion detected by fluorescence in situ hybridization. J Med Genet 1996; 33: 69–72.

McGahan JP, Grix A, Gerscovich EO. Prenatal diagnosis of lissencephaly: Miller–Dieker syndrome. J Clin Ultrasound 1994; 22: 560–3.

van Zelderen-Bhola SL, Breslau-Siderius EJ, Beverstock GC, et al. Prenatal and postnatal investigation of a case with Miller–Dieker syndrome due to a familial cryptic translocation t(17;20)(p13.3;q13.3) detected by fluorescence in situ hybridization. Prenat Diagn 1997; 17: 173–9.

Mohr Syndrome (Orofaciodigital Syndrome Type II)

Definition: This is a group of disorders consisting of postaxial polydactyly of the hands, polysyndactyly involving the great toe, lapping of the tongue, hyperplasia of the frenulum, typical facial expression, growth restriction, and deafness.

First described in 1941 by Mohr.

Origin: Autosomal-recessive inheritance.

Ultrasound findings: Ultrasound scanning shows *postaxial polydactyly, brachydactyly, syndactyly and clinodactyly of the hands*, as well as *doubling of the great toe*. Anomalies of the tongue such as splitting and overlapping, as well as thickening of the frenulum, are barely recognizable on scanning. *Facial features* of the fetus are abnormal: hypertelorism, broad nasal bridge, occasionally a median upper lip cleft, hypoplasia of the jaw. Additional cerebral anomalies such as widening of the ventricles, porencephaly, encephalocele, agenesis of the corpus callosum may be evident. Renal anomalies may also occur. This syndrome has been diagnosed at 21 weeks, due to detection of hydramnios, hydrocephalus, microgenia, club feet, and polydactyly.

Other clinical features: Absence of the middle incisors, raised palate, cleft palate, short or wide metatarsal.

Differential diagnosis: Orofaciodigital syndrome type I (only in girls), orofaciodigital syndrome types III–IX, Carpenter syndrome, hydrolethalus, Majewski syndrome, Meckel–Gruber syndrome, Smith–Lemli–Opitz syndrome.

Prognosis: Life expectancy is normal. However, mental development may be restricted if there are intracranial anomalies.

References

Adám Z, Papp Z. Prenatal diagnosis of orofaciodigital syndrome Varadi–Papp type [letter; comment]. J Ultrasound Med 1996; 15: 714.

Balci S, Guler G, Kale G, Soylemezoglu F, Besim A. Mohr syndrome in two sisters: prenatal diagnosis in a 22-week-old fetus with post-mortem findings in both. Prenat Diagn 1999; 19: 827–31.

Benson CB, Pober BR, Hirsh MP, Doubilet PM. Sonography of Nager acrofacial dysostosis syndrome in utero. J Ultrasound Med 1988; 7: 163–7.

Iaccarino M, Lonardo F, Giugliano M, Della BM. Prenatal diagnosis of Mohr syndrome by ultrasonography. Prenat Diagn 1985; 5: 415–8.

Suresh S, Rajesh K, Suresh I, Raja V, Gopish D, Gnanasoundari S. Prenatal diagnosis of orofaciodigital syndrome: Mohr type. J Ultrasound Med 1995; 14: 863–6.

Multiple Pterygium Syndrome

Definition: This is a heterogeneous group of syndromes with pterygium of the neck and joints. Two forms have been described: fatal and nonfatal forms. The fatal form is accompanied by fetal hydrops, diaphragmatic hernia, and pulmonary hypoplasia due to immobile thorax.

Incidence: Rare.

Sex ratio: M : F = 1 : 1.

Clinical history/genetics: Heterogeneous inheritance is known. The fatal forms are mostly sporadic, but autosomal-dominant and autosomal-recessive modes have also been reported. The fatal type is inherited in autosomal-recessive or X-chromosome-recessive forms.

Teratogen: Not known.

Origin: It is postulated that pterygium forms at the joints, which are for some reason not sufficiently mobile. Production of collagen and fibrous tissue is possibly abnormal, causing disturbance in lymph drainage and muscle development.

Ultrasound findings: *Nuchal edema or hygroma colli* are evident in the first trimester. *Multiple joint contractures:* the arms are constantly bent, the legs are bent at the hip joint, and in many cases the knees are in a fixed position. Fetal movement is reduced considerably, or may be totally absent. Hydramnios and fetal hydrops may develop. The following malformations may

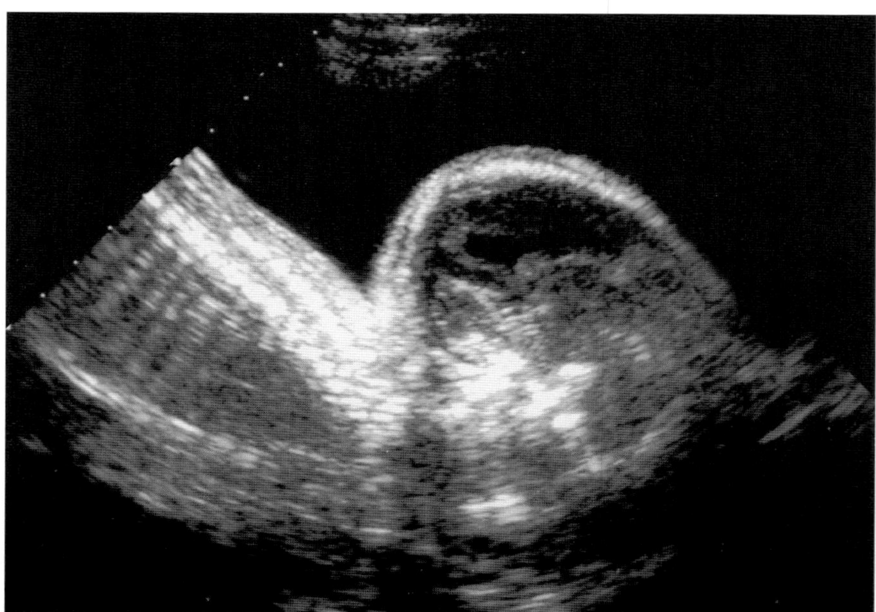

Fig. 11.**27** **Multiple pterygium syndrome** (MPS). A dorsoanterior longitudinal section of the fetal neck at 24 + 5 weeks. The head is fixed in a retroverted position in MPS.

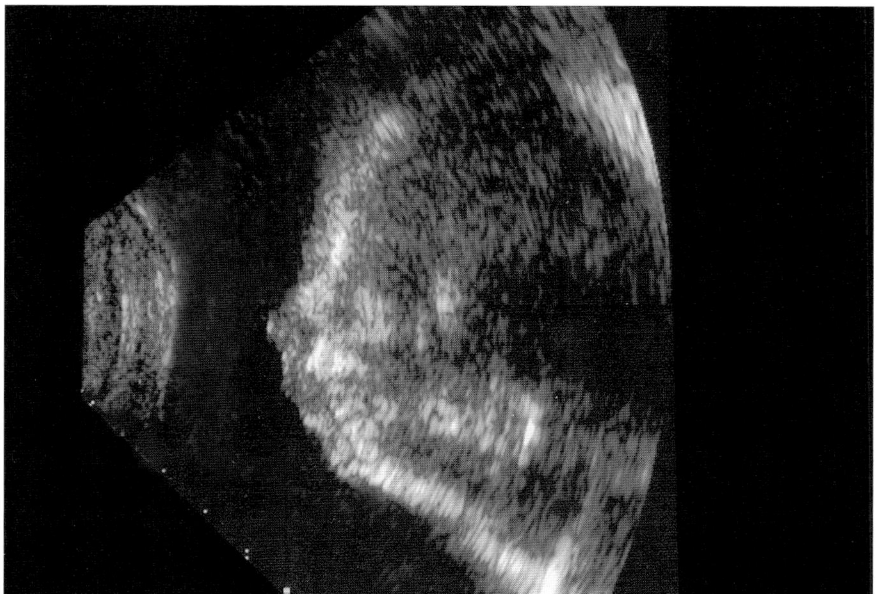

Fig. 11.**28** **Multiple pterygium syndrome** (MPS). Fetal profile at 24 + 5 weeks.

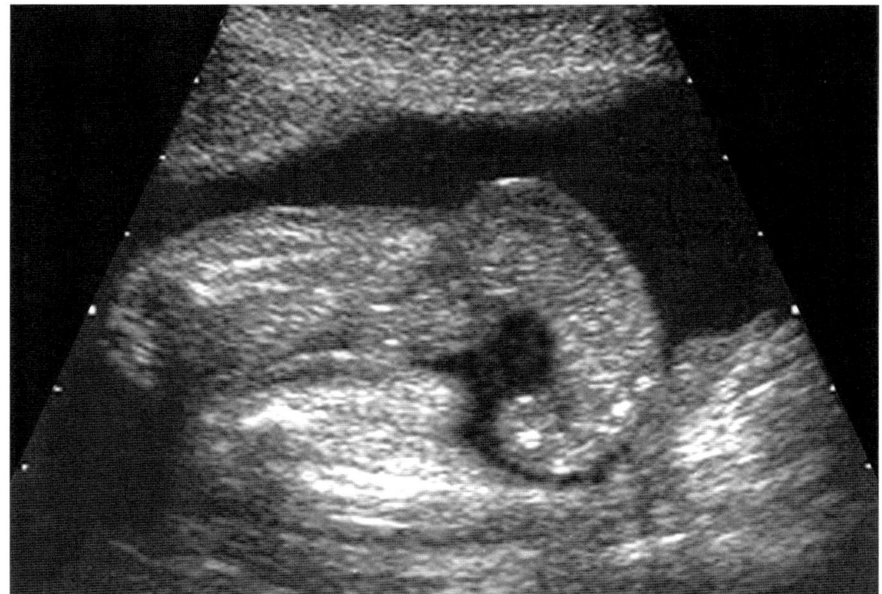

Fig. 11.**29** **Multiple pterygium syndrome** (MPS). Deformed pes equinovarus at 24 + 5 weeks.

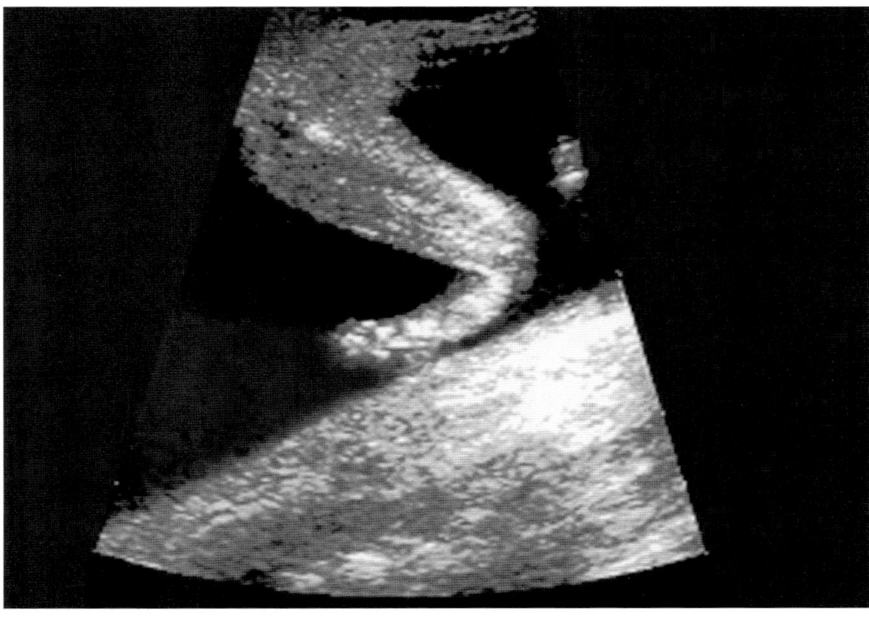

Fig. 11.**30** **Multiple pterygium syndrome** (MPS). Malpositioning of the fetal hand at 24 + 5 weeks.

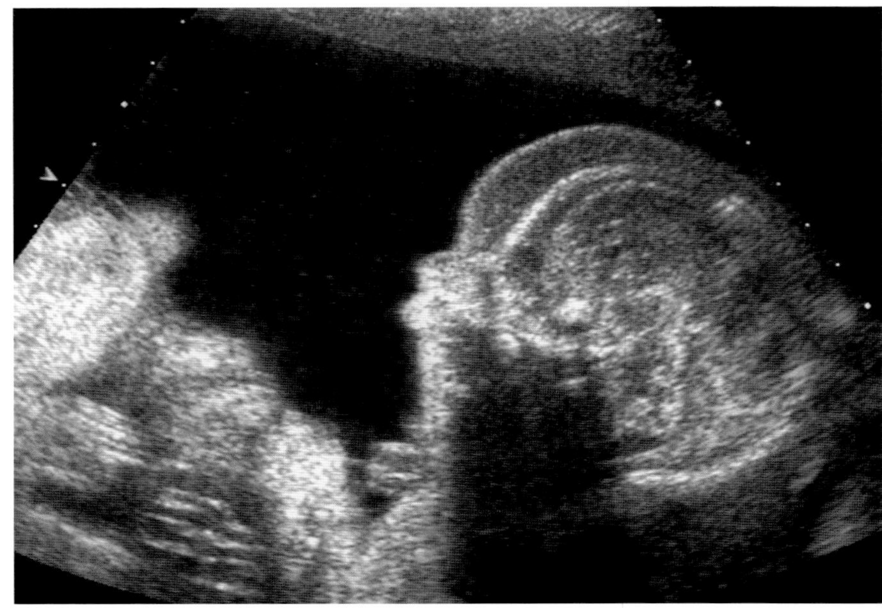

Fig. 11.**31** **Multiple pterygium syndrome** (MPS). Fetal profile at 21 + 6 weeks, demonstrating retrogenia and edema of the forehead.

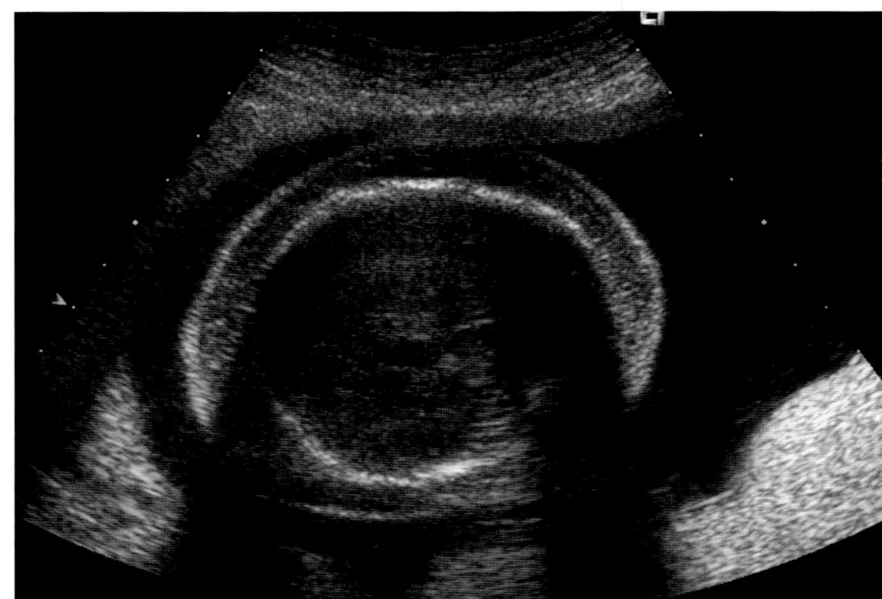

Fig. 11.**32** **Multiple pterygium syndrome** (MPS). Same fetus. Cross-section of the fetal head: anasarca in a case of nonimmune hydrops fetalis (NIHF) associated with fetal MPS.

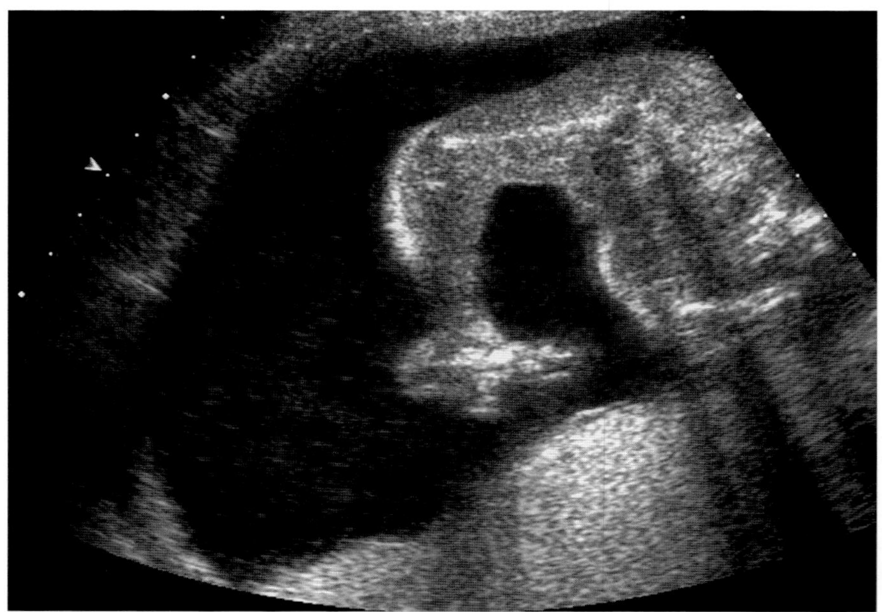

Fig. 11.**33** **Multiple pterygium syndrome** (MPS). Same fetus. The scan shows a fetal hand in a fixed, deformed position.

also be associated: microgenia, cleft palate, hypertelorism, microcephaly, widening of cerebral ventricles, omphalocele, cardiac defects, diaphragmatic hernia, hydronephroses, club feet, and syndactyly. Diagnosis has been possible at 13 weeks.

Differential diagnosis: Over 25 syndromes have been described involving the formation of pterygium over various joints. Amniotic band sequence, arthrogryposis, caudal regression syndrome, Cornelia de Lange syndrome, Freeman–Sheldon syndrome, Neu–Laxova syndrome, Pena–Shokeir syndrome, Roberts syndrome, Seckel syndrome, neurological and muscular impairment, triploidy, and trisomy 18.

Clinical management: Further screening, including fetal echocardiography. Karyotyping. The issue of obstetric management due to fetal distress should be discussed with the parents, and the extent of malformations should be taken into account.

Procedure after birth: The fatal forms lead to death in the early neonatal period. The infants die due to respiratory failure, as pulmonary hypoplasia results from the fixed thoracic cavity. Surviving infants with the nonfatal forms require orthopedic surgery to correct contraction deformities.

Prognosis: Infants with nonfatal forms have normal intelligence and life expectancy. Physical handicap continues to be a problem, despite orthopedic corrections. The fatal forms result in intrauterine fetal demise due to severe fetal hydrops, or early neonatal death due to respiratory failure.

References

Entezami M, Runkel S, Kunze J, Weitzel HK, Becker R. Prenatal diagnosis of a lethal multiple pterygium syndrome type II: case report. Fetal Diagn Ther 1998; 13: 35–8.

Lockwood C, Irons M, Troiani J, Kawada C, Chaudhury A, Cetrulo C. The prenatal sonographic diagnosis of lethal multiple pterygium syndrome: a heritable cause of recurrent abortion. Am J Obstet Gynecol 1988; 159: 474–6.

Sciarrone A, Verdiglione P, Botta G, Franceschini P, Todros T. Prenatal diagnosis of lethal multiple pterygium syndrome in mid-pregnancy [letter]. Ultrasound Obstet Gynecol 1998; 12: 218–9.

Yfantis H, Nonaka D, Castellani R, Harman C, Sun CC. Heterogeneity in fetal akinesia deformation sequence (FADS): autopsy confirmation in three 20–21-week fetuses. Prenat Diagn 2002; 22: 42–7.

Zeitune M, Fejgin MD, Abramowicz J, Ben Aderet N, Goodman RM. Prenatal diagnosis of the pterygium syndrome. Prenat Diagn 1988; 8: 145–9.

MURCS Association

Definition: This is the acronym for *mü*llerian duct aplasia, *r*enal aplasia, and dysplasia of the *c*ervicothoracic *s*omites.

First described in 1979.

Ultrasound findings: *Anomalies of the vertebral bodies* are seen at the border of neck and thoracic region. *Renal agenesis* or *ectopic kidney* is also evident. Genital anomalies such as hypoplasia of the uterus and the upper vagina are not detectable at the prenatal stage. Other malformations may also be present: cerebellar cysts, facial dysmorphisms such as cleft palate and lip, microgenia, dysplasia of the ear; anomalies of the ribs, and malformation of the upper limbs and shoulder. This syndrome has been diagnosed at 22 weeks after detection of severe oligohydramnios, dilated urinary bladder, urachal cysts, and anomalies of the vertebral bodies.

Differential diagnosis: Apert syndrome, Goldenhar syndrome, Gorlin syndrome, Jarcho–Levin syndrome, Klippel–Feil sequence, Noonan syndrome.

Prognosis: This is favorable in most cases. The well-known Rokitansky–Küster–Mayer syndrome is probably a variation of the MURCS association. It is characterized by hypoplasia of the uterus and external genitals and infertility. Sexual intercourse can be made possible by surgical correction. The prognosis mainly depends on renal anomalies and pulmonary hypoplasia.

References

Fernandez CO, McFarland RD, Timmons C, Ramus R, Twickler DM. MURCS association: ultrasonographic findings and pathologic correlation. J Ultrasound Med 1996; 15: 867–70.

Geipel A, Berg C, Germer U, et al. Diagnostic and therapeutic problems in a case of prenatally detected fetal hydrocolpos. Ultrasound Obstet Gynecol 2001; 18: 169–72.

Kubik HR, Wisser J, Stallmach T, Ladd ME, Meier A, Marincek B. Prenatal diagnosis of fetal malformations by ultrafast magnetic resonance imaging. Prenat Diagn 1998; 18: 1205–8.

Nager Syndrome (Acrofacial Dysostosis)

Definition: This disorder consists of mandibulofacial dysostoses with hypoplasia of the extremities, especially involving the upper limbs.

Incidence: Very rare; only 70 cases have been described.

Origin/genetics: Sporadic occurrence is the most frequent form. Autosomal-dominant forms with variable expression, as well as autosomal-recessive forms, are possible.

Clinical features: Growth restriction is common; mild to moderate mental impairment, respiratory and feeding disturbances such as those seen in Pierre Robin sequence are also possible. Facial dysmorphism (mandibulofacial dysostosis) is characteristic: deep-set and malformed ears, relative deafness, cleft lip and palate. Anomalies of the thumb (triphalangia, hypoplasia, aplasia), hypoplasia of the radius, radioulnar synostoses, and phocomelia may be evident. Maldevelopment of the lower limbs is also possible. Additional anomalies of the heart and kidneys are rare.

Ultrasound findings: According to one report, diagnosis was possible at 30 weeks on the basis of hydramnios, hypoplasia of the radius, and mandibular anomalies.

Differential diagnosis: Treacher–Collins syndrome, acrofacial dysostosis of the postaxial type and other mandibular or acrofacial dysostosis, Cornelia de Lange syndrome, EEC syndrome, Fanconi anemia, femur–fibula–ulna syndrome, Holt–Oram syndrome, multiple pterygium syndrome, Mohr syndrome, Pena–Shokeir syndrome, Pierre Robin sequence, Roberts syndrome, TAR syndrome, trisomy 18.

Prognosis: Facial features may become less marked as the infant gets older. Surgical treatment may help improve disturbed hearing. Respiratory complications such as those seen in Pierre Robin sequence may be evident at the neonatal stage.

Self-Help Organization

Title: Foundation for Nager and Miller Syndromes

Description: Networking for families that are affected by Nager or Miller Syndromes. Provides referrals, library of information, phone support, newsletter, brochures, scholarships for Camp About Face.

Scope: International

Founded: 1989

Address: 1827 Grove St., Glenview, IL 60025–2913, United States

Telephone: 1–800–507–3667

Fax: 847–724–6449

E-mail: fnms@interaccess.com

Web: http://www.fnms.net

References

Benson CB, Pober BR, Hirsh MP, Doubilet PM. Sonography of Nager acrofacial dysostosis syndrome in utero. J Ultrasound Med 1988; 7: 163–7.

Hecht JT, Immken LL, Harris LF, Malini S, Scott CI Jr. The Nager syndrome. Am J Med Genet 1987; 27: 965–9.

Satoh S, Takashima T, Takeuchi H, Koyanagi T, Nakano H. Antenatal sonographic detection of the proximal esophageal segment: specific evidence for congenital esophageal atresia. J Clin Ultrasound 1995; 23: 419–23.

Zori RT, Gray BA, Bent-Williams A, Driscoll DJ, Williams CA, Zackowski JL. Preaxial acrofacial dysostosis (Nager syndrome) associated with an inherited and apparently balanced X;9 translocation: prenatal and postnatal late replication studies. Am J Med Genet 1993; 46: 379–83.

Neu–Laxova Syndrome

Definition: This is a fatal disorder consisting of microcephaly, lissencephaly, exophthalmos, growth restriction, and subcutaneous edema.

Origin: Autosomal-recessive inheritance.

Ultrasound findings: A range of anomalies can be found on scanning: early severe growth restriction, hydramnios, small placenta, edema of the subcutaneous tissue, microcephaly, lissencephaly, agenesis of the corpus callosum, hypoplasia of the cerebellum, hypertelorism, cataracts, microphthalmia and exophthalmos, microgenia, short neck, genital hypoplasia, short limbs, syndactyly, edema of the hands and feet, flexion contractures. In addition, the following may be seen in combination with the above: cardiac anomalies, facial clefts, Dandy–Walker malformations, widening of the cranial ventricles. The earliest diagnosis was possible at 22 weeks after detection of growth restriction, microcephaly, hydramnios, exophthalmos, cataract, hygroma colli, syndactyly, and club feet.

Differential diagnosis: Miller–Dieker syndrome, Walker–Warburg syndrome, arthrogryposis, multiple pterygium syndrome, Pena–Shokeir syndrome, chromosomal anomalies, Cornelia de Lange syndrome, Freeman–Sheldon syndrome, rubella, Seckel syndrome, Smith–Lemli–Opitz syndrome, toxoplasmosis.

Prognosis: The outcome is fatal; this syndrome results in intrauterine demise or death in the neonatal period.

Self-Help Organization

Title: The Lissencephaly Network

Description: Support for families affected by lissencephaly or other neuronal migration disorders, and their families. Helps relieve the stress of caring for an ill child. Research updates, newsletter, database of affected children. Networking of parents.

Scope: International network

Founded: 1991

Address: 10408 Bitterroot Ct., Ft. Wayne, IN 46804, United States

Telephone: 219–432–4310

Fax: 219–432–4310

E-mail: DianneFitz@aol.com

Web: http://www.lissencephaly.org

References

Aslan H, Gul A, Polat I, Mutaf C, Agar M, Ceylan Y. Prenatal diagnosis of Neu–Laxova syndrome: a case report. BMC Pregnancy Childbirth 2002; 2: 1.

Driggers RW, Isbister S, McShane C, Stone K, Blakemore K. Early second trimester prenatal diagnosis of Neu–Laxova syndrome. Prenat Diagn 2002; 22: 118–20.

Durr-e-Sabih, Khan AN, Sabih Z. Prenatal sonographic diagnosis of Neu–Laxova syndrome. J Clin Ultrasound 2001; 29: 531–4.

Gülmezoglu AM, Ekici E. Sonographic diagnosis of Neu–Laxova syndrome. J Clin Ultrasound 1994; 22: 48–51.

Rode ME, Mennuti MT, Giardine RM, Zackai EH, Driscoll DA. Early ultrasound diagnosis of Neu–Laxova syndrome [review]. Prenat Diagn 2001; 21: 575–80.

Tolmie JL, Mortimer G, Doyle D, McKenzie R, McLaurin J, Neilson JP. The Neu–Laxova syndrome in female sibs: clinical and pathological features with prenatal diagnosis in the second sib. Am J Med Genet 1987; 27: 175–82.

Noonan Syndrome (Turner-Like Syndrome)

Definition: This syndrome is a combination of malformations and growth restriction, and consists of facial dysmorphism, dwarfism, and anomalies of the heart and various other organs.

Incidence: One in 2500–10 000 births.

Origin/genetics: A normal set of chromosomes is present. Autosomal-dominant inheritance with variable expression is found (gene locus: 12 q24). Sporadic occurrence is frequent. The risk of recurrence is 5%. The condition may become manifest after birth.

Clinical features: Symmetrical short stature; mental impairment may be mild to moderate. *Typical facial features:* widening of the interorbital distance, epicanthus, axis of the eyelids pointing downwards (antimongoloid), ptosis, microgenia. In addition, a low neck hairline, pterygium (differential diagnosis: Turner syndrome), cutis laxa, deep-set ears, raised palate. *Thorax:* shield chest, pectus excavatum; pulmonary stenosis, and other cardiac anomalies, pigment anomalies such as café-au-lait spots. Occasionally, lymphedema of the hands and feet.

Ultrasound findings: In the first trimester, nuchal edema is the most typical feature, and it may also present as cystic hygroma. Cardiac anomalies such as pulmonary stenosis are well diagnosed. If *a cystic hygroma* is detected in a fetus with *a normal set of chromosomes*, then the diagnosis of Noonan syndrome is most likely.

Differential diagnosis: Ulrich–Turner syndrome, LEOPARD syndrome, Aarskog syndrome, neurofibromatosis–Noonan syndrome, trisomy 18, trisomy 21, achondrogenesis, Apert syndrome, Cornelia de Lange syndrome, EEC syndrome, Joubert syndrome, Kniest syndrome, multiple pterygium syndrome, Pena–Shokeir syndrome, Roberts syndrome, Smith–Lemli–Opitz syndrome.

Clinical management: Further ultrasound screening, including fetal echocardiography. Genitals should be inspected carefully. Karyotyping.

Prognosis: This depends on the severity of the cardiac lesion and mental development. Only mild mental impairment is expected in 25% of cases. The affected individuals often have a tendency to bleed easily. In some cases, the diagnosis is confirmed in the mother after the birth of a severely affected infant.

Self-Help Organization

Title: Noonan Syndrome Support Group

Description: Provides information for persons with Noonan syndrome, their families, and other interested individuals. Networks individuals together for peer support. Information and referrals, speakers bureau, telephone helpline.

Scope: International network

Founded: 1996

Address: P.O. Box 145, Upperco, MD 21 155, United States

Telephone: 1-888-686-2224 or 410-374-5245

E-mail: info@noonansyndrome.org

Web: http://www.noonansyndrome.org

References

Benacerraf BR, Greene ME Holmes LB. The prenatal sonographic features of Noonan's syndrome. J Ultrasound Med 1989; 8: 59–63.

Bradley E, Kean L, Twining P, James D. Persistent right umbilical vein in a fetus with Noonan's syndrome: a case report. Ultrasound Obstet Gynecol 2001; 17: 76–8.

Cullimore AJ, Smedstad KG, Brennan BG. Pregnancy in women with Noonan syndrome: report of two cases. Obstet Gynecol 1999; 93: 813–6.

Grote W, Weisner D, Janig U, Harms D, Wiedemann HR. Prenatal diagnosis of a short-rib-polydactylia syndrome type Saldino–Noonan at 17 weeks' gestation. Eur J Pediatr 1983; 140: 63–6.

Hiippala A, Eronen M, Taipale P, Salonen R, Hiilesmaa V. Fetal nuchal translucency and normal chromosomes: a long-term follow-up study. Ultrasound Obstet Gynecol 2001; 18: 18–22.

Hill LM, Leary J. Transvaginal sonographic diagnosis of short-rib polydactyly dysplasia at 13 weeks' gestation. Prenat Diagn 1998; 18: 1198–201.

Menashe M, Arbel R, Raveh D, Achiron R, Yagel S. Poor prenatal detection rate of cardiac anomalies in Noonan syndrome [review]. Ultrasound Obstet Gynecol 2002; 19: 51–5.

Zarabi M, Mieckowski GC, Mazer J. Cystic hygroma associated with Noonan's syndrome. JCU J Clin Ultrasound 1983; 11: 398–400.

Pena–Shokeir Syndrome (Pseudotrisomy 18)

Definition: Originally this is a heterogeneous complex of malformations, with a similar phenotype to trisomy 18. It consists of growth restriction, hydramnios, joint contractures, facial dysmorphism and aplasia of the lungs.

Incidence: This is estimated at one in 12 000 births.

First described in 1974 by Pena and Shokeir.

Origin/genetics: Heterogeneous, mostly autosomal-recessive inheritance; sporadic cases are also known. X-chromosomal inheritance has also been described. The risk of recurrence lies at 10–15 %.

Ultrasound findings: Severe growth restriction, with hydramnios, a short umbilical cord, very thin cerebral cortex, widening of the cerebral ventricles, polymicrogyria. *Craniofacial anomalies* such as hypertelorism, microgenia, webbed neck, deep-set ears, hooked nose. *Anomalies of the extremities:* clenched fist as in trisomy 18, short limbs, abnormally shaped fingers and toes (cylindrical shape), rocker-bottom feet, reduced bone density. Anomalies that are not charac-

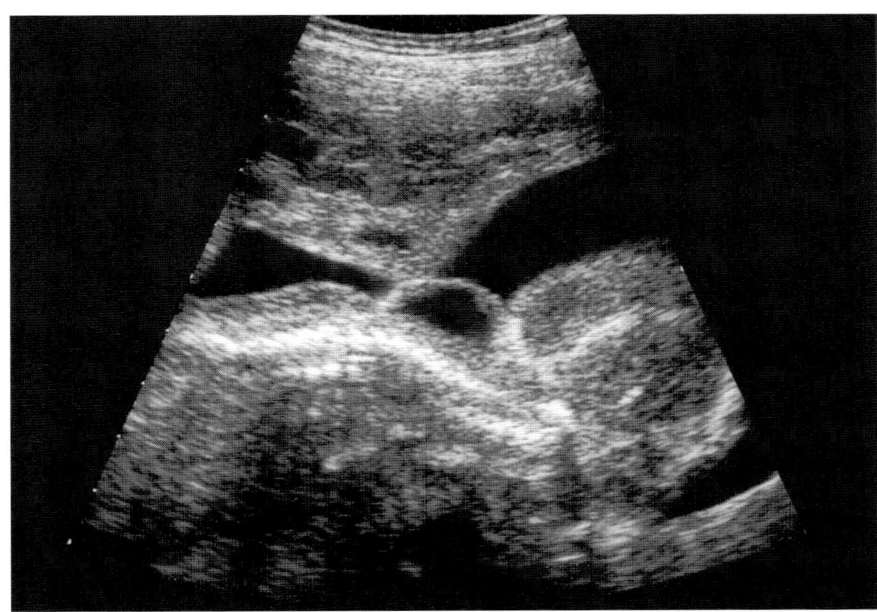

Fig. 11.**34** **Pena–Shokeir syndrome.** Fetal neck, showing cystic hygroma at 20 + 4 weeks.

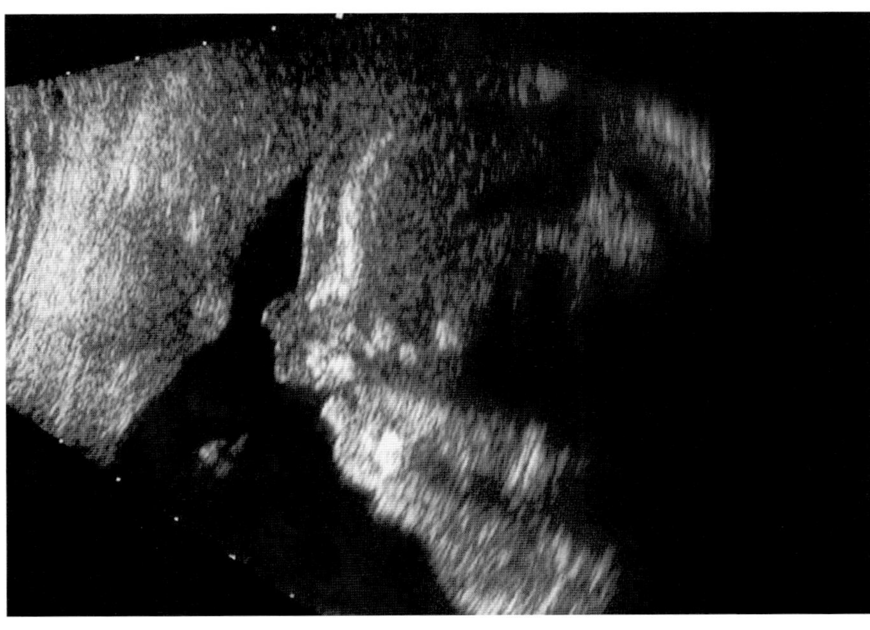

Fig. 11.**35** **Pena–Shokeir syndrome.** Fetal profile, demonstrating retrogenia at 20 + 4 weeks in a fetus with Pena–Shokeir syndrome.

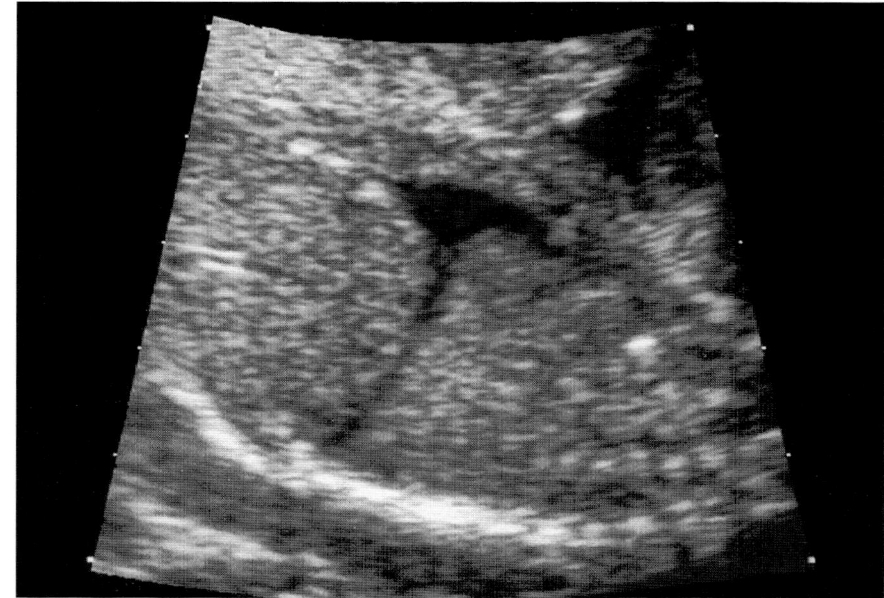

Fig. 11.**36** **Pena–Shokeir syndrome.** Fetal hydrothorax at 20 + 4 weeks.

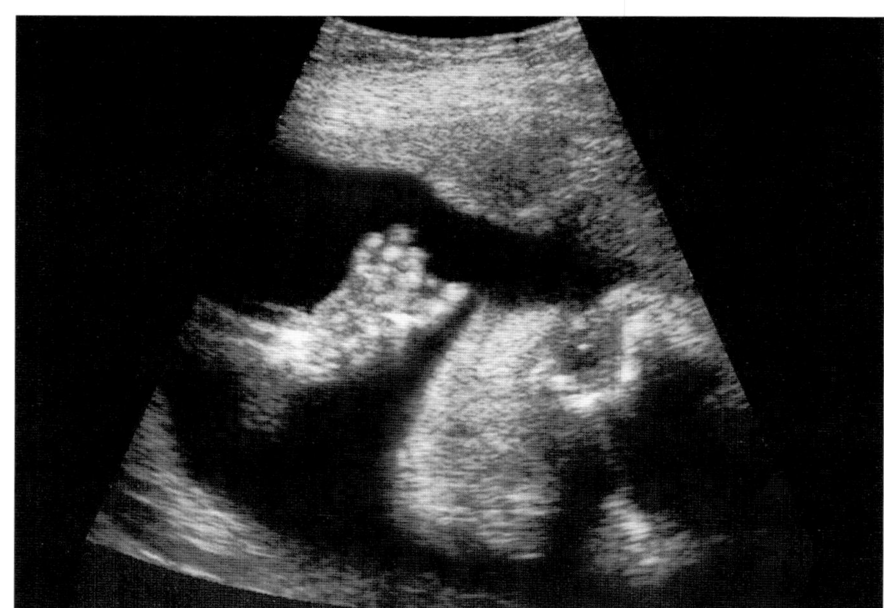

Fig. 11.**37** **Pena–Shokeir syndrome.** Clinodactyly of the hand at 20 + 4 weeks.

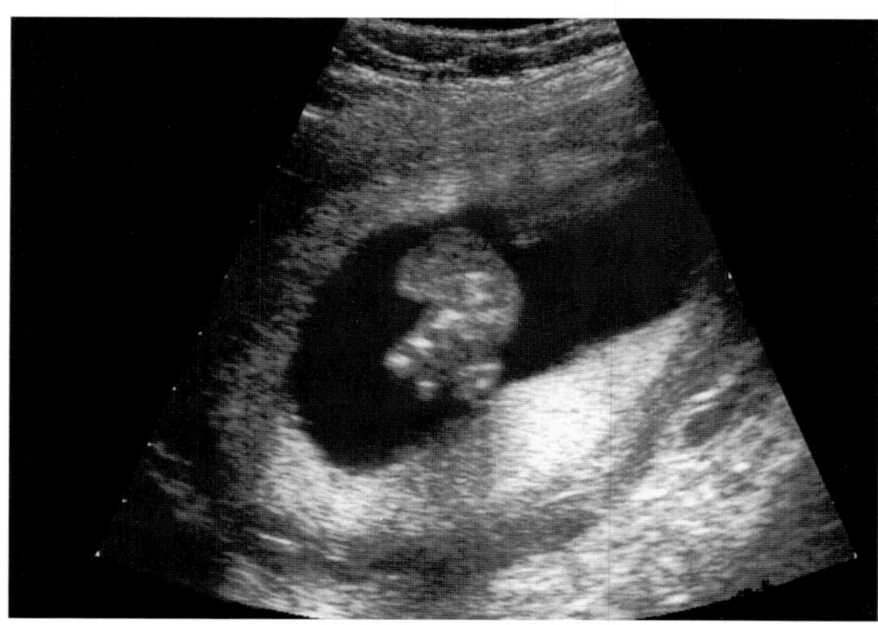

Fig. 11.**38** **Pena–Shokeir syndrome.** Malpositioning of the foot at 20 + 4 weeks.

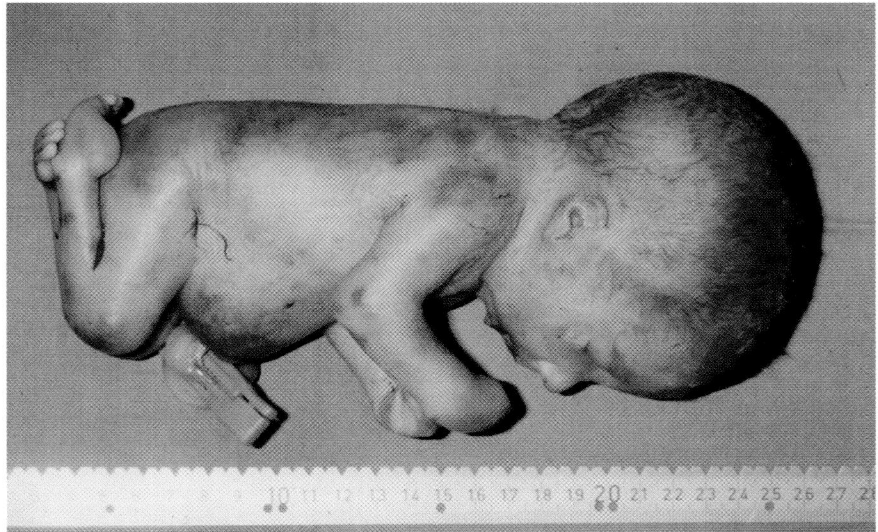

Fig. 11.**39** **Pena–Shokeir syndrome.** Profile view of the fetus after termination of pregnancy.

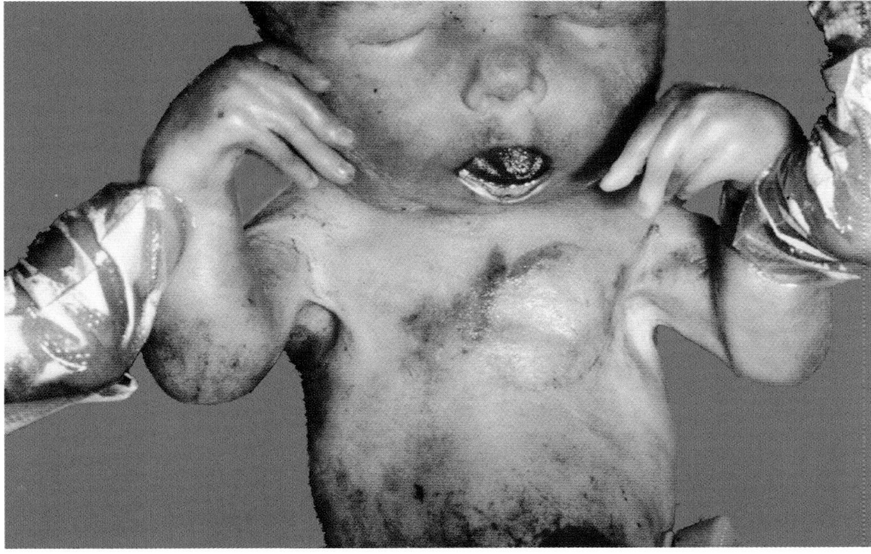

Fig. 11.**40** **Pena–Shokeir syndrome.** Same fetus, frontal view. The extremities are fixed and immobile, and the mouth is open.

teristic, but may be present, include: facial clefts, underdeveloped mandible, hypoplasia, hygroma colli, pterygium over joints, cardiac and renal anomalies, choanal atresia, stenosis of the larynx, bowel malformations, hypoplasia of the lungs and muscular atrophy. The earliest diagnosis was made at 15 weeks, due to abnormal fetal movements and malpositioning of the limbs.

Differential diagnosis: Trisomy 18, cerebro-oculofacial-skeletal syndrome (COFS), arthrogryposis, Freeman–Sheldon syndrome, multiple pterygium syndrome, Smith–Lemli–Opitz syndrome.

Prognosis: Fatal; 30% are stillborn, 40% die within the first 2 weeks of life, and the remainder mostly die within the first 4 months.

References

Ajayi RA, Keen CE, Knott PD. Ultrasound diagnosis of the Pena–Shokeir phenotype at 14 weeks of pregnancy. Prenat Diagn 1995; 15: 762–4.

Cardwell MS. Pena–Shokeir syndrome: prenatal diagnosis by ultrasonography. J Ultrasound Med 1987; 6: 619–21.

Genkins SM, Hertzberg BS, Bowie JD, Blow o. Pena–Shokeir type I syndrome: in utero sonographic appearance. JCU J Clin Ultrasound 1989; 17: 56–61.

Herva R, Leisti J, Kirkinen P, Seppanen U. A lethal autosomal recessive syndrome of multiple congenital contractures. Am J Med Genet 1985; 20: 431–9.

Muller LM, de Jong G. Prenatal ultrasonographic features of the Pena–Shokeir I syndrome and the trisomy 18 syndrome. Am J Med Genet 1986; 25: 119–29.

Ochi H, Kobayashi E, Matsubara K, Katayama T, Ito M. Prenatal sonographic diagnosis of Pena–Shokeir syndrome type I. Ultrasound Obstet Gynecol 2001; 17: 546–7.

Ohlsson A, Fong KW, Rose TH, Moore DC. Prenatal sonographic diagnosis of Pena–Shokeir syndrome type I, or fetal akinesia deformation sequence. Am J Med Genet 1988; 29: 59–65.
Paladini D, Tartaglione A, Agangi A, Foglia S, Martinelli P, Nappi C. Pena–Shokeir phenotype with variable onset in three consecutive pregnancies. Ultrasound Obstet Gynecol 2001; 17: 163–5.
Shenker L, Reed K, Anderson C, Hauck L, Spark R. Syndrome of camptodactyly, ankyloses, facial anomalies, and pulmonary hypoplasia (Pena–Shokeir syndrome): obstetric and ultrasound aspects. Am J Obstet Gynecol 1985; 152: 303–7.
Tongsong T, Chanprapaph P, Khunamornpong S. Prenatal ultrasound of regional akinesia with Pena–Shokeir phenotype. Prenat Diagn 2000; 20: 422–5.

Pierre Robin Sequence

Definition: Microgenia and retrogenia are typical features, presenting a high risk of respiratory obstruction.

Clinical history/genetics: Occurrence is mostly sporadic, however, autosomal-dominant and autosomal-recessive forms have also been reported.

Teratogens: Alcohol, amitriptyline, methotrexate, valproic acid.

Embryology: It is thought that underdevelopment of the mandible results in micrognathia and retrognathia.

Associated malformations: Cleft palate is the most frequent associated anomaly.

Ultrasound findings: This syndrome can be diagnosed in the second trimester on demonstration of *microgenia in a sagittal section of the fetal face.* Hydramnios may accompany this feature, especially in the third trimester. *Cleft palate* is not always detectable, as the posterior part of the palate is usually affected.

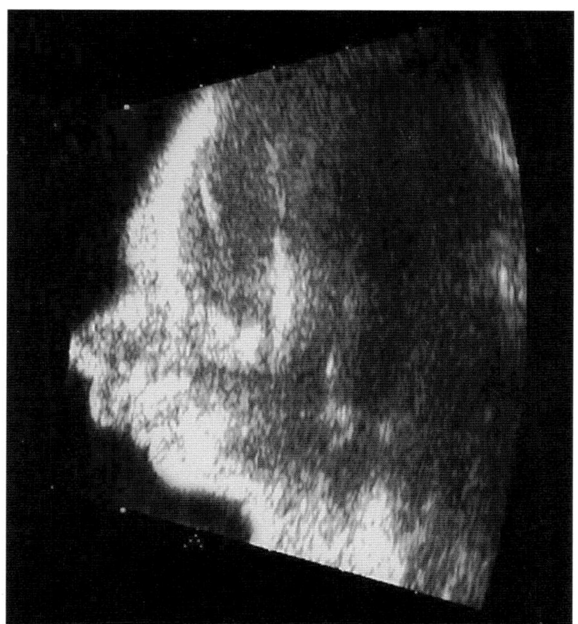

Fig. 11.**41** **Pierre Robin sequence.** Fetal profile at 21 + 4 weeks, demonstrating severe retrogenia.

Differential diagnosis: Pierre Robin sequence occurs as an isolated disorder. Microgenia is also found in achondrogenesis, amniotic banding, atelosteogenesis, camptomelic dysplasia, Carpenter syndrome, cerebrocostomandibular syndrome, CHARGE association, various chromosomal aberrations, Cornelia de Lange syndrome, Crouzon syndrome, diastrophic dysplasia, EEC syndrome, femur hypoplasia–unusual face syndrome, Fryns syndrome, Goldenhar syndrome, hydrolethalus, infantile polycystic kidney disease, Joubert syndrome, Meckel–Gruber syndrome, multiple pterygium syndrome, MURCS association, Nager syndrome, Neu–Laxova syndrome, Mohr syndrome, Pena–Shokeir syndrome, Roberts syndrome, Seckel syndrome, Shprintzen syndrome, Smith–Lemli–Opitz syndrome, Treacher–Collins syndrome.

Procedure after birth: Intubation of the newborn is often difficult; it can be facilitated by pulling the tongue out. Occasionally, an emergency tracheostomy is necessary. Respiratory obstruction leads to hypoxia and chronic infections, often resulting in cor pulmonale.

Prognosis: If the infants survive the neonatal stage, the prognosis is very good, as the microgenia often shows good remission. Associated anomalies may affect the prognosis.

Self-Help Organization

Title: Pierre Robin Network

Description: Support and education for individuals, parents, caregivers and professionals dealing with Pierre Robin syndrome or sequence. Literature, newsletter, information, advocacy. Online e-mail group and bulletin

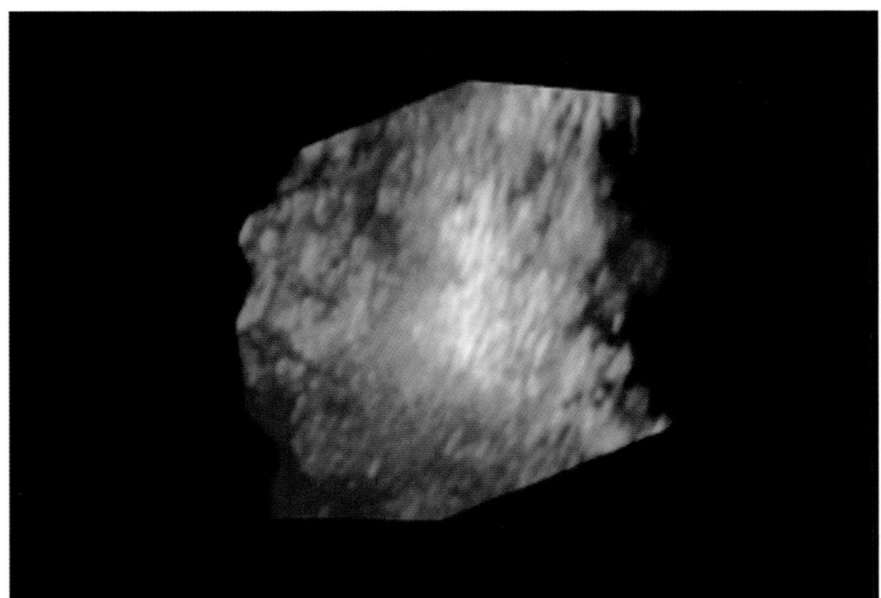

Fig. 11.**42** **Pierre Robin sequence.** Same fetus, showing a three-dimensional scan of the fetal face.

board. Outreach committee consisting of families available worldwide to correspond via mail, phone, in person, or by e-mail.

Scope: National network

Founded: 1999

Address: P.O. Box 3274, Quincy, IL 62305, United States

Telephone: 217-224-7480

Fax: 217-224-0292

E-mail: help@pierrerobin.org

Web: http://www.pierrerobin.org

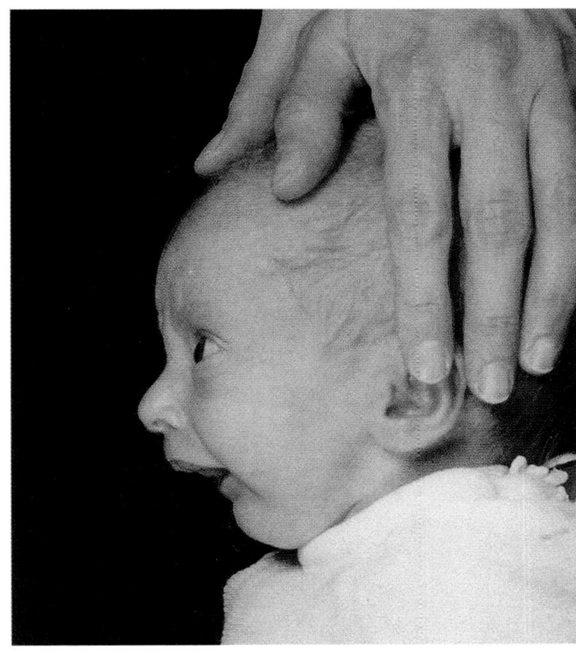

Fig. 11.**43** **Pierre Robin sequence.** Photograph taken after birth of the same fetus as in the previous figure.

References

Matsumoto M, Yanagihara T, Hanaoka U, et al. Antenatal three-dimensional sonographic features of Pierre Robin syndrome: case report. Gynecol Obstet Invest 2001; 51: 141–2.

Megier P, Ayeva DM, Esperandieu O, Aubry MC, Couly G, Desroches A. Prenatal ultrasonographic diagnosis of the cerebro-costo-mandibular syndrome: case report and review of the literature. Prenat Diagn 1998; 18: 1294–9.

Meizner I, Katz M, Bar ZJ, Insler V. Prenatal sonographic detection of fetal facial malformations. Isr J Med Sci 1987; 23: 881–5.

Morin G, Gekas J, Naepels P, et al. Cerebro-costo-mandibular syndrome in a father and a female fetus: early prenatal ultrasonographic diagnosis and autosomal-dominant transmission. Prenat Diagn 2001; 21: 890–3.

Pilu G, Romero R, Reece EA, Jeanty P, Hobbins JC. The prenatal diagnosis of Robin anomalad. Am J Obstet Gynecol 1986; 154: 630–2.

Rotten D, Levaillant JM, Martinez H, Ducou le Pointe H, Vicaut E. The fetal mandible: a 2D and 3D sonographic approach to the diagnosis of retrognathia and micrognathia. Ultrasound Obstet Gynecol 2002; 19: 122–30.

Soulier M, Sigaudy S, Chau C, Philip N. Prenatal diagnosis of Pierre Robin sequence as part of Stickler syndrome. Prenat Diagn 2002; 22: 567–8.

Winter RM, Crawfurd MA, Meire HB, Mitchell N. Osteopathia striata with cranial sclerosis: highly variable expression within a family including cleft palate in two neonatal cases. Clin Genet 1980; 18: 462–74.

Russell–Silver Syndrome

Definition: This is characterized by intrauterine and postnatal growth restriction, a large skull, small face, microgenia, asymmetrical body stature with short upper limbs as well as clinobrachydactyly of the small finger.

Incidence: Rare; only 200 cases have been reported.

Origin/genetics: Mostly sporadic; sex chromosomal dominant, autosomal-dominant or recessive inheritance appears in 10%. Gene locus: the long arm of chromosome 17 (17 q25). In 10% of cases, maternal uniparental disomy of chromosome 7, gene locus: 7 p12 –p11.2 is found. Variable expression.

Clinical features: Congenital short stature, relatively large skull (pseudohydrocephalus), small triangular face, short philtrum, mouth with thin lips, microretrogenia, adult height 150 cm. Premature puberty is possible due to high gonadotropin levels. Asymmetrical body development: the long bones are small and asymmetrical. Mental impairment is seen in 15%. In some cases, the disorder may first become manifest after birth.

Ultrasound findings: Biometric measurements in the second trimester demonstrate shortening of the long bones. The thoracic cavity appears narrow, and underdeveloped musculature may also be diagnosed. Careful ultrasound scanning may also reveal clinodactyly of the fifth finger as well as syndactyly of the second and third toes. Singular umbilical artery may be associated with this syndrome. The placenta may be enlarged.

Differential diagnosis: Floating Harbor syndrome, Rubinstein–Taybi syndrome, Dubowitz syndrome, SHORT syndrome.

Prognosis: This is mostly favorable. Normal mental development is common. Psychomotor developmental disturbances have been described. Short stature with a variable adult height is expected.

Self-Help Organization

Title: Russell–Silver Syndrome Support Network

Description: Network and exchange of information for parents of children with Russell–Silver syndrome. Information and referrals, phone support, pen pals, conferences, annual convention, literature. Newsletter.

Scope: National network

Founded: 1989

Address: c/o MAGIC Foundation, 1327 N. Harlem, Oak Park, IL 60303, United States

Telephone: 1–800–3-MAGIC-3 or 708–383–0808

Fax: 708–383–0899

E-mail: mary@magicfoundation.org

Web: http://www.magicfoundation.org

References

del Campo Casanelles M, Perez Jurado L. [Non-Mendelian genetics and growth: the Russell–Silver syndrome; in Spanish.] An Esp Pediatr 2001; 54: 531–5.

Martinez Nogueiras A, Teixeira Costeira M, Saraiva Moreira H, Araujo Antunes H. [Russell–Silver syndrome; in Spanish.] An Esp Pediatr 2001; 54: 591–4.

Parlato M, Del Core G. [Russell–Silver syndrome: aspects of odontomaxillofacial significance; in Italian.] Arch Stomatol (Napoli) 1989; 30: 461–6.

Peinado Garrido A, Borja Perez C, Narbona Lopez E, Contreras Chova F, Jerez Calero A, Miras Baldo M. [Intrauterine dwarfism and dysmorphic features: a case of Russell–Silver syndrome; in Spanish.] An Esp Pediatr 2001; 54: 588–90.

Shprintzen Syndrome (Velocardial Syndrome)

Definition: This is a disorder of malformations and growth restriction with moderate mental impairment, cleft palate, typical facial features and cardiovascular anomalies.

Incidence: Rare.
First described in 1978.

Origin/genetics: Autosomal-dominant inheritance with variable expression, microdeletion in chromosome 22q11.21–q11.23. An association with DiGeorge syndrome is possible.

Clinical features: Facial dysmorphism with a long and narrow face, microgenia, flat protruding nose, dysplasia of the auricle. Moderate mental impairment, with difficulty in learning and behavioral disorder, can be expected. Psychiatric disorders are diagnosed in 10% of adults. Typical anomalies are: cleft palate (possibly submucous), cardiac defects (VSD, tetralogy of Fallot, and others), and shortening of the long bones. Other malformations have also been associated with this syndrome: Pierre Robin sequence, holoprosencephaly, umbilical hernia, cryptorchism, and hypospadias.

Ultrasound findings: The diagnosis has been made at 17 weeks in a case in which a previous sibling had shown Pierre Robin sequence. Here a short femur, micrognathia and a VSD were detected. At 27 weeks, asymmetrical shortening of the radius and ulna was also diagnosed.

Differential diagnosis: Triploidy, trisomy 18, Cornelia de Lange syndrome, EEC syndrome, Fanconi anemia, femur–fibula–ulna syndrome, Holt–Oram syndrome, multiple pterygium syndrome, Neu–Laxova syndrome, Mohr syndrome, Roberts syndrome, Seckel syndrome, camptomelic dysplasia, diastrophic dysplasia, TAR syndrome.

Prognosis: This depends on the severity and type of cardiac anomaly and mental impairment. A decrease in muscle tone and speech and hearing disturbances dominate the clinical picture. Occasionally, disturbance of T-cell function and thymus anomalies have been found.

References

Fokstuen S, Vrticka K, Riegel M, Da Silva V, Baumer A, Schinzel A. Velofacial hypoplasia (Sedlackova syndrome): a variant of velocardiofacial (Shprintzen) syndrome and part of the phenotypical spectrum of del 22q11.2. Eur J Pediatr 2001; 160: 54–7.

Fryer AE. Goldberg–Shprintzen syndrome: report of a new family and review of the literature [review]. Clin Dysmorphol 1998; 7: 97–101.

Komatsu H, Kihara A, Komura E, et al. Combined trisomy 9P and Shprintzen syndrome resulting from a paternal t(9;22). Genet Couns 2001; 12: 137–43.

Olney AH, Kolodziej P. Velocardiofacial syndrome (Shprintzen syndrome, chromosome 22q11 deletion syndrome) [review]. Ear Nose Throat J 1998; 77: 460–1.

Robin HN, Shprintzen RJ. The heart and the ear. J Pediatr 1998; 133: 167–8.

Shprintzen RJ. Velocardiofacial syndrome. Otolaryngol Clin North Am 2000; 33: 1217–40.

Stratton RF, Payne RM. Frontonasal malformation with tetralogy of Fallot associated with a submicroscopic deletion of 22q11. Am J Med Genet 1997; 69: 287–9.

Smith–Lemli–Opitz Syndrome

Definition: This disorder involves small stature and delayed mental development in the presence of microcephaly, abnormal facial features, genital anomalies in the affected males, and other malformations.

Incidence: One in 20 000 births.
First described in 1964 by Smith.

Origin/genetics: Autosomal-recessive inheritance. Gene locus 11q12–q13, rarely 7q32.1. There is a defect in the biosynthesis of cholesterol. Differentiation into Smith–Lemli–Opitz types I and type II is questionable; it is more likely that these represent the same disorder with varying severity.

Clinical features: Microcephaly, growth restriction. *Facial dysmorphism:* blepharophimosis, ptosis, epicanthus, possibly squint, deep-set ears, nose resembling an electrical socket, small tongue, wide alveolar ridges, microgenia. *Geni-*

tals: underdevelopment of the penis, hypospadias, cryptorchism, occasionally pseudohermaphroditism. *Extremities:* Syndactyly of the second and third toes, possibly postaxial hexadactyly, malpositioning of the fingers and toes, pathological muscle tone. Other anomalies include: cataract, cleft palate, cranial, cardiac and urogenital anomalies. The affected individuals show hyperexcitability and tend to suffer from frequent infections.

Ultrasound findings: *Thickening of the nuchal fold* is a characteristic feature at 12 weeks. There is a discrepancy between the karyotype (male) and appearance of genitals on scanning (female); this may provide the first clue. In addition, microcephaly, growth restriction, facial and limb anomalies can be demonstrated during the progress of the pregnancy.

Differential diagnosis: Meckel–Gruber syndrome, Ellis–van Creveld syndrome, Joubert syndrome, Mohr syndrome, short rib–polydactyly syndrome, trisomy 13, Carpenter syndrome, CHARGE association, Cornelia de Lange syndrome.

Prognosis: This is unfavorable, especially regarding mental development. Frequently, death occurs soon after birth or in early infancy.

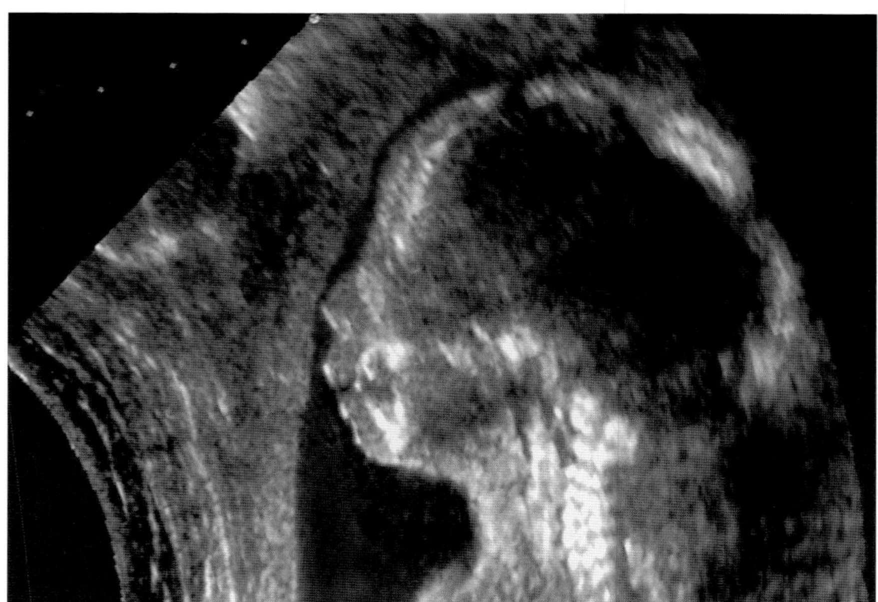

Fig. 11.**44** **Smith–Lemli–Opitz syndrome.** Fetal profile at 21 + 4 weeks (courtesy of Dr. Lebek).

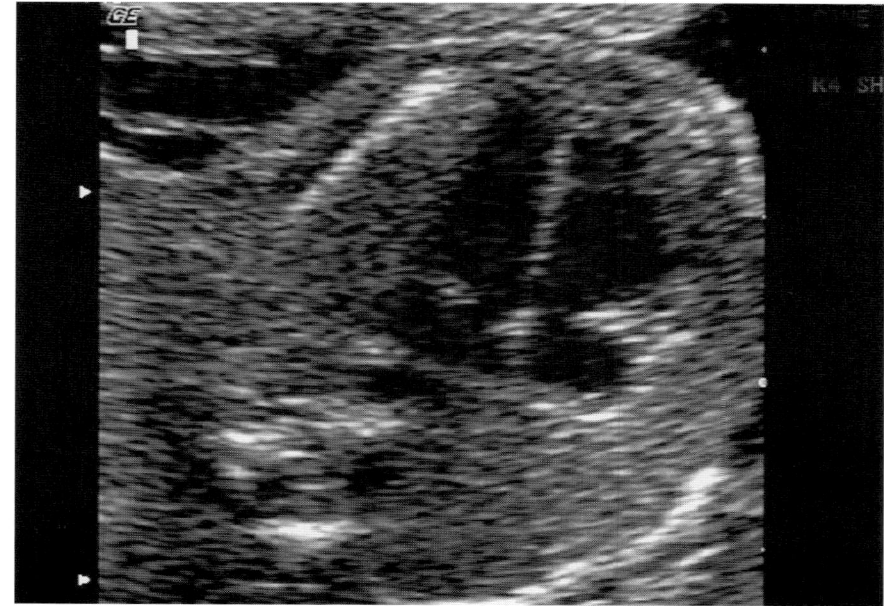

Fig. 11.**45** **Smith–Lemli–Opitz syndrome.** Fetal heart, showing a membranous VSD at 21 weeks in a fetus with Smith–Lemli–Opitz syndrome (courtesy of Dr. Lebek).

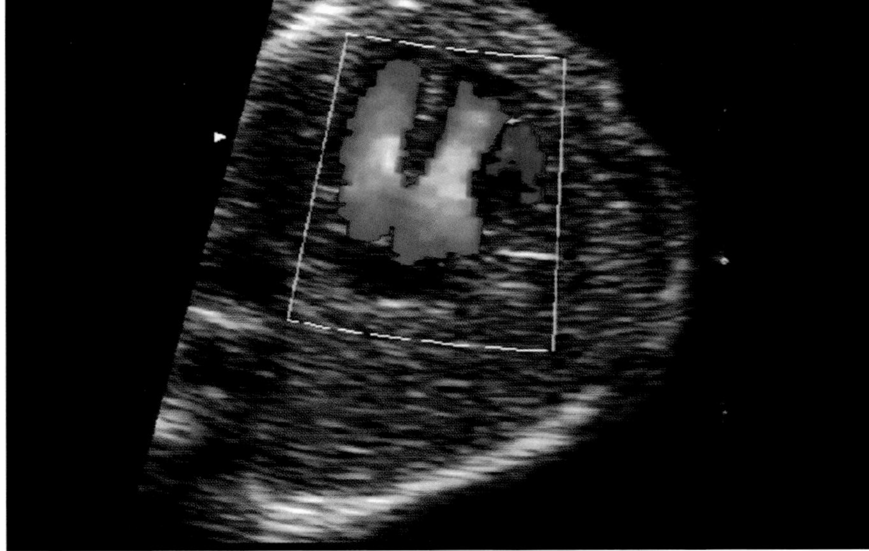

Fig. 11.**46** **Smith–Lemli–Opitz syndrome.** Color-coded Doppler imaging of the fetal heart, demonstrating the membranous VSD in Smith–Lemli–Opitz syndrome (courtesy of Dr. Lebek).

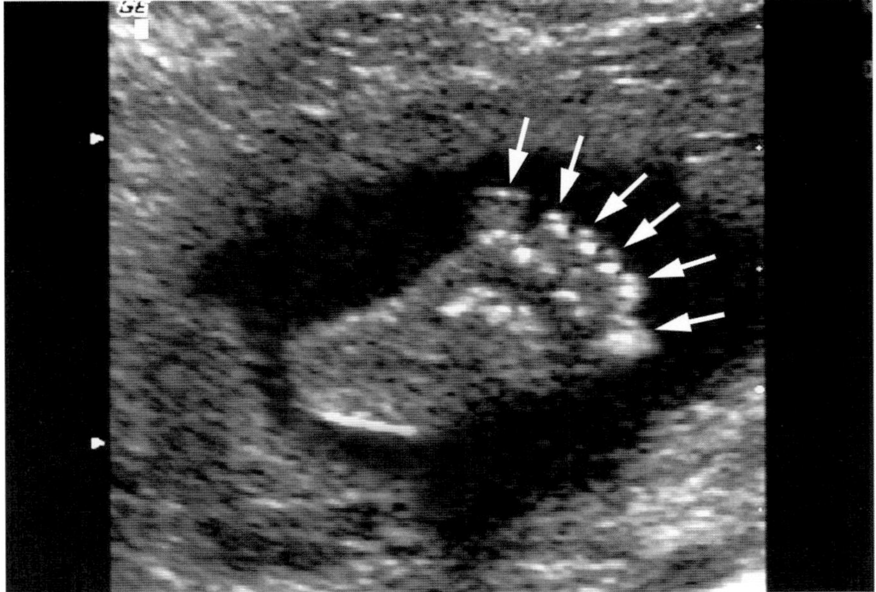

Fig. 11.**47** **Smith–Lemli–Opitz syndrome.** Hexadactyly of the foot (courtesy of Dr. Lebek).

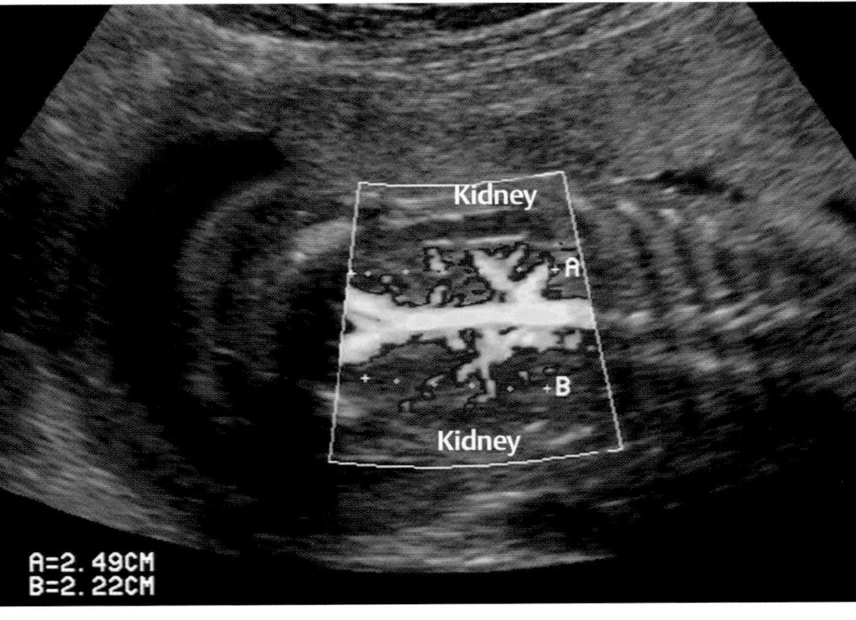

Fig. 11.**48** **Smith–Lemli–Opitz syndrome.** Demonstration of the renal artery, showing an atypical vascular pattern in a fetus with Smith–Lemli–Opitz syndrome at 21 weeks (courtesy of Dr. Lebek).

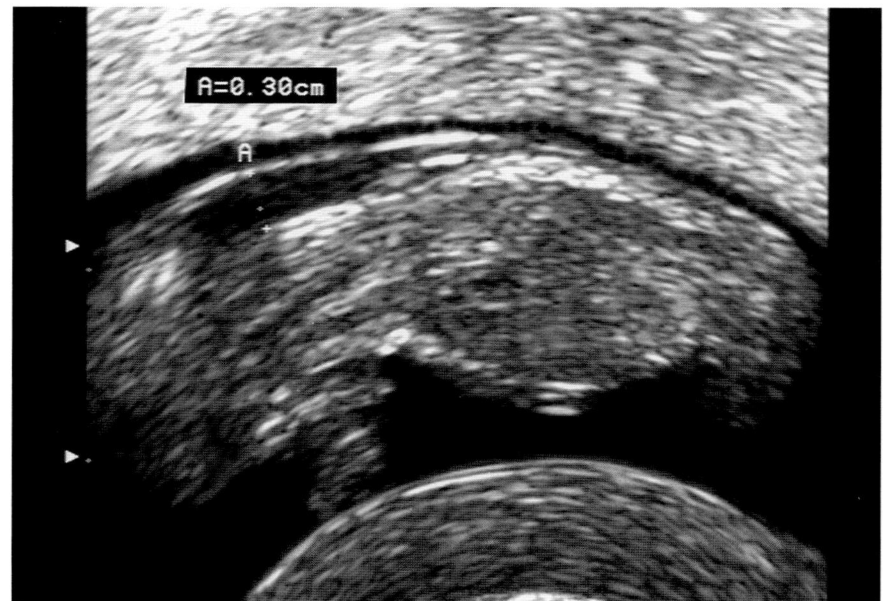

Fig. 11.**49** **Smith–Lemli–Opitz syndrome.** Cystic hygroma of the neck detected at 11 + 0 weeks (courtesy of Dr. Lebek).

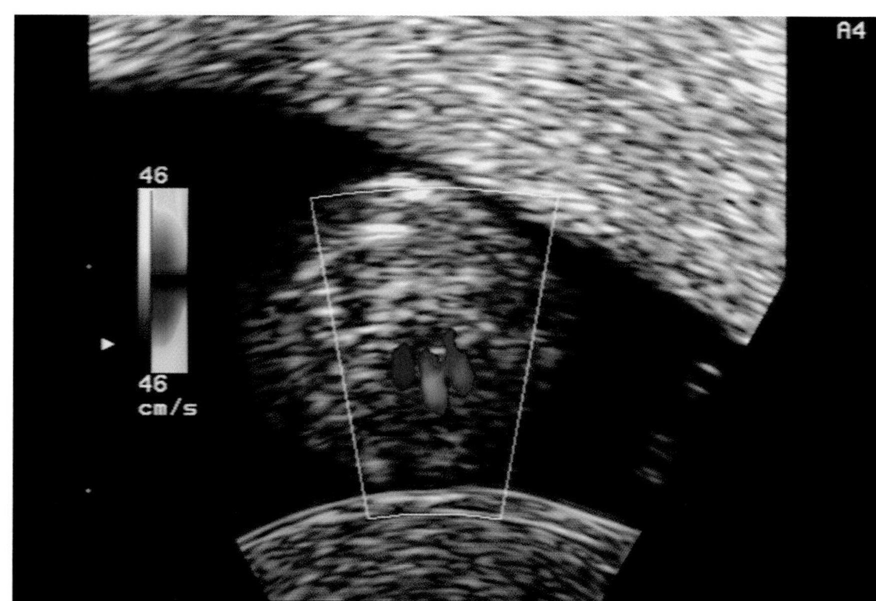

Fig. 11.**50** **Smith–Lemli–Opitz syndrome.** AV canal at 11 + 0 weeks (courtesy of Dr. Lebek).

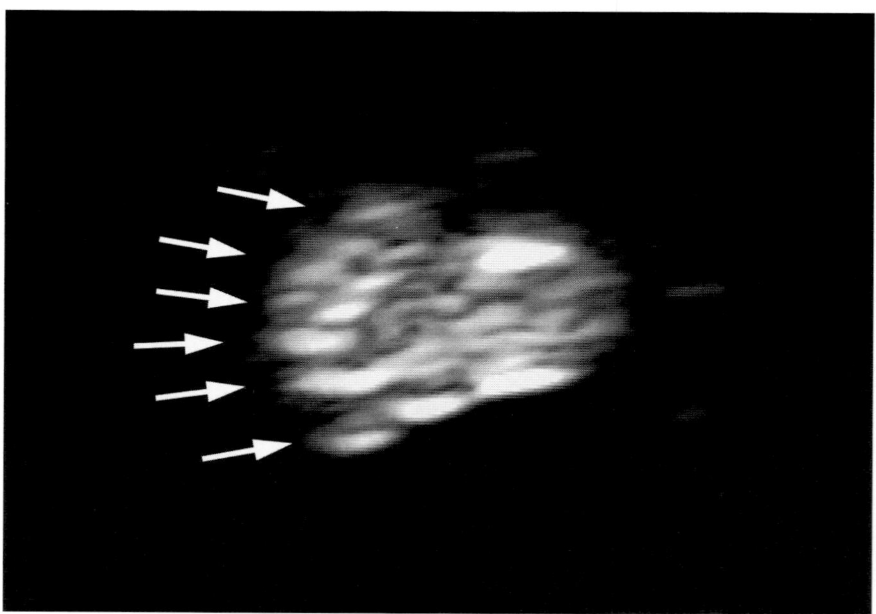

Fig. 11.**51** **Smith–Lemli–Opitz syndrome.** Hexadactyly of the foot, 11 + 0 weeks (courtesy of Dr. Lebek).

Self-Help Organization

Title: Smith–Lemli–Opitz Advocacy and Exchange

Description: Network of families with Smith–Lemli–Opitz children. Exchange of information, sharing of similar experiences, and correspondence between families. Provides education to medical community, new parents, and others. Phone support. Newsletter twice per year.

Scope: International

Founded: 1988

Address: 2650 Valley Forge Dr., Boothwyn, PA 19061, United States

Telephone: 610–485–9663

References

Angle B, Tint GS, Yacoub OA, Clark AL. Atypical case of Smith–Lemli–Opitz syndrome: implications for diagnosis. Am J Med Genet 1998; 80: 322–6.

Bick DP, McCorkle D, Stanley WS, et al. Prenatal diagnosis of Smith–Lemli–Opitz syndrome in a pregnancy with low maternal serum oestriol and a sex-reversed fetus. Prenat Diagn 1999; 19: 68–71.

Degenhardt F, Muhlhaus K. Delayed bone growth as a sonographic sign in the early detection of Smith–Lemli–Opitz syndrome. Z Geburtshilfe Perinatol 1988; 192: 169–72.

Greenberg F, Gresik MV, Carpenter RJ, Law SW, Hoffman LP, Ledbetter DH. The Gardner–Silengo–Wachtel or genito-palato-cardiac syndrome: male pseudohermaphroditism with micrognathia, cleft palate, and conotruncal cardiac defect. Am J Med Genet 1987; 26: 59–64.

Kratz LE, Kelley RI. Prenatal diagnosis of the RSH/Smith–Lemli–Opitz syndrome. Am J Med Genet 1999; 82: 376–81.

Lalatta F, Salmona S, Fogliani R, Rizzuti T, Nicolini U. Prenatal diagnosis of genetic syndromes may be facilitated by serendipitous findings at fetal blood sampling. Prenat Diagn 1998; 18: 834–7.

Loeffler J, Utermann G, Witsch-Baumgartner M. Molecular prenatal diagnosis of Smith–Lemli–Opitz syndrome is reliable and efficient. Prenat Diagn 2002; 22: 827–30.

Norgard M, Yankowitz J, Rhead W, Kanis AB, Hall BD. Prenatal ultrasound findings in hydrolethalus: continuing difficulties in diagnosis. Prenat Diagn 1996; 16: 173–9.

Nowaczyk MJ, Heshka T, Kratz LE, Kelley RE. Difficult prenatal diagnosis in mild Smith–Lemli–Opitz syndrome. Am J Med Genet 2000; 95: 396–8.

Nowaczyk MJ, Garcia DM, Eng B, Waye JS. Rapid molecular prenatal diagnosis of Smith–Lemli–Opitz syndrome. Am J Med Genet 2001; 102: 387–8.

Nowaczyk MJ, McCaughey D, Whelan DT, Porter FD. Incidence of Smith–Lemli–Opitz syndrome in Ontario, Canada. Am J Med Genet 2001; 102: 18–20.

Palomaki GE, Bradley LA, Knight GJ, Craig WY, Haddow JE. Assigning risk for Smith–Lemli–Opitz syndrome as part of 2nd trimester screening for Down's syndrome. J Med Screen 2002; 9: 43–4.

Sharp P, Haan E, Fletcher JM, Khong TY, Carey WE. First-trimester diagnosis of Smith–Lemli–Opitz syndrome. Prenat Diagn 1997; 17: 355–61.

Thrombocytopenia–Absent Radius (TAR) syndrome

Definition: This disorder combines bilateral radius aplasia with thrombocytopenia and possibly other malformations.

Incidence: Extremely rare: one in 500 000–1 000 000 births.

Origin/genetics: Autosomal-recessive inheritance, with variable penetrance.

Clinical features: Bilateral radius aplasia causing a fallen hand, thumbs are present. Often associated with humerus hypoplasia. *Thrombocytopenia* often leads to a severe tendency to bleed. Allergy to cow's milk may also be associated. Anemia due to hemolysis and bleeding; eosinophilia and leukocytosis are also evident. In one-third of the cases, heart defects are found (ASD, tetralogy of Fallot). Dwarfism. Rarely underdevelopment of the lower jaw and mid facial region, of shoulder region. Dysplasia of the hips, club feet, partly absent lower limbs (the fibula is missing in 50%), edema of the dorsal surface of the feet. Hypoplasia and bending of the ulna is possible. Other anomalies, such as hypoplasia of the cerebellar vermis, renal anomalies, and micrognathia, may also be associated.

Ultrasound findings: It has been possible to make the diagnosis in the early part of the first trimester. The *limb defects* have been demonstrated at the end of the first trimester.

Differential diagnosis: Aase syndrome, Holt–Oram syndrome, Fanconi anemia, thalidomide embryopathy, pseudothalidomide syndrome, trisomy 13, trisomy 18, Cornelia de Lange syndrome, Nager syndrome, radius aplasia, Roberts syndrome, VACTERL association.

Clinical management: Cesarean section may be necessary due to thrombocytopenia. The platelet count may be determined in the prenatal stage with umbilical venous sampling; if the platelet count lies above 50 000/mm^3, vaginal delivery is possible. Platelet transfusion may be given at the prenatal stage to allow vaginal delivery.

Procedure after birth: Platelet substitution is necessary, depending on laboratory values and clinical symptoms. Intensive-care treatment of the newborn is advisable.

Prognosis: The thrombocytopenia improves with the course of infant development. Normal values are found in adulthood. The mortality is very high in the first year of life; after this, a normal life expectancy is possible. Mental development is affected by possible intracranial bleeding occurring within the first 2 years of life.

Self-Help Organization

Title: Thrombocytopenia–Absent Radius Syndrome Association

Description: Information, networking and support for families children with thrombocytopenia–absent radius syndrome (a shortening of the arms), and for affected adults. (Does not include ITP). Newsletter, pen-pal program, phone network.

Scope: International

Founded: 1981

Address: 212 Sherwood Dr., Egg Harbor Township, NJ 08234–7658, United States

Telephone: 609–927–0418

Fax: 609–653–8639

E-mail: purinton@earthlink.net

References

Donnenfeld AE, Wiseman B, Lavi E, Weiner S. Prenatal diagnosis of thrombocytopenia absent radius syndrome by ultrasound and cordocentesis. Prenat Diagn 1990; 10: 29–35.

Ergur A, Yergok YZ, Ertekin A, Tayyar M, Yilmazturk A. Prenatal diagnosis of an uncommon syndrome: thrombocytopenia absent radius (TAR). Zentralbl Gynäkol 1998; 120: 75–8.

Shelton SD, Paulyson K, Kay HH. Prenatal diagnosis of thrombocytopenia absent radius (TAR) syndrome and vaginal delivery. Prenat Diagn 1999; 19: 54–7.

Tongsong T, Sirichotiyakul S, Chanprapaph P. Prenatal diagnosis of thrombocytopenia–absent radius (TAR) syndrome. Ultrasound Obstet Gynecol 2000; 15: 256–8.

Weinblatt M, Petrikovsky B, Bialer M, Kochen J, Harper R. Prenatal evaluation and in utero platelet transfusion for thrombocytopenia absent radii syndrome. Prenat Diagn 1994; 14: 892–6.

Tuberous Sclerosis

Definition: In this disorder, hamartomas develop in the brain, skin, heart, kidneys, and other organs.

Origin/genetics: Autosomal-dominant inheritance, genetically heterogeneous, mostly arising as new mutations in unaffected families. Gene locus: 9q32–34 and 16p13.3.

Clinical features: Typically, tumors are found in the brain, especially in the region of the basal ganglion and within the ventricles. These are probably not detectable in prenatal screening. The same applies to the more common skin tumors. Rhabdomyomas, however, can be demonstrated within the heart. Cystic degeneration of the bones and angiomyolipomas of the kidneys may also be present and as yet have not been detectable in prenatal screening.

Ultrasound findings: *Cardiac rhabdomyomas* are seen as echogenic tumors within the heart and may appear as thickened ventricular septum. They occasionally cause cardiac obstruction, leading to nonimmune fetal hydrops. It is difficult to differentiate isolated cardiac rhabdomyomas from tuberous scleroses; magnetic resonance imaging may be helpful, especially for detecting intracranial lesions.

Differential diagnosis: In tuberous sclerosis, the major finding in prenatal scanning is the demonstration of cardiac rhabdomyoma; in 50% of cases, these are associated with tuberous sclerosis. Cardiac rhabdomyoma should be differentiated from teratoma, myxoma, and fibroma.

Prognosis: Mental impairment and fits develop in 80% of cases. Spontaneous remission of the cardiac tumors is possible after birth (apoptosis). Surgical removal is occasionally required.

Self-Help Organization

Title: National Tuberous Sclerosis Alliance

Description: Dedicated to finding a cure for tuberous sclerosis while improving the lives of those affected. Provides research, support and education among individuals, families, and the helping professions. Newsletter, peer networking programs, conferences, information, audio tapes available.

Scope: National

Founded: 1974

Address: 801 Roeder Rd., Suite 750, Silver Spring, MD 20910–4467, United States

Telephone: 301–562–9890 or 1–800–225–6872

TTY: 301–562–9870

Fax: 301–459–0394

E-mail: linda.creighton@tsalliance.org

Web: http://www.tsalliance.org

References

D'Addario V, Pinto V, Di Naro E, Del Bianco A, Di Cagno L, Volpe P. Prenatal diagnosis and postnatal outcome of cardiac rhabdomyomas. J Perinat Med 2002; 30: 170–5.

Green KW, Bors KR, Pollack P, Weinbaum PJ. Antepartum diagnosis and management of multiple fetal cardiac tumors. J Ultrasound Med 1991; 10: 697–9.

Guerrini R, Carrozzo R. Epileptogenic brain malformations: clinical presentation, malformative patterns and indications for genetic testing. Seizure 2002; 11 (Suppl A): 532–43.

Gushiken BJ, Callen PW, Silverman NH. Prenatal diagnosis of tuberous sclerosis in monozygotic twins with cardiac masses. J Ultrasound Med 1999; 18: 165–8.

Holley DG, Martin GR, Brenner JI, et al. Diagnosis and management of fetal cardiac tumors: a multicenter experience and review of published reports. J Am Coll Cardiol 1995; 26: 516–20.

Journel H, Roussey M, Plais MH, Milon J, Almange C, Le Marec B. Prenatal diagnosis of familial tuberous sclerosis following detection of cardiac rhabdomyoma by ultrasound. Prenat Diagn 1986; 6: 283–9.

Krapp M, Baschat AA, Gembruch U, Gloeckner K, Schwinger E, Reusche E. Tuberous sclerosis with intracardiac rhabdomyoma in a fetus with trisomy 21: case report and review of literature. Prenat Diagn 1999; 19: 610–3.

Platt LD, Devore GR, Horenstein J, Pavlova Z, Kovacs B, Falk RE. Prenatal diagnosis of tuberous sclerosis: the use of fetal echocardiography. Prenat Diagn 1987; 7: 407–11.

Sonigo P, Elmaleh A, Fermont L, Delezoide AL, Mirlesse V, Brunelle F. Prenatal MRI diagnosis of fetal cerebral tuberous sclerosis. Pediatr Radiol 1996; 26: 1–4.

Stanford W, Abu YM, Smith W. Intracardiac tumor (rhabdomyoma) diagnosed by in utero ultrasound: a case report. JCU J Clin Ultrasound 1987; 15: 337–41.

van Oppen AC, Breslau SE, Stoutenbeek P, Pull TGA, Merkus JM. A fetal cystic neck mass associated with maternal tuberous sclerosis: case report and literature review. Prenat Diagn 1991; 11: 915–20.

VACTERL Association

Definition: This acronym refers to a combination of several anomalies: anomalies of the *v*ertebrae (60%), *a*nal atresia (60%), *c*ardiac anomalies (60%), *t*racheo-esophageal fistula with *e*sophageal atresia (85%), *r*enal anomalies (60%), and *l*imb defects (65%). At least three of the above should be present for a diagnosis of this disorder.

Incidence: Rare.

Sex ratio: M : F = 1 : 1.

Clinical history/genetics: Sporadic occurrence. Rarely, an autosomal-recessive form has been described, which is associated with a central nervous system anomaly such as hydrocephalus.

Origin: Early disturbance in the development of mesenchyme and blastogenesis has been postulated.

Ultrasound findings: The clinical signs vary considerably. The following anomalies may be found: *V (vertebra):* caudal regression, short vertebral column, scoliosis, hemivertebrae. *A (anus):* anal atresia; an attempt is made to demonstrate the anal fold. Dilation of the bowel secondary to this is evident, at the earliest, in the third trimester. *C (cor):* cardiac anomaly, mostly a VSD. *TE (tracheo-esophageal fistula):* the stomach appears small, or may be absent completely. Hydramnios is usually present. *R (renal):* hydronephrosis or unilateral polycystic kidneys. *L* *(limb):* polydactyly, underdeveloped or absent radius. Many other disorders have been added to this.

Differential diagnosis: Trisomy 13, trisomy 18, EEC syndrome, Fanconi anemia, Holt–Oram syndrome, Nager syndrome, TAR syndrome, Roberts syndrome, caudal regression syndrome, Jarcho–Levin syndrome, MURCS association, sirenomelia.

Clinical management: Karyotyping (differential diagnosis). Consultation with a pediatric surgeon to assess the diagnosis and to inform the parents. Hydramnios may lead to premature delivery. There is no advantage in delivering the mother by cesarean section in comparison with normal delivery.

Procedure after birth: This depends on the combination of anomalies. The prognosis is mostly influenced by the severity of the cardiac anomaly. If this is treatable, then the next clinical challenge is the correction of esophageal and anal atresia.

Prognosis: There is a 75% chance of survival; mental development is usually normal.

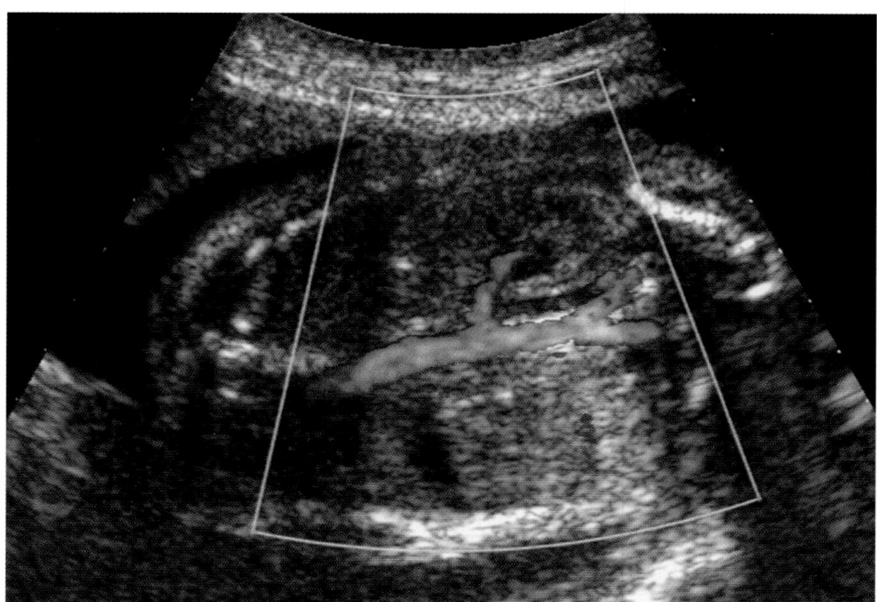

Fig. 11.**52** **VACTERL association.** Frontal view of the fetal abdominal retroperitoneum at 26 + 0 weeks, demonstrating the presence of only one renal artery and only one kidney: unilateral renal agenesis in VACTERL association.

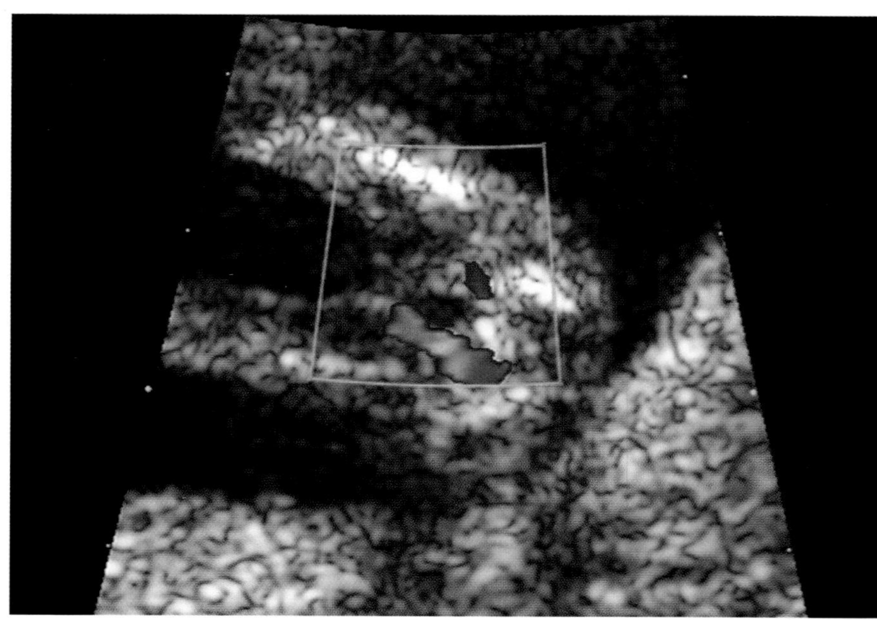

Fig. 11.**53** **VACTERL association.** Unilateral umbilical artery aplasia at 12 + 6 weeks.

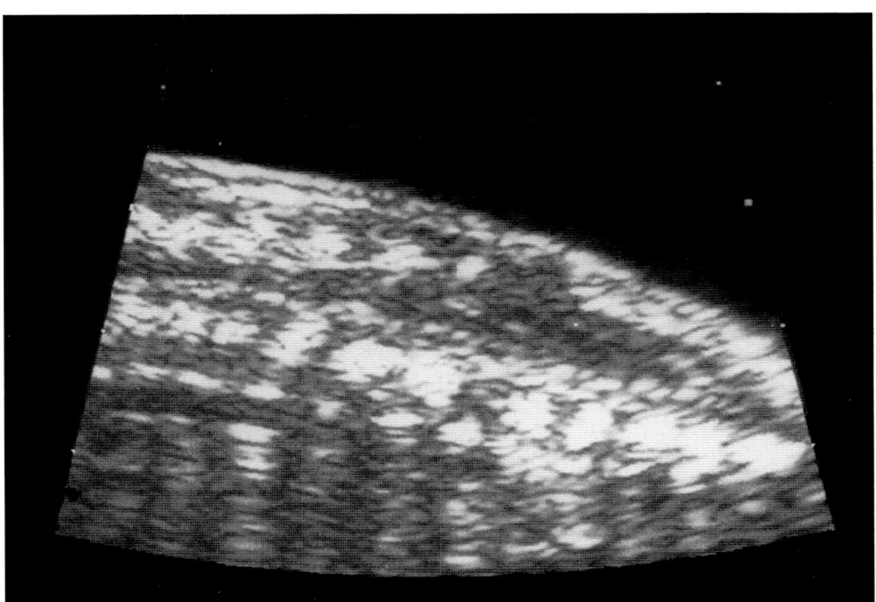

Fig. 11.**54** **VACTERL association.** A dorsoanterior longitudinal section through the lower vertebral canal at 30 + 3 weeks, demonstrating spina bifida occulta in a case of VACTERL association.

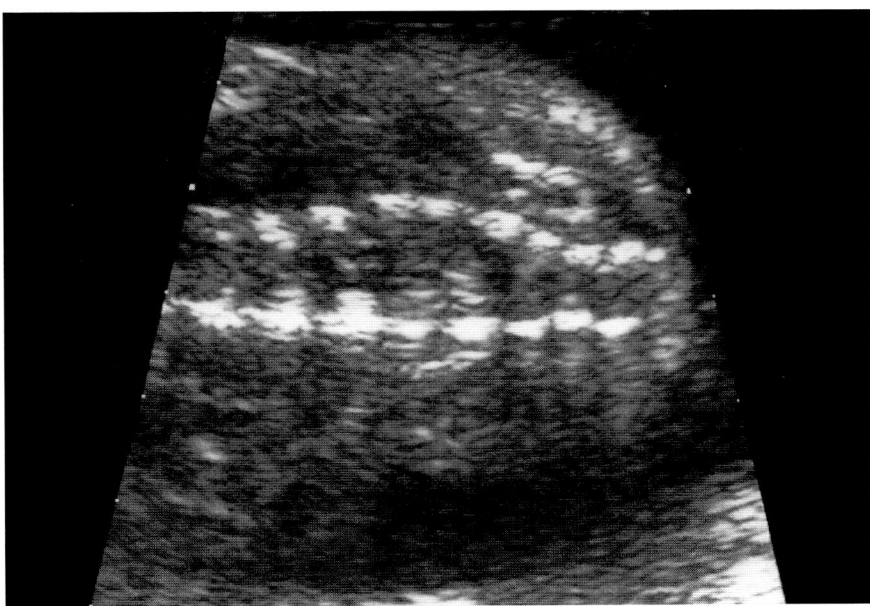

Fig. 11.**55** **VACTERL association.** Same situation, with a frontal view demonstrating the widening of the vertebral arch in the region of the neural tube defect.

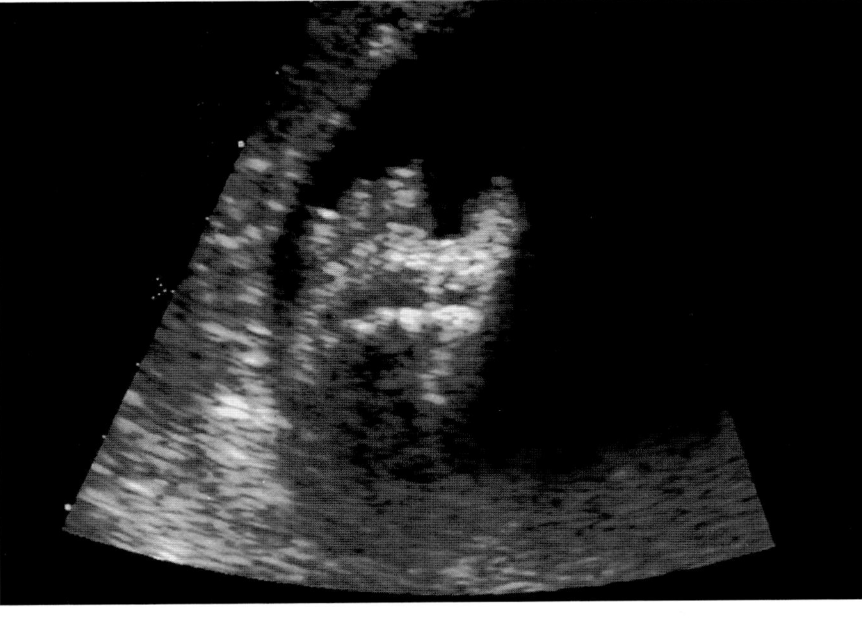

Fig. 11.**56** **VACTERL association.** Tetradactyly of the foot at 30 + 3 weeks.

Self-Help Organization

Title: VACTERL Association

Description: Support, encouragement and resources for parents, grandparents and siblings of children or adults with VACTERL association.

Scope: Online

Web: http://onelist.com/group/vacterlassn

Title: TEF/VATER Support Network (Connection)

Description: Offers support and encouragement for parents of children with tracheo-esophageal fistula, esophageal atresia, and VATER. Aims to bring current information to parents and the medical community. Newsletter, information and referrals, phone support.

Scope: International

Number of groups: Six groups

Founded: 1992

Address: The Vater Connection, 1722 Yucca Lane, Emporia, KS 66801, United States

Telephone: 316-342-6954

Web: http://www.vaterconnection.org

References

Blane CE, Barr M, DiPietro MA, Sedman AB, Bloom DA. Renal obstructive dysplasia: ultrasound diagnosis and therapeutic implications. Pediatr Radiol 1991; 21: 274–7.

Brons JT, van der Harten HJ, van Geijn HP, et al. Prenatal ultrasonographic diagnosis of radial-ray reduction malformations. Prenat Diagn 1990; 10: 279–88.

Cuschieri A. Anorectal anomalies associated with or as part of other anomalies. Am J Med Genet 2002; 110: 122–30.

Krapp M, Geipel A, Germer U, Krokowski M, Gembruch U. First-trimester sonographic diagnosis of distal urethral atresia with megalourethra in VACTERL association. Prenat Diagn 2002; 22: 422–4.

Miller OF, Kolon TF. Prenatal diagnosis of VACTERL association. J Urol 2001; 166: 2389–91.

Van Heurn LW, Cheng W, De Vries B, et al. Anomalies associated with oesophageal atresia in Asians and Europeans. Pediatr Surg Int 2002; 18: 241–3.

Walker–Warburg Syndrome (Lissencephaly Type II)

Definition: This is a fatal disorder consisting of *h*ydrocephalus, *a*gyria, *r*etinal *d*ysplasia, and *e*ncephalocele (HARDE syndrome).

Incidence: Extremely rare; only 70 cases have been reported, and one-third of these are familial.

First described in 1971 by Warburg.

Origin/genetics: It is either inherited in an autosomal-recessive form, or there is a sporadic occurrence in two-thirds of the cases. Gene locus: 9q31–33.

Clinical features: There is a severe restriction in development. Hydrocephalus is present in almost 100% of cases, mostly due to stenosis of the aqueduct. Dandy–Walker malformation (50%), agyria (lissencephaly type II), retinal dysplasia, microphthalmia (38%), cataract (35%), encephalocele (30%), microcephaly (16%). In addition, progressive congenital muscle dystrophy and increased levels of creatine kinase have been described. Other associated anomalies are: cataract, hypoplasia of the iris, optic coloboma, cleft lip and palate, glaucoma, microtia, absence of the external auditory canal, agenesis of the corpus callosum, hypoplasia of the white matter of the brain, and genital anomalies.

Ultrasound findings: In a case with a family history, the diagnosis was already made in the first trimester. Most of the cerebral anomalies are well demonstrated by ultrasound scanning. However, absence of the cerebral gyri and microcephaly are first diagnosed at a more advanced stage in the pregnancy.

Differential diagnosis: Miller–Dieker syndrome (lissencephaly type I), muscle–eye–brain disease, Fukuyama congenital muscular dystrophy, Fryns syndrome, Meckel–Gruber syndrome, Neu–Laxova syndrome, TORCH infections, trisomy 13, trisomy 18.

Prognosis: This disorder has a fatal prognosis; on average, most infants survive up to 9 months, and a few have survived for some years.

Self-Help Organization

Title: The Lissencephaly Network

Description: Support for families affected by lissencephaly or other neuronal migration disorders, and their families. Helps relieve the stress of caring for an ill child. Research updates, newsletter, database of affected children. Networking of parents.

Scope: International network

Founded: 1991

Address: 10408 Bitterroot Ct., Ft. Wayne, IN 46804, United States

Telephone: 219-432-4310

Fax: 219-432-4310

E-mail: DianneFitz@aol.com

Web: http://www.lissencephaly.org

References

Asano Y, Minagawa K, Okuda A, et al. A case of Walker–Warburg syndrome. Brain Dev 2000; 22: 454–7.

Bornemann A, Pfeiffer R, Beinder E, et al. Three siblings with Walker–Warburg Syndrome. Gen Diagn Pathol 1996; 141: 371–5.

Chitayat D, Toi A, Babul R, et al. Prenatal diagnosis of retinal nonattachment in the Walker–Warburg syndrome. Am J Med Genet 1995; 56: 357–8.

Crowe C, Jassani M, Dickerman L. The prenatal diagnosis of the Walker–Warburg syndrome. Prenat Diagn 1986; 6: 177–85.

Gasser B, Lindner V, Dreyfus M, et al. Prenatal diagnosis of Walker–Warburg syndrome in three sibs. Am j Med Genet 1998; 76: 107–10.

Monteagudo A, Alayon A, Mayberry P. Walker–Warburg syndrome: case report and review of the literature. J Ultrasound Med 2001; 20: 419–26.

Vohra N, Ghidini A, Alvarez M, Lockwood C. Walker–Warburg syndrome: prenatal ultrasound findings. Prenat Diagn 1993; 13: 575–9.

Cystic Fibrosis (Mucoviscidosis)

Definition: This is a metabolic disorder characterized by general dysfunction of mucous glands, with overproduction of mucous which has a high viscosity. This leads to chronic bronchial obstruction and recurrent infection of the respiratory tract, as well as to disturbance of exocrine pancreatic function. A high concentration of NaCl is found in the sweat.

Incidence: There is regional variation in the incidence; in Europe, it is one in 2000 births, making it the most common congenital metabolic disorder.

Origin/genetics: Autosomal-recessive inheritance; over 600 mutations of the cystic fibrosis gene are known. The most frequent gene defect is delta-F508 deletion. Using molecular-genetic diagnostic methods, it is possible to detect only the most frequent mutation, and thus about 85% of cases. Epithelial electrolyte transport is disturbed, causing a very thickened mucous production in the pancreas, intestines, and respiratory tract. There are alterations in the cystic fibrosis transmembrane conductance regulator.

Ultrasound findings: *Echogenic bowel* and *dilated loops of intestines* are occasionally seen in the second and third trimester. Meconium peritonitis and hydramnios may be detected. However, there are often no ultrasound signs that raise any suspicion. If anomalies are suspected on a prenatal scan, or if there is a positive family history, molecular-genetic evaluation should be performed using chorionic villus sampling or amniocentesis. In cases of bowel obstruction, cystic fibrosis appears to be the cause in about one-third of cases.

Differential diagnosis: Cytomegalovirus infection, trisomy 21, growth restriction, atresia of the bowel, idiopathic bowel perforation, volvulus.

Clinical management: Investigation of parents using molecular-genetic methods (is there a carrier?), prenatal diagnosis from amniotic fluid, chorion biopsy, or fetal blood (DNA analysis). Prenatal detection is not always possible, as a wide range of gene defects may be responsible.

Prognosis: This is a chronic and progressive disorder, which places a tremendous burden on the affected individuals and their families. The quality of life and life expectancy are considerably reduced. Today, it is possible to increase the life expectancy after combined heart–lung transplantation at around 20 years of age.

Self-Help Organization

Title: Cystic Fibrosis Foundation

Description: Provides information and referrals to individuals, families, and professionals on cystic fibrosis. Supports over 100 centers nationwide. Provides grants to researchers. Newsletter, literature, conferences.

Scope: National

Number of groups: 80 affiliated groups

Founded: 1955

Address: Cystic Fibrosis Foundation, 6931 Arlington Rd., Bethesda, MD 20814, United States

Telephone: 1-800-FIGHT-CF

Fax: 306-951-6378

E-mail: info@cff.org

Web: http://www.cff.org

References

Al-Kouatly HB, Chasen ST, Streltzoff J, Chervenak FA. The clinical significance of fetal echogenic bowel. Am J Obstet Gynecol 2001; 185: 1035–8.

Baeckert P, Mieth D, Schneider H, Schwöbel M. Meconium peritonitis: description of 3 cases with abnormal prenatal ultrasound findings. Helv Paediatr Acta 1987; 41: 539–44.

Hogge WA, Hogge JS, Boehm CD, Sanders RC. Increased echogenicity in the fetal abdomen: use of DNA analysis to establish a diagnosis of cystic fibrosis. J Ultrasound Med 1993; 12: 451–4.

Muller F, Boué C. Prenatal diagnosis of mucoviscidosis: biochemical technics and studies of affected fetuses. Chir Pediatr 1986; 27: 220–3.

Muller F, Simon-Bouy B, Girodon E, Monnier N, Malinge MC, Serre JL. Predicting the risk of cystic fibrosis with abnormal ultrasound signs of fetal bowel: results of a French molecular collaborative study based on 641 prospective cases. Am J Med Genet 2002; 110: 109–15.

Nyberg DA, Hastrup W, Watts H, Mack LA. Dilated fetal bowel: a sonographic sign of cystic fibrosis. J Ultrasound Med 1987; 6: 257–60.

Papp Z, Tóth Z, Szabó M, Szeifert GT. Early prenatal diagnosis of cystic fibrosis by ultrasound [letter]. Clin Genet 1985; 28: 356–8.

Scotet V, De Braekeleer M, Audrezet MP, et al. Prenatal detection of cystic fibrosis by ultrasonography: a retrospective study of more than 346 000 pregnancies. J Med Genet 2002; 39: 443–8.

Sipes SL, Weiner CP, Wenstrom KD, Williamson RA, Grant SS, Mueller GM. Fetal echogenic bowel on ultrasound: is there clinical significance? Fetal Diagn Ther 1994; 9: 38–43.

Yaron Y, Hassan S, Geva E, Kupferminc MJ, Yavetz H, Evans MI. Evaluation of fetal echogenic bowel in the second trimester. Fetal Diagn Ther 1999; 14: 176–80.

Other Causes of Fetal Disease and Anomalies

12 Fetal Hydrops

Nonimmune Hydrops Fetalis (NIHF)

Definition: Generalized accumulation of fluid in serous body cavities, such as the pleural, peritoneal, and pericardial spaces, as well as in fetal soft tissue (skin edema), which is not caused by rhesus incompatibility. In some reports, isolated fetal ascites has also been included in this definition.

Incidence: One in 2500–3500 live births.

Clinical history/genetics: Many different causes are known to be responsible for this condition, so that its occurrence may be sporadic or it may be associated with certain syndromes with a variable risk of recurrence. If no cause is found, then the risk of recurrence is empirically estimated at 5%.

Origin: The following disorders may cause fetal hydrops: cardiac insufficiency heads the list (anomalies, arrhythmia, volume overload due to AV anastomosis), followed by anemias (parvovirus B19, thalassemia), anomalies leading to decreased venous return to the heart (mediastinum shift due to diaphragmatic hernia or CCAM), as well as hypoproteinemia (infections, reduced protein synthesis in the liver, congenital nephrotic syndrome).

Associated syndromes and causative factors: Cystic hygroma colli, cardiac anomaly (25%), arrhythmias with bradycardia and tachycardia, fetal tumors (especially coccygeal tumor, tumors within the thoracic cavity, liver tumors), lymphangiomas, malformation of the lungs (CCAM), chorioangioma of the placenta, fetal infections such as cytomegalovirus, parvovirus B19, syphilis, toxoplasmosis, varicella. Chromosomal aberrations (15%) especially Down syndrome, other trisomies, and Turner syndrome. In twin pregnancy, twin-to-twin transfusion syndrome. Others include: fetomaternal bleeding, arteriovenous shunts, obstruction of the gastrointestinal tract. Rare syndromes: achondrogenesis, α-thalassemia, Fryns syndrome, disorder of glycogen metabolism, multiple pterygium syndrome, Neu–Laxova syndrome, Noonan syndrome.

Ultrasound findings: At least three of the following four findings should be detected: *fetal ascites, pleural effusion, pericardial effusion,* and *skin edema.* Pericardial effusion is often the first sign of a developing hydrops. Accompanying hydramnios is a common feature. The placenta may be swollen and thickened.

Clinical management: Further ultrasound screening, including fetal echocardiography. *Examination of the mother:* basic blood count, hemoglobin electrophoresis, Kleinhauer–Bethke test, infection serology (TORCH), including syphilis diagnosis. *Fetal examination:* fetal blood sampling (umbilical venous sampling) for determination of karyotype, blood count, possibly hemoglobin electrophoresis, serum albumin, IgM, infection serology (TORCH); other parameters may be necessary using polymerase chain reaction (PCR) and virus culture from amniotic fluid. Regular ultrasound examination is mandatory. Anemia (parvovirus B19) and tachycardia can be successfully treated. In cases of pulmonary disorder (CCAM), placement of a shunt has been promising in resolving fetal hydrops in isolated cases. Hydrops due to idiopathic causes has a high rate of fetal mortality. There is a high risk of fetal distress during labor, so that primary cesarean section is a preferred clinical option if maximum intensive care is to be given to the neonate. Aspiration of ascites or pleural effusion in the prenatal stage facilitates the primary care after birth.

Procedure after birth: Intensive care of the new born is needed, as they are usually severely distressed. Further treatment options depend on the cause of the hydrops.

Prognosis: This depends on the cause of hydrops. A fetal mortality rate of 50–90% has been reported.

References

Alter DN, Reed KL, Marx GR, Anderson CF, Shenker L. Prenatal diagnosis of congestive heart failure in a fetus with a sacrococcygeal teratoma. Obstet Gynecol 1988; 71: 978–81.

Anandakumar C, Biswas A, Wong YC, et al. Management of non-immune hydrops: 8 years' experience. Ultrasound Obstet Gynecol 1996; 8: 196–200.

Barss VA, Benacerraf BR, Greene MF, Phillippe M, Frigoletto FDJ. Sonographic detection of fetal hydrops: a report of two cases. J Reprod Med 1985; 30: 893–4.

Bollmann R, Chaoui R, Schilling H, Hoffmann H, Reiche M, Pahl L. [Prenatal diagnosis and management of fetal arrhythmias; in German.] Z Geburtshilfe Perinatol 1988; 192: 266–72.

Budorick NE, Pretorius DH, Leopold GR, Stamm ER. Spontaneous improvement of intrathoracic masses diagnosed in utero. J Ultrasound Med 1992; 11: 653–62.

Dillard JP, Edwards DK, Leopold GR. Meconium peritonitis masquerading as fetal hydrops. J Ultrasound Med 1987; 6: 49–51.

Engellenner W, Kaplan C, Van de Vegte GL. Pulmonary agenesis association with nonimmune hydrops. Pediatr Pathol 1989; 9: 725–30.

Entezami M, Becker R, Menssen HD, Marcinkowski M, Versmold H. Xerocytosis with concomitant intrauterine ascites: first description and therapeutic approach. Blood 1996; 87: 5392–3.

Fleischer AC, Shah DM, Jeanty P, Sacks GA, Boehm FH. Hydrops fetalis. Clin Diagn Ultrasound 1989; 25: 283–306.

Gloster ES, Godoy G, Burrows P, et al. Perinatal nonimmune hydrops: diagnostic ultrasonography and related aspects of management. J Perinatol 1989; 9: 430–6.

Jauniaux E, Ogle R. Color Doppler imaging in the diagnosis and management of chorioangiomas. Ultrasound Obstet Gynecol 2000; 15: 463–7.

Tongsong T, Wanapirak C, Srisomboon J, Piyamongkol W, Sirichotiyakul S. Antenatal sonographic features of 100 alpha-thalassemia hydrops fetalis fetuses. J Clin Ultrasound 1996; 24: 73–7.

Wafelman LS, Pollock BH, Kreutzer J, Richards DS, Hutchison AA. Nonimmune hydrops fetalis: fetal and neonatal outcome during 1983–1992. Biol Neonate 1999; 75: 73–81.

Rhesus Incompatibility

Definition: Fetal hemolytic disease caused by maternal antibodies to rhesus factors, particularly anti-D antibody.

Incidence: There are regional differences. About 1% of pregnant women were affected before the introduction of rhesus prophylaxis using anti-D immunoglobulin.

Origin: The mother produces IgG antibodies against rhesus system antigens that cross the placenta and destroy fetal erythrocytes. Despite increased synthesis of fetal erythrocytes, fetal anemia still results. If the hemoglobin values fall below 5–6 g%, fetal hydrops develops. The most common antigen leading to synthesis of maternal antibodies is antigen D, followed by C and E.

Ultrasound findings: *Fetal hydrops* is a classical feature of severe fetal anemia. *Hepatosplenomegaly* may also be evident. *Hydramnios* is often associated. The placenta is *swollen* and echogenic. *Growth restriction* is commonly seen. In subsequent pregnancies, the symptoms appear earlier and are more severe (boost). Today, rhesus incompatibility can be diagnosed using routine antibody testing during antenatal examination of the mother.

Clinical management: If the *antibody test is positive*, the titer and specific antibody should be further determined. The antibody titer should be controlled regularly during the course of the pregnancy. Serial scans should be carried out to detect early signs of hydrops. *Color-coded Doppler imaging of the ascending aorta and medial cerebral artery* should be performed to determine the *blood flow velocity*. Fetal anemia is often diagnosed if the maximum blood flow velocity (V_{max}) is increased. Values over 1 m/s in the aorta and 50 cm/s in the medial cerebral artery before 30 weeks of gestation are pathological. There are centile charts that show the range of velocities according to gestational age, and these should be taken into account for accurate diagnosis. Nowadays, *fetal blood sampling,* which allows direct estimation of fetal hemoglobin, is preferable to *amniocentesis,* which determines hemoglobin indirectly by photometric measurement of its breakdown products (Liley method). Extinction measurement of the amniotic fluid is inaccurate before 26 weeks, so that the Liley estimate has lost its importance as a diagnostic method. Nowadays, however, it is possible to detect *the fetal rhesus factor in amniotic fluid using polymerase chain reaction and to diagnose the fetal blood group by molecular-biological methods.* If the antibody titer remains constant, determination of the blood group and extinction measurements using amniotic fluid at 26 weeks may be a useful examination. Monitoring the pregnancy using Doppler flow imaging alone has not yet been sufficiently evaluated. The main disadvantage of repeated invasive procedures is the risk of *boosting* and thus *worsening* the initial condition.

Intrauterine transfusions of erythrocytes through the *umbilical vein* are indicated if the hemoglobin value falls below 8–10 g% (erythrocyte concentrate: O rhesus-negative, hematocrit 70%, cytomegalovirus-negative, irradiated to reduce the graft-versus-host reaction). The transfusion can be facilitated by administration of pancuronium (0.3 mg/kg estimated fetal weight) to relax the fetus. Once the transfusion has been carried out, repeated transfusions are usually required at 2–3-week intervals. The transfused erythrocytes cannot be destroyed by maternal antibodies, as they are O rhesus-negative. However, fetal erythropoiesis is suppressed due to these transfusions, so that at birth the percentage of erythrocytes in fetal blood with adult hemoglobin is almost 100%. If the transfusions are well tolerated, the pregnancy can be prolonged up to 37 weeks. In the absence of severe anemia and fetal hydrops, vaginal delivery is attempted.

Procedure after birth: Neonatal jaundice is seen frequently. Exchange transfusion is necessary if severe anemia and fetal hydrops are present.

Prognosis: The rate of survival after adequate therapy is 95%, and in case of hydrops 80–85%.

References

Andersen AS, Praetorius L, Jorgensen HL, Lylloff K, Larsen KT. Prognostic value of screening for irregular antibodies late in pregnancy in rhesus positive women. Acta Obstet Gynecol Scand 2002; 81: 407–11.

Dimer JA, David M, Dudenhausen JW. Intravenous drug abuse is an indication for antepartum screening for RH alloimmunization: a case report and review of literature. Arch Gynecol Obstet 1999; 263: 73–5.

Hohlfeld P, Wirthner D, Tissot JD. Perinatal hemolytic disease, 2: prevention and management. J Gynecol Obstet Biol Reprod (Paris) 1998; 27: 265–76.

Holzgreve W, Zhong XY, Burk MR, Hahn S. Enrichment of fetal cells and free fetal DNA from maternal blood: an insight into the Basel experience. Early Pregnancy 2001; 5: 43–4.

Moise KJ Jr. Management of rhesus alloimmunization in pregnancy [review]. Obstet Gynecol 2002; 100: 600–11.

Müller HI, Hackelber BJ, Kattner E. Pre- and postnatal diagnosis and treatment of hydrops fetalis: an interdisciplinary problem. Z Geburtshilfe Neonatol 1998; 202: 2–9.

Steiner EA, Judd WJ, Oberman HA, Hayashi RH, Nugent CE. Percutaneous umbilical blood sampling and umbilical vein transfusions: rapid serologic differentiation of fetal blood from maternal blood. Transfusion 1990; 30: 104–8.

Whitecar PW, Depcik-Smith ND, Strauss RA, Moise KJ. Fetal splenic rupture following transfusion. Obstet Gynecol 2001; 97: 824–5.

13 Infections

Congenital Syphilis

Definition: Maternal infection with the spirochete *Treponema pallidum*, which can be transmitted to the fetus.

Incidence: There is regional variation, about one in 100 000 births, most frequently in maternal stage II.

Origin: Contrary to many assumptions, this pathogen can cross the placental barrier at any time during the course of pregnancy.

Ultrasound findings: Hydramnios, enlarged placenta, hepatosplenomegaly, ascites; in severe cases, fetal hydrops, bent long bones.

Clinical features: Skin and bones are affected. Meningitis, nephritis, hepatosplenomegaly. In untreated cases, fetal demise or stillbirth occur in 50% of cases.

Differential diagnosis: Cytomegalovirus infection, meconium peritonitis, parvovirus, trisomy 21, Turner syndrome.

Clinical management: Maternal blood for serological testing (FTA-ABS). The pathogen can be identified either in amniotic fluid or in fetal blood samples. The mother should be treated with antibiotics. Fetal damage that may already have occurred is irreversible.

Procedure after birth: Cardiac and respiratory difficulties are often present. Blood and other secretions are highly infectious. Penicillin is given for 10 days.

Prognosis: At the time of birth, the neonate may appear clinically normal, but may show signs and symptoms of syphilitic disease at a later stage. Mental impairment, blindness, and sensorineural deafness are possible late sequelae. Infants with hydrops have a particularly unfavorable prognosis.

References

Conde-Agudelo A, Belizan JM, Diaz-Rossello JL. Epidemiology of fetal death in Latin America. Acta Obstet Gynecol Scand 2000; 79: 371–8.

Crino JP. Ultrasound and fetal diagnosis of perinatal infection. Clin Obstet Gynecol 1999; 42: 71–80.

Gust DA, Levine WC, St Louis ME, Braxton J, Berman SM. Mortality associated with congenital syphilis in the United States, 1992–1998. Pediatrics 2002; 109: E79–9.

Hollier LM, Harstad TW, Sanchez PJ, Twickler DM, Wendel GD Jr. Fetal syphilis: clinical and laboratory characteristics. Obstet Gynecol 2001; 97: 947–53.

Narducci F, Switala I, Rajabally R, Decocq J, Delahousse G. Maternal and congenital syphilis. J Gynecol Obstet Biol Reprod (Paris) 1998; 27: 150–60.

Newell ML, Thorne C, Pembrey L, Nicoll A, Goldberg D, Peckham C. Antenatal screening for hepatitis B infection and syphilis in the UK. Br J Obstet Gynaecol 1999; 106: 66–71.

Vieker S, Siefert S, Lemke J, Pust B. [Congenital syphilis after reactivation of "healed" maternal primary infection; in German.] Klin Pädiatr 2000; 212: 336–9.

Walker GJ. Antibiotics for syphilis diagnosed during pregnancy [review]. Cochrane Database Syst Rev 2001; 3: CD001143.

Zelop C, Benacerraf BR. The causes and natural history of fetal ascites. Prenat Diagn 1994; 14: 941–6.

5

Congenital Varicella

Definition: Infection with varicella zoster virus. This is a DNA virus belonging to the family of herpesviruses. The primary infection causes chickenpox; reactivation of the virus at a later stage from the sensory roots of the posterior horn of the spinal cord is responsible for the clinical symptoms of herpes zoster.

Incidence: Maternal infection during pregnancy, one in 2000–10 000. The risk of congenital infection to the fetus is low; congenital malformations result in less than 5% of cases.

Origin: The virus affects the nervous system, causing neurological impairment of fetal structures. Infections in the first trimester cause the most severe damage.

Clinical features: Focal ulceration of the skin and anomalies described in the following section.

Ultrasound findings: Rarely, the following are detected: growth restriction, hydramnios, microphthalmia, hydrocephalus, or microcephaly; ascites, pleural effusions and even full-fledged fetal hydrops; hepatic calcification, club feet and other limb anomalies, reduction in fetal movements. These anomalies develop only in the most severely affected cases, about 3–12 weeks after maternal infection.

Clinical management: Serology of maternal blood; fetal IgM is detectable from 20 weeks, amniotic fluid culture, chorionic villus sampling and polymerase chain reaction, regular scanning controls (is hydrocephalus developing?). IgG may be given to the mother within 72–96 h if the mother has been in contact with an infected individual and is not immune.

Procedure after birth: Acyclovir may be given after birth.

Prognosis: The infants usually do not show any symptoms. Fetal anomalies appear in 1–2% of cases if infection occurs before 20 weeks of gestation. About one-third of the most severely affected infants die in the early neonatal stage; in the surviving infants, mental impairment and fits may occur.

References

Dufour P, de Bièvre P, Vinatier D, et al. Varicella and pregnancy. Eur J Obstet Gynecol Reprod Biol 1996; 66: 119–23.
Harger JH, Ernest JM, Thurnau GR, et al. Frequency of congenital varicella syndrome in a prospective cohort of 347 pregnant women. Obstet Gynecol 2002; 100: 260–5.
Kerkering KW. Abnormal cry and intracranial calcifications: clues to the diagnosis of fetal varicella-zoster syndrome [review]. J Perinatol 2001; 21: 131–5.
Lecuru F, Taurelle R, Bernard JP, et al. Varicella zoster virus infection during pregnancy: the limits of prenatal diagnosis. Eur J Obstet Gynecol Reprod Biol 1994; 56: 67–8.
Mets MB. Eye manifestations of intrauterine infections [review]. Ophthalmol Clin North Am 2001; 14: 521–31.
Petignat P, Vial Y, Laurini R, Hohlfeld P. Fetal varicella-herpes zoster syndrome in early pregnancy: ultrasonographic and morphological correlation. Prenat Diagn 2001; 21: 121–4.
Pons JC, Vial P, Rozenberg F, et al. Prenatal diagnosis of fetal varicella in the second trimester of pregnancy. J Gynecol Obstet Biol Reprod (Paris) 1995; 24: 829–38.
Taylor WG, Walkinshaw SA, Thomson MA. Antenatal assessment of neurological impairment. Arch Dis Child 1993; 68: 604–5.
Yaron Y, Hassan S, Geva E, Kupferminc MJ, Yavetz H, Evans MI. Evaluation of fetal echogenic bowel in the second trimester. Fetal Diagn Ther 1999; 14: 176–80.

Parvovirus B19

Definition: Infection with parvovirus B19, a DNA virus causing erythema infectiosum. The disease is often asymptomatic in both children and adults. Infection of the fetus may lead to fetal anemia and hydrops.

Incidence: Some 50–75% of adult women are immune. There is a 10–20% risk of transmission to the fetus through the placenta, and it is most likely to occur in the first and second trimesters.

Clinical history: Joint pain and small areas of erythema may be the only clinical symptoms of this infection.

Origin: The infection destroys host cells, particularly those that have a high rate of mitosis and divide quickly, such as erythrocyte precursors.

Ultrasound findings: Severe cases show hydramnios, placentomegaly, ascites, pleural effusions, cardiomegaly, possibly reduced fetal movements. In addition, there may be hepatosplenomegaly and fetal hydrops. These findings are detected 3–13 weeks after maternal infection. If untreated, fetal demise or neonatal death results.

Differential diagnosis: Isoimmune parvoviruses, fetomaternal transfusion, arteriovenous shunts, bradycardia, cardiomyopathy, cardiac anomalies, tachycardia, chromosomal aberrations, tumors within the thoracic cavity causing compression of the mediastinum, chorioangiomas, cystic hygroma, obstruction of the gastrointestinal tract, hepatic tumors, lymphangiomas, teratomas, cytomegalovirus infection, syphilis, toxoplasmosis, varicella, achondrogenesis, alpha thalassemia, Fryns syndrome, glycogen storage disease, multiple pterygium syndrome, Neu–Laxova syndrome, Noonan syndrome, Pena–Shokeir syndrome, short rib–polydactyly syndrome types I and III.

Clinical management: Maternal serology; umbilical venous sampling to determine blood count; IgM, PCR. If the fetal hemoglobin falls below 8 g/dl, an intrauterine erythrocyte transfusion is necessary. If recent infection of the mother is confirmed, weekly scan controls are mandatory for up to the next 13 weeks to detect the development of fetal anemia. Even in case of severe fetal anemia, only a few transfusions are needed, as fetal erythropoiesis recovers quickly. In the absence of fetal hydrops, normal vaginal delivery is possible. In case of fetal hydrops, aspiration of excess fluids from the affected body cavities (such as pleural effusion, ascites) facilitates the immediate care of the neonate.

Procedure after birth: Apart from the difficulties posed by fetal hydrops, no other specific complications are expected.

Prognosis: There is a 10% risk of intrauterine fetal death due to anemia and hydrops.

References

Delle Chiaie L, Buck G, Grab D, Terinde R. Prediction of fetal anemia with Doppler measurement of the middle cerebral artery peak systolic velocity in pregnancies complicated by maternal blood group alloimmunization or parvovirus B19 infection. Ultrasound Obstet Gynecol 2001; 18: 232–6.

Goodear M, Hayward C, Crowther C. Foetal intracardiac transfusion for the treatment of severe anaemia due to human parvovirus B-19 infection. Australas Radiol 1998; 42: 275–7.

Ismail KM, Martin WL, Ghosh S, Whittle MJ, Kilby MD. Etiology and outcome of hydrops fetalis. J Matern Fetal Med 2001; 10: 175–81.

Karunajeewa H, Siebert D, Hammond R, Garland S, Kelly H. Seroprevalence of varicella zoster virus, parvovirus B19 and *Toxoplasma gondii* in a Melbourne obstetric population: implications for management. Aust N Z J Obstet Gynaecol 2001; 41: 23–8.

Naides SJ, Weiner CP. Antenatal diagnosis and palliative treatment of non-immune hydrops fetalis secondary to fetal parvovirus B19 infection. Prenat Diagn 1989; 9: 105–14.

Smulian JC, Egan JF, Rodis JF. Fetal hydrops in the first trimester associated with maternal parvovirus infection. J Clin Ultrasound 1998; 26: 314–6.

Suchet I, Ens W, Suchet R. Parvovirus B19 infection in utero: natural history and spectrum of sonographic manifestations in 7 cases. Can Assoc Radiol J 2000; 51: 198–204.

von Kaisenberg CS, Bender G, Scheewe J, et al. A case of fetal parvovirus B19 myocarditis, terminal cardiac heart failure, and perinatal heart transplantation. Fetal Diagn Ther 2001; 16: 427–32.

Yaron Y, Hassan S, Geva E, Kupferminc MJ, Yavetz H, Evans MI. Evaluation of fetal echogenic bowel in the second trimester. Fetal Diagn Ther 1999; 14: 176–80.

Zelop C, Benacerraf BR. The causes and natural history of fetal ascites. Prenat Diagn 1994; 14: 941–6.

Zerbini M, Gentilomi GA, Gallinella G, et al. Intrauterine parvovirus B19 infection and meconium peritonitis. Prenat Diagn 1998; 18: 599–606.

Toxoplasmosis

Definition: This is a parasite infection with *Toxoplasma gondii.* Maternal infection follows consumption of raw meat, raw milk products, or contamination through cat excrement. There is transplacental infection of the fetus, most severe during the first and second trimesters. Most congenital infections result after transmission in the third trimester.

Incidence: One in 100–1000 pregnancies. Fetal transmission occurs in 40% if it is a primary infection of the mother during the pregnancy. Seventy-five percent of these fetuses show no symptoms, whereas 10% are severely affected.

Origin: Fetal cells are destroyed by this infection.

Clinical features: Chorioretinitis, hydrocephalus, cataract, thrombocytopenia, anemia, and hydrops.

Ultrasound findings: *Intracranial calcifications* are a typical feature, and are distributed randomly (in contrast to cytomegalovirus infection). *Hepatosplenomegaly* with echogenic structures within the liver is detected. *Dilation of cerebral ventricles*, the posterior horns of the lateral ventricles are the first to be affected. Ascites, pleural effusion, and full-fledged hydrops may result. Following this, hydramnios, placentomegaly with echogenic structures and growth restriction are frequent findings.

Differential diagnosis: Cytomegalovirus infection.

Clinical management: Toxoplasmosis serology from maternal and fetal blood samples: the fetal IgM is first detectable after 20 weeks of gestation. Amniotic fluid PCR. Antibiotics should be given to the mother.

Procedure after birth: Blood and other secretions of the newborn may be infectious. Moderate jaundice, anemia, and hepatosplenomegaly are often present. The infant should be treated with antibiotics for a period of 1 year.

Prognosis: Most congenital toxoplasmosis infections do not show any clinical symptoms. In severe cases, the mortality may be as high as 12%. The central nervous system and eyes are affected in about 80% of infants, with severe infection causing mental impairment, fits, cerebral palsy, hydrocephalus and sensorineural hearing loss. Infections at an early stage of gestation affect the fetus most severely and often result in intrauterine fetal demise or severe central nervous system anomalies. Even in asymptomatic children, chorioretinitis and neurological injury may develop during the later course (up to the age of 10).

References

Al-Kouatly HB, Chasen ST, Streltzoff J, Chervenak FA. The clinical significance of fetal echogenic bowel. Am J Obstet Gynecol 2001; 185: 1035–8.

Bader TI, Macones GA, Asch DA. Prenatal screening for toxoplasmosis. Obstet Gynecol 1997; 90: 457–64.

Couvreur J. Problems of congenital toxoplasmosis: evolution over four decades. Presse Méd 1999; 28: 753–7.

Daffos F, Forestier F, Capella PM, et al. Prenatal management of 746 pregnancies at risk for congenital toxoplasmosis. N Engl J Med 1988; 318: 271–5.

Desmonts G, Daffos F, Forestier F, Capella PM, Thulliez P, Chartier M. Prenatal diagnosis of congenital toxoplasmosis. Lancet 1985; i: 500–4.

Eskild A, Magnus P. Little evidence of effective prenatal treatment against congenital toxoplasmosis: the implications for testing in pregnancy. Int J Epidemiol 2001; 30: 1314–5.

Favre R, Grange G, Gasser B. Congenital toxoplasmosis in twins: a case report. Fetal Diagn Ther 1994; 9: 264–8.

Foulon W, Naessens A, Mahler T, de Waele M, de Catte L, de Meuter F. Prenatal diagnosis of congenital toxoplasmosis. Obstet Gynecol 1990; 76: 769–72.

Garin JP, Mojon M, Piens MA, Chevalier NI. [Monitoring and treatment of toxoplasmosis in the pregnant woman, fetus and newborn; in French.] Pédiatrie 1989; 44: 705–712.

Gilbert RE, Gras L, Wallon M, Peyron F, Ades AE, Dunn DT. Effect of prenatal treatment on mother to child transmission of *Toxoplasma gondii:* retrospective cohort study of 554 mother–child pairs in Lyons, France. Int J Epidemiol 2001; 30: 1303–8.

Gras L, Gilbert RE, Ades AE, Dunn DT. Effect of prenatal treatment on the risk of intracranial and ocular lesions in children with congenital toxoplasmosis. Int J Epidemiol 2001; 30: 1309–13.

Mayer HO, Fast C, Hofmann H, Karpf EF, Stünzner D. Severe fetopathy: *Toxoplasma* despite serologic screening: a case report. Geburtshilfe Frauenheilkd 1989; 49: 504–5.

Pedreira DA, Diniz EM, Schultz R, Faro LB, Zugaib M. Fetal cataract in congenital toxoplasmosis. Ultrasound Obstet Gynecol 1999; 13: 266–7.

Pelloux H, Fricker-Hidalgo H, Pons JC, et al. [Congenital toxoplasmosis: prevention in the pregnant woman and management of the neonate; in French; review.] Arch Pediatr 2002; 9: 206–12.

Pratlong F Boulot P, Villena I, et al. Antenatal diagnosis of congenital toxoplasmosis: evaluation of the biological parameters in a cohort of 286 patients. Br J Obstet Gynaecol 1996; 103: 552–7.

Thulliez P. Commentary: Efficacy of prenatal treatment for toxoplasmosis: a possibility that cannot be ruled out. Int J Epidemiol 2001; 30: 1315–6.

Cytomegalovirus Infection

Definition: Infection with cytomegalovirus, a DNA virus belonging to the group of herpesviruses. In adults, this infection occurs without major symptoms. Infection of the fetus, however, can lead to severe damage. Transmission is through the placenta.

Incidence: Some 1–3% of newborn infants excrete cytomegalovirus, but only 5% of these show any symptoms in the neonatal period. About 1–4% of pregnant women are infected with cytomegalovirus; the primary infection during pregnancy causes fetal infection in 30%. Long-term damage may result in 10–15%, particularly if the primary infection occurs in the first trimester.

Origin: Cytomegalovirus destroys the infected cells.

Ultrasound findings: *Intracranial calcifications, microcephaly and obstructive hydrocephalus* are characteristic features. The calcifications are typically situated on the outside edge of the lateral cerebral ventricles and in the region of the basal ganglia. Additional findings are hepatic calcifications and echogenic bowel. Other anomalies may also be evident: growth restriction, fetal hydrops due to anemia, cardiomegaly, tachycardia, bradycardia, hepatosplenomegaly, hydronephrosis, hydramnios, possibly oligohydramnios and placentomegaly.

Differential diagnosis: Cystic fibrosis, trisomy 21, tuberous sclerosis, other intrauterine infections.

Clinical management: Maternal serology, amniotic fluid culture and PCR; evaluation of amniotic fluid is more useful than fetal blood. Fetal blood analysis may still be needed for blood count (thrombocytopenia, anemia, IgM). Serial scans are recommended for early detection of anomalies such as fetal hydrops, hydrocephalus, microcephaly, and growth restriction.

Procedure after birth: The neonate's body fluids are infectious. PCR diagnosis from urine or other secretions is possible. Treatment with the antiviral agent ganciclovir is probably ineffective, as organ damage has already occurred in the intrauterine stage.

Prognosis: Ninety-five percent of the infants do not show any clinical symptoms. Of the remainder, 80% will develop neurological symptoms at a later stage and 30% die in infancy. Of the asymptomatic infants, some may develop visual and hearing defects and neurological impairment.

References

Achiron R, Pinhas HO, Lipitz S, Heiman Z, Reichman B, Mashiach S. Prenatal ultrasonographic diagnosis of fetal cerebral ventriculitis associated with asymptomatic maternal cytomegalovirus infection. Prenat Diagn 1994; 14: 523–6.

Azzarotto T, Guerra B, Spezzacatena P, et al. Prenatal diagnosis of congenital cytomegalovirus infection. J Clin Microbiol 1998; 36: 3540–4.

Chaoui R, Zodan-Marin T, Wisser J. Marked splenomegaly in fetal cytomegalovirus infection: detection supported by three-dimensional power Doppler ultrasound. Ultrasound Obstet Gynecol 2002; 20: 299–302.

Choong KK, Gruenewald SM, Hodson EM. Echogenic fetal kidneys in cytomegalovirus infection. J Clin Ultrasound 1993; 21: 128–32.

Donner C, Liesnard C, Content J, Busine A, Aderca J, Rodesch F. Prenatal diagnosis of 52 pregnancies at risk for congenital cytomegalovirus infection. Obstet Gynecol 1993; 82: 481–6.

Henrich W, Meckies J, Dudenhausen JW, Vogel M, Enders G. Recurrent cytomegalovirus infection during pregnancy: ultrasonographic diagnosis and fetal outcome. Ultrasound Obstet Gynecol 2002; 19: 608–11.

Hohlfeld P, Vial Y, Maillard BC, Vaudaux B, Fawer CL. Cytomegalovirus fetal infection: prenatal diagnosis. Obstet Gynecol 1991; 78: 615–8.

Lipitz S, Achiron R, Zalel Y, Mendelson E, Tepperberg M, Gamzu R. Outcome of pregnancies with vertical transmission of primary cytomegalovirus infection. Obstet Gynecol 2002; 100: 428–33.

Mazeron MC, Cordovi VL, Perol Y. Transient hydrops fetalis associated with intrauterine cytomegalovirus infection: prenatal diagnosis. Obstet Gynecol 1994; 84: 692–4.

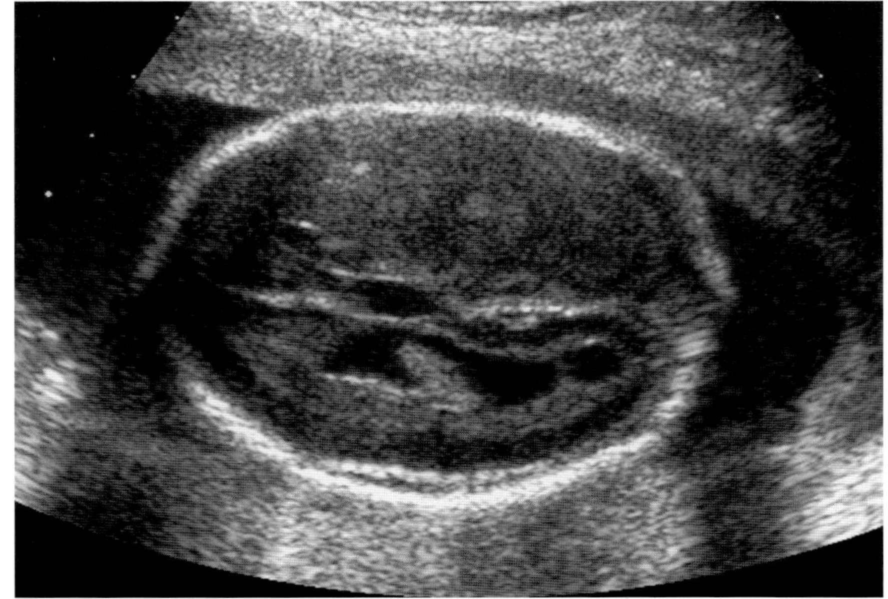

Fig. 13.**1** **Cytomegalovirus infection.** Fetal head at 24 + 0 weeks, showing slight widening of the ventricles and thickening of the edges with echogenicity, in fetal cytomegalovirus infection.

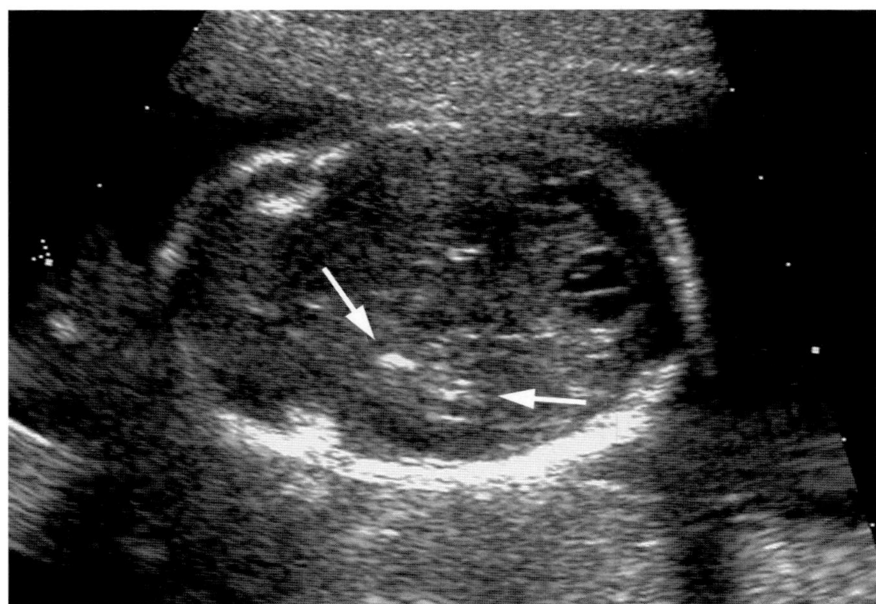

Fig. 13.**2** **Cytomegalovirus infection.** Cross-section of a fetal head, showing echogenic calcifications.

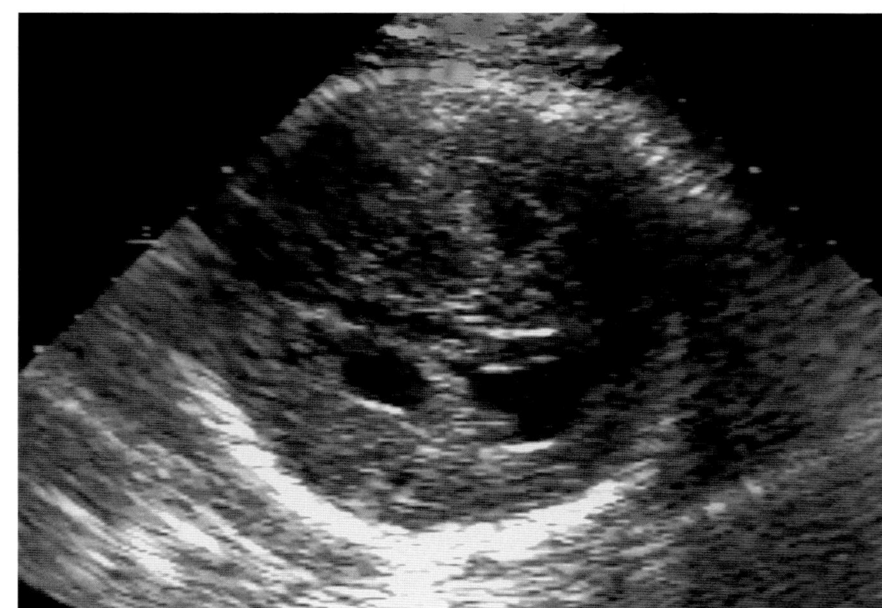

Fig. 13.**3** **Cytomegalovirus infection.** Cross-section of a fetal head at 38 + 4 weeks. Dilation of both lateral ventricles up to 14 mm in a fetus with congenital cytomegalovirus infection.

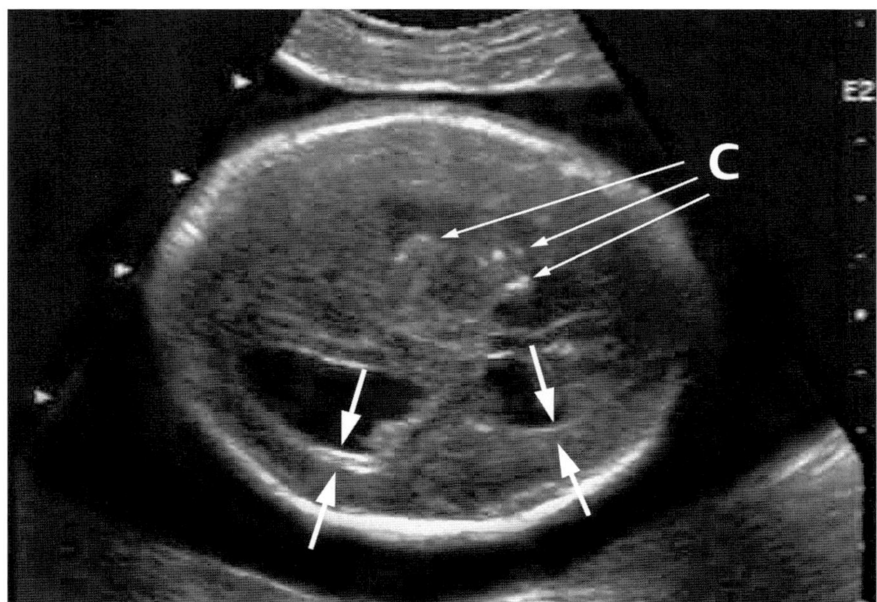

Fig. 13.**4** **Cytomegalovirus infection.** Cross-section of a fetal head at 30 + 5 weeks. Widening of the lateral ventricles and echogenic calcifications (C and arrows) in a case of cytomegalovirus infection.

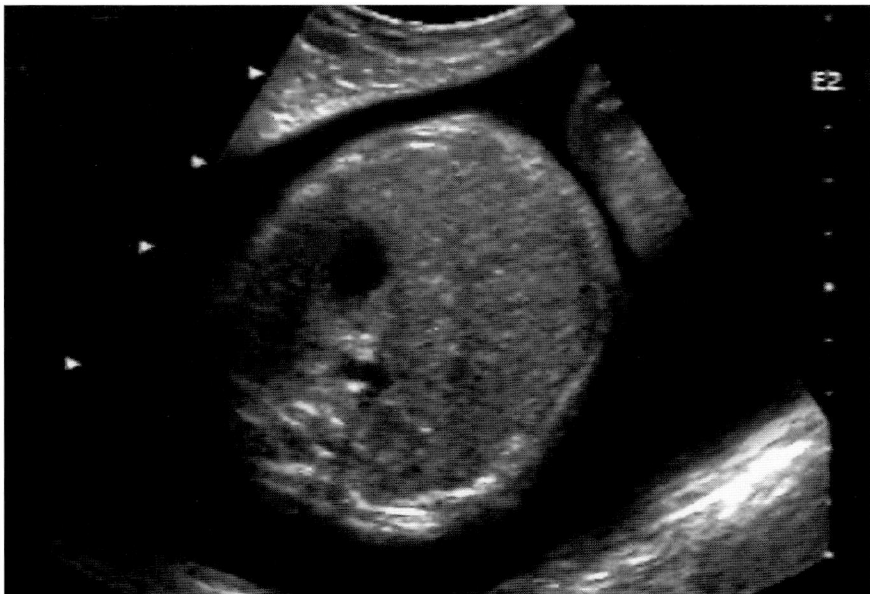

Fig. 13.**5** **Cytomegalovirus infection.** Cross-section of the fetal abdomen in the same fetus. The liver shows multiple calcifications.

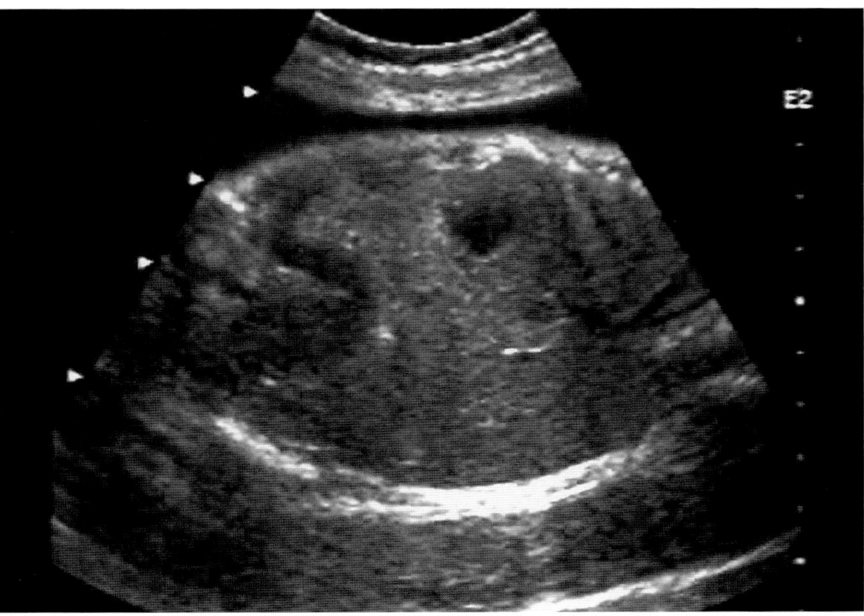

Fig. 13.**6** **Cytomegalovirus infection.** Same case, longitudinal section.

Miller H, Briese V. New methods for diagnosing infection in pregnancy. Zentralbl Gynäkol 1992; 114: 441–9.

Nigro G, La Torre R, Sali E, et al. Intraventricular haemorrhage in a fetus with cerebral cytomegalovirus infection. Prenat Diagn 2002; 22: 558–61.

Revello MG, Gerna G. Diagnosis and management of human cytomegalovirus infection in the mother, fetus, and newborn infant. Clin Microbiol Rev 2002; 15: 680–715.

Tomà P, Magnano GM, Mezzano P, Lazzini F, Bonacci W, Serra G. Cerebral ultrasound images in prenatal cytomegalovirus infection. Neuroradiology 1989; 31: 278–9.

Ville Y. The megalovirus [editorial]. Ultrasound Obstet Gynecol 1998; 12: 151–3.

Watt MM, Laifer SA, Hill LM. The natural history of fetal cytomegalovirus infection as assessed by serial ultrasound and fetal blood sampling: a case report. Prenat Diagn 1995; 15: 567–70.

Yaron Y, Hassan S, Geva E, Kupferminc MJ, Yavetz H, Evans MI. Evaluation of fetal echogenic bowel in the second trimester. Fetal Diagn Ther 1999; 14: 176–80.

14 Placenta, Cord, and Amniotic Fluid

Chorioangioma

Definition: Benign vascular tumors of the placenta, usually single, encapsulated and round-shaped tumors situated within the placenta.

Incidence: This is the most frequent placenta tumor, detected histologically in 1% of all placentas.

Clinical history/genetics: Sporadic occurrence.

Ultrasound findings: The fetus usually shows normal development. Rarely, fetal hydrops may result secondary to arteriovenous shunting within the tumor, which causes increased volume overload to the fetal heart. The earliest signs are hepatosplenomegaly and pericardial effusion. Pleural effusion, ascites, and skin edema may also result. Hydramnios is frequently present. Subsequent fetal anemia often leads to growth restriction. Chorioangioma can be detected as a vascular tumor within the placenta, located mostly near the insertion of the umbilical cord, and protruding into the amniotic cavity. Chorioangiomas causing hemodynamic complications are usually larger than 6 cm. They may even develop in the later stages of pregnancy.

Clinical management: Regular scans are recommended to detect the development of fetal hydrops and growth restriction as early as possible. Chorioangioma may even regress spontaneously during the course of pregnancy. The resulting hydramnios may lead to premature labor and delivery.

Procedure after birth: Unexpected neonatal anemia may be due to chorioangioma.

Prognosis: Most chorioangiomas do not have any pathophysiological relevance. Very rarely, vessel anastomosis within the tumor overload the fetal heart, causing fetal hydrops.

References

Bashiri A, Maymon E, Wiznitzer A, Maor E, Mazor M. Chorioangioma of the placenta in association with early severe polyhydramnios and elevated maternal serum HCG: a case report. Eur J Obstet Gynecol Reprod Biol 1998; 79: 103–5.

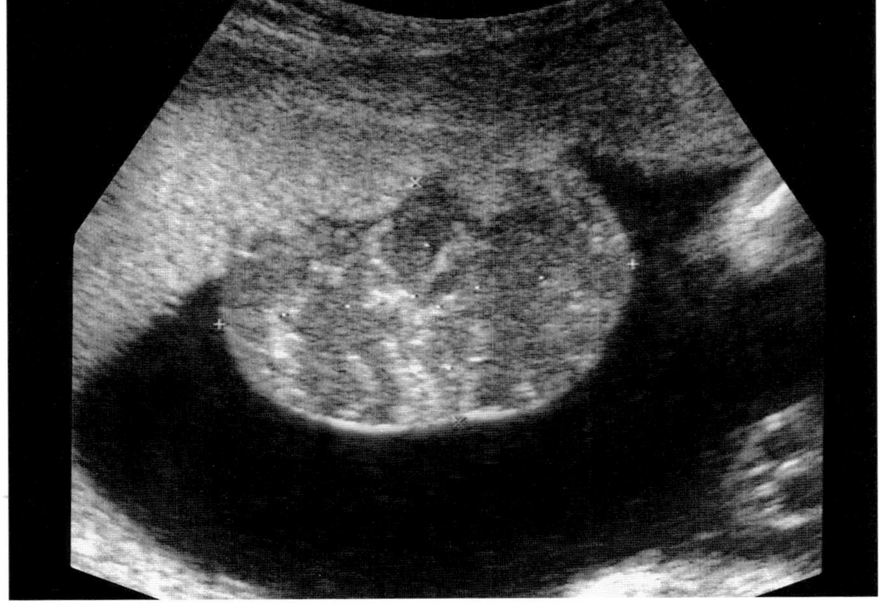

Fig. 14.1 **Chorioangioma.** A large chorioangioma on the surface of placenta at 30 weeks' gestation.

5

Bromley B, Benacerraf BR. Solid masses on the fetal surface of the placenta: differential diagnosis and clinical outcome. J Ultrasound Med 1994; 13: 883–6.
Cardwell MS. Antenatal management of a large placental chorioangioma: a case report. J Reprod Med 1988; 33: 68–70.
D'Ercole C, Cravello L, Boubli L, et al. Large chorioangioma associated with hydrops fetalis: prenatal diagnosis and management. Fetal Diagn Ther 1996; 11: 357–60.
Gitsch G, Deutinger J, Bernaschek G. Prenatal diagnosis of placental tumor using Doppler sonography. Geburtshilfe Frauenheilkd 1990; 50: 986–8.
Khong TY. Chorangioma with trophoblastic proliferation. Virchows Arch 2000; 436: 167–71.
Lampe S, Butterwegge M, Krech RH. Chorioangiomatosis of the placenta: diagnosis and obstetrical management. Zentralbl Gynäkol 1995; 117: 101–4.
Lopez HB, Kristoffersen SE. Chorioangioma of the placenta. Gynecol Obstet Invest 1989; 28: 108–10.
Noack F, Germer U, Gembruch U, Feller AC, Horny HP. [Uteroplacental insufficiency in chorangiomatosis; in German]. Zentralbl Gynäkol 2002; 124: 116–9.
Ogino S, Redline RW. Villous capillary lesions of the placenta: distinctions between chorangioma, chorangiomatosis, and chorangiosis. Hum Pathol 2000; 31: 945–54.
Reinhart RD, Wells WA, Harris RD. Focal aneurysmal dilatation of subchorionic vessels simulating chorioangioma. Ultrasound Obstet Gynecol 1999; 13: 147–9.

Hydramnios

Definition: Increased amount of amniotic fluid: amniotic fluid index (AFI) above 25 cm, or largest depot above 8 cm. At the due date, the amniotic fluid volume is more than 2 L.

Incidence: About 1 % of all pregnancies.

Clinical history/genetics: Diabetes mellitus.

Etiology: Fetal anomalies are responsible in up to 20% of cases: atresia of the esophagus, duodenal stenosis, jejunal stenosis, disturbance of swallowing reflex due to muscular or neural causes, displacement of the mediastinum as in CCAM or diaphragmatic hernia, some fetal syndromes (Pena–Shokeir syndrome, and rarely Neu–Laxova syndrome). It may also occur in association with fetal hydrops and congenital infections.

Ultrasound findings: Amniotic fluid index of above 25 cm, or the largest depot measuring above 8 cm. Development of hydramnios is rare prior to 24–25 weeks, even if fetal anomalies are present.

Clinical management: Detailed scan is mandatory. Maternal diabetes mellitus should be excluded. Search for infections (TORCH), possibly karyotyping. Therapeutic amniocentesis for aspiration of amniotic fluid is recommended to relieve maternal abdominal pressure and prevent premature delivery, if there is dyspnea or premature contractions, which affect cervical competence.

Prognosis: This depends on the causative factor. The perinatal mortality rate is increased due to premature birth and complications arising during labor (dystocia, umbilical cord prolapse).

References

Chitty LS, Goodman J, Seller MJ, Maxwell D. Esophageal and duodenal atresia in a fetus with Down's syndrome: prenatal sonographic features. Ultrasound Obstet Gynecol 1996; 7: 450–2.
Dashe JS, McIntire DD, Ramus RM, Santos-Ramos R, Twickler DM. Hydramnios: anomaly prevalence and sonographic detection. Obstet Gynecol 2002; 100: 134–9.
Hendricks SK, Conway L, Wang K, et al. Diagnosis of polyhydramnios in early gestation: indication for prenatal diagnosis? Prenat Diagn 1991; 11: 649–54.
Hill LM. Resolving polyhydramnios: a sign of improved fetal status. Am J Perinatol 1988; 5: 61–3.
Hill LM, Breckle R, Thomas ML, Fries JK. Polyhydramnios: ultrasonically detected prevalence and neonatal outcome. Obstet Gynecol 1987; 69: 21–5.
Linder R, Grumbrecht C, Soder A, Stosiek U, Maier WA. Abnormalities of the upper gastrointestinal tract diagnosed prenatally by ultrasound. Ultraschall Med 1984; 5: 148–51.
Myles TD, Santolaya-Forgas J. Normal ultrasonic evaluation of amniotic fluid in low-risk patients at term. J Reprod Med 2002; 47: 621–4.
Panting-Kemp A, Nguyen T, Castro L. Substance abuse and polyhydramnios. Am J Obstet Gynecol 2002; 187: 602–5.
Queisser-Luft A, Stolz G, Wiesel A, Schlaefer K, Spranger J. Malformations in newborn: results based on 30 940 infants and fetuses from the Mainz congenital birth defect monitoring system (1990–1998). Arch Gynecol Obstet 2002; 266: 163–7.
Quinlan RW, Cruz AC, Martin M. Hydramnios: ultrasound diagnosis and its impact on perinatal management and pregnancy outcome. Am J Obstet Gynecol 1983; 145: 306–11.
Shulman A, Mazkereth R, Zalel Y, et al. Prenatal identification of esophageal atresia: the role of ultrasonography for evaluation of functional anatomy. Prenat Diagn 2002; 22: 669–74.

Cysts of the Umbilical Cord

Definition: Cysts of the umbilical cord arising from the remains of the allantoic duct (urachus) or omphalomesenteric duct (vitelline duct).

Incidence: Rare.

Clinical history/genetics: Mostly sporadic occurrence, but may also be found in trisomy 18 and other chromosomal aberrations. Umbilical cord cysts are also associated with nonchromosomal anomalies.

Associated malformation: Omphalocele, urachal cysts.

Ultrasound findings: One or more echo-free cysts without a septum arising from the umbilical cord. They are mostly located at the fetal abdomen, near the insertion of the cord. Their size may vary from a few millimeters to 5 cm.

Clinical management: Karyotyping.

Prognosis: Isolated cysts have no clinical significance, but may be associated with fetal anoma-

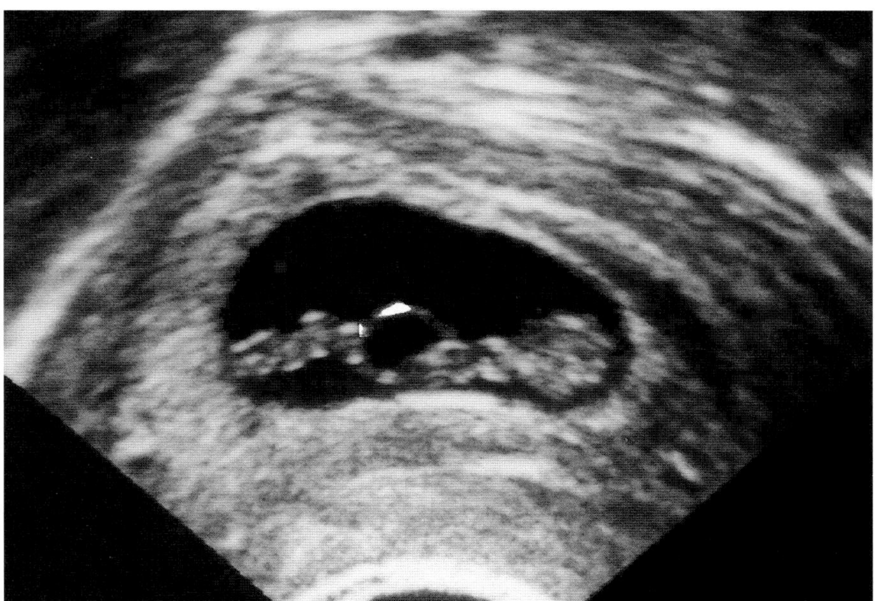

Fig. 14.2 **Umbilical cord cysts,** at 10 weeks' gestation.

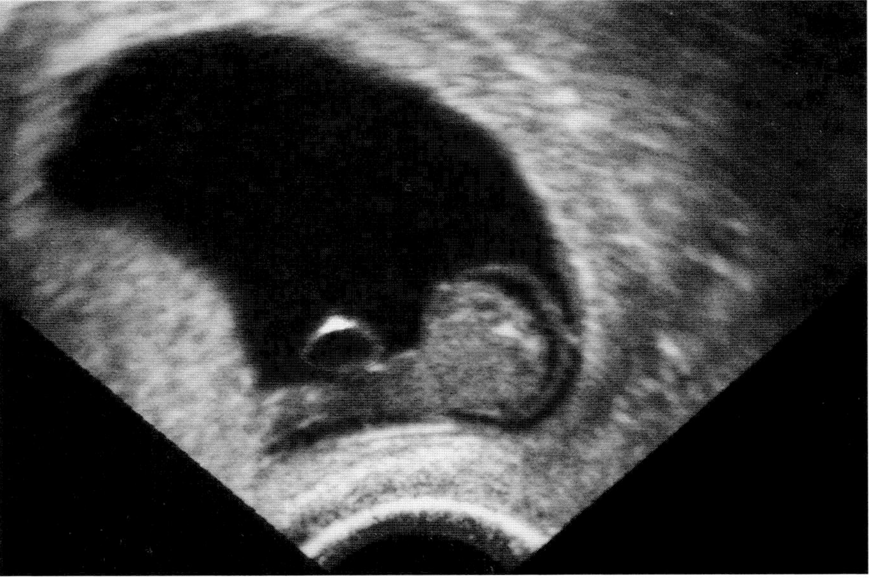

Fig. 14.3 **Umbilical cord cysts.** Early hydrops is also seen in a case of intrauterine death (missed abortion) at 11 weeks.

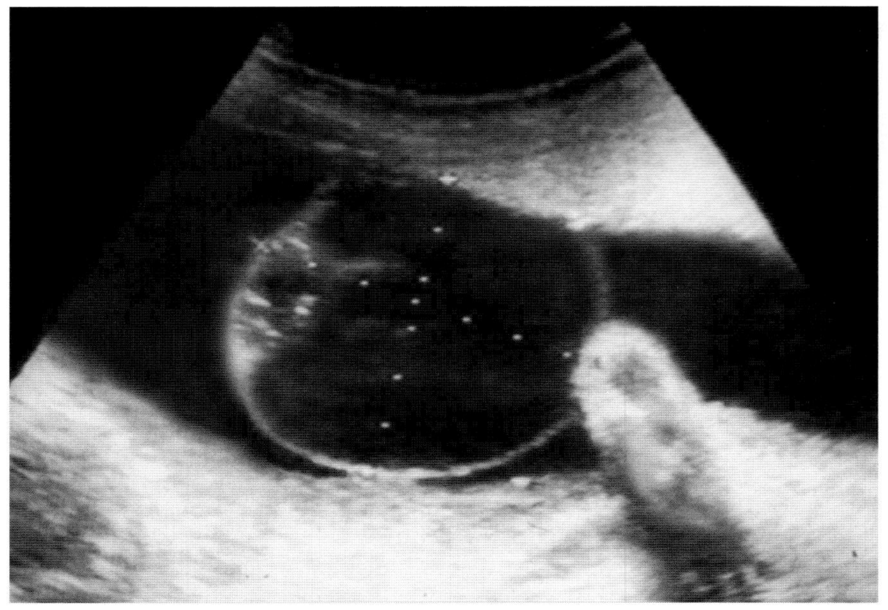

Fig. 14.**4** **Large umbilical cord cyst,** in a case of trisomy 18 at 31 weeks of gestation.

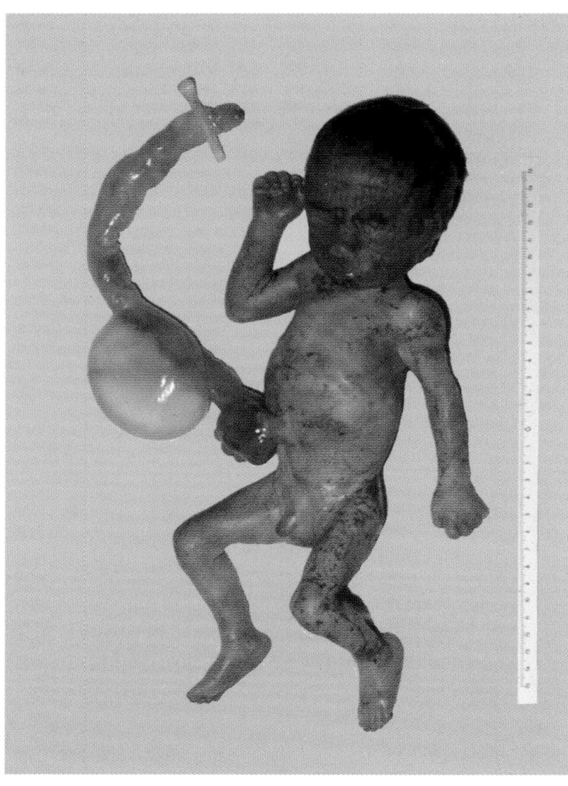

Fig. 14.**5** **Large umbilical cord cyst.** Trisomy 18. Findings after termination of the pregnancy.

lies and chromosomal aberrations, and thus may be an important clinical finding.

References

Babay ZA, Lange IR, Elliott PD, Hwang WS. A case of varix dilatation of the umbilical vein and review of the literature. Fetal Diagn Ther 1996; 11: 221–3.

Brown R, Nicolaides K. Umbilical cord hematoma associated with an umbilical cord cyst and fetal death at 28 weeks of gestation. J Ultrasound Med 2000; 19: 223–5.

Chen CP, Jan SW, Liu FF, et al. Prenatal diagnosis of omphalocele associated with umbilical cord cyst. Acta Obstet Gynecol Scand 1995; 74: 832–5.

Jacquemyn Y, Markov D, Beckstedde I. Umbilical cord cyst in a monochorionic twin pregnancy: an experiment of nature for the treatment of twin–twin transfusion syndrome. Fetal Diagn Ther 2002; 17: 233–5.

Kalter CS, Williams MC, Vaughn V, Spellacy WN. Sonographic diagnosis of a large umbilical cord pseudocyst. J Ultrasound Med 1994; 13: 487–9.

Kirkinen P, Jouppila P. Intrauterine membranous cyst: a report of antenatal diagnosis and obstetric aspects in two cases. Obstet Gynecol 1986; 67: 26 S– 30 S.

Rempen A. Sonographic first-trimester diagnosis of umbilical cord cyst. JCU J Clin Ultrasound 1989; 17: 53–5.

Sepulveda W, Bower S, Dhillon HK, Fisk NM. Prenatal diagnosis of congenital patent urachus and allantoic cyst: the value of color flow imaging. J Ultrasound Med 1995; 14: 47–51.

Sepulveda W, Gutierrez J, Sanchez J, Be C, Schnapp C. Pseudocyst of the umbilical cord: prenatal sonographic appearance and clinical significance. Obstet Gynecol 1999; 93: 377–81.

Stella A, Babbo GL. Omphalocele and umbilical cord cyst: prenatal diagnosis [review]. Minerva Ginecol 2000; 52: 213–6.

Tennstedt C, Chaoui R, Bollmann R, Dietel M. Angiomyxoma of the umbilical cord in one twin with cystic degeneration of Wharton's jelly: a case report. Pathol Res Pract 1998; 194: 55–8.

Oligohydramnios

Definition: Decrease in the volume of amniotic fluid; oligohydramnios is diagnosed if the diameter of the largest amniotic fluid depot is below 2 cm, or if the amniotic fluid index lies below 5.1 cm. The amniotic fluid index (AFI) is defined as the sum of the largest vertical diameters of the amniotic fluid depots measured in all four quadrants of the uterus. The normal average volume of the amniotic fluid at 16 weeks of gestation is 250 mL; it increases to 800 mL at 28 weeks and further to 1000 mL at 38 weeks, decreasing slightly to 800 mL at 40 weeks.

Incidence: Oligohydramnios is diagnosed in 0.5–4.0% of all pregnancies, depending on how it is defined.

Teratogen: Indomethacin.

Etiology: Reduced urine production, premature rupture of the membranes.

Ultrasound findings: The reduced amount of amniotic fluid makes ultrasound examination difficult. Renal diseases, such as bilateral renal agenesis, cystic anomalies of the kidneys, dysplasia, and obstructive uropathy may be causative factors. In addition, severe growth restriction and premature rupture of the membranes may also be considered. Oligohydramnios over a long period of time causes club feet and other anomalies.

Clinical management: Amnioinfusion is carried out in severe cases to allow sonographic diagnosis of fetal anomalies and to exclude rupture of the membranes. In the later stages of the second trimester and in the third trimester, Doppler flow imaging of the fetal and maternal vessels is used to detect signs of placental insufficiency.

Prognosis: This is favorable if oligohydramnios develops late in pregnancy. Detection of oligohydramnios in the first trimester or early second trimester is a bad sign and is an indication of severe underlying anomalies. In these cases, the prognosis is poor due to pulmonary hypoplasia secondary to oligohydramnios.

References

Bastide A, Manning F, Harman C, Lange I, Morrison I. Ultrasound evaluation of amniotic fluid: outcome of pregnancies with severe oligohydramnios. Am J Obstet Gynecol 1986; 154: 895–900.

Fisk NM, Ronderos DD, Soliani A, Nicolini U, Vaughan J, Rodeck CH. Diagnostic and therapeutic transabdominal amnioinfusion in oligohydramnios. Obstet Gynecol 1991; 78: 270–8.

Ghosh G, Marsal K, Gudmundsson S. Amniotic fluid index in low-risk pregnancy as an admission test to the labor ward. Acta Obstet Gynecol Scand 2002; 81: 852–5.

Kassanos D, Christodoulou CN, Agapitos E, Pavlopoulos PM, Pagalos N. Prenatal ultrasonographic detection of the tracheal atresia sequence. Ultrasound Obstet Gynecol 1997; 10: 133–6.

Kilbride HW, Thibeault DW. Strategies of cardiovascular and ventilatory management in preterm infants with prolonged rupture of fetal membranes and oligohydramnios. J Perinatol 2002; 22: 510.

Mandsager NT, Bendon R, Mostello D, Rosenn B, Miodovnik M, Siddiqi TA. Maternal floor infarction of the placenta: prenatal diagnosis and clinical significance. Obstet Gynecol 1994; 83: 750–4.

Poulain P, Odent S, Maire I, et al. Fetal ascites and oligohydramnios: prenatal diagnosis of a sialic acid storage disease (index case). Prenat Diagn 1995; 15: 864–7.

Queisser-Luft A, Stolz G, Wiesel A, Schlaefer K, Spranger J. Malformations in newborn: results based on 30,940 infants and fetuses from the Mainz congenital birth defect monitoring system (1990–1998). Arch Gynecol Obstet 2002; 266: 163–7.

Sherer DM. A review of amniotic fluid dynamics and the enigma of isolated oligohydramnios [review]. Am J Perinatol 2002; 19: 253–66.

Shipp TD, Bromley B, Pauker S, Frigoletto FDJ, Benacerraf BR. Outcome of singleton pregnancies with severe oligohydramnios in the second and third trimesters. Ultrasound Obstet Gynecol 1996; 7: 108–13.

Stiller RJ, Pinto M, Heller C, Hobbins JC. Oligohydramnios associated with bilateral multicystic dysplastic kidneys: prenatal diagnosis at 15 weeks' gestation. JCU J Clin Ultrasound 1988; 16: 436–9.

Swinford AE, Bernstein J, Toriello HV, Higgins JV. Renal tubular dysgenesis: delayed onset of oligohydramnios. Am J Med Genet 1989; 32: 127–32.

Takeuchi K, Moriyama T, Funakoshi T, Maruo T. Prenatal diagnosis of fetal urogenital abnormalities with oligohydramnios by magnetic resonance imaging using turbo spin echo technique. J Perinat Med 1998; 26: 59–61.

Williams K, Wittmann BK, Dansereau J. Correlation of subjective assessment of amniotic fluid with amniotic fluid index. Eur J Obstet Gynecol Reprod Biol 1992; 46: 1–5.

Yaron Y, Heifetz S, Ochshorn Y, Lehavi O, Orr-Urtreger A. Decreased first trimester PAPP-A is a predictor of adverse pregnancy outcome. Prenat Diagn 2002; 22: 778–82.

Zimmer EZ, Divon MY. Sonographic diagnosis of IUGR-macrosomia. Clin Obstet Gynecol 1992; 35: 172–84.

15 Multiple Pregnancy

Determination of Zygosity

Perinatal mortality is still three times higher in twin gestations than in singleton pregnancies. The reason for this appears to be a considerably higher incidence of premature birth, placental insufficiency, and congenital malformations in twins than in singleton pregnancies. According to the *Hellin rule,* the frequency of twin pregnancies is one in 85 pregnancies, that of triplets one in 85^2, and that of quadruplets one in 85^3. These data apply to Caucasian populations. The frequency of twin pregnancies varies considerably in relation to geography and ethnic origin. In Japan, there is one twin pregnancy to 155 singletons, about half of that expected in Caucasians. By contrast, there are regions of Nigeria in which one twin pregnancy occurs for 25 singletons—about three times higher than the rate predicted by Hellin.

It is important to differentiate between dizygotic and monozygotic twins, as risks in pregnancy differ accordingly. Two-thirds of multiple pregnancies are dizygotic and one-third are monozygotic. The geographical variation in the rate of twins is due only to the differing frequency of dizygotic twins; the incidence of monozygotic twins remains constant throughout the world, at one in 250 pregnancies.

This natural incidence of twin pregnancies has dramatically changed in recent years due to advances in fertility therapies. Twin pregnancies and multiple gestations are seen more frequently today due to follicle stimulation, ovulation treatments, and artificial insemination therapies. This primarily affects dizygotic twins. *Monozygotic pregnancies* arise from a single fertilized ovum that splits at various times during the first 2 weeks of embryogenesis. Depending on the stage of embryogenesis at which the zygote splits, four types of identical twins can result:

1. Dichorionic, diamniotic twins result from the division of the zygote within the first 3 days after fertilization. Each fetus has its own placenta and is surrounded by two layers—the chorion and amnion—and is thus separated from the other fetus by four layers. In the prenatal stage, these twins can not be differentiated from dizygotic twins if they are of the same sex. This applies to about 30% of monozygotic twin pregnancies.

2. Cellular division occurring between 3 and 8 days after fertilization results in monochorionic, diamniotic twins. Although there are two amniotic cavities, the placenta is shared by the two fetuses. The twins are separated by only two layers—the amnions of each twin. This constellation is present in about 70% of monozygotic twin pregnancies.

3. Monochorionic, monoamniotic twins occur with division between the 8th and 13th day after fertilization. The twins are not separated by membranes. This pattern constitutes about 1% of monozygotic pregnancies. It is associated with a high rate of intrauterine mortality of almost 50%, resulting from umbilical cord complications.

4. Conjoined twins are caused by incomplete division of the embryonic disk after day 13. The incidence is one in 70 000 completed pregnancies.

In monochorionic diamniotic twins (which always arise from a single ovum), there is a special risk that has to be considered, that of *twin-to-twin transfusion syndrome (TTTS).* Blood is transfused from one twin (donor) to the other (recipient), due to vascular shunts within the joined placenta. Three forms of vascular shunt have been described: connections between two arteries (arterioarterial), between two veins (venovenous), and between one artery and one vein (arteriovenous). Although these vessel anastomoses are present in 85% of monochorionic pregnancies, clinical manifestation of twin–twin transfusion syndrome occurs only in 10–15% of cases. This means that blood transfusion between twins is a common phenomenon and not an exception. *Chronic twin-to-twin transfusion syndrome* is found only when there is an imbalance of transfusion from one twin to the other; arteriovenous shunts are responsible for this. In addition to this chronic TTTS, there is also an *acute twin–twin transfusion* syndrome arising during birth in monochorionic twins. This may have fatal consequences, leading to the death of one or both twins.

The *chronic twin-to-twin transfusion syndrome*, if untreated, results in high morbidity and mortality rates. The mortality can be as high as 90%, and diagnosis and management of this syndrome is therefore a challenge to modern prenatal and pediatric medicine. The morbidity associated with chronic TTTS is also high; one-third of the affected children show neurological damage at a later age.

The *characteristic clinical features* of chronic TTTS are: 1, disparity in fetal size, the recipient being larger than the donor; and 2, the amount of amniotic fluid differs considerably between the two amniotic cavities.

In the second half of pregnancy, fetal urine production is mainly responsible for the formation of amniotic fluid. In TTTS, the *donor twin* has a lower blood volume and fluid load compared to the *recipient twin*. Thus, there is a reduction or complete absence of diuresis, leading to oligohydramnios or in severe cases to anhydramnios. In contrast to this, due to a higher volume load in the *recipient twin*, there is increased diuresis and thus development of hydramnios.

In addition, fetal hydrops develops in the *recipient twin* due to cardiac overload, causing ascites, skin edema, pleural effusion and pericardial effusion. In contrast to this, it is often difficult to detect the urinary bladder of the *donor twin*, due to the absence of diuresis.

It is important to differentiate TTTS from *placental insufficiency* in one of the twins. This also results in disparity of fetal size; the affected twin is smaller, and there may be oligohydramnios. However, the larger twin, does not show hydramnios, as long as other causative factors for the development of it are absent.

To calculate the risk of developing TTTS, it is of the utmost importance to know whether the twin pregnancy is monochorionic or dichorionic. TTTS is virtually unique to monochorionic twin gestations and almost never occurs in dichorionic gestations.

Early ultrasound examination in the first trimester provides the best opportunity to identify zygosity antenatally. This scan is included in routine antenatal screening in Germany. At this gestational age, the chorion is thick and surrounds the amniotic cavity completely, while the amnion is a very thin layer. The layer separating the two cavities is easily recognizable in dichorionic pregnancies, as it is at least 2–3 mm thick. In monochorionic gestations, this layer is detected as a very thin rim consisting of the two amnion membranes. After the first trimester, it is not easy to distinguish between the two forms of pregnancy, as the chorionic layer degenerates and does not appear as thick as in early pregnancy, so that even in dichorionic gestations the separation barely differs from that in monochorionic twins. At this stage of pregnancy, a search has to be made for the lambda sign (a lambda-shaped connection between the fetal membranes and placenta). However, the diagnosis cannot be made with certainty.

Monochorionic gestation can be diagnosed easily in the first part of the pregnancy; this is a spot diagnosis and can be detected even by less experienced sonographers if basic principles are followed. This means that it is possible to assess or exclude a risk of developing TTTS at an early stage.

The prognosis in TTTS is mostly very poor, and there are no standard treatment protocols. Premature delivery is opted for if the gestational age is adequate. After 28 weeks of gestation, this is almost always the preferred choice of treatment. For gestations below 28 weeks, *four different therapeutic interventions* are possible:

1. Repeated aspiration of amniotic fluid from the *recipient twin* every few days, to relieve the polyhydramnios. This reduces the risk of premature labor and/or intrauterine death and also improves placental perfusion by decreasing uterine pressure. This procedure makes it possible to reduce TTTS mortality by 50%. However, one-third of the survivors will still suffer late neurological damage.

2. Administration of digitalis to the mother and thus indirectly through the placenta to the fetus. The aim of this treatment is to prevent and treat cardiac failure in the *recipient twin*, which is struggling to cope with the volume overload.

3. As a last resort, selective fetocide of one twin, usually the donor, has also been tried, to improve the chances of survival of the second twin.

4. Endoscopic laser ablation of vascular shunts is now the most important treatment option, if available. In recent years, this method has been used in the treatment of severe TTTS. Its main disadvantage is the high rate of fetal demise, up to 50%. However, recent studies show that if successfully applied, late neurological complications occur in only 5% of surviving infants.

It is possible to differentiate very early in pregnancy between a high-risk monochorionic pregnancy and low-risk dichorionic twin gestation. Monochorionic pregnancies should be monitored with serial ultrasound assessments at short intervals.

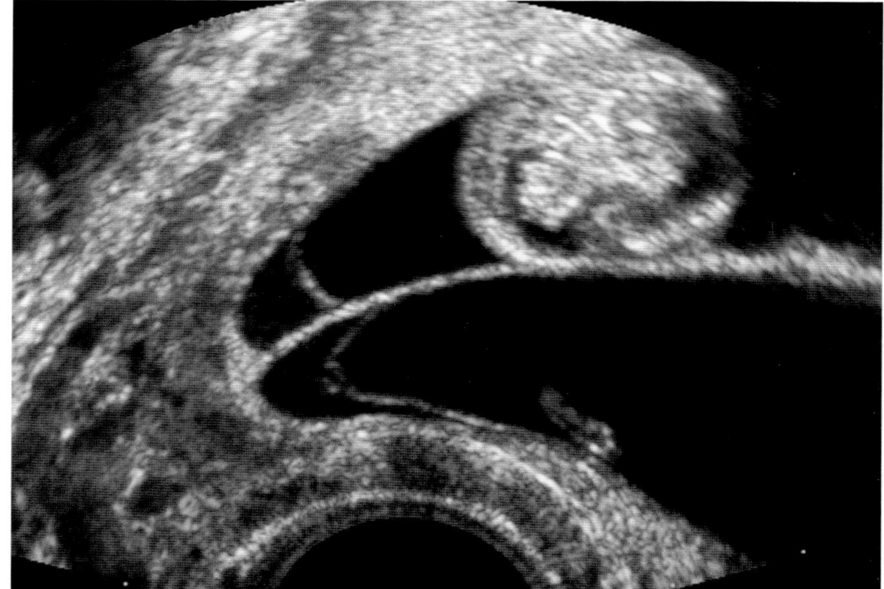

Fig. 15.**1** **Twins.** Vaginal scan demonstrating the "lambda sign" in diamniotic dichorionic twins at 12 + 1 weeks. There is a thick membrane (chorion) separating the two amniotic cavities; thin layers of amnion are also seen.

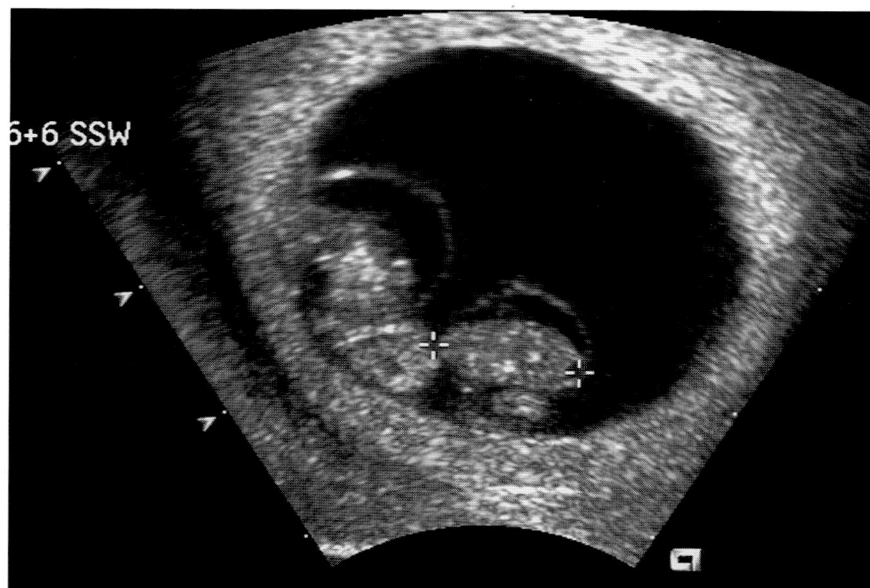

Fig. 15.**2** **Twins.** Vaginal scan at 6 + 6 weeks of gestation in diamniotic monochorionic (and thus monozygotic) twins.

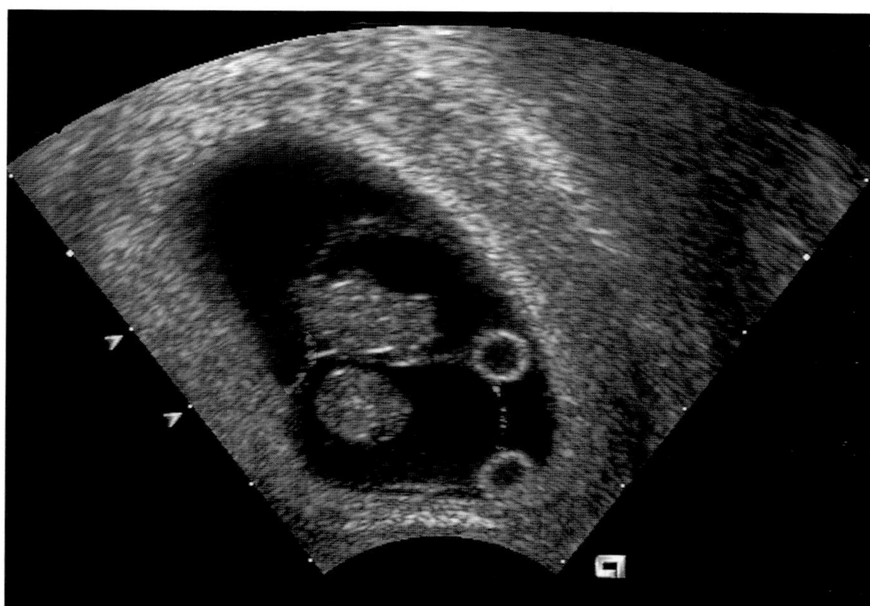

Fig. 15.**3** **Twins.** Monochorionic diamniotic (monozygotic) twins at 7 + 6 weeks, demonstrating the amnion and both yolk sacs.

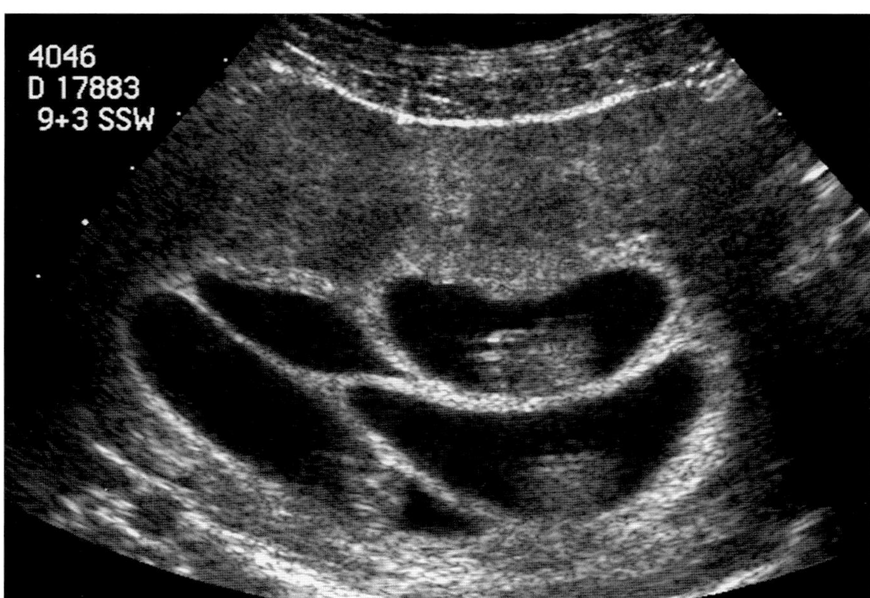

Fig. 15.4 **Quadruplets.** Tetra-amniotic, tetrachorionic quadruplets at 9 + 3 weeks.

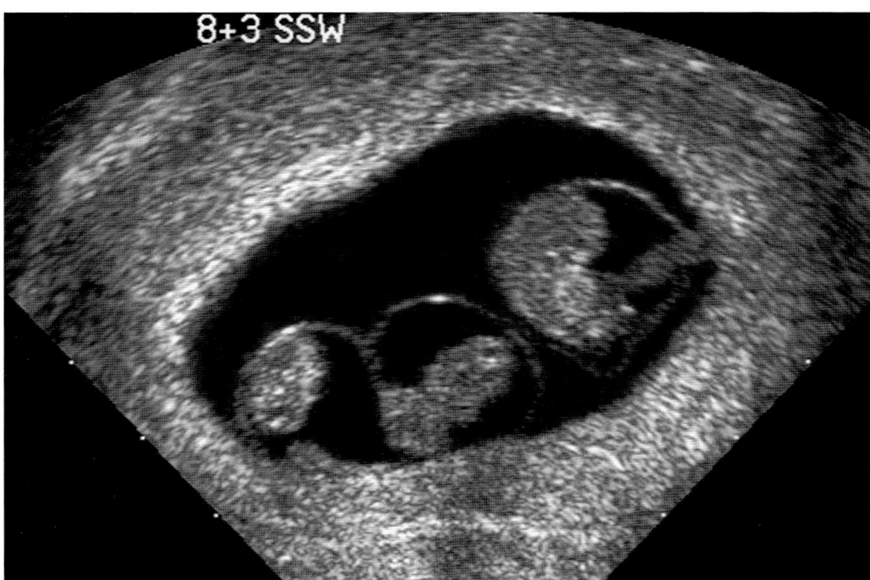

Fig. 15.5 **Triplets.** Triamniotic, monochorionic triplets at 8 + 3 weeks. There is a thin membrane (only amnion, with no chorion) separating the amniotic cavities.

Measurement of nuchal translucency at 13 weeks also allows risk evaluation of TTTS. In early TTTS, fluid accumulation in the recipient twin causes nuchal edema, and nuchal translucency measurements are significantly higher than in the donor twin. If there is no significant difference in nuchal translucency measurements between the two twins, then the risk of developing TTTS is assumed to be low.

From 16 weeks onwards, regular ultrasound assessment of fetal growth and amniotic fluid volume is necessary. Early warning signs of TTTS development can be detected in this way, and various therapy options can then be considered. It may even be necessary to hospitalize the mother.

To improve the prognosis of TTTS, continuous assessment during the whole of the pregnancy is advisable. The complications foreseen can be discussed with a pediatrician to ensure the best clinical management for the twins in this very precarious situation.

In summary, ultrasound examination in early pregnancy is a simple and reliable method of detecting zygosity and thus whether there is a high-risk pregnancy—allowing for risk-adjusted antenatal management of twin pregnancies.

Self-Help Organizations

Title: National Organization of Mothers of Twins Clubs

Description: Opportunity for mothers of multiple births share information, concerns, and advice on dealing with their unique problems and joys. Literature, quarterly newspaper,

5

group development guidelines, quarterly newsletter, bereavement support, pen-pal program. Membership through local clubs.

Scope: National

Number of groups: 475 clubs

Founded: 1960

Address: P.O. Box 438, Thompson Station, TN 37179–0438, United States

Telephone: 1–877–540–2200 (referrals only) or 615–595–0936

E-mail: nomotc@aol.com

Web: http://www.nomotc.org/

Title: Triplet Connection

Description: Network of caring and sharing for families of multiple birth. The emphasis is on providing quality information regarding pregnancy management and preterm birth prevention for high-risk multiple pregnancies. Expectant parents' package, quarterly newsletter, phone support, and resources.

Scope: International

Founded: 1982

Address: P.O. Box 99571, Stockton, CA 95209, United States

Telephone: 209–474–0885

Fax: 209–474–2233

E-mail: tc@tripletconnection.org

Web: http://www.tripletconnection.org

Title: MOST (Mothers of Super Twins)

Description: Support network of families who are expecting, or are already the parents of, triplets or more. Provides information, support, resources, and empathy during pregnancy, infancy, toddlerhood, and school age. Magazine, networking, phone and online support, catalogue. Specific resource persons for individual challenges. Help in starting groups.

Scope: National

Number of groups: 50 + affiliated groups

Founded: 1987

Address: P.O. Box 951, Brentwood, NY 11717–0627, United States

Telephone: 631–859–1110

Fax: 631–859–3580

E-mail: mostmom@nyc.pipeline.com

Web: http://www.MOSTonline.org

Conjoined Twins

Definition: Incomplete separation of monozygotic twins; in 70% of cases, the thoracic region is affected (thoracopagus).

Incidence: One in 70 000 births; one in 300 monozygotic twin pregnancies.

Sex ratio: M < F.

Embryology: Incomplete division of the embryonic disk at a later developmental stage of the blastocyte (at least 13 days after fertilization) in a monozygotic twin pregnancy.

Ultrasound findings: Conjoined twins are always associated with monochorionic, monozygotic twin pregnancies. The fetuses lie in the immediate proximity of one another and are unable to move away from each other. They may be joined at the head (craniopagus, less than 2%), at the hips (ischiopagus, 5%), at the thorax (thoracopagus, 70%), or at various other body parts. *Dicephalus* is a special form of conjoined twins: one body and two heads. Hydramnios is frequently present.

Clinical management: Further ultrasound screening, including fetal echocardiography. Pediatricians and pediatric surgeons should be consulted regarding the prognosis. Serial ultrasound scans are advised for detection of fetal hydrops and monitoring of growth. Intrauterine fetal death occurs in 30% of cases. If the mother decides to continue with the pregnancy, primary

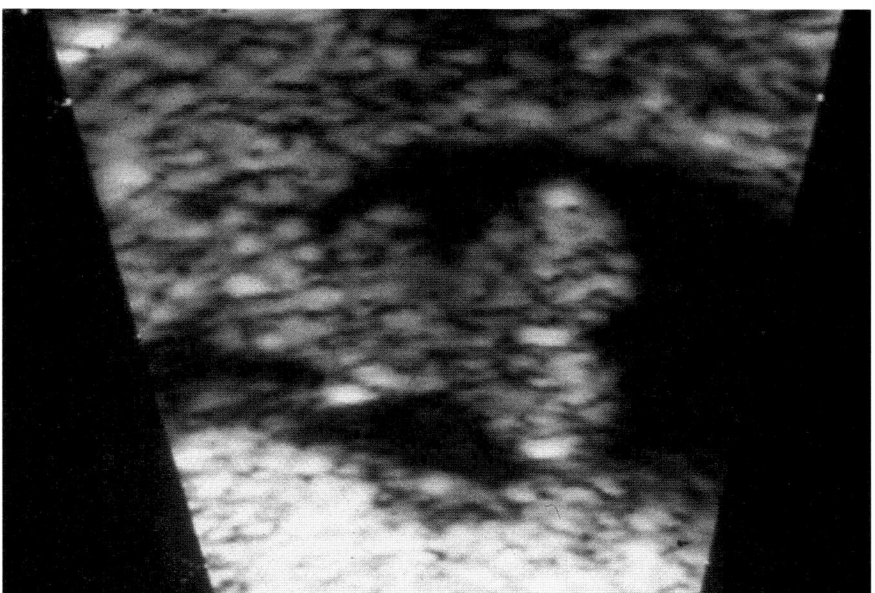

Fig. 15.6 **Conjoined twins.** Vaginal scan of dicephalus twin pregnancy at 10 + 1 weeks.

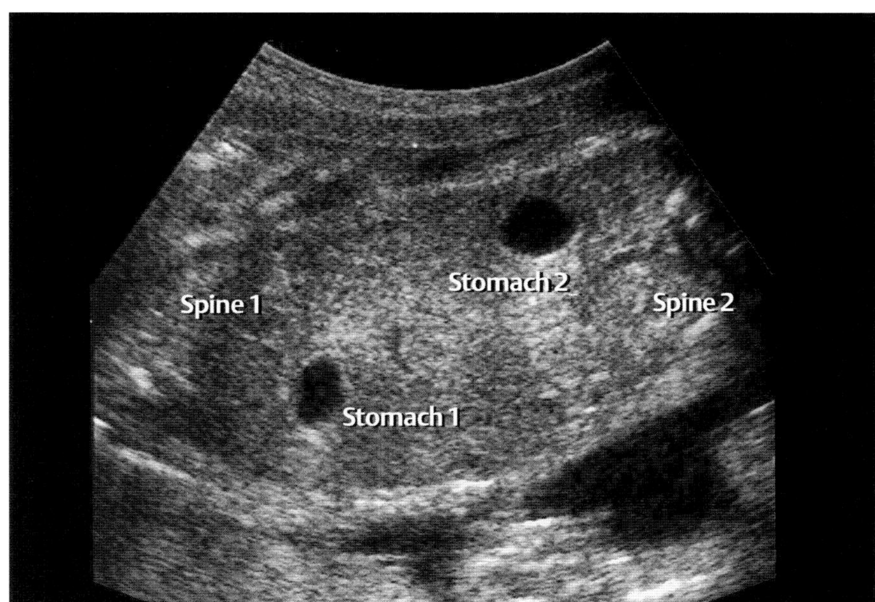

Fig. 15.7 **Conjoined twins.** Cross-section through a fetal double thorax in a thoracopagus twin pregnancy at 24 + 2 weeks.

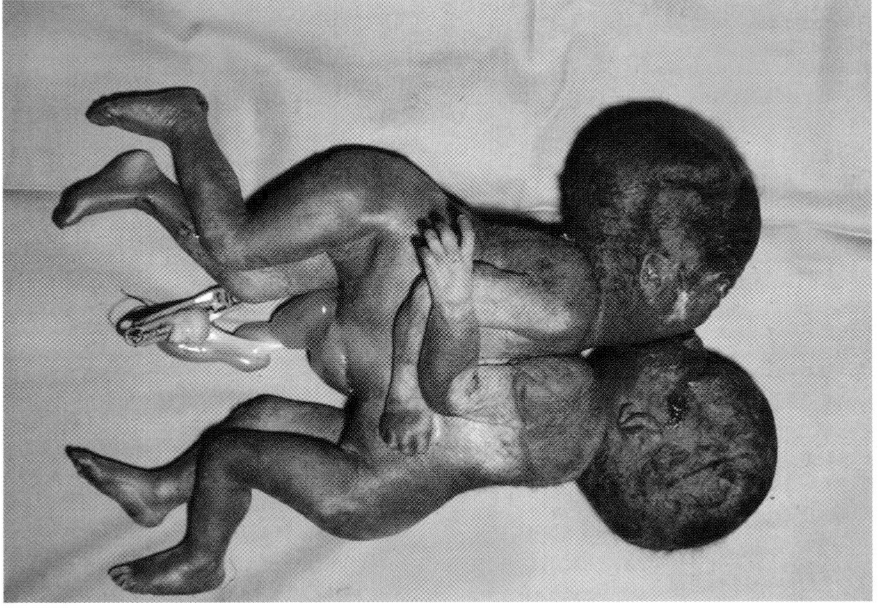

Fig. 15.8 **Conjoined twins.** Thoracopagus: findings after birth at 27 weeks of gestation.

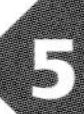

cesarean section is indicated for the benefit of both the mother and the twins.

Procedure after birth: Immediate care of the neonates can prove to be extremely difficult, especially if respiratory distress is present. Cardiac massage is impossible in thoracopagus twins. Surgical intervention is more successful if there is sufficient time for optimal preparation and if it can be performed at a much later stage, rather than in the immediate neonatal period. The main aim of the operation is to separate the twins.

Prognosis: This depends on the location and length of fusion. The prognosis also depends on the presence of vital organs such as the liver and heart in both twins. If surgical separation is absolutely necessary in the first 3 weeks after birth, there is a high mortality rate of almost 50%. Surgical separation performed between 4 and 14 weeks after birth has a 90% survival rate.

Self-Help Organization

Title: Conjoined Twins International

Description: Support for conjoined twins, their families, and professionals. Offers peer support, professional counseling, crisis intervention, telephone helpline, pen-pal network, videos. Information and referrals. Peer counseling speakers bureau. Registry of affected families. Quarterly newsletter. Membership directory.

Scope: International network

Founded: 1996

Address: P.O. Box 10 895, Prescott, AZ 86 304–0895, United States

Telephone: 520–445–2777

References

Barth RA, Filly RA, Goldberg JD, Moore P, Silverman NH. Conjoined twins: prenatal diagnosis and assessment of associated malformations [published erratum appears in Radiology 1991; 178: 287]. Radiology 1990; 177: 201–7.
Cazeneuve C, Nihoul FEC, Adafer M, et al. Conjoined omphalopagous twins separated at fifteen days of age. Arch Pediatr 1995; 2: 452–5.
Chatterjee MS, Weiss RR, Verma UL, Tejani NA, Macri J. Prenatal diagnosis of conjoined twins. Prenat Diagn 1983; 3: 357–61.
De Ugarte DA, Boechat MI, Shaw WW, Laks H, Williams H, Atkinson JB. Parasitic omphalopagus complicated by omphalocele and congenital heart disease. J Pediatr Surg 2002; 37: 1357–8.
Hubinont C, Kollmann P, Malvaux V, Donnez J, Bernard P. First-trimester diagnosis of conjoined twins. Fetal Diagn Ther 1997; 12: 185–7.
Intödy Z, Pálffy I, Hajdu K, Hajdu Z, Török M, Laszlo J. Prenatal diagnosis of thoracopagus in the 19th week of pregnancy. Zentralbl Gynäkol 1986; 108: 57–61.
Karsdorp VH, van den Linden JC, Sobotka PM, Prins H, van den Harten JJ, van VugtJM. Ultrasonographic prenatal diagnosis of conjoined thoracopagus twins: a case report. Eur J Obstet Gynecol Reprod Biol 1991; 39: 157–61.
Skupski DW, Streltzoff J, Hutson JM, Rosenwaks Z, Cohen J, Chervenak FA. Early diagnosis of conjoined twins in triplet pregnancy after in vitro fertilization and assisted hatching. J Ultrasound Med 1995; 14: 611–5.
Spitz L, Kiely EM. Experience in the management of conjoined twins. Br J Surg 2002; 89: 1188–92.
Weingast GR, Johnson ML, Pretorius DH, et al. Difficulty in sonographic diagnosis of cephalothoracopagus. Ultrasound Med 1984; 3: 42–3.
Wenzl R, Schurz B, Amann G, Eppel W, Schon HJ, Reinolc E. Diagnosis of cephalothoracopagus: a case report. Ultraschall Med 1992; 13: 199–201.

Twin Reversed Arterial Perfusion (TRAP sequence)

Definition: This is a complex malformation arising exclusively in monochorionic twins. In this case, a rudimentary twin, without head (acranius) or heart (acardius), is being provided by the healthy second twin.

Incidence: One in 35 000 births; about one in 150 monozygotic twins.

Laboratory parameters: Alpha fetoprotein is elevated in serum and in amniotic fluid. Acetylcholinesterase test results are positive in amniotic fluid.

Embryology: This probably arises due to vessel anastomoses between monozygotic twins within the placenta. The communicating vessels may lead to reverse perfusion in one twin. The perfused twin receives blood with a lower oxygen content. The resulting hypoxia is responsible for aplasia or hypoplasia of the heart, head, and upper extremities. The twin providing the blood supply is usually healthy. However, cardiac failure and hydrops may develop in this twin, leading to intrauterine fetal death.

Ultrasound findings: A *second twin* is found in addition to a normal fetus (the providing or "pump twin"), in which a *heart or a heart beat* cannot be demonstrated. The recipient is usually *hydropic*, and has a pulse identical to that of the "pump twin." In the affected twin, the head or brain are usually absent (*acranius* or *anencephaly*). Occasionally, the upper extremities are also missing. *Club feet* are frequently detected. Despite the absence of head and heart, the recipient fetus demonstrates movements. Signs of *cardiac failure or fetal hydrops* may develop in the "pump twin" (hepatosplenomegaly, pleural and pericardial effusion, skin edema, cardiomegaly, enlargement of the right atrium). Hydramnios is a frequent finding. Oligohydramnios or anhydramnios is found in the recipient. The recipient fetus also has a singular umbilical artery in 50% of cases. *Color-coded Doppler imaging* of the umbilical artery near the bladder is the best method of demonstrating reversed blood flow in the recipient fetus.

Clinical management: There is a high risk of premature labor due to hydramnios. Serial scanning

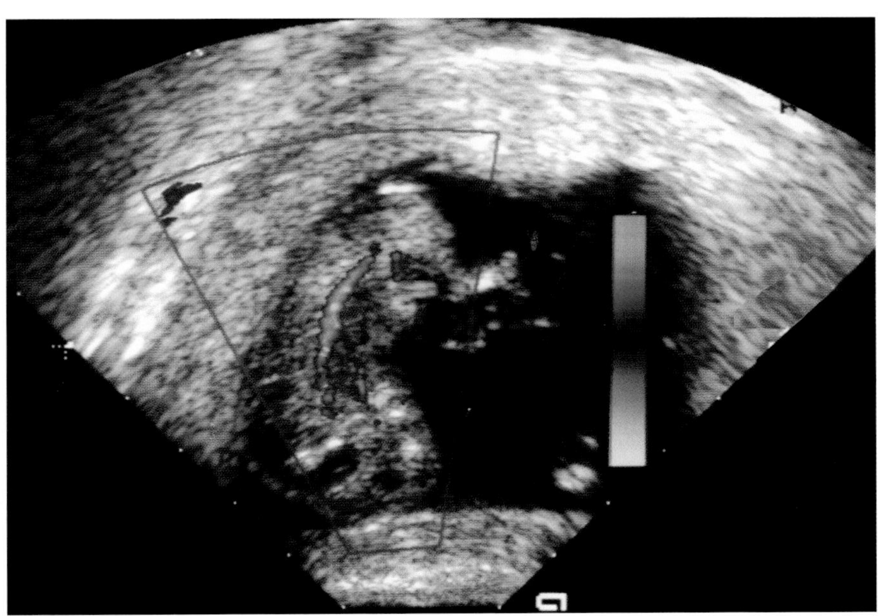

Fig. 15.**9** **Twin reversed arterial perfusion (TRAP sequence).** The recipient in TRAP sequence at 11 + 6 weeks. Color-coded Doppler scanning demonstrates the direction of blood flow from the lower body parts to the thorax and head.

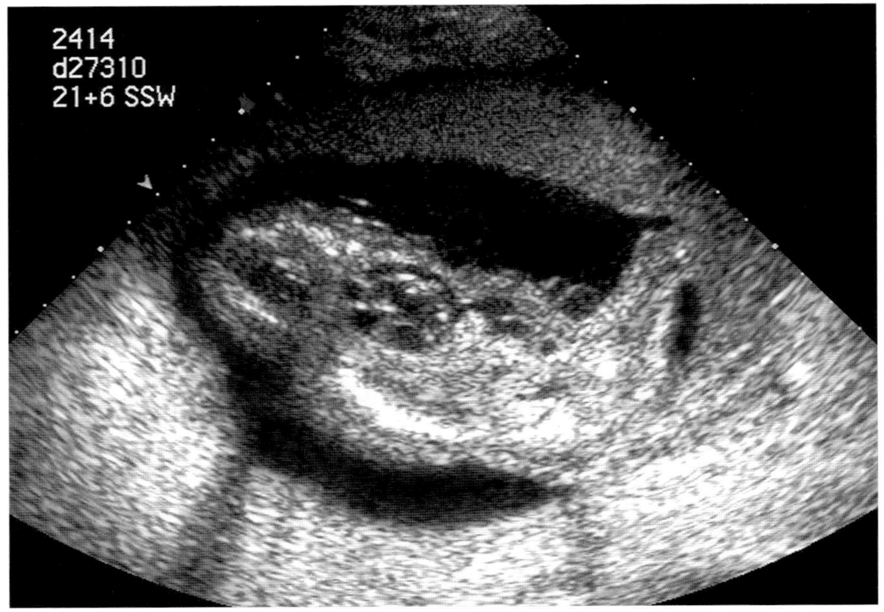

Fig. 15.**10** **Twin reversed arterial perfusion (TRAP sequence).** The recipient in TRAP sequence at 21 + 6 weeks. The fetal head is small and severely deformed. In this case, in addition to reverse perfusion, bradycardia was detected in the recipient ("acranius cardius").

5

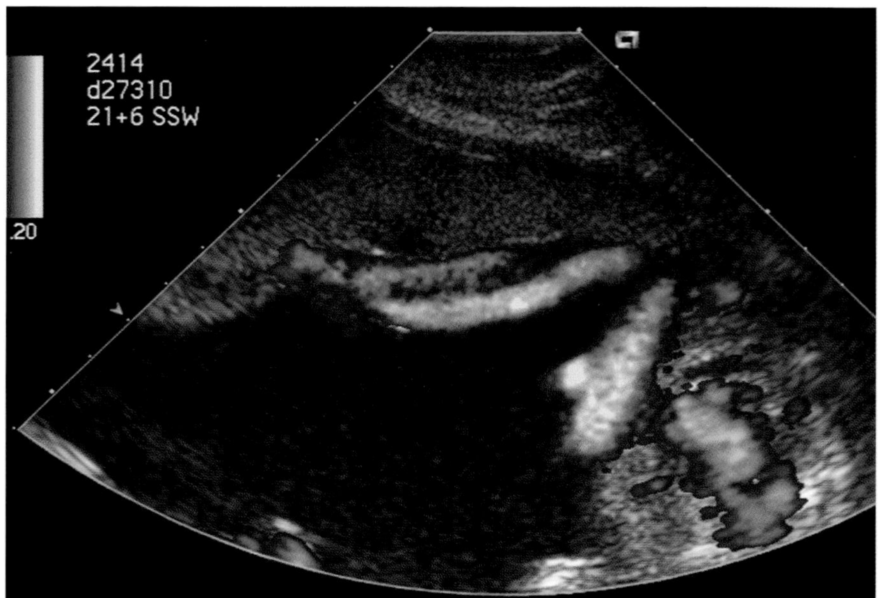

Fig. 15.**11** **Twin reversed arterial perfusion (TRAP sequence).** This demonstrates the site of communication of the two fetal circulations on the placental surface.

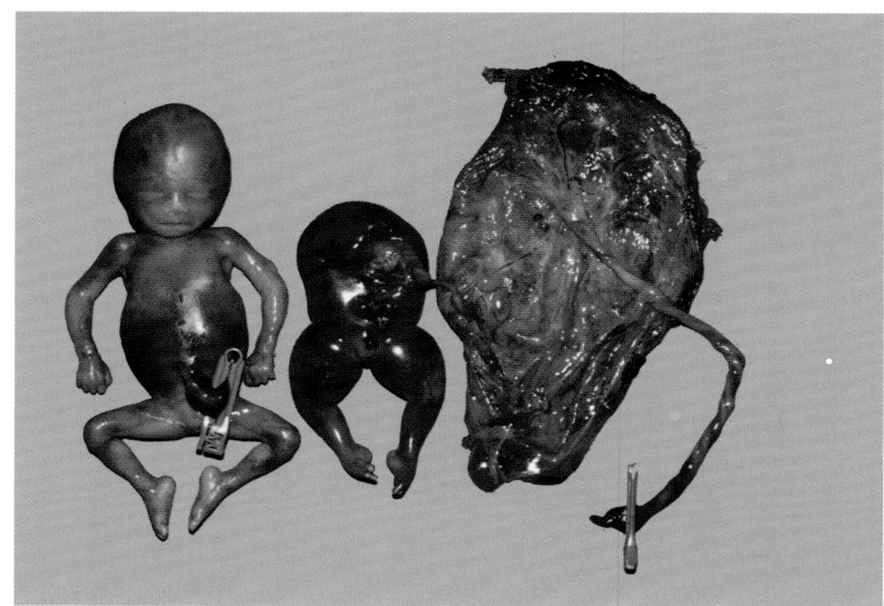

Fig. 15.**12** **Twin reversed arterial perfusion (TRAP sequence).** The placenta and fetus after abortion at 22 weeks of gestation.

at short intervals is recommended. It is important to exclude fetal hydrops and cardiac failure in the "pump twin." The following therapeutic options are available: 1, administration of digitalis to the mother; 2, amniotic fluid aspiration to reduce polyhydramnios; 3, fetoscopic ligation of the umbilical cord of the recipient twin. Administration of indomethacin may also help in case of hydramnios.

Procedure after birth: Intensive treatment of the newborn is required, depending on the gestational age and presence of cardiac insufficiency or hydrops.

References

Borrell A, Pesarrodona A, Puerto B, Deulofeu P, Fuster JJ, Fortuny A. Ultrasound diagnostic features of twin reversed arterial perfusion sequence. Prenat Diagn 1990; 10: 443–8.

Gembruch U, Viski S, Bagamery K, Berg C, Germer U. Twin reversed arterial perfusion sequence in twin-to-twin transfusion syndrome after the death of the donor co-twin in the second trimester. Ultrasound Obstet Gynecol 2001; 17: 153–6.

Mohanty C, Mishra OP, Singh CP, Das BK, Singla PN. Acardiac anomaly spectrum. Teratology 2000; 62: 356–9.

Osborn P, Gross TL, Shah JJ, Ma L. Prenatal diagnosis of fetal heart failure in twin reversed arterial perfusion syndrome. Prenat Diagn 2000; 20: 615–7.

Sanjaghsaz H, Bayram MO, Qureshi F. Twin reversed arterial perfusion sequence in conjoined, acardiac, acephalic twins associated with a normal triplet: a case report. J Reprod Med 1998; 43: 1046–50.

Schwarzler P, Ville Y, Moscosco G, Tennstedt C, Bollmann R, Chaoui R. Diagnosis of twin reversed arterial perfusion sequence in the first trimester by transvaginal color Doppler ultrasound. Ultrasound Obstet Gynecol 1999; 13: 143–6.
Sepulveda W, Sfeir D, Reyes M, Martinez J. Severe polyhydramnios in twin reversed arterial perfusion sequence: successful management with intrafetal alcohol ablation of acardiac twin and amniodrainage. Ultrasound Obstet Gynecol 2000; 16: 260–3.
Tanawattanacharoen S, Tantivatana J, Charoenvidhya D, et al. Occlusion of umbilical artery using a Guglielmi detachable coil for the treatment of TRAP sequence. Ultrasound Obstet Gynecol 2002; 19: 313–5.

Twin-to-Twin Transfusion Syndrome (TTTS)

Definition: This syndrome is unique to monochorionic twin pregnancies, and represents an unbalanced arteriovenous placental shunt leading to vascular compromise of the fetuses. The donor gives blood to the recipient twin, resulting in growth restriction of the donor and volume overload of the recipient. The recipient twin may consequently develop cardiac failure. There is a high rate of intrauterine death of both twins.

Incidence: This occurs in 5–10% of all twin pregnancies. About 5% of monochorionic pregnancies are severely affected.

Associated symptoms: "*Donor*": anemia, growth restriction, oligohydramnios, or anhydramnios ("stuck twin"). "*Recipient*": macrosomia, hydramnios, cardiac failure, fetal hydrops, postnatal plethora.

Ultrasound findings: Monochorionic, diamniotic twin pregnancies showing severe disparity in fetal growth. The fetuses are always of the same gender (monozygotic). The larger, "recipient" twin may develop signs of cardiac insufficiency and hydrops (pleural effusion, pericardial effusion, ascites, skin edema, hepatosplenomegaly) as well as hydramnios. Oligohydramnios or even anhydramnios ("stuck twin") is the case in "donor" twin. There is disparity in the circumference of the umbilical cord. Marginal or velamentous insertion is frequently seen in the donor twin. To detect whether there is significant blood transfusion between the twins, the donor is given a muscle relaxant (pancuronium) through its umbilical vein; if there is TTTS, relaxation of the recipient twin will also occur. However, vascular anastomoses are found in over 85% of monochorionic placentas, so that relaxation of the recipient twin does not necessarily indicate clinically significant transfusion due to vascular shunts. The placenta, especially of the recipient twin, may be thick and swollen. Fetal echocardiography frequently shows incompetence of the AV valve in the recipient, due to volume overload. Rare cases have been reported in which there is a reversal in the role of the donor and recipient twins during the progress of the pregnancy.

Clinical management: The diagnosis is confirmed on the basis of the ultrasound findings. The higher frequency of chromosomal aberrations and anomalies in monochorionic twins also has to be taken into account. Detection of TTTS prior to 20 weeks of gestation has an unfavorable prognosis. The poor prognosis and high neurological morbidity associated with early detection should be explained to the parents, and the option of pregnancy termination should be discussed. Serial ultrasound scanning and fetal echocardiography at short intervals are necessary to detect the development of cardiac insufficiency. Administration of digitalis to the mother and repeated aspiration of amniotic fluid to relieve hydramnios may be considered as therapeutic options. In recent years, coagulation of vascular anastomoses using endoscopic laser surgery has been successful in reducing the late neurological morbidity. If one twin dies during the course of pregnancy, the surviving twin has a very high risk of developing brain damage; there is a surge of thromboplastic substances that may cause cerebral infarcts, hydrocephalus, and periventricular leukomalacia. In this case, it is difficult to determine whether early delivery of the surviving twin has a benefit. In the United Kingdom, where fetocide is socially acceptable as an option for terminating pregnancy, it is being debated whether the pregnancy should be continued for 3–4 weeks after the intrauterine death of one twin, retaining the option of fetocide if severe neurological signs appear in the surviving twin. In severe cases of

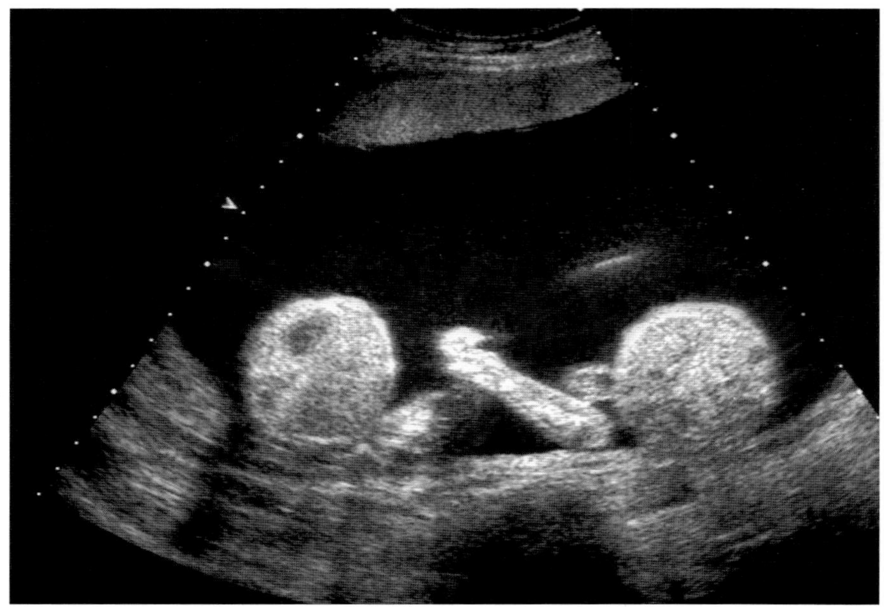

Fig. 15.**13** **Twin-to-twin transfusion syndrome.** Abdominal scan, showing a monoamniotic twin pregnancy at 21 + 3 weeks with twin-to-twin transfusion syndrome and severe hydramnios. Intrauterine fetal death followed.

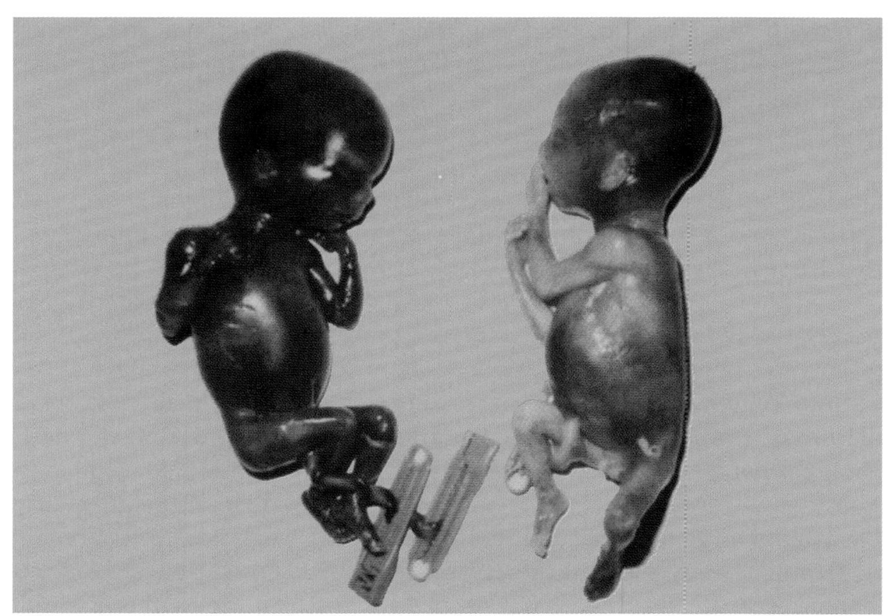

Fig. 15.**14** **Twin-to-twin transfusion syndrome.** Twins after intrauterine fetal demise following twin-to-twin transfusion syndrome.

TTTS, cesarean section should be the mode of delivery.

Procedure after birth: Intensive medical treatment of both twins is required. The recipient shows polycythemia and the donor twin anemia (difference in hemoglobin concentration of more than 5 g%). Ultrasound of the fetal skull at the early neonatal stage is advisable to detect prenatal infarction or periventricular leukomalacia.

Prognosis: There is a high mortality rate of 50–90% in severe cases. Intrauterine death of one or both twins may occur. Complications arise due to premature birth. If intrauterine death of one twin occurs, the surviving twin has a high risk of neurological morbidity.

Self-Help Organizations

Title: Twin-to-twin Transfusion Syndrome Foundation

Description: Soley dedicated to providing immediate and life-saving educational, emotional, and financial support for families, medical professionals, and caregivers before, during, and after pregnancy with twin-to-twin transfusion syndrome. Dedicated to saving the babies, improving their future health and care, furthering medical research, providing neonatal intensive care, and support for special needs and bereavement. Pen pals, newsletter, literature, phone support, visitation, conferences. Guidelines for professionals on multiple birth loss during pregnancy. Help in starting new chapters. International registry.

Scope: International

Founded: 1992

Address: 411 Longbeach Parkway, Bay Village, OH 44140, United States

Telephone: 440-899-8887

E-mail: tttsfound@aol.com

Web: http://www.tttsfoundation.org

Title: Twin Hope

Description: Voluntary, non-profit organization dedicated to serving the needs of families affected by twin-to-twin transfusion syndrome and other twin-related diseases. Support for group meetings, phone support. Information and referrals, conferences, fundraising, current treatment options, biannual newsletter, library. Educates the public. Assistance in starting new groups.

Scope: International

Number of groups: Three affiliated groups

Founded: 1994

Address: 2592 W. 14th St., Cleveland, OH 44113, United States

Telephone: 502-243-2110 or 440-327-8335

E-mail: twinhope@twinhope.com

Web: http://www.twinhope.com

References

Berghella V, Kaufmann M. Natural history of twin–twin transfusion syndrome [review]. J Reprod Med 2001; 46: 480–4.

Blaicher W, Ulm B, Ulm M, Kuhle S, Deutinger J, Bernaschek G. The twin–twin transfusion syndrome: an unsolved problem. Ultraschall Med 2002; 23: 108–12.

Entezami M, Runkel S, Becker R, Weitzel HK, Arabin B. Feto-feto-fetal triplet transfusion syndrome (FFFTTS). J Matern Fetal Med 1997; 6: 334–7.

Feldstein VA, Machin GA, Albanese CT, et al. Twin–twin transfusion syndrome: the 'Select' procedure. Fetal Diagn Ther 2000; 15: 257–61.

Giles WB, Trudinger BJ, Cook CM. Doppler sonography findings of the umbilical arteries in eight cases of twin transfusion syndrome [letter; comment]. J Ultrasound Med 1989; 8: 531–2.

Hecher K, Diehl W, Zikulnig L, Vetter M, Hackeloer BJ. Endoscopic laser coagulation of placental anastomoses in 200 pregnancies with severe mid-trimester twin-to-twin transfusion syndrome. Eur J Obstet Gynecol Reprod Biol 2000; 92: 135–9.

Hubinont C, Bernard P, Pirot N, Biard J, Donnez J. Twin-to-twin transfusion syndrome: treatment by amniodrainage and septostomy [review]. Eur J Obstet Gynecol Reprod Biol 2000; 92: 141–4.

Jones JM, Sbarra AJ, Cetrulo CL. Twin transfusion syndrome: reassessment of ultrasound diagnosis. J Reprod Med 1996; 41: 11–4.

Lees CC, Schwarzler P, Ville Y, Campbell S. Stuck twin syndrome without signs of twin-to-twin transfusion. Ultrasound Obstet Gynecol 1998; 12: 211–4.

Mari G, Detti L, Levi DA, Kern L. "Pseudo" twin-to-twin transfusion syndrome and fetal outcome. J Perinatol 1998; 18: 399–403.

Matias A, Montenegro N, Areias JC. Anticipating twin–twin transfusion syndrome in monochorionic twin pregnancy: is there a role for nuchal translucency and ductus venosus blood flow evaluation at 11–14 weeks? Twin Res 2000; 3: 65–70.

Nicolaides KH, Heath V, Cicero S. Increased fetal nuchal translucency at 11–14 weeks [review]. Prenat Diagn 2002; 22: 308–15.

Ohno Y, Ando H, Tanamura A, Kurauchi O, Mizutani S, Tomoda Y. The value of Doppler ultrasound in the diagnosis and management of twin-to-twin transfusion syndrome. Arch Gynecol Obstet 1994; 255: 37–42.

Sebire NJ, Talbert D, Fisk NM. Twin-to-twin transfusion syndrome results from dynamic asymmetrical reduction in placental anastomoses: a hypothesis [review]. Placenta 2001; 22: 383–91.

Sohn C, Wallwiener D, Kurek R, Hahn U, Schiesser M, Bastert G. Treatment of the twin–twin transfusion syndrome: initial experience using laser-induced interstitial thermotherapy. Fetal Diagn Ther 1996; 11: 390–7.

van Gemert MJ, Vandenbussche FP, Schaap AH, et al. Classification of discordant fetal growth may contribute to risk stratification in monochorionic twin pregnancies. Ultrasound Obstet Gynecol 2000; 16: 237–44.

Weiner CP, Ludomirski A. Diagnosis, pathophysiology, and treatment of chronic twin-to-twin transfusion syndrome. Fetal Diagn Ther 1994; 9: 283–90.

Yamada A, Kasugai M, Ohno Y, Ishizuka T, Mizutani S, Tomoda Y. Antenatal diagnosis of twin–twin transfusion syndrome by Doppler ultrasound. Obstet Gynecol 1991; 78: 1058–61.

Growth Restriction in Twins

Definition: Growth restriction is diagnosed if the sonographically estimated fetal weight lies below the 5th percentile. This is usually associated with disparity in the size of the twins. The values measured are compared with the standard fetal weight charts for twins.

Incidence: Occurs in 12–47% of twin pregnancies.

Ultrasound findings: One or both twins are small for gestational age; the thoracoabdominal circumference is most frequently affected. Oligohydramnios is a frequent accompanying feature. Twin-to-twin transfusion syndrome has to be considered in the differential diagnosis, but this can be excluded if the pregnancy is not monochorionic (TTTS occurs almost exclusively in monochorionic pregnancy). If the pregnancy is monochorionic, then an absence of hydramnios, cardiac failure, and hydrops (characteristic for the recipient twin in TTTS) in the larger twin excludes TTTS.

Clinical management: Karyotyping, search for infections (TORCH). The high frequency of chromosomal and structural anomalies in twin pregnancies has to be taken into account. Frequent scanning of fetal growth using color-coded Doppler imaging and echocardiography at short intervals. Premature delivery may be an option, depending on the gestational age and severity. Administration of cortisone to promote maturation of the lungs has not shown any clear benefit in twin pregnancies. Some studies have reported a beneficial effect of additional administration of thyrotropin-releasing hormone (TRH).

Procedure after birth: Fetal distress during labor and respiratory insufficiency in the immediate neonatal stage are frequent complications. In addition, polycythemia, hypoglycemia, and hyperbilirubinemia may be present.

Prognosis: Growth-restricted infants have a higher morbidity and mortality.

References

Ananth CV, Vintzileos AM, Shen-Schwarz S, Smulian JC, Lai YL. Standards of birth weight in twin gestations stratified by placental chorionicity. Obstet Gynecol 1998; 91: 917–24.

Audibert F, Boullier M, Kerbrat V, Vial M, Boithias C, Frydman R. [Growth discordance in dichorionic twin pregnancies: risk factors, diagnosis and management; in French.] J Gynecol Obstet Biol Reprod (Paris) 2002; 31 (Suppl 1): 215–24.

Blickstein I, Goldman RD, Mazkereth R. Risk for one or two very low birth weight twins: a population study. Obstet Gynecol 2000; 96: 400–2.

Bruner JP, Wheeler TC, Bliton MJ. Sectio parva for fetal preservation [review]. Fetal Diagn Ther 1999; 14: 254–6.

Demissie K, Ananth CV, Martin J, Hanley ML, MacDorman MF, Rhoads GG. Fetal and neonatal mortality among twin gestations in the United States: the role of intrapair birth weight discordance. Obstet Gynecol 2002; 100: 474–80.

Gaziano EP, Gaziano C, Terrell CA, Hoekstra RE. The cerebroplacental Doppler ratio and neonatal outcome in diamnionic monochorionic and dichorionic twins. J Matern Fetal Med 2001; 10: 371–5.

Jakobovits AA. Twin birth weight discordance and the risk of preterm birth. Am J Obstet Gynecol 2001; 185: 256.

Khong TY, Hague WM. Biparental contribution to fetal thrombophilia in discordant twin intrauterine growth restriction. Am J Obstet Gynecol 2001; 185: 244–5.

Zhang J, Brenner RA, Klebanoff MA. Differences in birth weight and blood pressure at age 7 years among twins. Am J Epidemiol 2001; 153: 779–82.

Zuppa AA, Maragliano G, Scapillati ME, Crescimbini B, Tortorolo G. Neonatal outcome of spontaneous and assisted twin pregnancies. Eur J Obstet Gynecol Reprod Biol 2001; 95: 68–72.

16 Growth Disturbance

Macrosomia

Definition: Birth weight above 4000 g or estimated fetal weight above the 95th centile for the given gestational age. It is important to differentiate between a constitutionally large fetus ("large for gestational age") and a fetus with characteristic diabetic macrosomia (normal head circumference, increase in abdominal circumference, increased subcutaneous fat tissue).

Incidence: 1–2% of births; if the percentile curves were correct, 5% of births would be detected.

Clinical history: Genetically determined; parental heights. Pathological glucose tolerance test. Gestational diabetes. Macrosomia occurs frequently in consecutive pregnancies.

Associated syndromes: Macrosomia is seen in Beckwith–Wiedemann syndrome, Weaver syndrome, and Sotos syndrome.

Ultrasound findings: Fetal parameters, mainly the abdominal circumference, lie above the 95th centile. Estimating fetal weight, especially in macrosomia, is relatively inaccurate (maximum sensitivity 70%, positive predictive value 60 %). The abdominal circumference is possibly the best parameter for detecting macrosomia. The quotient of femur length and abdominal circumference (normally > 20%) is not a reliable parameter either (sensitivity 60%). Mild hydramnios is frequently present. Typically, the neck region and cheeks (cheek-to-cheek distance as measured using Abramowicz's method) appear swollen, but this is due to fat tissue rather than edema.

Clinical management: Glucose tolerance test, serial ultrasounds, possibly early delivery at 38 weeks of gestation. If the estimated fetal weight is above 4500 g, the benefit of primary cesarean section to avoid shoulder dystocia is disputed, as weight estimation in macrosomia is frequently not very accurate.

Procedure after birth: A pediatrician should be present at delivery. Fetal distress and hypoglycemia are often observed.

Prognosis: Normal, unless there are complications and injuries arising from delivery (for example, shoulder dystocia).

References

Benson CB, Coughlin BF, Doubilet PM. Amniotic fluid volume in large-for-gestational-age fetuses of nondiabetic mothers. J Ultrasound Med 1991; 10: 149–51.

Best G, Pressman EK. Ultrasonographic prediction of birth weight in diabetic pregnancies. Obstet Gynecol 2002; 99: 740–4.

Delpapa EH, Mueller HE. Pregnancy outcome following ultrasound diagnosis of macrosomia. Obstet Gynecol 1991; 78: 340–3.

Elliott JP, Garite TI, Freeman RK, McQuown DS, Patel IM. Ultrasonic prediction of fetal macrosomia in diabetic patients. Obstet Gynecol 1982; 60: 159–62.

Landon MB, Mintz MC, Gabbe SG. Sonographic evaluation of fetal abdominal growth: predictor of the large-for-gestational-age infant in pregnancies complicated by diabetes mellitus. Am J Obstet Gynecol 1989; 160: 115–21.

Levine AB, Lockwood CJ, Brown B, Lapinski R, Berkowitz RL. Sonographic diagnosis of the large for gestational age fetus at term: does it make a difference? Obstet Gynecol 1992; 79: 55–8.

Lurie S, Zalel Y, Hagay ZJ. The evaluation of accelerated fetal growth. Curr Opin Obstet Gynecol 1995; 7: 477–81.

Miller JMJ, Brown HL, Khawli OF, Korndorffer FA, Gabert HA. Fetal weight estimates in diabetic gravid women. JCU J Clin Ultrasound 1988; 16: 569–72.

Miller JMJ, Kissling GE, Brown HL, Nagel PM, Korndorffer FA, Gabert HA. In utero growth of the large-for-menstrual-age fetus. JCU J Clin Ultrasound 1989; 17: 15–7.

Taylor R, Lee C, Kyne-Grzebalski D, Marshall SM, Davison JM. Clinical outcomes of pregnancy in women with type 1 diabetes (1). Obstet Gynecol 2002; 99: 537–41.

Van Assche FA, Holemans K, Aerts L. Long-term consequences for offspring of diabetes during pregnancy [review]. Br Med Bull 2001; 60: 173–82.

Wong SF, Chan FY, Cincotta RB, Oats JJ, McIntyre HD. Sonographic estimation of fetal weight in macrosomic fetuses: diabetic versus non-diabetic pregnancies. Aust N Z J Obstet Gynaecol 2001; 41: 429–32.

Growth Restriction

Definition: Varying limits have been defined: birth weight lower than the 10th, 5th, or 3rd centile. It is important to differentiate between infants who are small as a result of placental insufficiency and those who are small due to genetic disposition.

Incidence: Depending on the definition (see above), 3–10% of pregnancies, if correct birth weight percentiles are applied.

Clinical history: The birth weight depends on genetic factors. There are families in which small infants are more frequent and these cases are not the result of inadequate placental function. Genuine placental insufficiency causing growth restriction occurs, usually repeatedly, in mothers who have certain underlying diseases—for example, kidney disease, hypertension, or thrombophilic disorders. Other important factors for placental insufficiency include smoking and alcohol consumption during pregnancy.

Embryology: Growth restriction may be the result of uteroplacental insufficiency, environmental factors, drugs, maternal infections, or genetic disposition to small stature. Asymmetrical growth restriction is characteristic for placenta insufficiency: the head circumference and femur length are larger than the abdominal circumference, which is considerably smaller for the gestational age.

Associated syndromes: Cornelia de Lange syndrome, Russell–Silver syndrome (asymmetrical growth restriction with normal head circumference and dwarfism), Seckel syndrome, Smith–Lemli–Opitz syndrome, Miller-Dieker syndrome, Neu–Laxova syndrome, Freeman–Sheldon syndrome, osteopetrosis (autosomal-recessive disease with diffuse sclerosis of the skeletal system, increased bone density, bone fractures, widening of cranial ventricles and shortening of the long bones), Wolf–Hirschhorn syndrome, Jacobsen syndrome (11 q deletion), triploidy, trisomy 9, trisomy 10, trisomy 18, Harlequin syndrome (autosomal-recessive disease with callus formation and characteristic facial features: "clown-like face").

Ultrasound findings: Fetal measurements lie below the expected values for the gestational age. For accurate diagnosis of fetal growth restriction, early measurements of crown–rump length at 8–12 weeks of gestation are indispensable.

There are two types of growth restriction: 1, *symmetrical*: in this type, the measurements of head and abdominal circumference and femur length are all below the expected values; and 2, *asymmetrical*: the head circumference is normal, but the abdominal circumference and length of the extremities are too small. Oligohydramnios is a common feature when there is placental insufficiency. Using color-coded Doppler imaging, pathological values are obtained in fetal vessels and also in maternal vessels (increased vascular resistance).

Clinical management: In severe forms of growth restriction (below the 5th centile), especially if the growth restriction is symmetrical and diagnosed early in pregnancy and the Doppler values are normal, karyotyping and exclusion of maternal infections (TORCH) are necessary. Serial ultrasound assessment, including Doppler measurements, are indicated. If the maternal hematocrit is high, hemodilution can be carried out. Some centers have tried to nurture the fetus artificially by infusions of amino acids or glucose into the amniotic fluid or umbilical vein, but without much success. Premature delivery is often opted for, in severe cases by cesarean section. A very high perinatal mortality rate of 75% is caused by intrauterine fetal death and results from severe placental insufficiency. Very early premature delivery—as early as 24 or 25 weeks of gestation—may be necessary to prevent intrauterine mortality. When placental insufficiency occurs repeatedly and very early, or if there is a clinical history of fetal demise in a previous pregnancy, anticardiolipin antibody, lupus anticoagulant, or thrombophilic disorders may be the causative factors. In such cases, early therapy with low-dose acetylsalicylic acid and possibly heparin may be needed.

Procedure after birth: A pediatrician should be present at birth. There is a high incidence of fetal distress during labor and delivery.

Prognosis: There is a fourfold to eightfold increase in perinatal mortality in severe cases of growth restriction (below the third centile). The survivors have a neonatal morbidity of up to 50%, but the long-term neurological morbidity rate is usually low.

References

Achiron R, Mazkereth R, Orvieto R, Kuint J, Lipitz S, Rotstein Z. Echogenic bowel in intrauterine growth restriction fetuses: does this jeopardize the gut? Obstet Gynecol 2002; 100: 120–5.

Antovic JP, Rafik Hamad R, Antovic A, Blomback M, Bremme K. Does thrombin activatable fibrinolysis inhibitor (TAFI) contribute to impairment of fibrinolysis in patients with preeclampsia and/or intrauterine fetal growth retardation? Thromb Haemost 2002; 88: 644–7.

Benson CB, Doubilet PM. Doppler criteria for intrauterine growth retardation: predictive values. J Ultrasound Med 1988; 7: 655–9.

DeVore GR, Platt LD. Diagnosis of intrauterine growth retardation: the use of sequential measurements of fetal growth parameters. Clin Obstet Gynecol 1987; 30: 968–84.

Houlton MC, Marivate M, Philpott RH. The prediction of fetal growth retardation in twin pregnancy. Br J Obstet Gynaecol 1981; 88: 264–73.

Jahn A, Razum O, Berle P. Routine screening for intrauterine growth retardation in Germany: low sensitivity and questionable benefit for diagnosed cases. Acta Obstet Gynecol Scand 1998; 77: 643–8.

Johnson MR, Anim-Nyame N, Johnson P, Sooranna SR, Steer PJ. Does endothelial cell activation occur with intrauterine growth restriction? BJOG Br J Obstet Gynecol 2002; 109: 836–9.

Klockenbusch W, Rath W. [Prevention of preeclampsia by low-dose acetylsalicylic acid: a critical appraisal; in German.] Z Geburtshilfe Neonatol 2002; 206: 125–30.

La Batide-Alanore A, Tregouet DA, Jaquet D, Bouyer J, Tiret L. Familial aggregation of fetal growth restriction in a French cohort of 7,822 term births between 1971 and 1985. Am J Epidemiol 2002; 156: 180–7.

Ott WJ. Sonographic diagnosis of intrauterine growth restriction. Clin Obstet Gynecol 1997; 40: 787–95.

Persson PH, Kullander S. Long-term experience of general ultrasound screening in pregnancy. Am J Obstet Gynecol 1983; 146: 942–7.

Reece EA, Goldstein I, Pilu G, Hobbins JC. Fetal cerebellar growth unaffected by intrauterine growth retardation: a new parameter for prenatal diagnosis. Am J Obstet Gynecol 1987; 157: 632–8.

Rochelson B, Bracero LA, Porte J, Farmakides G. Diagnosis of intrauterine growth retardation as a two-step process with morphometric ultrasound and Doppler umbilical artery velocimetry. J Reprod Med 1992; 37: 925–9.

Sarmandal P, Grant JM. Effectiveness of ultrasound determination of fetal abdominal circumference and fetal ponderal index in the diagnosis of asymmetrical growth retardation. Br J Obstet Gynaecol 1990; 97: 118–23.

Selbing A, Wichman K, Ryden G. Screening for detection of intra-uterine growth retardation by means of ultrasound. Acta Obstet Gynecol Scand 1984; 63: 543–8.

17 Diabetes Mellitus

Definition: Maternal diabetes mellitus is considered to be a very significant risk factor in pregnancy and is responsible for a high rate of perinatal mortality (4%). It is important to differentiate *pre-existing diabetes mellitus* from *gestational diabetes*. In the pre-existing form, in addition to fetal macrosomia and immaturity of organs, there is an increased incidence of fetal malformations, especially if glycemic control has not been optimal during the pre-conception and early first-trimester stages.

Incidence: Gestational diabetes is seen in up to 3% of pregnancies.

Associated symptoms: These may include macrosomia and hydramnios (late second trimester), and—when there is maternal vascular damage—growth restriction (Doppler ultrasonography of the uterine vessels at 22 weeks).

Associated malformations: Anencephaly, holoprosencephaly, neural tube defects (2%), microcephaly. Caudal regression syndrome, cardiac anomalies (2–4%) such as transposition of great vessels, VSD, tetralogy of Fallot. Bowel atresia, renal anomalies such as renal hypoplasia or hydronephrosis.

Differential diagnosis: Syndromes associated with macrosomia: Beckwith–Wiedemann syndrome, Marshall–Smith syndrome, Sotos syndrome, Weaver syndrome.

Clinical management: Oral glucose tolerance test, profile of blood glucose levels for 1 day, tight glycemic control (fasting values below 100 mg%, peak values not exceeding 130 mg%). If dietetic measures are insufficient, therapy with insulin is required. Serial Doppler assessments.

Procedure after birth: A pediatrician should be present at delivery. Monitoring of blood glucose values to prevent neonatal hypoglycemia (hyperinsulinemia of the newborn).

Prognosis: There is an increased risk of intrauterine fetal death, especially in late pregnancy. Risk of shoulder dystocia during delivery. Immaturity of the lungs despite large fetal size and weight.

References

Benson CB, Doubilet PM, Saltzman DH, Greene MF, Jones TB. Femur length/abdominal circumference ratio: poor predictor of macrosomic fetuses in diabetic mothers. J Ultrasound Med 1986; 5: 141–4.

Brundage SC. Preconception health care. Am Fam Physician 2002; 65: 2507–14.

Hahmann K, Issel EP Assessment of fetal growth using the humerus and femur in ultrasound fetometry. Zentralbl Gynäkol 1988; 110: 370–82.

Landon MB, Mintz MC, Gabbe SG. Sonographic evaluation of fetal abdominal growth: predictor of the large-for-gestational-age infant in pregnancies complicated by diabetes mellitus. Am J Obstet Gynecol 1989; 160: 115–21.

Landon MB, Sonek J, Foy P, Hamilton L, Gabbe SG. Sonographic measurement of fetal humeral soft tissue thickness in pregnancy complicated by GDM. Diabetes 1991; 40 (Suppl 2): 66–70.

Langer O, Langer N. Diabetes in women older than 40 years of age: social and medical aspects. Obstet Gynecol Clin North Am 1993; 20: 299–311.

Meyer WM, Simpson JM, Sharland GK. Incidence of congenital heart defects in fetuses of diabetic mothers: a retrospective study of 326 cases. Ultrasound Obstet Gynecol 1996; 8: 8–10.

Miller JMJ, Kissling GE, Brown HL, Nagel PM, Korndorffer FA, Gabert HA. In utero growth of the large-formenstrual-age fetus. JCU J Clin Ultrasound 1989; 17: 15–7.

Mostello D, Catlin TK, Roman L, Holcomb WL Jr, Leet T. Preeclampsia in the parous woman: who is at risk? Am J Obstet Gynecol 2002; 187: 425–9.

Ogata ES, Sabbagha R, Metzger BE, Phelps RL, Depp R, Freinkel N. Serial ultrasonography to assess evolving fetal macrosomia: studies in 23 pregnant diabetic women. JAMA 1980; 243: 2405–8.

Pachi A, Fallucca F, Gerlini GF, Maggi E, La Torre R. Relationship between ultrasound findings in pregnancy and neonatal morbidity. Acta Endocrinol Suppl (Copenh) 1986; 277: 145–9.

Pedra SR, Smallhorn JF, Ryan G, et al. Fetal cardiomyopathies: pathogenic mechanisms, hemodynamic findings, and clinical outcome. Circulation 2002; 106: 585–91.

Pijlman BM, de Koning WB, Wladimiroff JW, Stewart PA. Detection of fetal structural malformations by ultrasound in insulin-dependent pregnant women. Ultrasound Med Biol 1989; 15: 541–3.

Taylor R, Lee C, Kyne-Grzebalski D, Marshall SM, Davison JM. Clinical outcomes of pregnancy in women with type 1 diabetes (1). Obstet Gynecol 2002; 99: 537–41.

Van Assche FA, Holemans K, Aerts L. Long-term consequences for offspring of diabetes during pregnancy [review]. Br Med Bull 2001; 60: 173–82.

Wong SF, Chan FY, Cincotta RB, Oats JJ, McIntyre HD. Routine ultrasound screening in diabetic pregnancies. Ultrasound Obstet Gynecol 2002; 19: 171–6.

18 Drugs

Anticonvulsive Drugs

Substances: Phenytoin, carbamazepine, valproic acid, phenobarbiturate.

Definition: Effects of anticonvulsive drugs with a known teratogenic effect on the fetus. In the presence of epilepsy, there is a two- to threefold increase in the risk of fetal anomalies, even without the effects of medication.

Incidence: The risk of fetal malformations lies at 10% if medications are given in early pregnancy. In patients with an autosomal-recessively inherited deficiency in epoxide hydrolase (a metabolic enzyme), the risk of fetal anomalies under the influence of anticonvulsive drugs is extremely high.

Associated malformations: Phenytoin and carbamazepine may cause facial dysmorphism, microcephaly, finger hypoplasia, nail hypoplasia, growth restriction, and mental impairment. Valproic acid and carbamazepine increase the risk of neural tube defects to 1%.

Clinical features: *Central nervous system anomalies:* microcephaly, holoprosencephaly, myelomeningocele. *Facial anomalies:* hypertelorism, cleft lip and palate, stubby nose, wide nasal bridge. *Skeletal anomalies:* hypoplasia of the distal phalanges, ulnar deviation of the thumb, hip dysplasia, short neck, pterygium of the neck, anomalies of the ribs and sternum. *Cardiac malformations:* VSD, pulmonary stenosis, aortic stenosis. *Anomalies of the urogenital system:* ambiguous genitalia, renal anomalies. Growth restriction and oligohydramnios.

Clinical management: Karyotyping (differential diagnosis). Measurement of epoxide hydrolase in amniotic fluid; this is still experimental. There is an increased risk of cranial bleeding if medications belonging to the hydantoin group are used. In this situation, vitamin K should be administered to the mother before the start of labor.

Procedure after birth: When the mother is receiving hydantoin, vitamin K should be given. Intracranial bleeding should be excluded. With carbamazepine, growth restriction and developmental disturbances are frequently expected at the neonatal stage.

Prognosis: Over 90% of women suffering from fits have normal children. The prognosis depends on the type and severity of fetal malformation.

Self-Help Organization

Title: Epilepsy Foundation

Description: Information and support for people with epilepsy, their families and friends. Pharmaceutical program, newsletter for members. Affiliates' development kit. Referrals to local affiliates (many of which have employment-related programs). Information and referrals.

Scope: National (English/Spanish)

Number of groups: 60 + affiliates

Founded: 1967

Address: 4351 Garden City Dr., Landover, MD 20785, United States

Telephone: Information 800-332-1000; library 800-332-4050; catalog sales 800-213-5821; 301-459-3700

Fax: 301-577-4941

E-mail: postmaster@efa.org

Web: http://www.epilepsyfoundation.org

References

Buehler BA, Delimont D, van Waes M, Finnell RH. Prenatal prediction of risk of the fetal hydantoin syndrome. N Engl J Med 1990; 322: 1567–72.

Ceci O, Loizzi P, Caruso G, Caradonna F, Clemente R, Ferreri R. Fetal malformations in an epileptic pregnant woman treated with carbamazepine. Zentralbl Gynäkol 1996; 118: 169–71.

Dean JC, Hailey H, Moore SJ, Lloyd DJ, Turnpenny PD, Little J. Long term health and neurodevelopment in children exposed to antiepileptic drugs before birth. J Med Genet 2002; 39: 251–9.

Giardina S, Contarini A, Becca B. Maternal diseases and congenital malformations. Ann Ist Super Sanita 1993; 29: 69–76.

Holmes LB. Looking for long-term effects from prenatal exposures to anticonvulsants. Teratology 2001; 64: 175–6.

Janz D. Pregnancy and fetal development in epileptic women. Geburtshilfe Frauenheilkd 1984; 44: 428–34.

Koch S, Losche G, Jager R, et al. Major and minor birth malformations and antiepileptic drugs. Neurology 1992; 42: 83–8.

Kroes HY, Reefhuis J, Cornel MC. Is there an association between maternal carbamazepine use during pregnancy and eye malformations in the child? [review]. Epilepsia 2002; 43: 929–31.

Lowe SA. Drugs in pregnancy: anticonvulsants and drugs for neurological disease [review]. Best Pract Res Clin Obstet Gynaecol 2001; 15: 863–76.

McAuley JW, Anderson GD. Treatment of epilepsy in women of reproductive age: pharmacokinetic considerations [review]. Clin Pharmacokinet 2002; 41: 559–79.

Olafsson E, Hallgrimsson JT, Hauser WA, Ludvigsson P, Gudmundsson G. Pregnancies of women with epilepsy: a population-based study in Iceland. Epilepsia 1998; 39: 887–92.

Omtzigt JG, Los FJ, Grobbee DE, et al. The risk of spina bifida aperta after first-trimester exposure to valproate in a prenatal cohort. Neurology 1992; 42: 119–25.

Samrén EB, van Duijn CM, Koch S, et al. Maternal use of antiepileptic drugs and the risk of major congenital malformations: a joint European prospective study of human teratogenesis associated with maternal epilepsy. Epilepsia 1997; 38: 981–90.

Shankaran S, Papile LA, Wright LL, et al. Neurodevelopmental outcome of premature infants after antenatal phenobarbital exposure. Am J Obstet Gynecol 2002; 187: 171–7.

Yerby MS. Risks of pregnancy in women with epilepsy. Epilepsia 1992; 33 (Suppl 1): S23 –S26.

Fetal Alcohol Syndrome

Definition: A complex syndrome developing in the fetus due to chronic maternal alcohol abuse.

Incidence: Estimated at one in 1000 births. The risk of fetal alcohol syndrome in mothers with chronic alcohol abuse is 20–40%.

Embryology: Alcohol and its metabolites cross the placenta and disturb or destroy fetal cell growth.

Clinical features: Facial dysmorphism (hypoplasia of mid-facial region, epicanthus, smooth philtrum with short upper lip, ear anomalies); cardiac anomalies (70%), CNS anomalies, microcephaly (80%), neural tube defects, cleft lip and palate; skeletal anomalies, urogenital anomalies (10%).

Ultrasound findings: Growth restriction. Associated anomalies are: *cardiac anomalies:* VSD, ASD, double-outlet right ventricle (DORV), pulmonary atresia, dextrocardia, tetralogy of Fallot. *CNS anomalies:* Microcephaly, neural tube defects. *Facial anomalies:* micrognathia, cleft lip and palate, underdevelopment of upper jaw. *Urogenital anomalies:* hypoplasia of external genitalia, oligohydramnios. Others: pectus excavatum, vertebral anomalies in the neck region, diaphragmatic hernia. These anomalies are mostly diagnosed in the third trimester.

Clinical management: Karyotyping; TORCH serology; maternal metabolic disorders should be excluded (phenylketonuria). Taking a detailed clinical history is important. Additional screening of fetal organs, including fetal echocardiography. Serial ultrasounds (growth restriction).

Procedure after birth: The pediatrician should be present at the time of birth, as fetal distress is frequently seen. Alcohol withdrawal syndrome may develop in infancy.

Prognosis: This depends on how much and over what period of time the mother has been consuming alcohol. The average intelligence quotient of affected children is 65. Neurodevelopmental disorders may frequently develop.

Self-Help Organizations

Title: Fetal Alcohol Network

Description: Mutual support for parents of children with fetal alcohol syndrome. Interested in advocacy, educational issues, behavioral problems and accessing community services. Newsletter, conferences. Group development guidelines.

Scope: International

Founded: 1990

Address: 158 Rosemont Ave., Coatesville, PA 19320, United States

Telephone: 610-384-1133

E-mail: 72157.564@compuserve.com

Title: Fetal Alcohol Syndrome Family Resource Institute

Description: Grassroots coalition of families and professionals concerned with fetal alcohol syndrome/effects. Educational programs, brochures, information packets. Regional representatives being identified. Support group meetings. Advocacy, information and referrals, phone support, conferences.

Scope: International

Founded: 1990

Address: P.O. Box 2525, Lynnwood, WA 98070, United States

Telephone: 1-800-999-3429 (in WA); 253-531-2878 (outside WA)

Fax: 425-640-9155

E-mail: vicfas@h

Web: html://fetalalcoholsyndrome.org

References

[Anonymous]. Alcohol-exposed pregnancy: characteristics associated with risk. Am J Prev Med 2002; 23: 166.

Bagheri MM, Burd L, Martsolf JT, Klug MG. Fetal alcohol syndrome: maternal and neonatal characteristics. J Perinat Med 1998; 26: 263–9.

Bookstein FL, Sampson PD, Connor PD, Streissguth AP. Midline corpus callosum is a neuroanatomical focus of fetal alcohol damage. Anat Rec 2002; 269: 162–74.

Cadle RG, Dawson T Hall BD. The prevalence of genetic disorders, birth defects and syndromes in central and eastern Kentucky. J Ky Med Assoc 1996; 94: 237–41.

Church MW, Kaltenbach JA. Hearing, speech, language and vestibular disorders in the fetal alcohol syndrome: a literature review. Alcohol Clin Exp Res 1997; 21: 495–512.

Ernhart CB. Clinical correlations between ethanol intake and fetal alcohol syndrome. Recent Dev Alcohol 1991; 9: 127–50.

Halmesmaki E. Alcohol counselling of 85 pregnant problem drinkers: effect on drinking and fetal outcome. Br J Obstet Gynaecol 1988; 95: 243–7.

Keppen LD, Pysher T, Rennert OM. Zinc deficiency acts as a co-teratogen with alcohol in fetal alcohol syndrome. Pediatr Res 1985; 19: 944–7.

Lemoine P. Outcome of children of alcoholic mothers (study of 105 cases followed to adult age) and various prophylactic findings. Ann Pediatr (Paris) 1992; 39: 226–35.

Ornoy A. The effects of alcohol and illicit drugs on the human embryo and fetus. Isr J Psychiatry Relat Sci 2002; 39: 120–32.

Pauli RM, Feldman PF. Major limb malformations following intrauterine exposure to ethanol: two additional cases and literature review. Teratology 1986; 33: 273–80.

Polygenis D, Wharton S, Malmberg C, et al. Moderate alcohol consumption during pregnancy and the incidence of fetal malformations: a meta-analysis. Neurotoxicol Teratol 1998; 20: 61–7.

Spohr HL, Willms J, Steinhausen HC. Prenatal alcohol exposure and long-term developmental consequences. Lancet 1993; 341: 907–10.

Verdoux H. Long-term psychiatric and behavioural consequences of prenatal exposure to psychoactive drugs. J Therapie 2002; 57: 181–5.

Zachman RD, Grummer MA. The interaction of ethanol and vitamin A as a potential mechanism for the pathogenesis of Fetal Alcohol syndrome. Alcohol Clin UP Res 1998; 22: 1544–56.

Cocaine and Heroin

Definition: Influence of cocaine and/or of heroin on fetal malformation and development.

Incidence: This varies; teratogenic effect of these drugs are rare.

Embryology: Cocaine and heroin may cause an increase in maternal blood pressure. This results in disturbance of placental perfusion and may lead to fetal growth restriction. Reduction in blood pressure following an increase may further worsen the situation due to vasoconstriction and insufficient placental perfusion.

Associated malformations: Urogenital anomalies, craniofacial anomalies, cardiac malformations, CNS anomalies, limb defects, anomalies affecting the eye and growth restriction.

Ultrasound findings: Most fetuses exposed to these drugs show normal development. The following anomalies have been observed: *CNS anomalies:* cerebral infarcts and intracranial bleeding, porencephaly, hydrocephalus, hydranencephaly, microcephaly, agenesis of the corpus callosum, encephalocele and others. In addition, shortening or amputation of limbs, intestinal atresia, meconium peritonitis; cleft lip and palate; growth restriction and oligohydramnios; premature rupture of membranes.

Clinical management: Karyotyping (differential diagnosis). Further ultrasound screening including fetal echocardiography. Serial scans (growth restriction). Increased risk of placental abruption.

Procedure after birth: Increased risk of fetal distress during labor. Necrotizing enterocolitis is seen frequently in newborns after maternal cocaine abuse. Neonatal withdrawal syndrome occurs after heroin abuse.

Prognosis: Perinatal mortality is high due to premature delivery, placental abruption and growth restriction.

References

Bennett DS, Bendersky M, Lewis M. Children's intellectual and emotional-behavioral adjustment at 4 years as a function of cocaine exposure, maternal characteristics, and environmental risk. Dev Psychol 2002; 38: 648–58.

Chasnoff IJ, Chisum GM, Kaplan WE. Maternal cocaine use and genitourinary tract malformations. Teratology 1988; 37: 201–4.

Chiriboga CA, Brust JC, Bateman D, Hauser WA. Dose-response effect of fetal cocaine exposure on newborn neurologic function. Pediatrics 1999; 103: 79–85.

Church MW, Crossland WJ, Holmes PA, Overbeck GW, Tilak JP. Effects of prenatal cocaine on hearing, vision, growth, and behavior. Ann N Y Acad Sci 1998; 846: 12–28.

Fantel AG, Macphail BJ. The teratogenicity of cocaine. Teratology 1982; 26: 17–9.

Hume RFJ, Martin LS, Bottoms SF, et al. Vascular disruption birth defects and history of prenatal cocaine exposure: a case control study. Fetal Diagn Ther 1997; 12: 292–5.

Hunter ES, Kotch LE, Cefalo RC, Sadler TW. Effects of cocaine administration during early organogenesis on prenatal development and postnatal growth in mice. Fundam Appl Toxicol 1995; 28: 177–86.

Jacobson SW, Chiodo LM, Sokol RJ, Jacobson JL. Validity of maternal report of prenatal alcohol, cocaine, and smoking in relation to neurobehavioral outcome. Pediatrics 2002; 109: 815–25.

Joseph H, Stancliff S, Langrod J. Methadone maintenance treatment (MMT): a review of historical and clinical issues [review]. Mt Sinai J Med 2000; 67: 347–64.

Lipshultz SE, Frassica JJ, Orav EJ. Cardiovascular abnormalities in infants prenatally exposed to cocaine. J Pediatr 1991; 118: 44–51.

Loebstein R, Koren G. Pregnancy outcome and neurodevelopment of children exposed in utero to psychoactive drugs: the Motherisk experience. J Psychiatry Neurosci 1997; 22: 192–6.

Lutiger B, Graham K, Einarson TR, Koren G. Relationship between gestational cocaine use and pregnancy outcome: a meta-analysis. Teratology 1991; 44: 405–14.

Morgan RE, Garavan HP, Mactutus CF, Levitsky DA, Booze RM, Strupp BJ. Enduring effects of prenatal cocaine exposure on attention and reaction to errors. Behav Neurosci 2002; 116: 624–33.

Morild I, Stajic M. Cocaine and fetal death. Forensic Sci Int 1990; 47: 181–9.

Oats JN, Beischer NA, Breheny JE, Pepperell RJ. The outcome of pregnancies complicated by narcotic drug addiction. Aust N Z J Obstet Gynaecol 1984; 24: 14–6.

Ornoy A, Segal J, Bar-Hamburger R, Greenbaum C. Developmental outcome of school-age children born to mothers with heroin dependency: importance of environmental factors. Dev Med Child Neurol 2001; 43: 668–75.

Rizk B, Atterbury JL, Groome LJ. Reproductive risks of cocaine. Hum Reprod Update 1996; 2: 43–55.

Yanai J, Steingart RA, Snapir N, Gvaryahu G, Rozenboim II, Katz A. The relationship between neural alterations and behavioral deficits after prenatal exposure to heroin. Ann NY Acad Sci 2000; 914: 402–11.

Zuckerman B, Frank DA, Mayes L. Cocaine-exposed infants and developmental outcomes: "crack kids" revisited. JAMA 2002; 287: 1990–1.

19 Appendix

Further Reading

Benacerraf BR. Ultrasound of fetal syndromes. Philadelphia: Churchill Livingstone, 1998.

Bisset RAL, Khan AN, Thomas NB. Differential diagnosis in obstetric and gynecologic ultrasound. Philadelphia: Saunders, 1997.

Chervenak FA, Isaacson GC, Campbell S. Ultrasound in obstetrics and gynecology. Boston: Little, Brown, 1993.

Gilbert-Barnes E. Potter's pathology of the fetus and infant. St. Louis: Mosby, 1997.

Hickey J, Goldberg F. Ultrasound review of obstetrics and gynecology. Philadelphia: Lippincott–Raven, 1996.

Hofmann V, Deeg KH, Hoyer PF. Ultraschalldiagnostik in Pädiatrie and Kinderchirurgie. Stuttgart: Thieme, 1996.

Leiber B. Die klinischen Syndrome. 8th ed. Munich: Urban and Schwarzenberg, 1996.

O'Rahilly R, Müller F. Human embryology and teratology. 3rd ed. New York: Wiley-Liss, 2001.

Sanders RC. Structural fetal abnormalities: the total picture. St. Louis: Mosby, 1996.

Snijders RJM, Nicolaides KH. Ultrasound markers for fetal chromosomal defects. London: Parthenon, 1996.

Sohn C, Holzgreve W. Ultraschall in Gynäkologie and Geburtshilfe. Stuttgart: Thieme, 1995.

Skandalakis JE, Gray SW. Embryology for surgeons. 2nd ed. Baltimore: Williams and Wilkins, 1994.

Stevenson RE, Hall JG, Goodman RM. Human malformations and related anomalies. New York: Oxford University Press, 1993.

Wiedemann HR, Kunze J. Atlas der klinischen Syndrome. 4th ed. Stuttgart: Schattauer, 1995.

Wittkowski R, Prokop O, Ullrich E. Lexikon der Syndrome and Fehlbildungen. Berlin: Springer, 1995.

List of Abbreviations and Acronyms

AFI	amniotic fluid index
ASD	atrial septal defect
AV	atrioventricular
AVM	atrioventricular malformation
BPD	biparietal diameter
CCAM	congenital cystic adenomatoid malformation
CFM	color flow mapping
CHARGE	*c*oloboma, *h*eart disease, *a*tresia of choanae, *r*etarded mental development, *g*enital hypoplasia, *e*ar anomalies and deafness
CNS	central nervous system
COFS	cerebro-oculofacial-skeletal syndrome
CRL	crown–rump length
DORV	double-outlet right ventricle
ECG	electrocardiography
ECMO	extracorporeal membrane oxygenation
EEC	ectrodactyly–ectodermal dysplasia–clefting
FAIT	fetal alloimmune thrombocytopenia
FFU	femur–fibula–ulna (syndrome)
FISH	fluorescent in-situ hybridization
FOD	frontal occipital diameter
FTA-ABS	*f*luorescent *t*reponemal *a*ntibody, *abs*orbed (test)
HARDE	*h*ydrocephalus, *a*gyria, *r*etinal *d*ysplasia, and *e*ncephalocele (syndrome)
β-HCG	α-human chorionic gonadotropin
ITP	idiopathic thrombocytopenic purpura
IUGR	intrauterine growth retardation
LEOPARD	*l*entigines, *E*CG abnormalities, *o*cular hypertelorism, *p*ulmonary stenosis, *a*bnormalities of genitalia, *r*etardation of growth, and *d*eafness (syndrome)

MURCS	*m*üllerian duct aplasia, *r*enal aplasia, and dysplasia of the *c*ervicothoracic *s*omites
NT	nuchal translucency
PANDAS	*p*ediatric *a*utoimmune *n*europsychiatric *d*isorders *a*ssociated with *s*treptococcal infection
PAPP-A	pregnancy-associated plasma protein-A
PCR	polymerase chain reaction
PDA	patent ductus arteriosus
PRF	pulse repetition frequency
SHORT	*s*hort stature, *h*yperextensibility of joints or hernia or both, *o*cular depression, *R*ieger anomaly, and *t*eething delayed (syndrome)
SLO	Smith–Lemli–Opitz (syndrome)
SRPS	short rib–polydactyly syndrome
SUA	single umbilical artery
TAR	thrombocytopenia–absent radius (syndrome)
TGA	transposition of the great arteries
TORCH	*t*oxoplasmosis, *o*ther (congenital syphilis and viruses), *r*ubella, *c*ytomegalovirus, and *h*erpes simplex virus
TRH	thyrotropin-releasing hormone
TSH	thyroid-stimulating hormone
TTTS	twin-to-twin transfusion syndrome
VACTERL	*v*ertebral abnormalities, *a*nal atresia, *c*ardiac abnormalities, *t*racheo-*e*sophageal fistula, *r*enal agenesis and dysplasia, and *l*imb defects
VATER	*v*ertebral defects, imperforate *a*nus, *t*racheo-*e*sophageal fistula, and *r*adial and renal dysplasia
VSD	ventricular septal defect

Table 19.**1** Differential diagnosis at the second screening

Fetoplacental unit		
Fetus/placenta		
✔ Number of fetuses?		
✔ Position of fetus?		
✔ Site of placenta?	Placenta previa	
Amniotic fluid volume		
✔ Oligohydramnios?	Growth restriction, premature rupture of membranes, obstructive uropathy	
✔ Polyhydramnios?	"Idiopathic" in 60–70% of cases, diabetes mellitus, esophageal atresia, other gastrointestinal atresias and stenosis, cardiac insufficiency, fetal anemia, disturbance in swallowing due to CNS damage, fetal hydrops, CCAM, diaphragmatic hernia, infections, chromosomal aberrations	
Birth canal		
✔ Length of cervical canal?		
✔ Funneling of internal cervical os?		

Continue ▶

Table 19.1 (Continue)

Fetal biometric assessment		
	✔ Biparietal head circumference?	
	✔ Fronto-occipital circumference?	*Below 5th centile:* Due date accurate? Microcephaly? *Above 95th centile:* Due date? Hydrocephalus?
	✔ Width of cerebral ventricles?	*Over 8–10 mm:* Obstructive hydrocephalus? Other indications of chromosomal aberrations? Prenatal infection? Serial ultrasound assessment
	✔ Size of cerebellum?	
	✔ Cisterna magna? (optional)	
	✔ Femur length?	*Below 5th centile:* Other stigmata of chromosomal disorders? Shortening of other long bones? Signs of skeletal dysplasia? Early sign of growth restriction? Possibly assessment of humerus, ulna and tibia
	✔ Thorax measurements?	Thorax circumference: Below 5th centile: correct estimation of delivery date? Early evidence of growth restriction?
	✔ Cardiac assessment: Ventricles? Great vessels?	Normal crossing over of the great vessels? Transposition of great arteries? Asymmetry of cardiac ventricles? Obstruction of outflow tract (Hypoplasia of the left heart? Pulmonary stenosis? Pulmonary atresia?)
Color flow Doppler imaging		
	✔ Resistance in umbilical artery?	*Increased:* Sign of early growth restriction?
	✔ Resistance in uterine arteries at the crossing of external iliac artery, uterine notch?	Increased resistance index with notch in both arteries? Increased resistance in only one artery with notching when the placenta is located laterally?
Screening of fetal organs and body regions		
	Central nervous system and eye	
	✔ Head shape normal?	
	✔ Brachycephaly?	Other signs of chromosomal aberrations?
	✔ Dolichocephaly?	Due to fetal position: (breech or transverse lie), widening of the cisterna magna, stigmata for trisomy 18
	✔ "Lemon sign"?	Neural tube defect? Within normal variation? (In approx. 1% of fetuses; also visualized as an artefact)
	✔ Cerebral ventricles: width? Symmetry?	
	✔ Hydrocephalus?	Neural tube defect, obstructive hydrocephalus, Dandy-Walker malformation, agenesis of the corpus callosum, hydranencephaly, holoprosencephaly, arachnoidal cysts, porencephaly, prenatal infection
	✔ Choroid plexus cysts?	Other signs of chromosomal aberrations?
	✔ Is the mid-echo normal?	Asymmetrical cranial malformation? Holoprosencephaly?
	✔ Cerebellar diameter?	*Below 5th centile:* Correct due date?
	✔ Is cisterna magna widened?	
	✔ Arnold-Chiari malformation?	Hypoplasia of the cerebellum? "Banana sign"?
	✔ Dandy-Walker cysts?	
	✔ Is the corpus callosum visible?	Agenesis of the corpus callosum? Other anomalies?
	✔ Is the cavum septi pellucidi visible?	Agenesis of the corpus callosum?
	✔ Eyes?	*Anophthalmia:* Trisomy 13, Goltz syndrome, Fraser syndrome, Goldenhar syndrome, Lenz microphthalmia syndrome, Waardenburg syndrome?

Continue ▶

Table 19.1 (Continue)

Screening of fetal organs and body regions		
	Face and neck	
	✔ Is the nose too small?	Chromosomal anomaly, holoprosencephaly
	✔ Mouth and jaw normal?	Cleft lip and cleft palate, isolated finding, chromosomal disorder?
	✔ Chin and facial profile normal?	Retrogenia? Within normal variation? Further anomalies?
	✔ Is the neck normal?	Chromosomal aberration? Pierre Robin sequence?
	✔ Cystic hygroma detected?	Trisomy 21, trisomy 18, trisomy 13, Turner syndrome and other anomalies
	✔ Evidence of goiter?	
	Thorax	
	✔ Position of the heart?	Altered due to diaphragmatic hernia (enterothorax)? Effected by cardiac anomalies and pulmonary malformations? Situs inversus?
	✔ Structure of the lungs?	
	✔ Intrathoracic cysts?	Teratoma, bronchogenic cysts, cystic dilation of the bronchus, diaphragmatic hernia, pericardial cysts, CCAM, hemangioma/lymphangioma, pulmonary sequestrum, pulmonary cysts, neuroblastoma, dilation of the blind end of esophagus in esophageal atresia, mediastinal meningocele, neuroenteric cysts
	✔ Hydrothorax?	Immune and nonimmune fetal hydrops, chylothorax, diaphragmatic hernia, CCAM, Pena–Shokeir syndrome, trisomy 21, Turner syndrome, Noonan syndrome, cardiac failure, hypoalbuminemia, infections
	The heart	
	✔ Is the heartbeat rhythmic?	Extrasystoles, tachycardia, ventricular flutter, atrial bigeminus, AV block with bradycardia, sinus bradycardia
	✔ Axis of the heart?	
	✔ Pericardial effusion?	
	✔ Four-chamber view?	*Left ventricle small or absent:* Left heart hypoplasia? Mitral atresia? Aortic atresia? Aortic stenosis? Coarctation of the aorta? *Right ventricle small or absent:* Pulmonary atresia? Tricuspid atresia? *Enlarged right ventricle:* Tricuspid incompetence? Pulmonary stenosis? Coarctation of the aorta? Constriction of ductus arteriosus (Botallo's duct)? Restrictive foramen ovale? Growth restriction? *Enlarged right atrium:* Ebstein anomaly? Tricuspid incompetence? Pulmonary stenosis? Pulmonary vein anomaly? Cardiac failure? *Absence of AV valve level:* AV canal with a large ASD/VSD?
	✔ Ventricular septum?	
	✔ Atrial septum/foramen ovale?	
	✔ AV valves?	
	✔ Great vessels, valves, vessel crossings?	*Small pulmonary artery:* Tetralogy of Fallot? Pulmonary atresia? Communicating trunk? *Small aortic bridge:* Aortic atresia? Coarctation of the aorta? Interruption of aortic arch? *Absence of vessel crossing:* Transposition of great arteries?
	✔ Is the arch of aorta visible?	Hypoplasia (coarctation of the aorta)? Interruption in continuity?

Continue ▶

Table 19.**1** (Continue)

Screening of fetal organs and body regions	
The abdomen	
✔ Ascites?	Pseudoascites (artefact), fetal hydrops, infections, meconium peritonitis, megacystis, cardiac insufficiency
✔ The abdominal wall?	Cord insertion normal? Abdominal wall continuous?
✔ "Tumor" in front of the abdomen?	Omphalocele, gastroschisis, bladder exstrophy, pentalogy of Cantrell
✔ Stomach?	*Stomach bubble absent:* transitory (reassessment); Esophageal atresia? VACTERL association? Diaphragmatic hernia?
✔ Bowel?	"Double bubble": transitory (peristaltic wave of the stomach)? Atresia or stenosis of the duodenum? Jejunal atresia? Annular pancreas? Stomach and an additional cystic lesion within the abdomen?
✔ Liver?	*Hepatomegaly:* infections, hemolysis, cardiac failure, hepatic tumors (hemangiomas, hamartomas, adenomas and others), metabolic disease, Beckwith–Wiedemann syndrome, Zellweger syndrome?
✔ Cystic lesions?	Mesenterial cysts, bowel duplication, cysts of the choledochus, hepatic hemangioma, hepatic cysts, pancreatic cysts, splenic cysts, ovarian cysts, bowel atresia, ileus
Urogenital tract	
✔ Kidneys?	Renal agenesis, ectopic kidneys, horse-shoe kidneys, hydronephrosis (obstructive), renal cysts, cystic kidneys, reflux
✔ Urinary bladder?	*Absence of the bladder:* repeat scan (has the bladder just been emptied?); bilateral renal agenesis, or bilateral renal dysplasia? Bladder exstrophy? *Megacystis:* urethral valve syndrome? Urethral atresia? Megacystis–microcolon syndrome? Prune belly sequence? Caudal regression syndrome?
✔ Umbilical vessels?	Three vessels? Singular umbilical artery? Renal anomalies? Other organ anomalies or signs of chromosomal disorders?
✔ Genitals?	*Genital anomalies:* Hydrocele of the testis? Ambiguous genitalia? Cloacal anomalies?
Skeleton	
✔ Vertebral column?	Normal? Neural tube defect? (Cranial signs of hydrocephalus, "banana sign," "lemon sign"?) Scoliosis?
✔ Extremities?	*Shortening of the long bones:* Familial disposition? Asymmetric growth restriction? Skeletal dysplasia syndrome?
✔ Symmetry of limbs?	Aplasia or dysplasia of the radius: Turner syndrome, Roberts syndrome, Holt–Oram syndrome, Fanconi anemia, VACTERL association, amniotic band sequence, TAR syndrome, Baller–Gerold syndrome, Levy–Hollister syndrome, fetal valproic acid syndrome?
✔ Hands/fingers?	Normal appearance? Absence of hand or fingers? Hexadactyly?
✔ Feet/toes?	*Club feet:* chromosomal disorders, skeletal dysplasia, neural tube defect, teratogens

Table 19.**2** Summary of differential diagnoses of fetal anomalies, in order of organs involved or body region affected

Disorder	Skull/vertebral column	Central nervous system	Facial findings	Neck/hygroma colli	Extremities, skeleton
Aarskog syndrome	Craniosynostosis or anomalies of cervical vertebrae		Round face, hypertelorism, mid face hypoplasia, short, broad nose, nostrils pointing to the front		Slim hands and feet, hypoplasia of end-phalanges, very short 5th finger
Aase syndrome			Occ. cleft lip and palate	Fetal hydrops in presence of anemia	Thumb with three phalanges, radius aplasia
Achondrogenesis, p. 147	Large head, reduction or absence of ossification in skull and vertebral column		Microgenia	Hygroma colli, possibly hydrops	Short limbs, short ribs, reduced mineralization, of the bones, narrow thorax
Achondroplasia, p. 148	Frontal bossing, large head, increased lumbar lordosis	Occ. widening of ventricles	Flattened nasal bridge		Short femurs and humerus, trident hands, fingers equally long
Adrenogenital syndrome type 3					
Alpha-thalassemia (Hb Bart)				Hydrops	
Amnion band sequence, p. 149		Encephalocele, anencephaly	Microgenia, facial clefts		Asymmetric amputation of limbs, occ. only constriction ring, club feet, clenched fist
Apert syndrome, p. 236	Craniosynostosis, brachycephaly, acrocephaly, flattened skull, fusion of cervical vertebrae 5 and 6	Agenesis of corpus callosum, widening of ventricles	Flat face, hypertelorism	1st trimester	Syndactyly (2nd, 3rd, and 4th fingers), broad thumb and toe, occ. anomalies of long bones
Arthrogryposis multiplex congenita, p. 150	Occ. microcephaly	Occ. widening of ventricles, lissencephaly, agenesis of corpus callosum and vermis			Fixed limbs, mostly bent, overextended knees, club feet, clenched fist, overlapping index finger, reduced movement
Asphyxiating thorax dysplasia (Jeune)					Shortening of long bones (2nd–/3rd trimester), narrow thorax, short ribs, occ. polydactyly

Cardiac findings	Thoraco-abdominal anomalies	Urogenital tract	Growth restriction	Other disorders	Prognosis
	Occasionally anomalies of the navel	Cryptorchism, penis surrounded by folds of scrotal tissue	Short stature, usually first evident after birth, long torso		Favorable; short stature; occasionally mild mental impairment
Occ. VSD			Growth restriction	Anemia due to reduced erythropoiesis in bone marrow	Favorable; occ. mild mental impairment
					Fatal (pulmonary hypoplasia)
					Fatal only in homozygous disease. Otherwise normal mental development and life expectancy, short stature up to 140 cm
		In girls. ambiguous genitalia at birth			In two-thirds, salt depletion syndrome; fatal without therapy, favorable if treated adequately
Cardiomegaly, pericardial effusion	Hepato-splenomegaly, pleural effusion				Hb Bart fatal; others courses range from asymptomatic to severe hemolytic anemia
	Gastroschisis, omphalocele				Depends on the severity of malformations
	Occ. cystic kidneys, hydronephrosis, cryptorchism				Variable; high mortality in the first years of life, sometimes mental impairment
		Occ. renal anomalies			Very variable, ranging from fatal forms to those with minimal handicap and normal life expectancy
					Usually fatal; after improvement of pulmonary damage, renal failure and small stature in survivors

Continue ▶

Table 19.**2** (Continue)

Disorder	Skull/vertebral column	Central nervous system	Facial findings	Neck/hygroma colli	Extremities, skeleton
Atelosteogenesis	Abnormal vertebral bodies, platyspondyly, narrow thorax		Depressed nasal bridge, microgenia		Short limbs, reduced mineralization, bent long bones, absence of fibula, club feet, contractures
Baller–Gerold syndrome	Craniosynostosis, vertebral body malformation	Occ. hydrocephalus, polymicrogyria, agenesis of corpus callosum	Hypertelorism, pronounced nasal bridge, microgenia or progenia, cleft palate		Mostly symmetrical anomaly of radius, hypoplasia of ulna, club hand, absence of thumb
Beckwith–Wiedemann syndrome, p. 239			Macroglossia		
Camptomelic dysplasia, p. 157	Occ. large biparietal	Dilation of ventricle	Cleft palate, hypertelorism, occ. microgenia, depressed nasal bridge		Bent femurs and tibias, fibula hypoplasia, club feet, bell-shaped thorax, hypoplasia of scapula
Cantrell's pentalogy	Occ. neural tube defects		Occ. facial anomalies	Hygroma colli	
Carpenter syndrome	Craniosynostosis, brachycephaly, acrocephaly (often asymmetrical)		Depressed nasal bridge, microgenia, deep-set ears		Clinodactyly, syndactyly, polydactyly
Caudal dysplasia (caudal regression syndrome), p. 250	Agenesis or dysgenesis of os sacrum, anomalies of lumbar vertebrae, pelvis defects, occ. neural tube defects		Occ. facial clefts		Femur hypoplasia, club feet, flexion contractures of lower limbs, reduced movements of lower limbs
CHARGE association, p. 241		Occ. widening of ventricle, Dandy–Walker variant	Hypoplasia of nose, occ. ear anomalies, microgenia, cleft lip or palate, hypertelorism, microphthalmia		
Chondrodysplasia punctata	Occ. microcephaly		Cataracts		Symmetrical shortening of proximal long bones, joint contractures, increased dotted mineralization of epiphysis

Cardiac findings	Thoraco-abdominal anomalies	Urogenital tract	Growth restriction	Other disorders	Prognosis
		Rarely, renal anomalies			Fatal outcome in neonatal stage
Occ. VSD, Fallot, aortic stenosis		Occ. ectopic kidneys, hydronephrosis, unilateral renal agenesis			Frequently sudden infant death, mental impairment in 30%
Cardiomegaly	Omphalocele, hepato-splenomegaly	Occ. cryptorchism, hypospadias		Hypoglycemia, frequent occurrence of blastoma in infancy, macrosomia	Perinatal mortality rate up to 20%
Occ. cardiac anomaly	Pulmonary hypoplasia	Occ. large kidneys, hydronephrosis, ambiguous genitalia		Hydramnios	Mostly fatal in the neonatal stage, otherwise chronic pulmonary disease
Cardiac anomaly, e.g. Fallot	Large abdominal wall defect with omphalocele and ectopia cordis				Unfavorable
Cardiac anomaly (ASD, VSD, Fallot, transposition)	Omphalocele	Hypogonadism, cryptorchism			Occ. developmental retardation
Occ. cardiac anomalies	Occ. pulmonary hypoplasia, anal atresia	Occ. renal anomalies, renal agenesis		Associated with maternal diabetes	Normal intelligence; prognosis depends on the severity of renal anomalies
Cardiac defects (Fallot, DORV, AV canal, VSD, ASD)	Occ. anal atresia, omphalocele, esophageal atresia	Micropenis, undescended testis, occ. renal anomalies			Perinatal mortality extremely high, mental impairment frequent
			Growth restriction	Ichthyosis of skin	Depending on the type, ranges from poor to relatively good, slightly short stature at a later stage

Continue ▶

Table 19.**2** (Continue)

Disorder	Skull/vertebral column	Central nervous system	Facial findings	Neck/hygroma colli	Extremities, skeleton
Cleidocranial dysplasia	Macrocephaly		Occ. hypoplasia of mid-face, hypertelorism		Shortening or absence of clavicle, hypoplasia of bony pelvis
COFS (cerebro-oculofacioskeletal syndrome, Pena–Shokeir II)	Microcephaly	Lissencephaly, agenesis of corpus callosum	Anophthalmia, microphthalmia, cataract, microgenia		Clenched fist, rocker-bottom feet, joint contractures
Conradi–Hünermann syndrome (chondrodysplasia punctata)	Kyphoscoliosis		Flattened nasal bridge, partial visual loss		Asymmetrical shortening of limbs, pathological calcification of femoral and humeral epiphysis
Cornelia de Lange syndrome, p. 243	Brachycephaly, microcephaly		Microgenia	First trimester	Micromelia, ulnar dysplasia, contractures of upper limbs, syndactyly, oligodactyly
Crouzon syndrome, p. 244	Craniosynostosis, abnormally shaped skull, cloverleaf skull	Occ. widening of ventricle, agenesis of corpus callosum	Beaked nose, microgenia, hypertelorism, hypotelorism, exophthalmos, cleft lip and palate		
Cystic fibrosis, p. 283					
Diastrophic dysplasia, p. 155	Kyphoscoliosis		Microgenia, cleft lip		Shortening of long bones, club feet, “hitchhiker thumb”
Di George sequence (see Shprintzen syndrome)					
EEC syndrome		Occ. semilobular holoprosencephaly	Cleft lip, possible cleft palate, facial clefts, occ. choanal atresia, microgenia, ear anomalies		Syndactyly, ectrodactyly
Ellis van Creveld syndrome, p. 244		Occ. Dandy–Walker cysts			Shortening of long bones, occ. club feet, polydactyly of hands, occ. of feet, small thorax, short ribs

Cardiac findings	Thoraco-abdominal anomalies	Urogenital tract	Growth restriction	Other disorders	Prognosis
					Short stature, normal intelligence
		Renal anomalies	Growth restriction		Fatal; life expectancy of up to 3 years
				Affected females show skin changes	Fatal in the neonatal stage; survivors have small stature
VSD, ASD		Maldescended testis, hypospadias	After 20 weeks of gestation		Mild to moderate mental impairment, growth restriction
					Mostly normal mental development, hearing loss and atrophy of optic nerve possible
	Echogenic bowel, dilated loops of bowel and meconium peritonitis (3rd trimester)				Chronic disease progression; as yet no effective therapy
Cardiac anomaly					Rarely, fatal outcome in neonatal stage; usually normal intelligence and life expectancy
		Megaureter, ureterocele, hydronephrosis, renal aplasia, genital anomalies			Anomalies of teeth, eye problems; intelligence usually normal
Cardiac malformations		Occ. cryptorchism			Infant mortality up to 50 %, normal intelligence; adult height 105–160 cm

Continue ▶

Table 19.2 (Continue)

Disorder	Skull/vertebral column	Central nervous system	Facial findings	Neck/hygroma colli	Extremities, skeleton
Fanconi anemia	Occ. microcephaly	Occ. widening of ventricles, agenesis of corpus callosum			Short radius, finger anomalies
Femur–fibula–ulna (FFU) complex					Hypoplasia or absence of femur and fibula, especially unilateral; absence of arms, finger anomalies, missing fingers
Femur hypoplasia–facial dysmorphism syndrome	Anomalies of vertebral bodies, sacral dysplasia		Microgenia, cleft palate, deep-set ears		Shortened and bent femur (also unilateral), occ. humeral hypoplasia, club feet
Fraser syndrome			Cryptophthalmus, anomalies of nose and ear, stenosis or atresia of larynx, facial clefts		Syndactyly
Freeman–Sheldon syndrome (whistling face), p. 245	Microcephaly, kyphoscoliosis		Raised forehead, narrow nose, deep-set ears, long philtrum, small mouth		Ulna deviation of hands, flexion deformities of fingers, contractures of hips and knees, club feet
Fryns syndrome		Widening of ventricles, Dandy–Walker cysts, agenesis of corpus callosum	Microgenia, cleft lip, cleft palate, ear anomalies, occ. microphthalmia	Occ. cystic hygroma, fetal hydrops	Occ. hypoplasia of fingers
Goldenhar symptom complex, p. 248	Hemivertebrae (cervical and thoracic)	Occ. widening of ventricles	Mandibular hypoplasia, facial asymmetry, microphthalmia, ear anomalies, facial clefts		
Goltz–Gorlin syndrome	Microcephaly, vertebral anomalies	Ventricle dilation, calcification of falx cerebri, occ. agenesis of corpus callosum			Short 4th metacarpal, rib deformities, scoliosis, syndactyly, polydactyly
Hallermann–Streiff syndrome	Vertebral anomalies, scoliosis		Microgenia		
Holt–Oram syndrome, p. 249	Occ. vertebral anomalies				Phocomelia, radial hypoplasia, humeral and ulnar anomalies, absent thumb, syndactyly, anomaly of clavicle

Cardiac findings	Thoraco-abdominal anomalies	Urogenital tract	Growth restriction	Other disorders	Prognosis
Occ. cardiac anomalies	Occ. gastro-intestinal obstruction	Urinary tract and genital anomalies		Pancytopenia from infancy	80% fatality up to 12 years of age; possibly subclinical course, small stature, developmental retardation
					Normal intelligence, normal life expectancy
		Anomalies of urinary tract		Associated with maternal diabetes	Normal intelligence
	Ascites	Genital anomalies, urinary tract malformations, renal agenesis			Mental handicap, increased rate of still birth
			Intrauterine growth restriction		Usually normal intelligence and life expectancy, short stature
Occ. cardiac anomalies	Diaphragmatic hernia, intestinal malrotation, pulmonary hypoplasia	Renal cysts, anomalies of uterus, cryptorchism, hypospadias	Large birth weight	Hydramnios	Fatal outcome in neonatal stage. Mental impairment expected in survivors
Occ. cardiac defects		Occ. renal anomalies			Frequently mental handicap
Occ. heart anomalies		Occ. renal anomalies		Affected females have focal dermal hypoplasia, ocular and dental anomalies	Mental impairment is frequent
					Small stature, premature aging
Cardiac anomalies: ASD, VSD, persistent Botallo's duct				Disturbance of cardiac conduction system	Depends on the severity of cardiac anomalies; normal intelligence

Continue ▶

Table 19.**2** (Continue)

Disorder	Skull/vertebral column	Central nervous system	Facial findings	Neck/hygroma colli	Extremities, skeleton
Hydrolethalus syndrome, p. 239	Neural tube defects	Widening of ventricle	Microgenia, cleft lip and palate, deep-set ears		Club feet, polydactyly, doubling of great toe
Hypochondroplasia, p. 156	Macrocephaly, occ. frontal bossing, narrowing of the lumbar spinal column		Occ. cataract		Mild shortening of long bones (3rd trimester), occ. polydactyly of feet
Infantile polycystic kidney disease			Microgenia		
Ivemark syndrome (II)		CNS anomalies			
Jarcho–Levin syndrome	Anomalies of vertebral bodies, kyphoscoliosis, absent or fused ribs, occ. neural tube defects				
Joubert syndrome		Dandy–Walker malformation	Microgenia	Hygroma colli	Polydactyly
Klippel–Feil sequence	Fused cervical vertebrae, kyphoscoliosis, spina bifida occulta	Occ. hydrocephalus	Short neck, occ. cleft palate, microphthalmia		Anomalies of ribs
Klippel–Trenaunay syndrome, p. 251			Occ. asymmetrical facial hypertrophy		Limb hypertrophy, asymmetry
Kniest dysplasia	Thoracic kyphoscoliosis		Exophthalmos, flattened nasal bridge, frequently cleft palate		Short limbs; appear to arise directly from joints
Larsen syndrome, p. 253	Dysraphia, scoliosis, vertebral anomalies		Depressed nose, cleft palate, hypertelorism, occ. cleft lip		Hyperextension of knee, dislocation of hip, knee and elbow, club feet
LEOPARD syndrome			Hypertelorism, progenia		Occ. skeletal anomalies

Cardiac findings	Thoraco-abdominal anomalies	Urogenital tract	Growth restriction	Other disorders	Prognosis
VSD, AV canal				Hydramnios	Fatal outcome in neonatal period
					Normal life expectancy; adult height varies, small stature due to shortening of short bones
Cardiac anomalies, e.g., VSD	Hepatic fibrosis	Enlarged echogenic kidneys, major symptom oligohydramnios			Renal failure in infancy, Potter sequence/neonatal death
Severe cardiac defect, situs inversus	Agenesis of spleen			Frequent sepsis	Depends on cardiac anomaly
	Protruding abdomen (short vertebral column); occ. single umbilical artery	Occ. genital anomalies, cryptorchism, hydronephrosis	Occ. intrauterine growth restriction		Disproportionate small stature, in severe form respiratory distress
		Multiple renal cysts			Neonatal respiratory distress, developmental retardation
Occ. cardiac anomaly		Often unilateral renal agenesis, hydronephrosis, ectopic kidney			Depends on the severity of malformations
	Occ. hemangioma, lymphectasia				Usually good; occ. severe cosmetic problems
				Myopia, hardness of hearing	Normal life expectancy with physical handicap, adult height 105–155 cm
Occ. cardiac defect	Occ. tracheomalacia				Normal intelligence, respiratory difficulty in newborn, secondary deformities of joints
Cardiac anomaly, e.g., pulmonary stenosis, aortic stenosis		Occ. genital dysplasia	Occ. short stature	Multiple spotting of skin, varying severity of hearing loss	Depends on the severity of the syndrome

Continue ▶

Table 19.2 (Continue)

Disorder	Skull/vertebral column	Central nervous system	Facial findings	Neck/hygroma colli	Extremities, skeleton
Majewski syndrome (SRPS type II)		Occ. hypoplasia of vermis	Facial clefts		Shortening of long bones, polydactyly, narrow thorax, short ribs
Meckel–Gruber syndrome, p. 169	Microcephaly	Widening of ventricles, posterior encephalocele, cerebellar hypoplasia, agenesis of corpus callosum, Dandy–Walker cysts, Arnold–Chiari malformation	Microgenia, cleft palate, microphthalmia		Polydactyly
Metatropic dysplasia	Large biparietal, platyspondyly, kyphoscoliosis	Occ. ventricle dilation			Shortened limbs with disproportionate long hands and feet, narrow thorax
Miller–Dieker syndrome, p. 258	Microcephaly (late)	Absence of gyri, dilation of ventricle			
Mohr syndrome (orofaciodigital syndrome type II) , p. 259		Occ. ventricular dilation, porencephaly, encephalocele, lipoma, agenesis of corpus callosum	Microgenia, facial clefts, broad nose, split nasal tip, tumors of tongue		Polysyndactyly, splitting of big toe, clinodactyly of 5th finger
Multiple pterygium syndrome, fatal	Occ. microcephaly	Occ. dilation of ventricle	Microgenia, hypertelorism, cleft palate	Hygroma colli, cystic pterygium colli, occ. hydrops	Flexion contractures of all limb joints, narrow thorax
MURCS association, p. 263	Vertebral anomalies of C5, T1, occ. rib deformities, scapula anomaly	Occ. cerebellar cysts, encephalocele	Occ. facial and ear anomalies, microgenia, cleft lip and palate		Occ. malformations of upper extremities
Muscle–eye–brain disease			Infantile glaucoma, congenital myopia		
Nager syndrome, p. 264	Occ. malformations of ribs and vertebrae		Microgenia, underdevelopment of lower jaw, ear anomalies, occ. cleft lip		Short radius, reduction defect of radial part of limb, club feet, syndactyly, clinodactyly
Neu–Laxova syndrome, p. 265	Microcephaly	Lissencephaly, corpus callosum agenesis, cerebral and cerebellar hypoplasia, occ. Dandy–Walker cysts, dilation of ventricles	Microgenia, hypertelorism, exophthalmos, absent eye lids, cataract, microphthalmia, occ. facial clefts	Short neck, rarely hydrops	Short limbs, edema of hands and feet, flexion contractures

Cardiac findings	Thoraco-abdominal anomalies	Urogenital tract	Growth restriction	Other disorders	Prognosis
		Occ. renal anomalies			Fatal outcome in neonatal stage (pulmonary hypoplasia)
Cardiac anomaly		Cystic renal dysplasia, cryptorchism			One-third of cases stillbirths, others die in neonatal stage
					If diagnosed prenatally, severe disease and high mortality
Cardiac anomaly	Duodenal atresia	Renal dysplasia	IUGR		Severe mental impairment
		Occ. renal anomalies			Normal life expectancy; prognosis depends on severity of cranial anomalies
Occ. cardiac defect		Occ. hydronephrosis			Fatal due to pulmonary hypoplasia; other nonfatal forms exist
		Renal agenesis or ectopy, hypoplasia of uterus and upper vagina			Depends on renal anomalies
			Macrosomia		Severe reduction in muscle tone, mental impairment
					Mostly favorable
Occ. heart defects		Hypoplasia of genitals	Early severe growth restriction	Hydramnios	Fatal; intrauterine fetal death or neonatal death

Continue ▶

Table 19.**2** (Continue)

Disorder	Skull/vertebral column	Central nervous system	Facial findings	Neck/hygroma colli	Extremities, skeleton
Noonan syndrome, p. 265	Hemivertebrae		Hypertelorism, deep-set ears	1st and 2nd trimester, cystic hygroma with hydrops	
Osteogenesis imperfecta, p. 159	Demineralization of skull, intercalated bone			Occ. hygroma colli	Short limbs, fractures, narrow thorax, possibly bell-shaped thorax, reduced fetal movements
Osteopetrosis	Macrocephaly	Hydrocephalus			
Otopalatodigital syndrome type I	Incomplete closure of arches of isolated vertebrae		Broad forehead, hypertelorism, supraorbital folds, broad nasal bridge, flat mid-face, microgenia, cleft palate		Short and stubby end phalanges of hands and feet (frog hand), swelling of large joints and reduction in movement
Otopalatodigital syndrome type II	Widening of cranial sutures		Cleft palate, microgenia, microstomia, hypertelorism		Clenched fist, short thumb, broad great toe
Pena–Shokeir syndrome, p. 267			Microgenia, depressed nasal bridge, hypertelorism, occ. cleft palate		Multiple joint contractures, ulnar deviation of hands, club feet, akinesia syndrome, thoracic hypoplasia, clenched hands, camptodactyly
Perlman syndrome					
Peters-plus syndrome	Occ. microcephaly	Occ. hydrocephalus, agenesis of corpus callosum	Microgenia, round, broad face, clouding of cornea		Short-limb dwarfism, clinodactyly of the 5th finger
Pfeiffer syndrome (acrofacial dysostosis)	Craniosynostosis, brachycephaly, acrocephaly, occ. cloverleaf skull, fused vertebral bodies	Occ. dilation of ventricle	Depressed nasal bridge, hypertelorism, occ. choanal atresia		Broad thumbs and big toes, partial syndactyly
Pierre Robin sequence, p. 270			Microgenia, cleft palate		
Potter sequence	Occ. neural tube defects	Occ. widening of ventricles			Narrow thorax

Cardiac findings	Thoraco-abdominal anomalies	Urogenital tract	Growth restriction	Other disorders	Prognosis
Pulmonary stenosis, VSD, ASD		Cryptorchism, micropenis	Short stature, frequently after birth		Varies; 25 % have mental impairment
					Type II fatal; otherwise variable physical handicap due to fractures, premature deafness; forms with blue sclera
	Hepato-splenomegaly			Pancytopenia, blindness, hardness of hearing	30 % live up to 6 years; improvement of prognosis after bone-marrow transplantation
			Occ. short stature	Hardness of hearing, almost always affects males	Normal life expectancy; mostly mild mental impairment
				Usually affects males	Mostly severe mental handicap
Occ. cardiac anomalies	Pulmonary hypoplasia	Cryptorchism		Hydramnios	Intrauterine or neonatal death
		Hypertrophy of organs	Macrosomia	Hydramnios	Frequently neonatal death
Occ. VSD, ASD		Urogenital anomalies		Occ. hydramnios, SUA	Initially delayed development, later normal intelligence, adult height 128–155 cm
	Occ. anomalies of trachea				Variable expression
					Increased neonatal mortality, thereafter favorable prognosis
Occ. cardiac anomalies	Pulmonary hypoplasia, occ. esophageal atresia, duodenal atresia, anal atresia	Absent or nonfunctioning kidneys			Fatal outcome

Continue ▶

Table 19.**2** (Continue)

Disorder	Skull/vertebral column	Central nervous system	Facial findings	Neck/hygroma colli	Extremities, skeleton
Prune belly sequence					
Roberts syndrome	Microcephaly, occ. craniosynostosis	Occ. widening of ventricles, encephalocele	Microgenia, cleft lip, hypertelorism, occ. microphthalmia, cataract	Occ. cystic hygroma	Phocomelia, short radius, hypoplasia or aplasia of femur, tibia and fibula, flexion contractures of all limb joints
Rokitansky–Küster–Mayer complex					
Russell–Silver syndrome, p. 272	Relative microcephaly		Frontal bossing		Asymmetry, shortened long bones, syndactyly (2nd and 3rd toes), clinodactyly
Saldino–Noonan and Naumoff syndrome (SRPS types I and III), p. 168		Occ. CNS anomalies	Cleft lip and palate, flattened nasal bridge		Micromelia, polydactyly, very short ribs, narrow thorax
Schinzel–Giedion syndrome	Shortened skull base, intercalated bone		Flattening of midface, choanal atresia		Postaxial polydactyly, club feet
Seckel syndrome	Microcephaly	Occ. agenesis of corpus callosum	Microgenia, prominent nose		Deformities of knee and hips, dislocation of joints (head of radius)
Shprintzen syndrome	Microcephaly	Occ. holoprosencephaly	Microgenia, cleft palate, occ. Pierre Robin sequence		Shortening of long bones
Simpson–Golabi–Behmel syndrome	Macrocephaly				Occ. hexadactyly
Sirenomelia	Anomalies of vertebrae (lumbar, sacrum)		Potter face		Severely deformed and fused lower limbs

Cardiac findings	Thoraco-abdominal anomalies	Urogenital tract	Growth restriction	Other disorders	Prognosis
	Defect of abdominal musculature (secondary)	Severe dilation of urinary bladder, megaureters, cryptorchism		Affects mostly males (95%)	Increased neonatal mortality due to pulmonary hypoplasia
Occ. heart anomalies		Occ. renal and genital anomalies			Stillbirth in 20%, mental impairment in about 50%
		Rudimentary uterus, renal anomalies			Primary sterility in normal female phenotype
			IUGR		Mostly normal intelligence
Cardiac anomalies (transposition, DORV, AV canal)	Intestinal atresia, anal atresia	Renal hypoplasia or polycystic kidneys, ambiguous genitalia			Fatal in neonatal stage (pulmonary hypoplasia)
Cardiac anomalies		Renal anomalies			Mostly fatal; otherwise severe developmental handicap
			Early growth restriction		Short stature, mentally handicapped
Cardiac anomalies (anomalies of trunk)	Occ. umbilical hernia	Occ. cryptorchism, hypospadias	Occ. growth restriction		Variable
Cardiac anomalies (VSD)	Enlargement of organs		Macrosomia		Increased early mortality; mental impairment possible
Cardiac anomalies	Defects of abdominal wall, anal atresia, thorax anomalies, pulmonary hypoplasia	Renal agenesis, absence of genitals			Depends on the severity of renal anomalies

Continue ▶

Table 19.**2** (Continue)

Disorder	Skull/vertebral column	Central nervous system	Facial findings	Neck/hygroma colli	Extremities, skeleton
Smith–Lemli–Opitz syndrome, p. 273	Microcephaly	Occ. hypoplasia of cerebellum	Occ. microgenia, cleft palate, cataract	1st trimester	Clenched fist, pes valgus, syndactyly (2nd and 3rd toes), polydactyly
Sotos syndrome	Macrocephaly	Discrete dilation of ventricles			Oversized hands and feet
Spondyloepiphyseal dysplasia	Shortening of vertebral column				Relatively long limbs, normal-sized hands and feet
Thanatophoric dysplasia, p. 171	Cloverleaf skull		Flattened nasal bridge		Bent and extreme shortening of long bones, fibulae shorter than tibiae, narrow thorax
Thrombocytopenia–absent radius syndrome, p. 277		Occ. vermis hypoplasia	Occ. microgenia		Bilateral absence of radii with hypoplasia or absence of ulnae in presence of thumbs, abnormal humerus, anomalies and dislocation of lower limbs
Townes–Brocks syndrome (anus–hand–ear)			Microtia, ear tags, occ. microgenia, cleft lip and palate		Polydactyly, thumb with three phalanges, absence of thumb, occ. absent toes, rarely aplasia of radius
Treacher–Collins syndrome			Microgenia, ear anomaly, ear tags, choanal atresia, cleft palate, notching of eyelids, underdevelopment of cheek bone		
Tuberous sclerosis, p. 278		Intracranial calcifications			
VACTERL association, p. 279	Hemivertebrae, scoliosis, occ. spinal dysraphism				Hypoplasia or aplasia of radius, occ. polydactyly, syndactyly, anomalies of lower limbs

Cardiac findings	Thoraco-abdominal anomalies	Urogenital tract	Growth restriction	Other disorders	Prognosis
Occ. cardiac anomalies		Hydronephrosis, renal cysts, renal hypoplasia; micropenis, cryptorchism, hypospadias, ambiguous genitalia	Late growth restriction		Increased infant mortality rate; mental impairment
Frequent cardiac anomalies			Macrosomia		Normal adult height; mental handicap
				Frequently myopia, retinal ablation	Adult height usually less than 140 cm; normal intelligence
Occ. cardiac anomaly		Occ. hydronephrosis			Fatal in neonatal stage (pulmonary hypoplasia)
Occ. cardiac anomalies: Fallot, ASD		Occ. renal malformations		Thrombocytopenia	High mortality in first year of life; mental development in survivors depends on neonatal intracranial bleeding
	Anal atresia	Urinary tract obstruction		Middle ear deafness	Depends on the severity of anomalies; normal intelligence
					Difficulty in hearing; normal intelligence
Rhabdomyomas		Occ. renal cysts			In 80%, fits and mental impairment
Cardiac defects	Esophageal atresia, anal atresia	Hydronephrosis, cystic kidneys, occ. anomalies of genitalia			Survival in 75%; mostly with normal intelligence

Continue ▶

Table 19.2 (Continue)

Disorder	Skull/vertebral column	Central nervous system	Facial findings	Neck/hygroma colli	Extremities, skeleton
Van der Woude syndrome			Cleft lip and palate, dimple in lower lip or protrusion, hypodontia		
Walker–Warburg syndrome, p. 282	Microcephaly	Agyria, lissencephaly, ventricle dilation, occipital encephalocele, Dandy–Walker cysts, agenesis of corpus callosum	Microphthalmia, cataract, occ. cleft lip		
Weaver syndrome	Macrocephaly	Occ. dilation of ventricles	Hypertelorism, broad nasal bridge, big ears		Club feet, clinodactyly of toes, camptodactyly of fingers
X-chromosomal hydrocephalus	Macrocephaly possible	Dilation of ventricles (lateral and third)			Adducted thumbs, occ. thumb hypoplasia

Cardiac findings	Thoraco-abdominal anomalies	Urogenital tract	Growth restriction	Other disorders	Prognosis
					Good
		Occ. anomalies of genitalia			Fatal in first years of life
				Macrosomia	Disturbance in mental development (not mandatory)
					Variable, mental impairment, spasticity

Table 19.3 Summary of differential diagnoses in chromosomal disorders

Chromosomal disorder	Skull/vertebral column	CNS	Facial findings	Hygroma colli/neck
4 p deletion (Wolf–Hirschhorn syndrome), p. 215	Cranial asymmetry, microcephaly	Agenesis of corpus callosum	Micrognathia, hypertelorism, cleft lip and/or cleft palate	
11 q deletion (Jacobsen syndrome), p. 175	Trigonocephaly, microcephaly	Occ. widening of ventricles, holoprosencephaly	Hypertelorism, flattened nasal bridge, micrognathia, ear anomalies	
Tetrasomy 12 p mosaicism (Pallister–Killian syndrome), p. 179		Hypoplasia of cerebellum	Facial dysmorphism, hypertelorism, deep-set ears	Hygroma colli
Triploidy, p. 180	Myelomeningocele	Dilation of ventricles, Dandy–Walker cysts, agenesis of corpus callosum, holoprosencephaly	Hypertelorism, microphthalmia, micrognathia	Cystic hygroma colli
Trisomy 9 mosaicism, p. 186	Microcephaly, neural tube defects	Anomaly of cerebellum	Cleft lip and/or cleft palate, micrognathia, microphthalmia	
Trisomy 10 mosaicism, p. 187			Hypertelorism, cleft lip and/or cleft palate, micrognathia	Hygroma colli
Trisomy 13 (Patau syndrome), p. 187	Microcephaly, neural tube defect	Holoprosencephaly, widening of ventricles, dilation of cisterna magna, agenesis of corpus callosum	Cleft lip and palate, hypoplasia of mid-face, cyclopia, hypotelorism, microphthalmia	Hygroma colli
Trisomy 18 (Edwards syndrome), p. 193	Occ. meningomyelocele	Agenesis of corpus callosum, cysts of choroid plexus, anomalies of posterior fossa, occ. ventricular dilation	Micrognathia, deep-set ears, hypertelorism, occ. cleft lip and palate	Cystic hygroma colli
Trisomy 21 (Down syndrome), p. 204	Brachycephaly	Widening of ventricles	Flat facial profile, small ears	Hygroma colli
Trisomy 22			Cleft lip and palate	Occ. hygroma colli
Turner syndrome (45, XO), p. 211				Cystic hygroma colli

Extremities, skeletal findings	Cardiac findings	Thoracoabdominal anomalies	Urogenital findings	Growth restriction
Club feet	Cardiac defect—e.g., VSD	Diaphragmatic hernia	Hypospadias, cryptorchism	Yes
Joint contractures, occ. clinodactyly of 5th finger	Cardiac anomaly		Hypospadias, cryptorchism, occ. renal anomalies	Yes
Shortening of femur and humerus, clinodactyly of 5th finger	Cardiac defects, dextrocardia	Diaphragmatic hernia, omphalocele, edema of torso	Hydronephrosis	
Club feet, syndactyly of 3rd and 4th fingers	Cardiac anomaly	Omphalocele	Hydronephrosis, hypospadias	Early severe growth restriction
Flexion deformities of fingers, malpositioning of foot	Cardiac anomaly	Diaphragmatic hernia	Multicystic renal disease, hydronephrosis, cryptorchism	Yes
Polydactyly, syndactyly of toes	Cardiac anomalies		Cryptorchism	Yes
Flexion deformities of fingers, aplasia of radius, polydactyly	Cardiac anomalies, “white spots”	Omphalocele, echogenic bowel	Echogenic, enlarged kidneys	
Clenched fist, overlapping index finger, club feet, rocker-bottom feet, short radius	Cardiac anomalies	Omphalocele, diaphragmatic hernia	Hydronephrosis, cryptorchism	Yes
Short femur and humerus, clinodactyly, short middle phalanx of 5th finger, wide angle of iliac bones	Cardiac anomaly, especially ASD, VSD, AV canal, Fallot, “white spots”	Duodenal atresia, echogenic bowel, SUA	Hydronephrosis	
Occ. hypoplasia of fingers	Cardiac anomaly	Bowel anomaly, anal atresia	Renal anomalies	
Short femur	Aortic isthmus stenosis	Hydrops	Horseshoe kidneys	

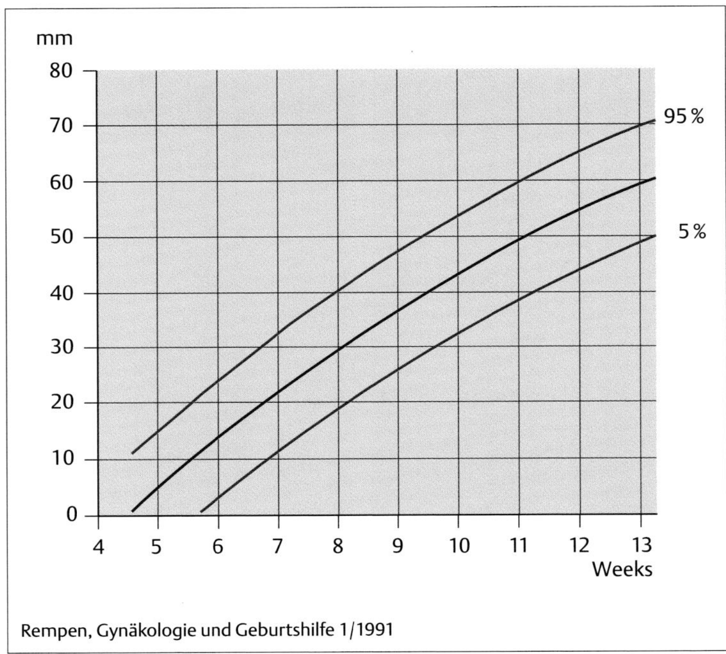

Fig. 19.**1** Gestational sac, average diameter.

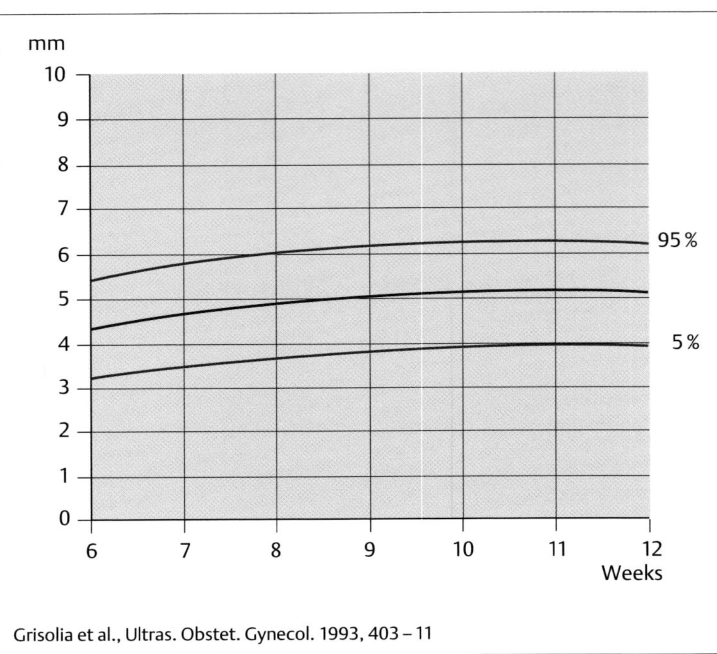

Fig. 19.**2** Yolk sac, average diameter.

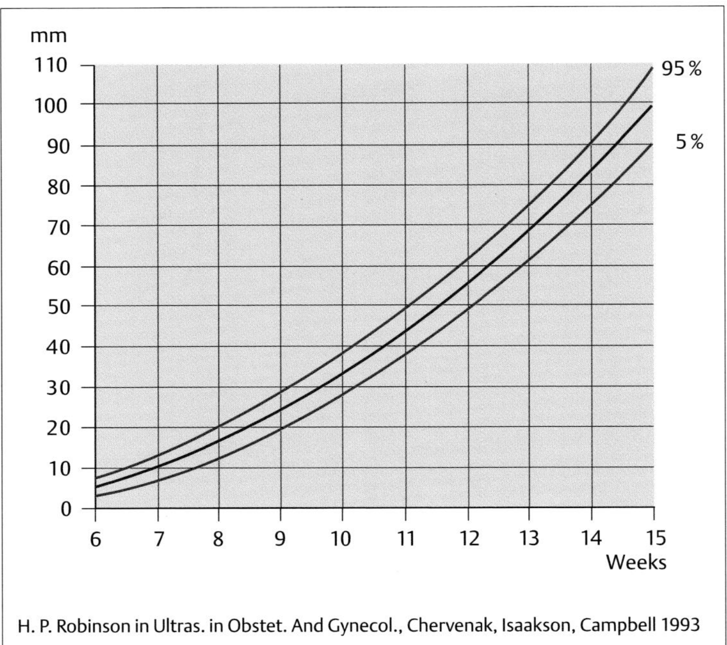

Fig. 19.**3** Crown–rump length.

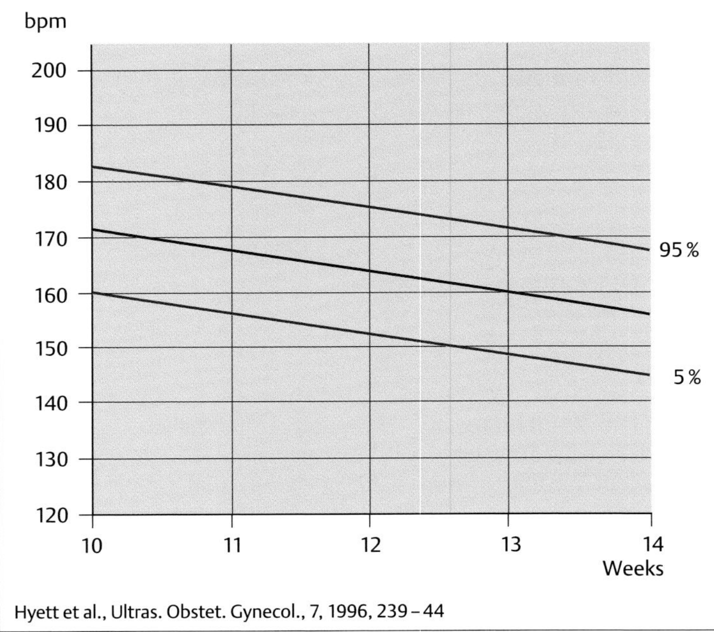

Fig. 19.**4** Fetal heart rate (1st trimester).

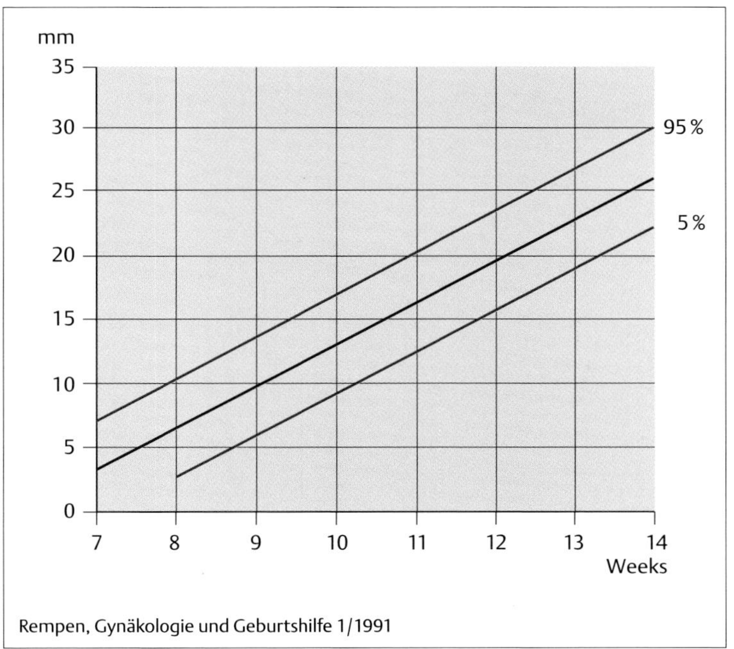

Fig. 19.**5** Biparietal diameter (1st trimester).

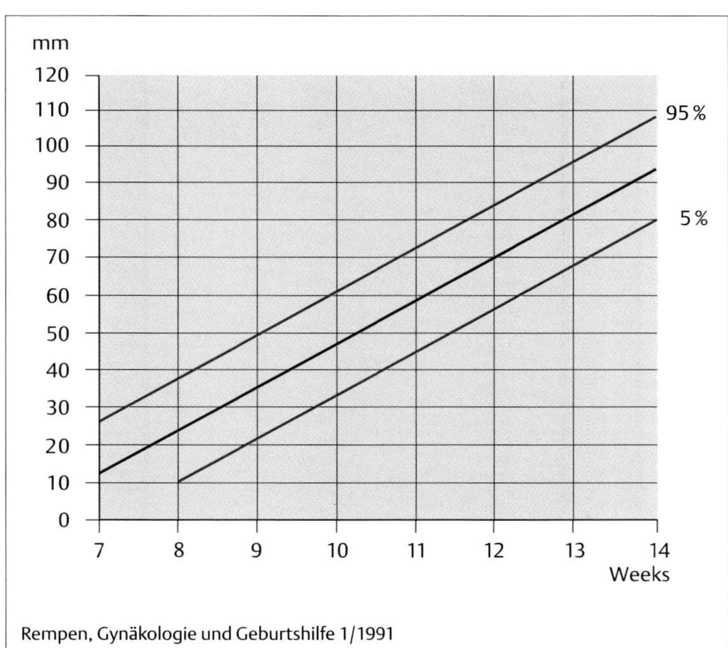

Fig. 19.**6** Head circumference (1st trimester).

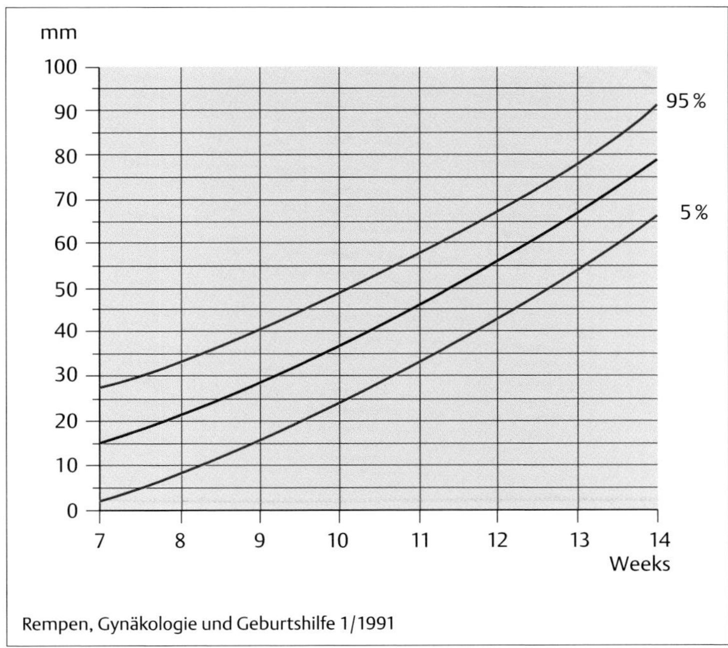

Fig. 19.**7** Abdominal circumference (1st trimester).

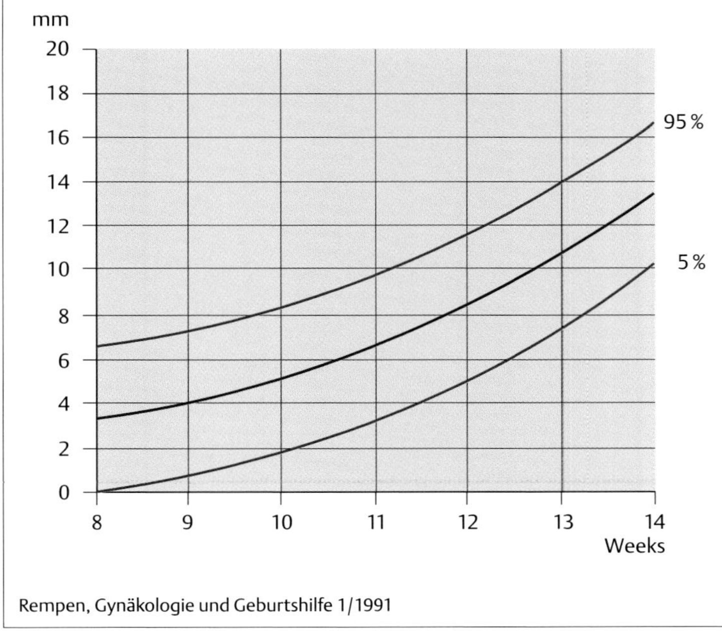

Fig. 19.**8** Femur length (1st trimester).

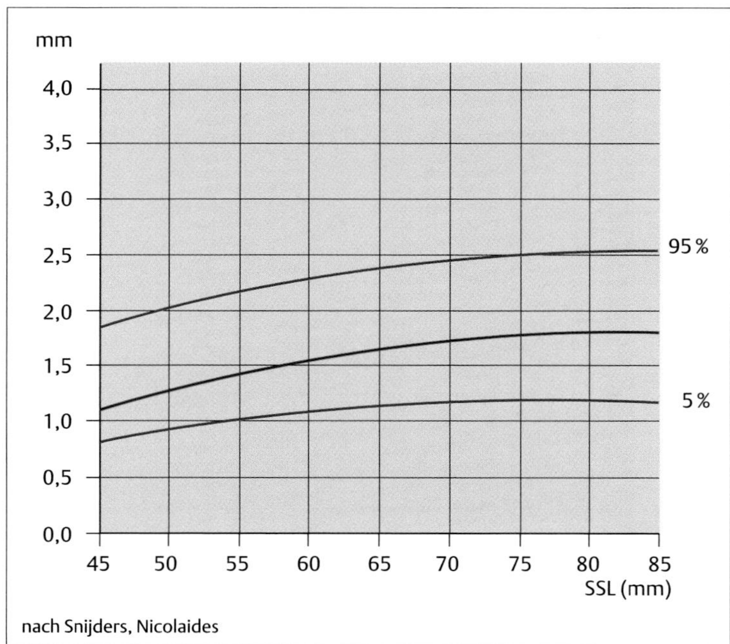

Fig. 19.**9** Nuchal translucency.

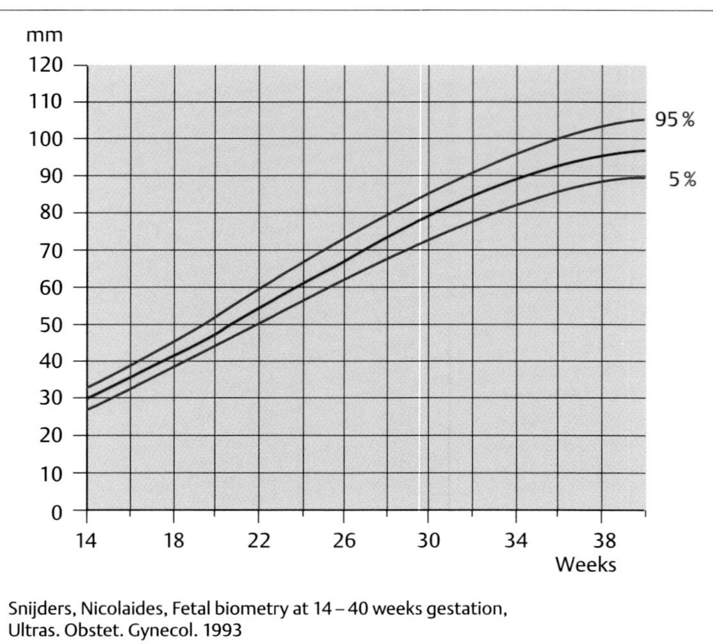

Fig. 19.**10** Biparietal diameter.

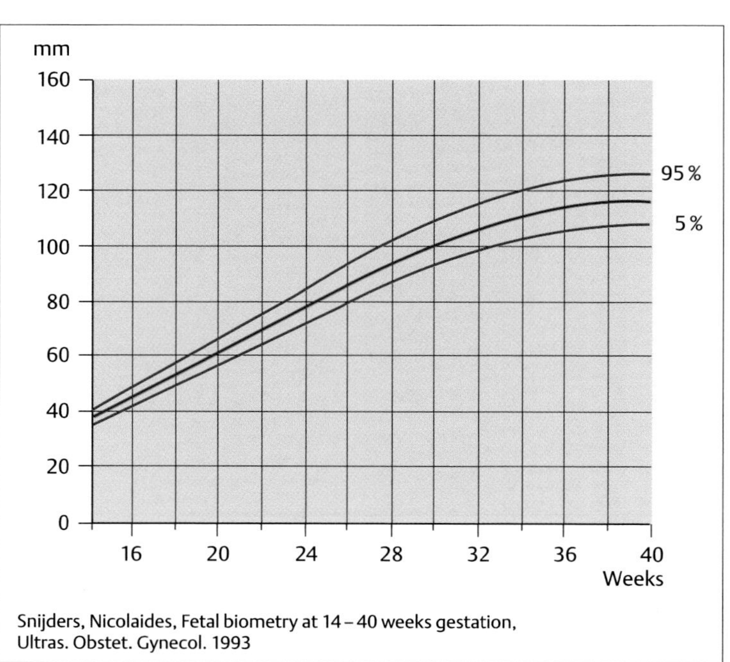

Fig. 19.**11** Fronto-occipital diameter.

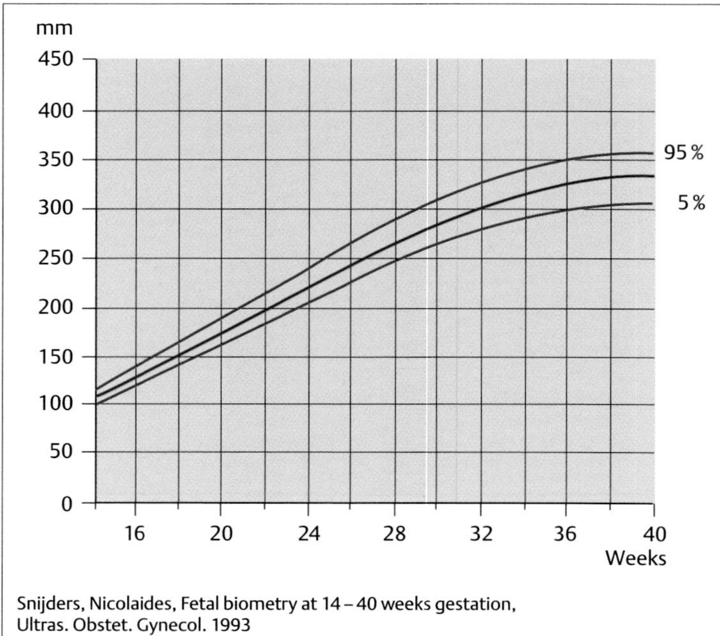

Fig. 19.**12** Head circumference.

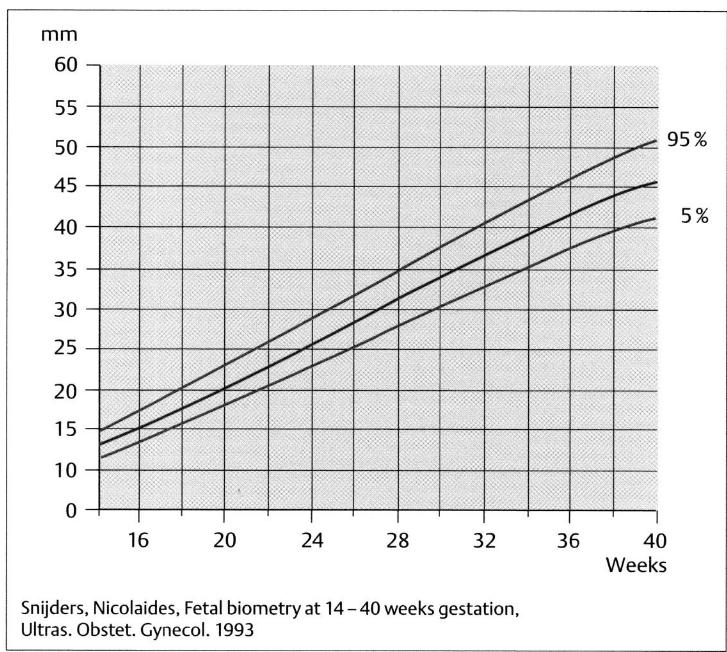

Fig. 19.**13** Transverse cerebellar diameter.

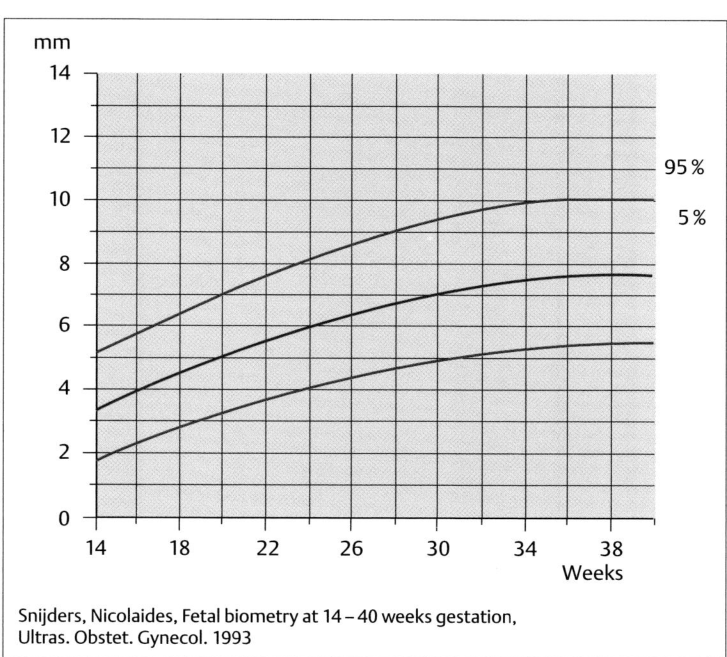

Fig. 19.**14** Cisterna magna diameter, anteroposterior.

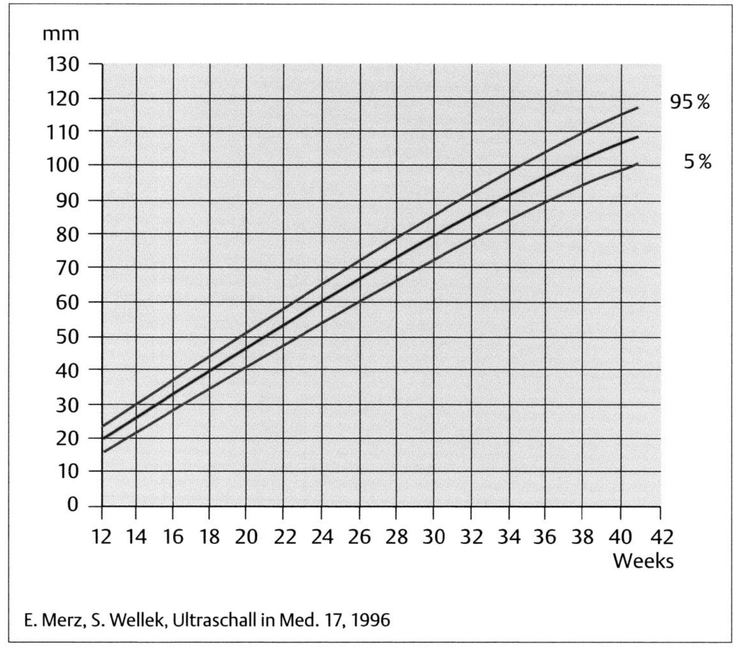

Fig. 19.**15** Thoracoabdominal diameter: transverse.

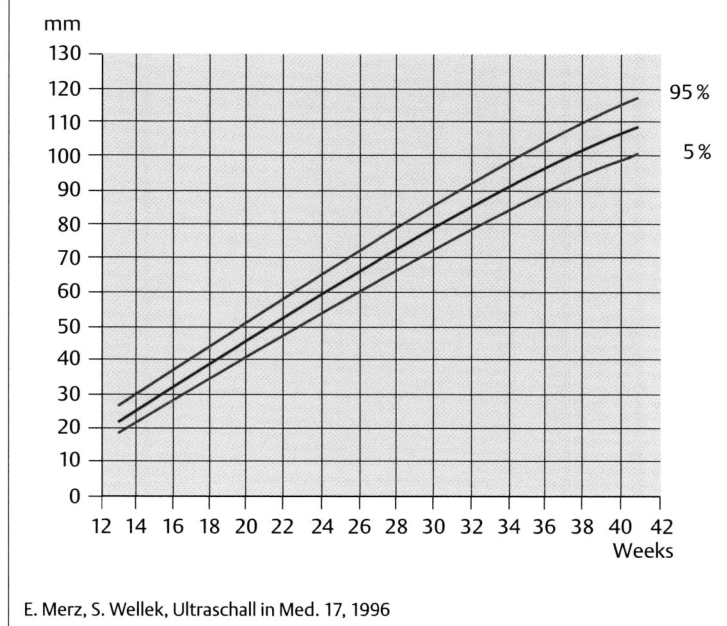

Fig. 19.**16** Thoracoabdominal diameter, anteroposterior.

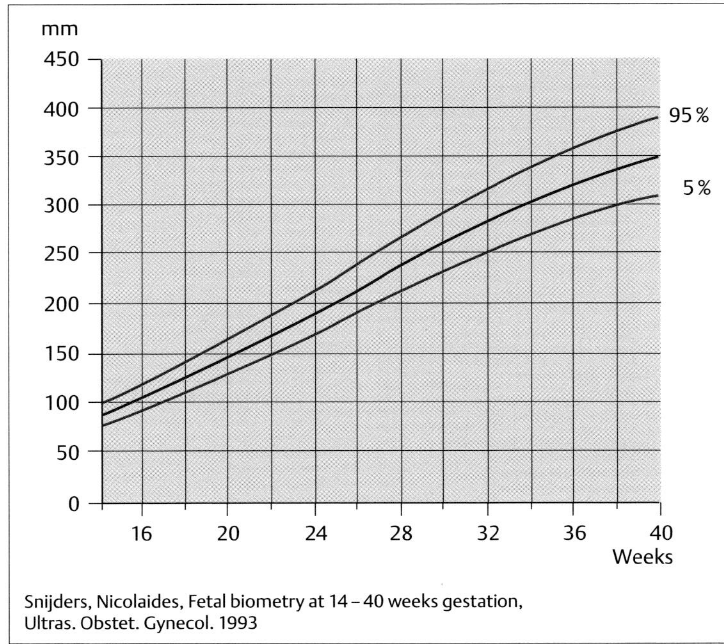

Fig. 19.**17** Thoracoabdominal circumference.

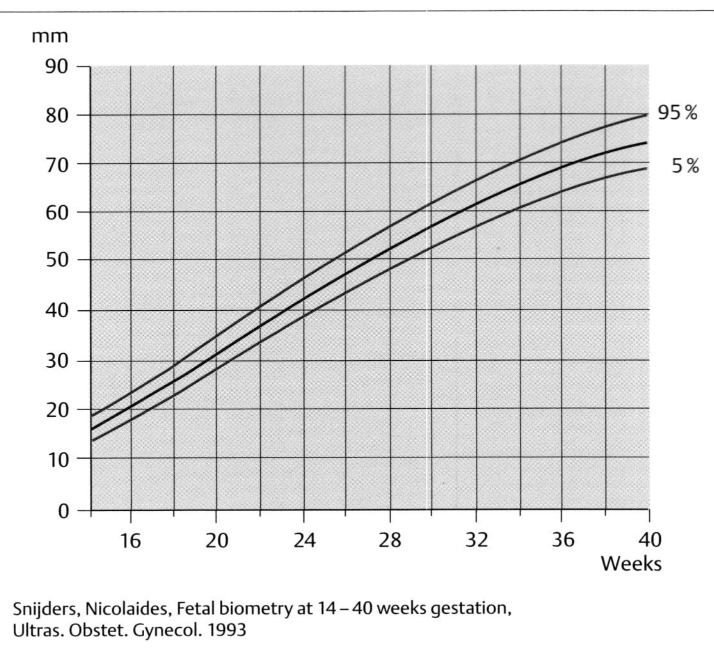

Fig. 19.**18** Femur length.

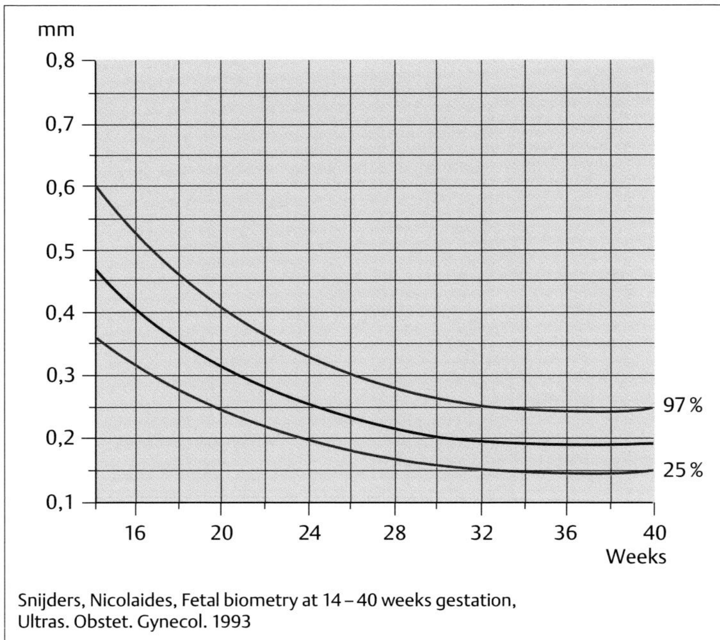

Fig. 19.**19** Lateral ventricle (posterior horn)/cerebral hemisphere width ratio.

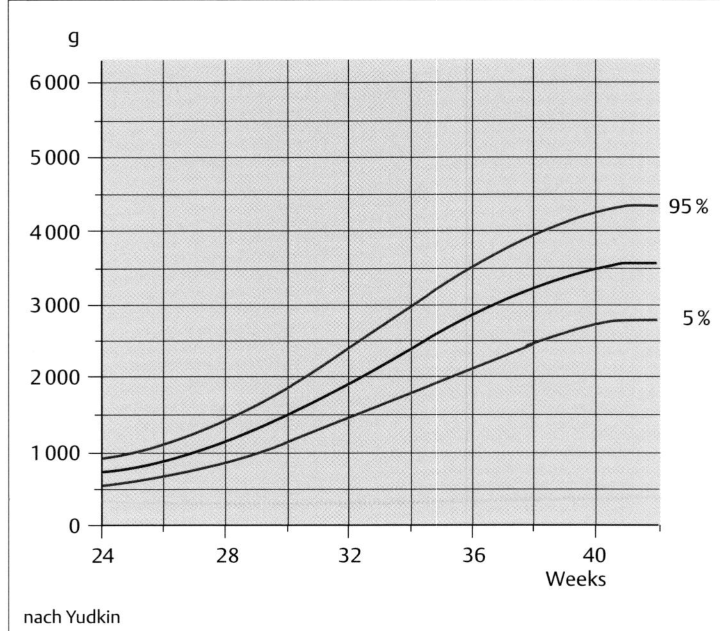

Fig. 19.**20** Estimated fetal weight (adapted from Yudkin).

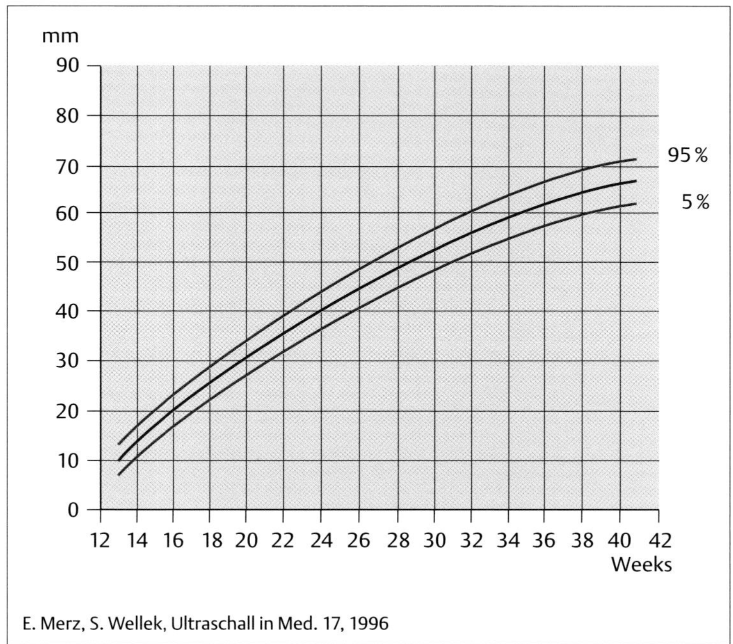

Fig. 19.**21** Humerus length.

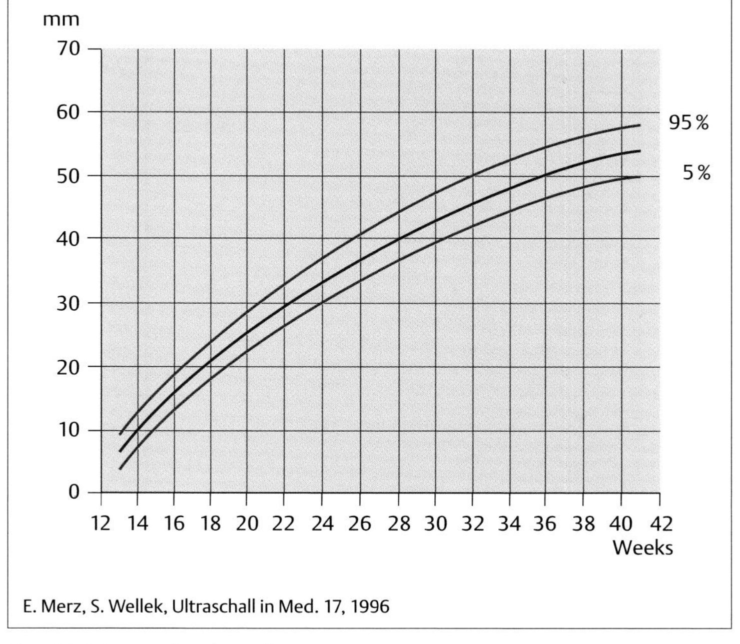

Fig. 19.**22** Radius length.

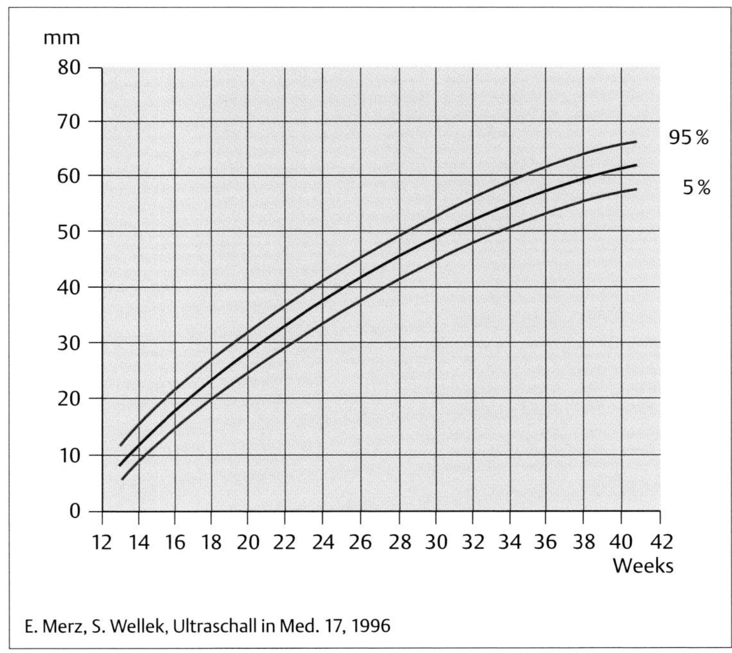

Fig. 19.**23** Ulna length.

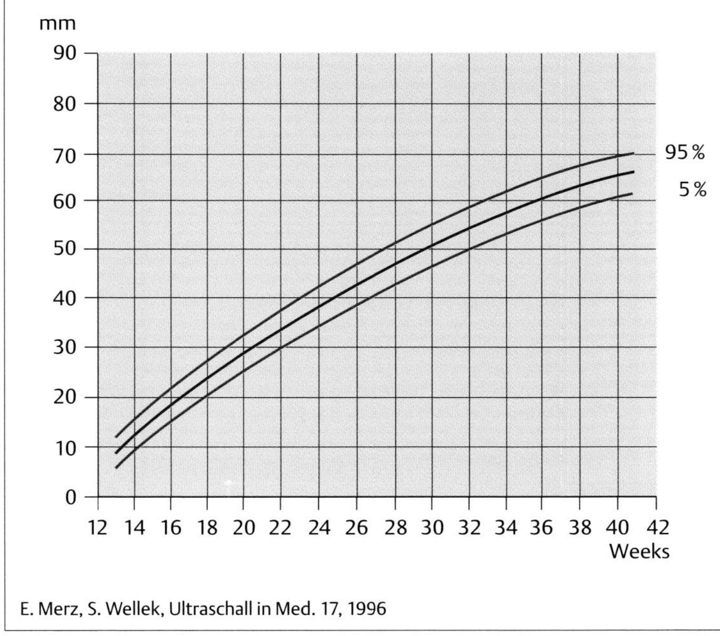

Fig. 19.**24** Tibia length.

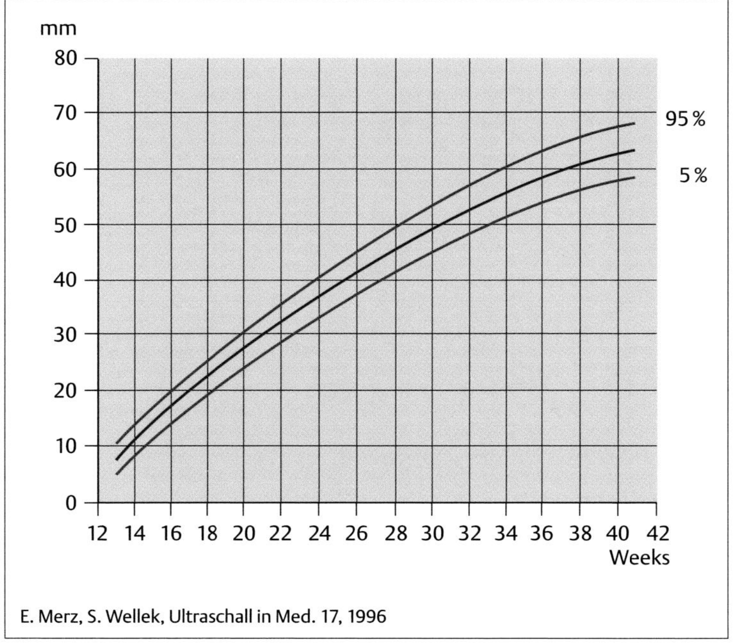

Fig. 19.**25** Fibula length.

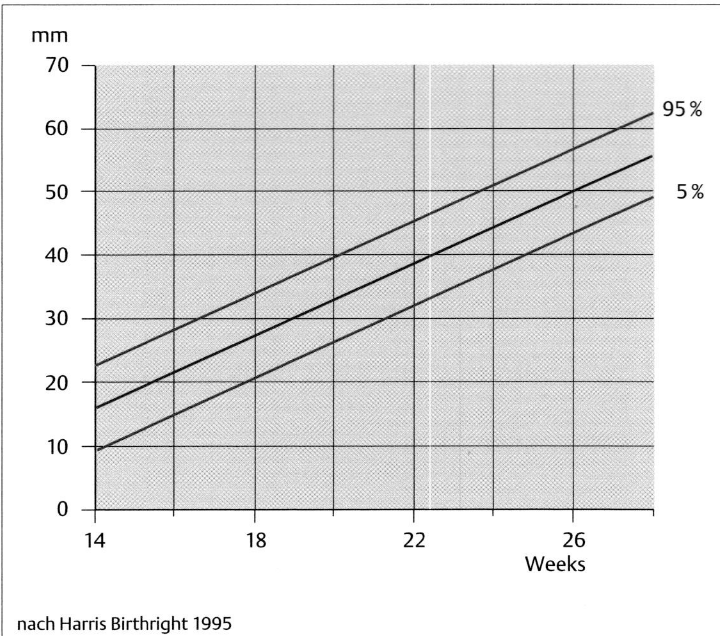

Fig. 19.**26** Foot length.

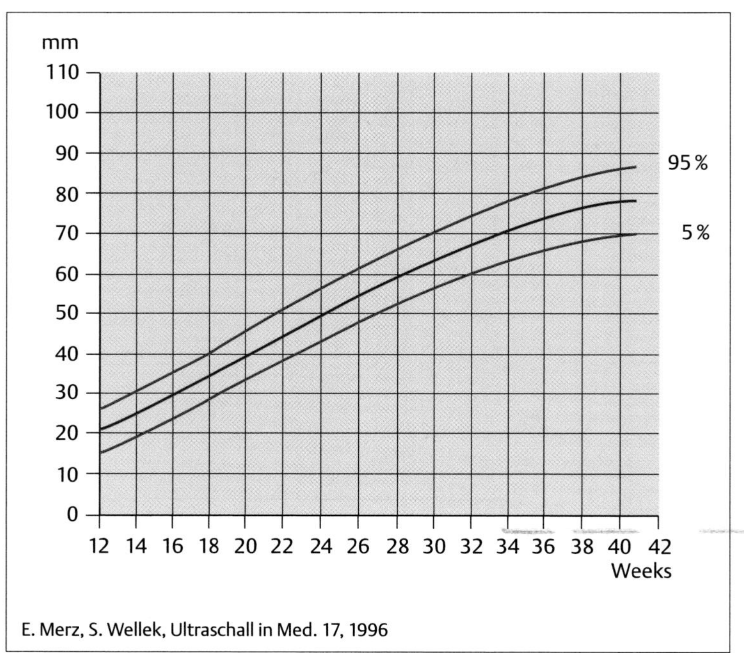

Fig. 19.**27** Transverse thoracic diameter (cardiac level).

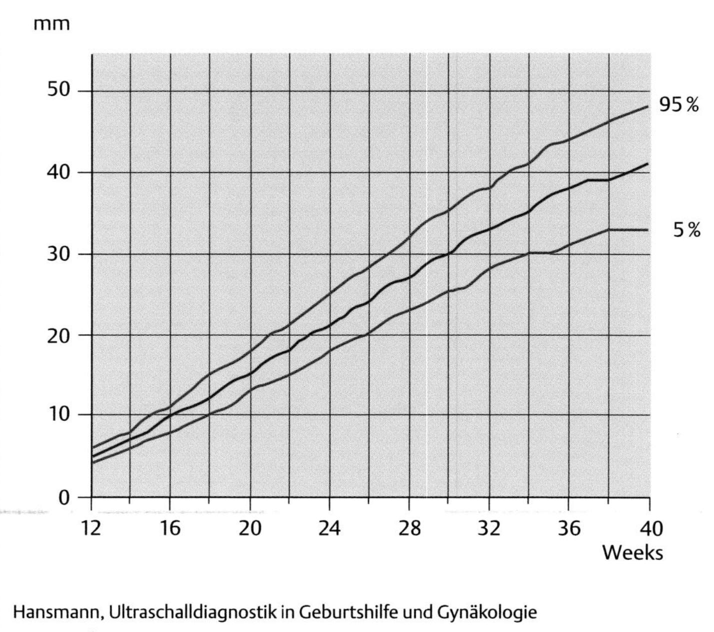

Fig. 19.**28** Transverse cardiac diameter (diastolic phase).

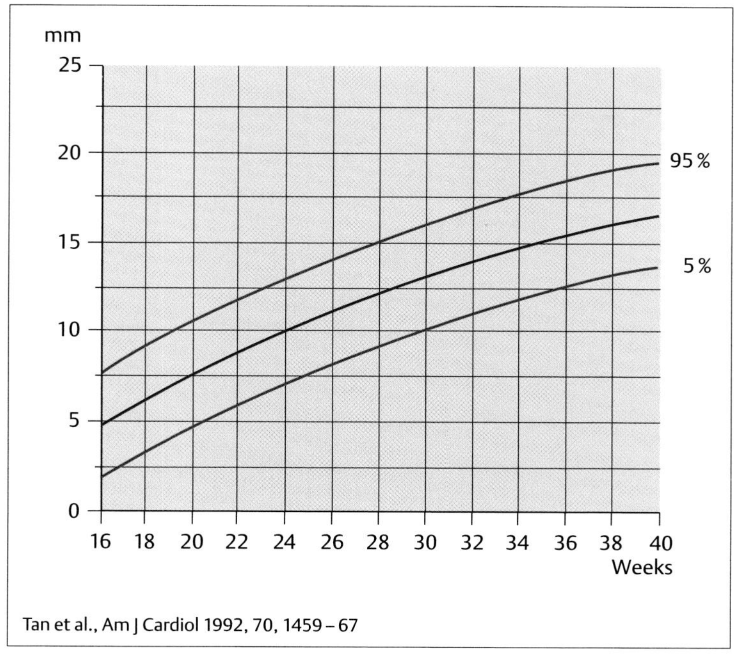

Fig. 19.**29** Transverse diameter of right cardiac ventricle (diastolic phase).

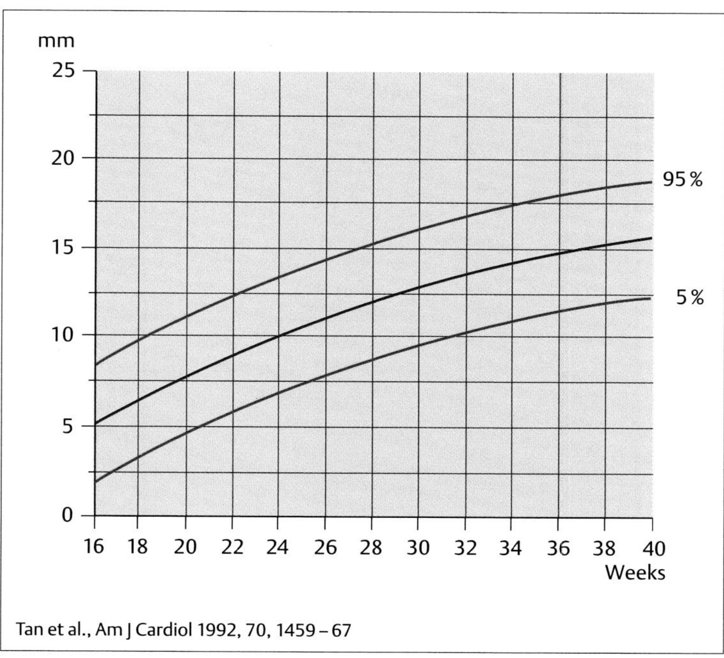

Fig. 19.**30** Transverse diameter of left cardiac ventricle (diastolic phase).

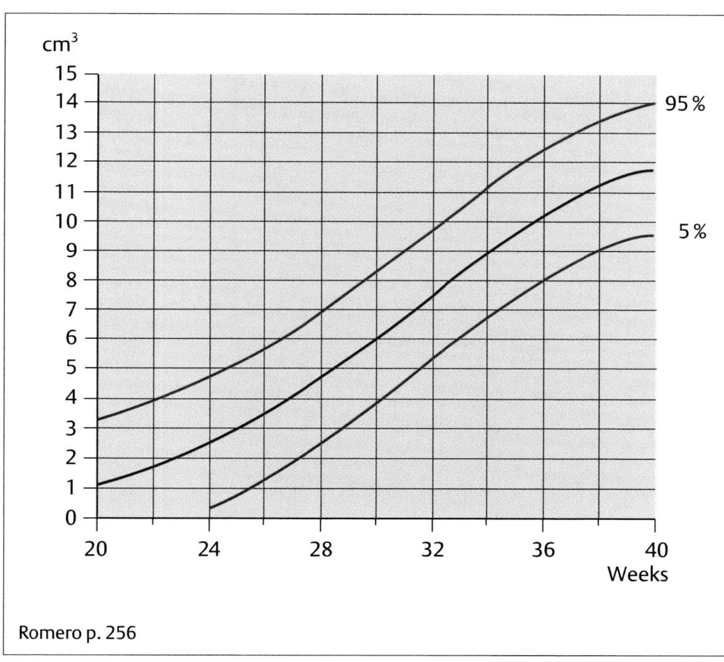

Fig. 19.**31** Renal volume.

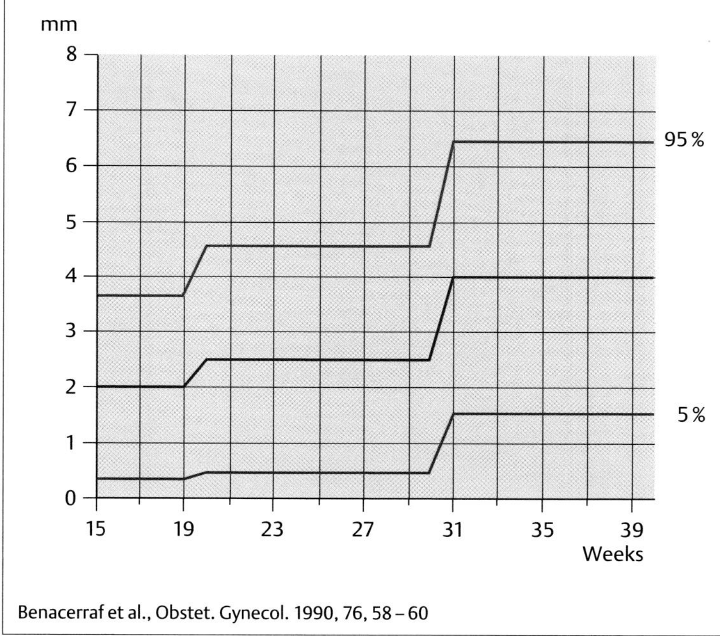

Fig. 19.**32** Renal pelvis diameter: anteroposterior.

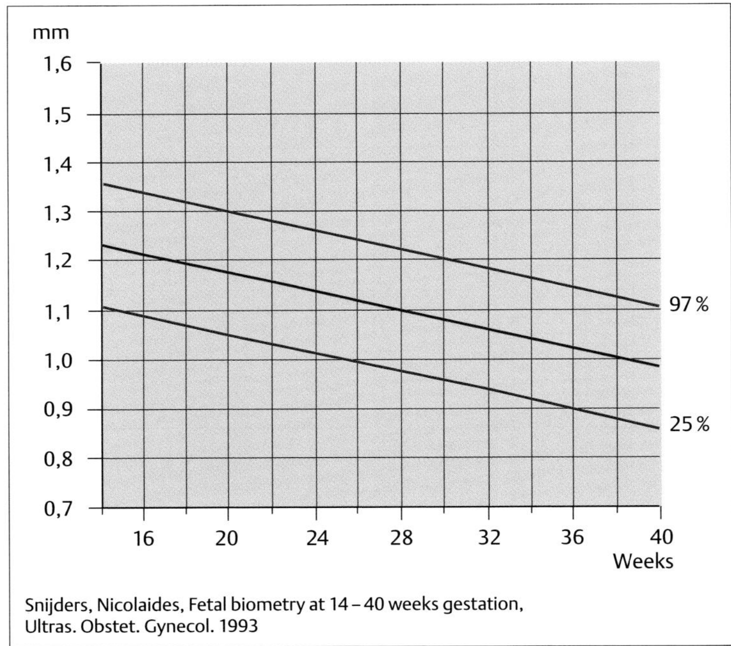

Fig. 19.**33** Head circumference/thoracoabdominal circumference ratio.

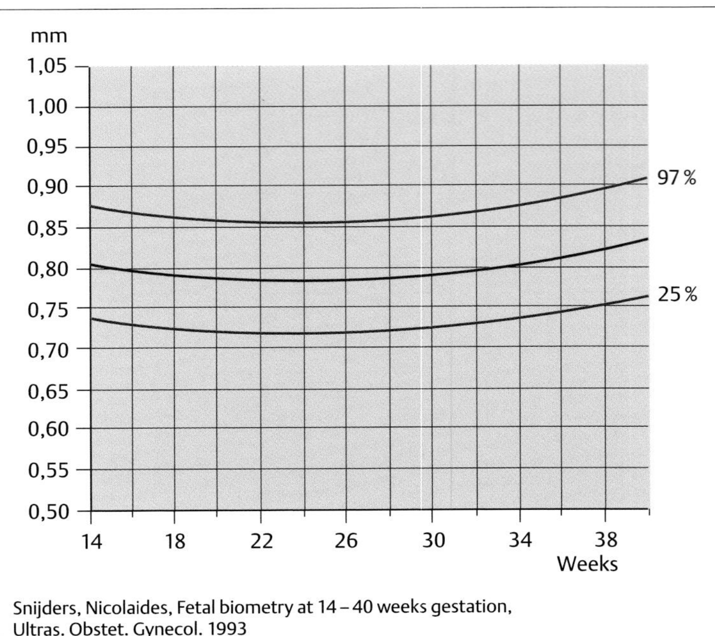

Fig. 19.**34** Biparietal diameter/fronto-occipital diameter ratio.

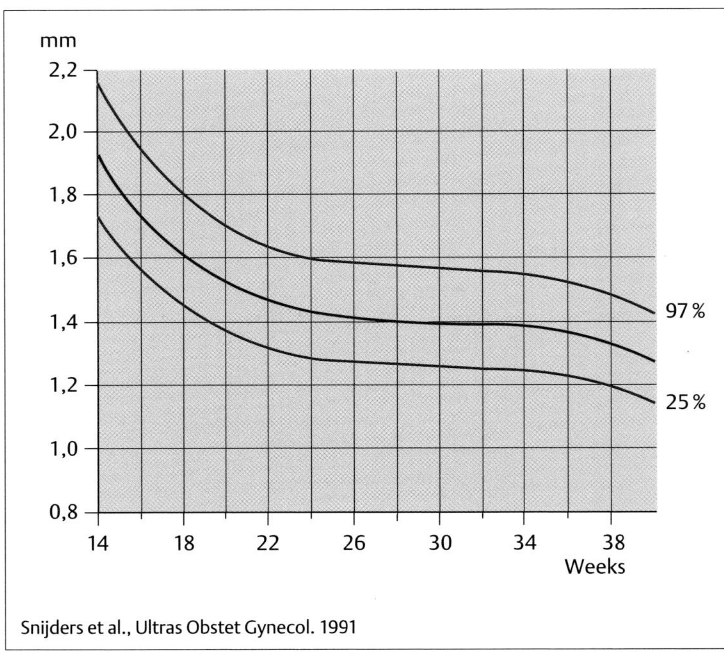

Fig. 19.**35** Biparietal diameter/femur length ratio.

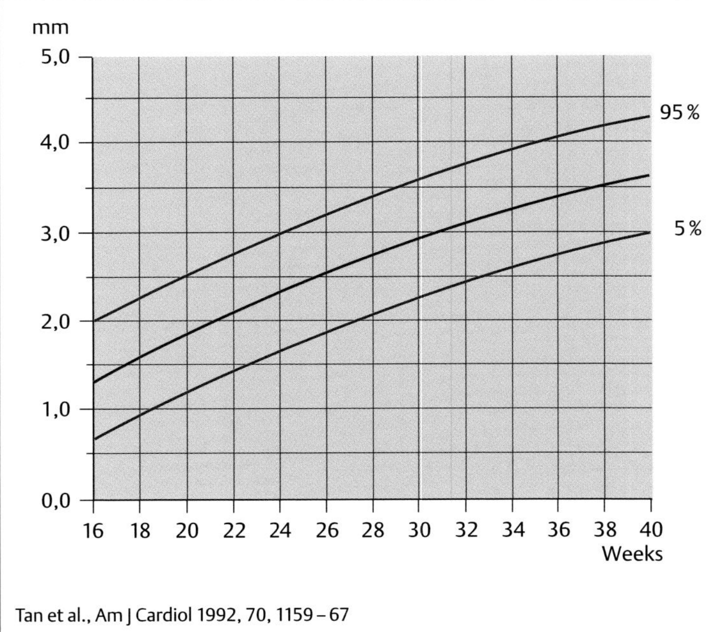

Fig. 19.**36** Ventricular septum width.

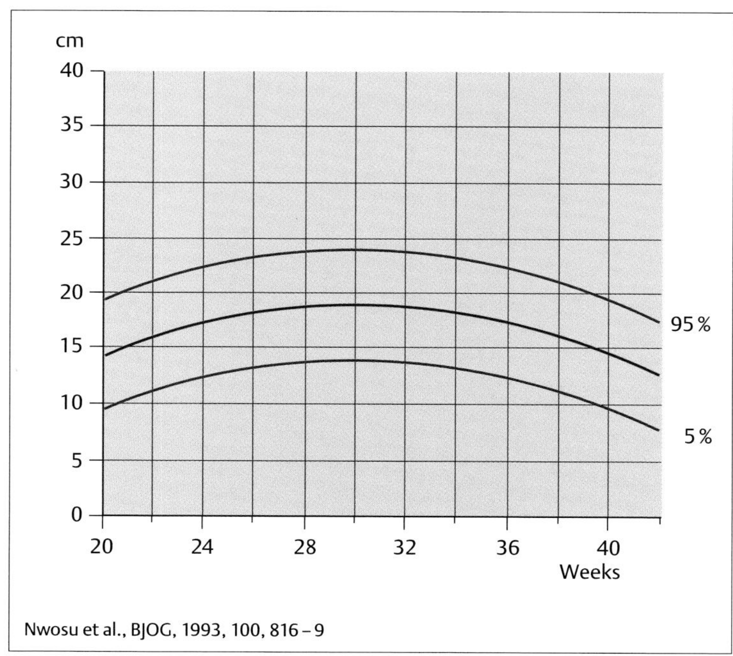

Fig. 19.**37** Amniotic fluid index.

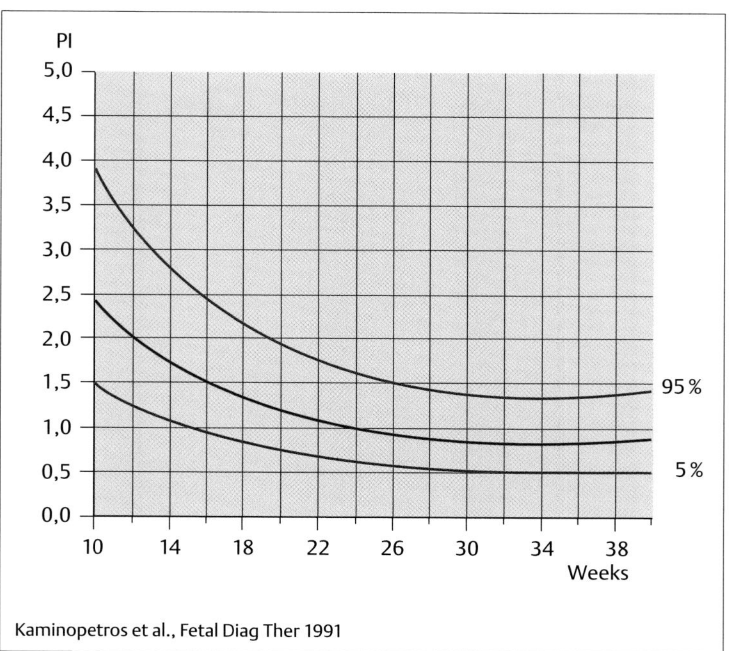

Fig. 19.**38** Pulsatility index: uterine artery.

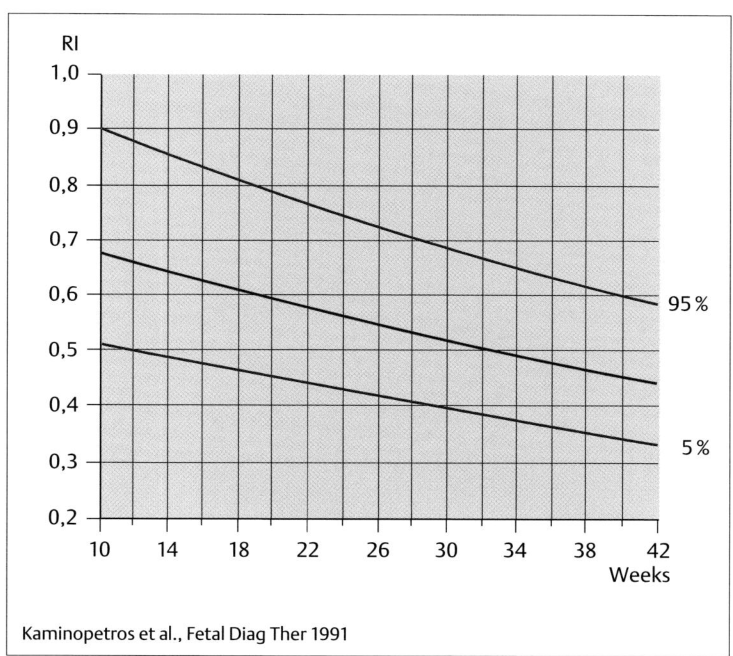

Fig. 19.**39** Resistance index: uterine artery.

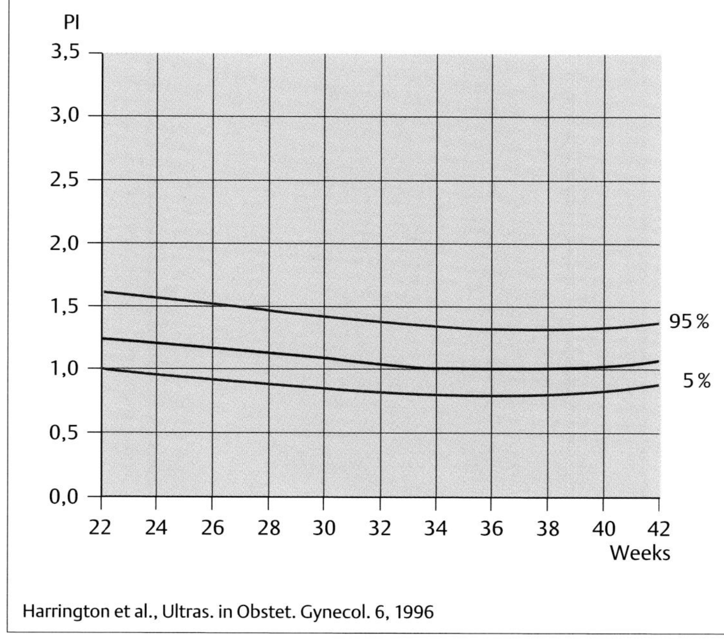

Fig. 19.**40** Pulsatility index: umbilical artery.

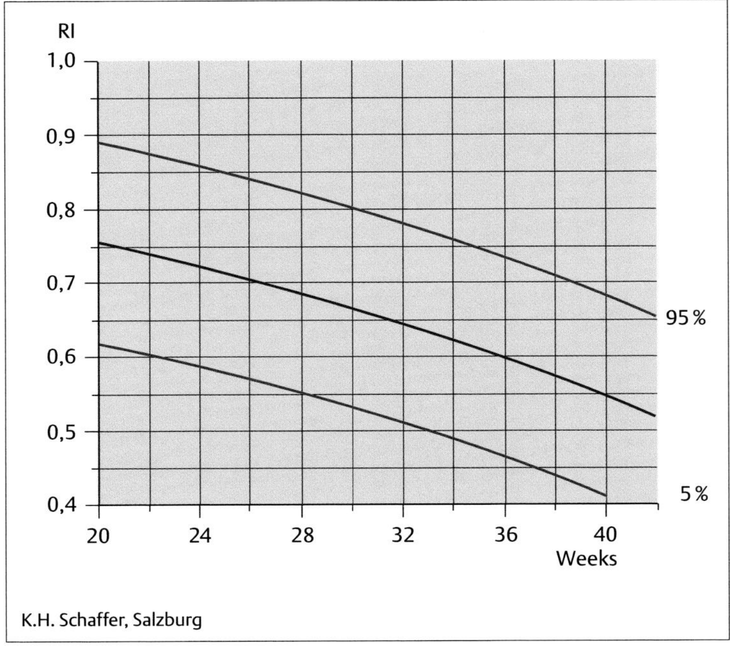

Fig. 19.**41** Resistance index: umbilical artery.

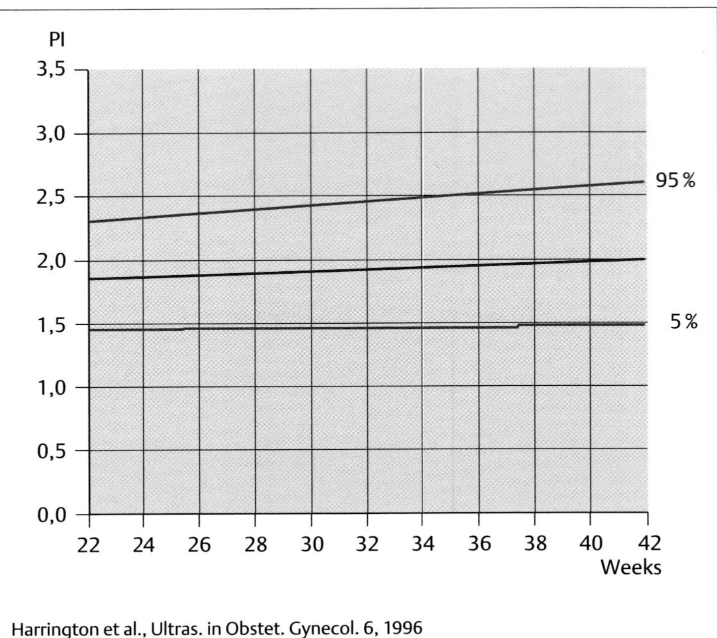

Fig. 19.**42** Pulsatility index: fetal abdominal aorta.

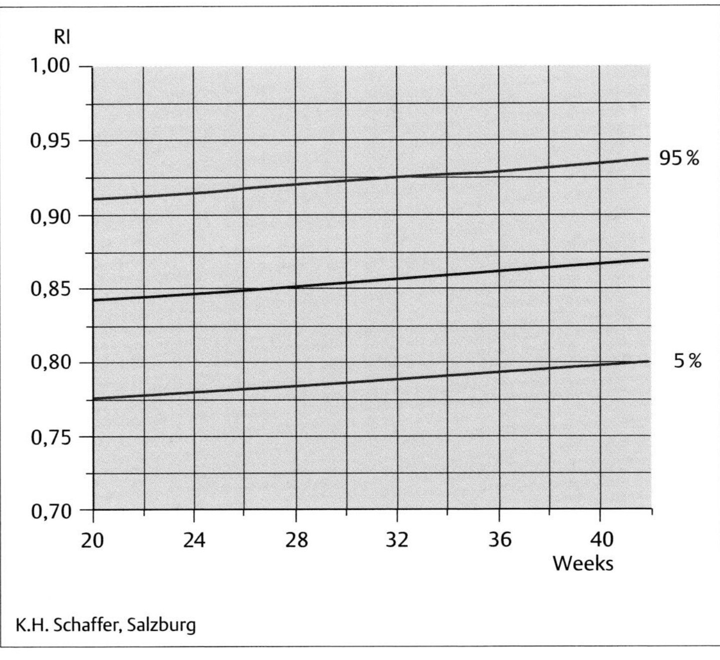

Fig. 19.**43** Resistance index: fetal abdominal aorta.

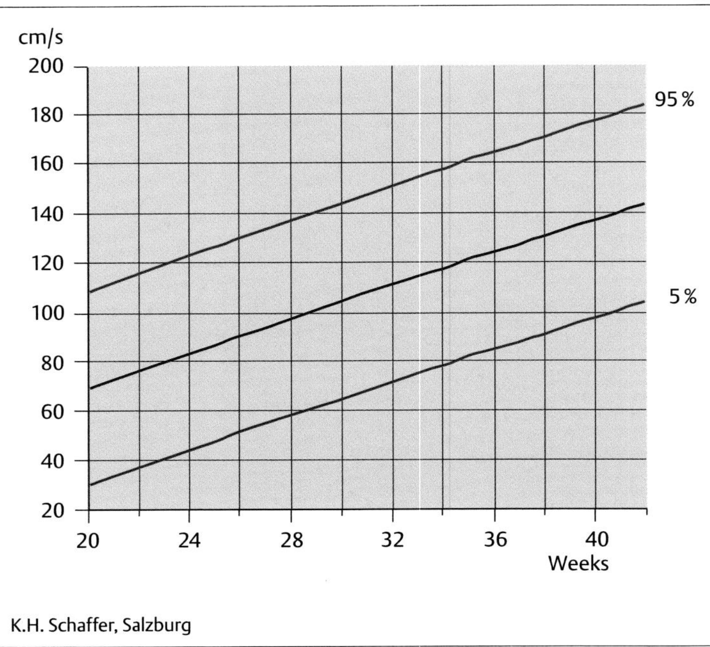

Fig. 19.**44** Maximum systolic flow velocity in the fetal thoracic aorta.

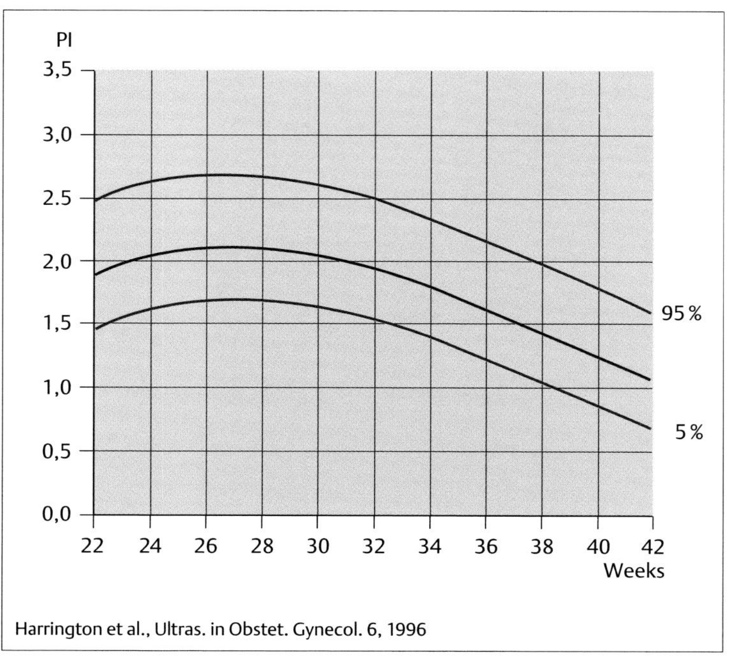

Fig. 19.**45** Pulsatility index: medial cerebral artery.

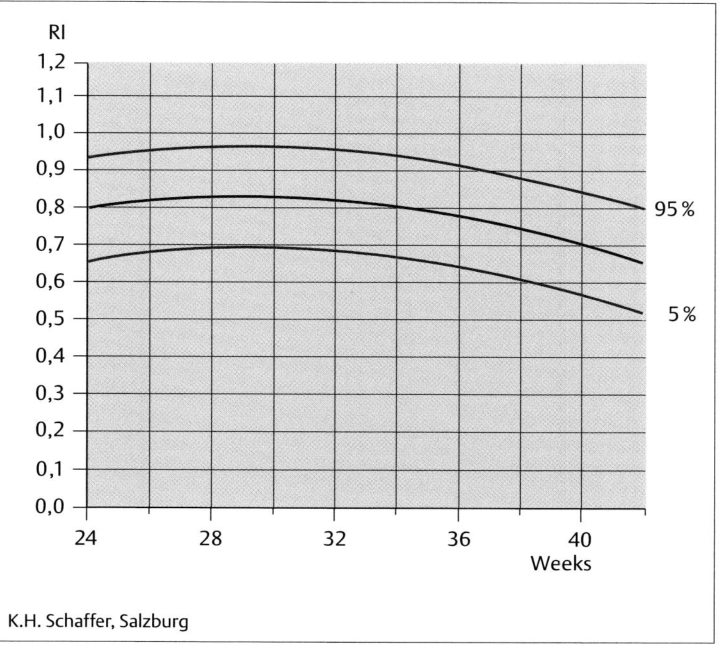

Fig. 19.**46** Resistance index: medial cerebral artery.

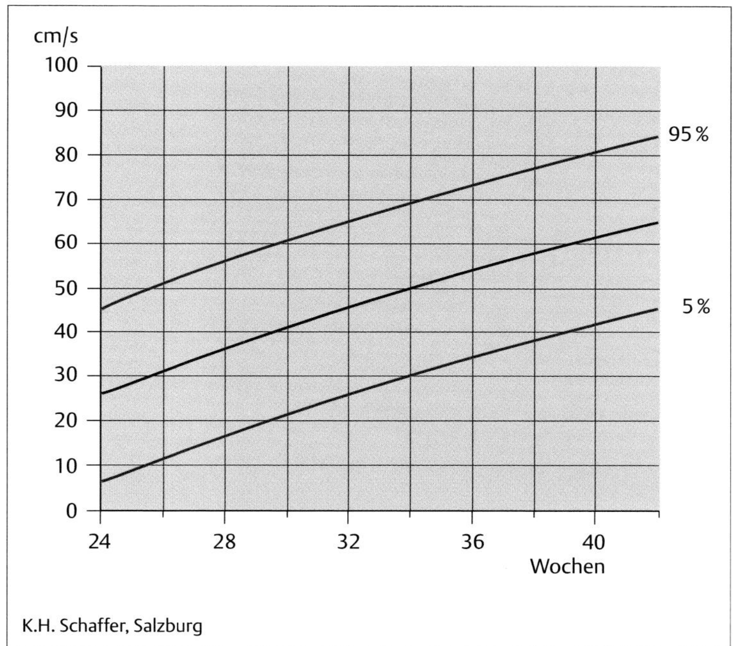

Fig. 19.**47** Maximum systolic flow velocity: middle cerebral artery

Index

Note: Named regions, organs and vessels are fetal unless stated otherwise. "Differential diagnosis" is indicated by "d.d.".
Page numbers in *italics* refer to figures and tables. Page numbers in **bold** type refer to major references.

D

G

H

N

O

P

Q

R

S

U

V

W

X

Y

Z